PROGRESS IN BRAIN RESEARCH

VOLUME 96

NEUROBIOLOGY OF ISCHEMIC BRAIN DAMAGE

Recent volumes in PROGRESS IN BRAIN RESEARCH

Volume 71: Neural Regeneration, by F.J. Seil, E. Herbert and B.M. Carlson (Eds.) – 1987.
Volume 72: Neuropeptides and Brain Function, by E.R. de Kloet, V.M. Wiegant and D. de Wied (Eds.) – 1987.
Volume 73: Biochemical Basis of Functional Neuroteratology, by G.J. Boer, M.G.P. Feenstra, M. Mirmiran, D.F. Swaab and F. van Haaren (Eds.) – 1988.
Volume 74: Transduction and Cellular Mechanisms in Sensory Receptors, by W. Hamann and A. Iggo (Eds.) – 1988.
Volume 75: Vision within Extrageniculo-Striate Systems, by T.B. Hicks and G. Benedek (Eds.) – 1988.
Volume 76: Vestibulospinal Control of Posture and Locomotion, by O. Pompeiano and J.H.J. Allum (Eds.) – 1988.
Volume 77: Pain Modulation, by H.L. Fields and J.-M. Besson (Eds.) – 1988.
Volume 78: Transplantation into the Mammalian CNS, by D.M. Gash and J.R. Sladek, Jr. (Eds.) – 1988.
Volume 79: Nicotinic Receptors in the CNS, by A. Nordberg, K. Fuxe, B. Holmstedt and A. Sundwall (Eds.) – 1989.
Volume 80: Afferent Control of Posture and Locomotion, by J.H.J. Allum and M. Hulliger (Eds.) – 1989.
Volume 81: The Central Neural Organization of Cardiovascular Control, by J. Ciriello, M.M. Caverson and C. Polosa (Eds.) – 1989.
Volume 82: Neural Transplantation: From Molecular Basis to Clinical Applications, by S. Dunnett and S.-J. Richards (Eds.) – 1990.
Volume 83: Understanding the Brain through the Hippocampus, by J. Storm-Mathisen, J. Zimmer and O.P. Ottersen (Eds.) – 1990.
Volume 84: Cholinergic Neurotransmission: Functional and Clinical Aspects, by S.-M. Aquilonius and P.-G. Gillberg (Eds.) – 1990.
Volume 85: The Prefrontal Cortex: Its Structure, Function and Pathology, by H.B.M. Uylings, C.G. van Eden, J.P.C. de Bruin, M.A. Corner and M.G.P. Feenstra (Eds.) – 1991.
Volume 86: Molecular and Cellular Mechanisms of Neuronal Plasticity in Normal Aging and Alzheimer's Disease, by P.D. Coleman, G.A. Higgins and C.H. Phelps (Eds.) – 1990.
Volume 87: Role of the Forebrain in Sensation and Behavior, by G. Holstege (Ed.) – 1991.
Volume 88: Neurobiology of the Locus Coeruleus, by C.D. Barnes and O. Pompeiano (Eds.) – 1991.
Volume 89: Protein Kinase C and its Brain Substrates: Role in Neuronal Growth and Plasticity, by W.H. Gispen and A. Routtenberg (Eds.) – 1991.
Volume 90: GABA in the Retina and Central Visual System, by R.R. Mize, R.E. Marc and A.M. Sillito (Eds.) – 1992.
Volume 91: Circumventricular Organs and Brain Fluid Environment, by A. Ermisch, R. Landgraf and H.-J. Rühle (Eds.) – 1992.
Volume 92: The Peptidergic Neuron, by J. Joosse, R.M. Buijs and F.J.H. Tilders (Eds.) – 1992.
Volume 93: The Human Hypothalamus in Health and Disease, by D.F. Swaab, M.A. Hofman, M. Mirmiran, R. Ravid and F.W. van Leeuwen (Eds.) – 1992.
Volume 94: Neuronal-Astrocytic Interactions: Implications for Normal and Pathological CNS Function, by A.C.H. Yu, L. Hertz, M.D. Norenberg, E. Syková and S. Waxman (Eds.) – 1992.
Volume 95: The Visually Responsive Neuron: from Basic Neurophysiology to Behavior, by T.P. Hicks, S. Molotchnikoff and T. Ono (Eds.) – 1993.

PROGRESS IN BRAIN RESEARCH

VOLUME 96

NEUROBIOLOGY OF ISCHEMIC BRAIN DAMAGE

EDITED BY

K. KOGURE

Department of Neurology, Institute of Brain Diseases, Tohoku University School of Medicine, Sendai, Japan

K.-A. HOSSMANN

Department of Experimental Neurology, Max-Planck-Institute for Neurological Research, Cologne, Germany

B.K. SIESJÖ

Laboratory for Experimental Brain Research, University of Lund, Lund, Sweden

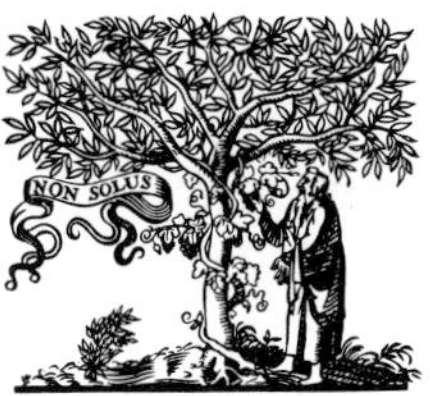

ELSEVIER
AMSTERDAM – LONDON – NEW YORK – TOKYO
1993

ISBN 0-444-89603-1 (volume)
ISBN 0-444-80104-9 (series)

This book is printed on acid-free paper.

Published by:
Elsevier Science Publishers B.V.
P.O. Box 211
1000 AE Amsterdam
The Netherlands

Printed in The Netherlands

List of Contributors

K. Abe, Department of Neurology, Institute of Brain Diseases, Tohoku University School of Medicine, 1-1 Seiryo-machi, Aoba-ku, Sendai 980, Japan.

G. Allan, LSU Eye Center and Neuroscience Center, Louisiana State University Medical Center School of Medicine, 2020 Gravier Street, Suite B, New Orleans, LA 70112, U.S.A.

H. Aoki, Department of Neurology, Institute of Brain Diseases, Tohoku University School of Medicine, 1-1 Seiryo-machi, Aoba-ku, Sendai 980, Japan.

N.G. Bazan, LSU Eye Center and Neuroscience Center, Louisiana State University Medical Center School of Medicine, 2020 Gravier Street, Suite B, New Orleans, LA 70112, U.S.A.

M. Berg, Molecular Neuropathology Unit and PharmaBiotec Research Center, Institute of Neuropathology, University of Copenhagen, 11 Frederik V's vej, DK-2100 Copenhagen, Denmark.

K. Bergstedt, Laboratory for Experimental Brain Research, Department of Neurobiology, Experimental Research Center, Lund University Hospital, S-221 85 Lund, Sweden.

T. Bruhn, Molecular Neuropathology Unit and PharmaBiotec Research Center, Institute of Neuropathology, University of Copenhagen, 11 Frederik V's vej, DK-2100 Copenhagen, Denmark.

A. Buchan, Neuroscience Research, Ottawa Civic Hospital, 1053 Carling Avenue, Ottawa, Ont. K1Y4E9, Canada.

R. Busto, Cerebral Vascular Disease Research Center, Department of Neurology, 11 University of Miami School of Medicine, P.O. Box 016960, Miami, FL 33101, U.S.A.

E. Carlson, Department of Pediatrics, University of California School of Medicine, San Francisco, CA 94143-0114, U.S.A.

P.H. Chan, Department of Neurology and Neurosurgery, University of California School of Medicine, San Francisco, CA 94143-0114, U.S.A.

S.F. Chen, Department of Neurology, University of California School of Medicine, San Francisco, CA 94143-0114, U.S.A.

D.W. Choi, Department of Neurology, Box 8111, Washington University School of Medicine, 660 South Euclid Ave., St. Louis, MO 63110, U.S.A.

M. Cleef, Department of Experimental Neurology, Max-Planck-Institute for Neurological Research, Gleueler Strasse 50, 5000 Cologne 41, Germany.

N.H. Diemer, Molecular Neuropathology Unit and PharmaBiotec Research Center, Institute of Neuropathology, University of Copenhagen, 11 Frederik V's vej, DK-2100 Copenhagen, Denmark.

W.D. Dietrich, Cerebral Vascular Disease Research Center, Department of Neurology, University of Miami School of Medicine, P.O. Box 016960, Miami, FL 33101, U.S.A.

U. Dirnagl, Department of Neurology, University of Munich, Klinikum Grosshadern, 8000 Munich 70, Germany.

A. Ekholm, Laboratory for Experimental Brain Research, Experimental Research Center, Lund University Hospital, S-221 85 Lund, Sweden.

C.J. Epstein, Department of Pediatrics and Biochemistry and Biophysics, University of California School of Medicine, San Francisco, CA 94143-0114, U.S.A.

S.M. Gentleman, Serious Mental Afflictions Research Team, Department of Anatomy and Cell Biology, St Mary's Medical School, Imperial College, Norfolk Place, London, W2 1PG, U.K.

M.D. Ginsberg, Cerebral Vascular Disease Research Center, Department of Neurology, University of Miami School of Medicine, P.O. Box 016960, Miami, FL 33101, U.S.A.

M.Y.-T. Globus, Cerebral Vascular Disease Research Center, Department of Neurology, University of Miami School of Medicine, P.O. Box 016960, Miami, FL 33101, U.S.A.

D.I. Graham, Department of Neuropathology, Institute of Neurological Sciences, Southern General Hospital, Glasgow, G51 4TF, U.K.

K. Hisanaga, Department of Neurology, University of California at San Francisco, and Veterans Affairs Medical Center, 4150 Clement Street, San Francisco, CA 94121, U.S.A.

K.-A. Hossmann, Department of Experimental Neurology, Max-Planck-Institute for Neurological Research, Gleueler Strasse 50, D-5000 Cologne 41, Germany.

B.R. Hu, Laboratory for Experimental Brain Research, Department of Neurobiology, Experimental Research Center Clinical Research Center, Lund University Hospital, S-221 85 Lund, Sweden.

S. Imaizumi, Department of Neurology, University of California School of Medicine, San Francisco, CA 94143-0114, U.S.A.

F.F. Johansen, Molecular Neuropathology Unit and PharmaBiotec Research Center, Institute of Neuropathology, University of Copenhagen, 11 Frederik V's vej, DK-2100 Copenhagen, Denmark.

M.B. Jørgensen, Molecular Neuropathology Unit and PharmaBiotec Research Center, Institute of Neuropathology, University of Copenhagen, 11 Frederik V's vej, DK-2100 Copenhagen, Denmark.

K. Katsura, Laboratory for Experimental Brain Research, Experimental Research Center, Lund University Hospital, S-221 85 Lund, Sweden.

H. Kinouchi, Department of Neurology, University of California School of Medicine, San Francisco, CA 94143-0114, U.S.A.

T. Kirino, Department of Neurosurgery, Teikyo University School of Medicine, 2-11-1 Kaga, Itabashi-ku, Tokyo 173, Japan.

K. Kogure, Department of Neurology, Institute of Brain Diseases, Tohoku University School of Medicine, 1-1 Seiryo-machi, Aoba-ku, Sendai 980, Japan.

J. Lundgren, Laboratory for Experimental Brain Research, Experimental Research Center, Lund University Hospital, S-221 85 Lund, Sweden.

P. Mellergård, Laboratory for Experimental Brain Research, Experimental Research Center, Lund University Hospital, S-221 85 Lund, Sweden.

M. Müller, Department of Neuromorphology, Institute for Neurobiology and Brain Research, Magdeburg, Germany.

T.S. Nowak Jr., Laboratory of Neuropathology and Neuroanatomical Sciences, National Institute of Neurological Disorders and Stroke, National Institutes of Health, Bethesda, MD 20892, U.S.A.

H. Onodera, Department of Neurology, Institute of Brain Diseases, Tohoku University School of Medicine, 1-1 Seiryo-machi, Aoba-ku, Sendai 980, Japan.

O.C. Osborne, Laboratory of Neuropathology and Neuroanatomical Sciences, National Institute of Neurological Disorders and Stroke, National Institutes of Health, Bethesda, MD 20892, U.S.A.

A.E.I. Pajunen, Biocenter and Department of Biochemistry, University of Oulu, Oulu, Finland.

W. Paschen, Department of Experimental Neurology, Max-Planck-Institute for Neurological Research, Gleueler Strasse 50, 5000 Cologne 41, Germany.

W. Pulsinelli, Cerebrovascular Disease Research Center, Department of Neurology and Neuroscience, Cornell University Medical College, 1300 York Avenue, New York, NY, U.S.A.

G.W. Roberts, Serious Mental Afflictions Research Team, Department of Anatomy and Cell Biology, St Mary's Medical School, Imperial College, Norfolk Place, London, W2 1PG, U.K.

E.B. Rodriguez de Turco, LSU Eye Center and Neuroscience Center, Louisiana State University Medical Center School of Medicine, 2020 Gravier Street, Suite B, New Orleans, LA 70112, U.S.A.

G. Röhn, Department of Experimental Neurology, Max-Planck-Institute for Neurological Research, Gleueler Strasse 50, 5000 Cologne 41, Germany.

A. Sarokin, Cerebrovascular Disease Research Center, Department of Neurology and Neuroscience, Cornell University Medical College, 1300 York Avenue, New York, NY, U.S.A.

B.K. Siesjö, Laboratory for Experimental Brain Research, Experimental Research Center, Lund University Hospital, S-221 85 Lund, Sweden.

M-L. Smith, Laboratory for Experimental Brain Research, Experimental Research Center, Lund University Hospital, S-221 85 Lund, Sweden.

S. Suga, Department of Neurosurgery, Keio University School of Medicine, 35 Shinanomachi, Shinjuku-ku, Tokyo 160, Japan.

E. Valente, Molecular Neuropathology Unit and PharmaBiotec Research Center, Institute of Neuropathology, University of Copenhagen, 11 Frederik V's vej, DK-2100 Copenhagen, Denmark.

B.D. Watson, Cerebral Vascular Disease Research Center, Department of Neurology, University of Miami

School of Medicine, P.O. Box 016960, Miami, FL 33101, U.S.A.
T. Wieloch, Laboratory for Experimental Brain Research, Department of Neurobiology, Experimental Research Center, Lund University Hospital, S-221 85 Lund, Sweden.

Preface

Nine years ago, the first Sendai symposium on ischemic brain damage was organized and held in Zao, Japan. The symposium was made possible by a generous educational grant from A.G. Sandoz in Basel, Switzerland. The focus in the symposium was on mechanisms of ischemic brain damage. Most of the participants of that meeting submitted manuscripts which, after editing, were collected in Volume 63 of Progress in Brain Research, published in 1985. The volume has been widely circulated and the articles frequently quoted. This probably reflects the novelty of the concept, *i.e.* of a symposium concentrating effort on the mechanisms leading to cell death.

Eight years after the first Sendai symposium, a second symposium was organized in Okinawa, again generously supported by A.G. Sandoz. In the years which had passed since the first one, the development in the research field had been very fast. For example, receptor physiology and pharmacology was now an intensely studied field, and the excitotoxic hypothesis of cell death had reached common acceptance. Furthermore, it had been recognized that ischemia and other insults give rise to a sustained depression of overall protein synthesis, yet leading to the expression of dormant genes and to synthesis of new proteins.

In view of this development, we felt the need to focus the symposium on cellular and molecular aspects of ischemic brain damage. Since the symposium seemed a timely event, attempts were made to collect a series of manuscripts both from the participants of the symposium, and from a few specially invited contributors. Again, we were lucky to get the volume accepted for publication in Progress in Brain Research. We hope that the volume will be of value and assistance to all those interested in the pathophysiology of ischemic and traumatic brain damage.

Kyuya Kogure
Konstantin-Alexander Hossmann
Bo K. Siesjö

Contents

K. Kogure, K.-A. Hossmann and B.K. Siesjö (Eds.)
Progress in Brain Research, Vol. 96

CHAPTER 1

A new perspective on ischemic brain damage?

B.K. Siesjö

University of Lund, Laboratory for Experimental Brain Research, Experimental Research Center, University Hospital, S-221 85 Lund, Sweden

Introduction

Research on mechanisms of ischemic brain damage has come to age. Initially, ischemia research was centered on changes in blood flow, water and electrolyte metabolism and oxygen delivery, justifying the expression "pathophysiology of hypoxic/ischemic damage". However, data relevant to the effect of ischemia on cellular energy homeostasis, as well as on carbohydrate, amino acid and lipid metabolism, were published several decades ago (Thorn et al., 1958; Lowry et al., 1964; Hinzen et al., 1970). In the years to follow, much additional information was collected on cellular metabolic responses to ischemia/hypoxia and, at the same time, attempts were made to systematize available information into hypothetical schemes of the pathogenetic mechanisms involved (Siesjö, 1978). In view of this development it seemed relevant to discuss the mechanisms involved under the heading "neurochemistry of ischemic brain damage". A review article published more than 10 years ago identified three mechanisms of putative importance: loss of cellular calcium homeostasis, excessive acidosis and enhanced production of free radicals (Siesjö, 1981). Progress during the last decade has born out such speculations and provided solid experimental support, particularly for the hypothesis of calcium-related damage (Choi, 1988; Siesjö, 1988, 1991). This is also the period in which the excitotoxic hypothesis of cell damage (Olney, 1978) was extended to encompass ischemia/hypoxia and hypoglycemia (Auer et al., 1984; Benveniste et al., 1984; Simon et al., 1984; Wieloch, 1985a,b). This hypothesis had a major impact on ischemia research since it revived the calcium hypothesis of cell death and provided new information on the channels which are involved in so called cell calcium overload.

Recent studies emphasize that additional pathogenetic mechanisms come into play, notably those related to a depressed or an altered protein synthesis and to the expression of new genes (Abe and Kogure, this volume; Hossmann, this volume; Nowak et al., this volume; Wieloch et al., this volume). These mechanisms are intimately related to changes in second messengers and to activation of protein kinases and phosphatases which affect membrane function, sometimes over long periods. The results of such studies hint that we are seeing the birth of a new and potentially very important research field, encompassing the molecular biology of brain damage. However, although both the tools used and the message delivered are new, the interpretations are, by necessity, based on concepts and ideas developed during the last 10 – 15 years of research in a field which is now perhaps best described by the term "neurobiology of ischemic brain damage".

In February 1991, a group of neurobiologists met in Okinawa to discuss molecular mechanisms of ischemic brain damage ("Sendai Forum II"). At that time, it was decided to collect a number of chapters on key issues into a comprehensive volume. Some of the participants of the Sendai Forum and several others were asked to contribute to the book which now appears as Volume 96 of *Progress in Brain Research.*

The objective of this brief introductory chapter is to attempt bridging the gap between research conducted during the early years and that of today. I will point out the central pathogenetic role played by cellular energy failure, emphasize the importance of distinguishing between two major types of ischemia, and discuss the pathogenetic importance of loss of calcium homeostasis and of production of free radicals.

Energy failure and cell death

Cell survival depends on the maintenance of an optimal phosphorylation potential, defined as the ratio $ATP \cdot ADP^{-1} \cdot P_i^{-1}$, where P_i stands for inorganic phosphate. This is because the phosphorylation potential modulates the balance between leak fluxes and active transport of physiological ions including calcium, as well as the balance between spontaneous or enzyme-catalyzed degradation of cell constituents including membranes, and their resynthesis or reassembly by ATP-dependent reactions. Thus, when the phosphorylation potential falls, the pump/leak relationship for calcium and other ions is disturbed and the degradation of cell structure is not properly matched by anabolic reactions. This is a precarious state which may not allow long-term recovery, either because it is associated with excessive activation of enzymes which degrade cell structure or with suppression of endergonic reactions such as protein synthesis.

One of the consequences of energy failure is an increase in the free cytosolic calcium concentration (Ca_i^{2+}). This is because energy failure affects both the ATP-dependent extrusion of calcium and its intracellular sequestration (Hansen, 1985; Siesjö and Bengtsson, 1989; Siesjö, 1991). However, Ca_i^{2+} is determined by both the pump and the leak. Since the latter is a function of the calcium permeability of plasma and intracellular membranes, Ca_i^{2+} can increase even though the phosphorylation potential has not decreased. This typically occurs during spreading depression (SD), a condition with a transient increase in membrane permeability to calcium, probably caused by presynaptic release of glutamate (Hansen, 1985).

On the basis of this concept, i.e., of a disturbed pump/leak relationship for calcium, we can discern three types of perturbations. One is primary pump failure observed in anoxia. Although anoxia primarily leads to a rise in Ca_i^{2+} because energy production fails, the leak is also enhanced, at least in part because glutamate and associated excitatory amino acids (EAAs) are released. The second condition is one in which the leak is transiently increased, as in SD. Since the pump function is intact the rise in Ca_i^{2+} is predictably less marked, and clearly transient. A third condition can be envisaged in which energy metabolism is compromised rather than disrupted, meaning that although the phosphorylation potential may be close to normal, the rate of ATP production is reduced. It seems likely that, in this condition, a transient increase in membrane permeability to calcium is associated with a more marked and more sustained rise in Ca_i^{2+}. This contention is supported by results showing that moderately severe hypoglycemia, a condition which does not reduce the phosphorylation potential of the tissue, is associated with prolonged calcium transients following depolarization-induced SD (Gidö et al., 1992).

The importance of energy failure is underscored by the fact that even relatively brief periods of ischemia cause damage to vulnerable cells (Smith et al., 1984a,b) whereas SDs can be elicited for hours without inflicting such damage on cells of non-ischemic subjects (Nedergaard and Hansen, 1988). It is tempting to assume that incipient energy failure exaggerates and prolongs the calcium transients. Clearly, if a rise in Ca_i^{2+} is a determinant of cell survival we can envisage that a twilight zone of energy failure exists, in which a reduced capacity to generate ATP is associated with depolarization-induced calcium transients of sufficient severity to cause cell damage.

Types of ischemia encountered

One of the major advances during the last 10 – 15 years of research in this field was the development of reproducible techniques for induction of global/forebrain ischemia (Pulsinelli and Brierley, 1979; Smith et al., 1984a,b) and focal ischemia (Tamura et al., 1981) in rats. In contrast to the gerbil, the rat lends itself to extensive physiological monitoring and, compared to cats and monkeys, it is a relatively inexpensive experimental animal. Nonetheless, caution should be exercised when results are extrapolated from rats to primates (Siesjö, 1992a). This is probably because in focal ischemia, due to middle cerebral artery occlusion, the collateral supply of blood from the anterior and posterior cerebral arteries is feeble in rats compared to cats and monkeys.

Ischemic brain damage incurred as a result of forebrain or global ischemia is clearly a different entity from that cause by MCA occlusion (Siesjö and Bengtsson, 1989; Siesjö et al., 1990). In the former, the ischemia is usually very dense (or complete) and commonly of brief duration. In terms of the pump/leak relationship discussed, this means that the pump has essentially ceased and that the leak is markedly enhanced. Furthermore, since multiple calcium conductances are activated it is not feasible pharmacologically to block calcium uptake by the energy-deprived cells.

Conditions are different in focal ischemia due to MCA occlusion. Thus, although the densely ischemic focus of such an insult probably behaves like the forebrain or the whole brain in forebrain or global ischemia, the perifocal or "penumbra" zone has a more subtle deterioration of cellular energy metabolism (for discussion and further literature, see Siesjö, 1992a,b). Essentially, this zone comprises all tissues which have a cerebral blood flow which is sufficiently reduced to put the cells "at risk". Thus, if recirculation is not achieved and pharmacological protection is not instituted the cells in the penumbra zone will die and the penumbra zone will become part of the final infarction.

The mechanisms which will lead to an extension of the infarct into the penumbra zone are under debate. One possible mechanism is constituted by repeated depolarizations which, when they occur in an energy-compromised tissue, could lead to cumulative calcium-related damage (Nedergaard, 1988; Siesjö and Bengtsson, 1989).

We recognize the conceptual difference between these two types of ischemia. In one, i.e., forebrain or global ischemia, the insult is brief and transient, and the damage incurred is conspicuously delayed. One intuitively feels that the (delayed) damage is the result of biochemical events which have been triggered during the insult but which "matures" in the recovery period, when oxygen supply has been restored. In the other type of ischemia, i.e., that due to MCA occlusion, the pathogenetically important events are the ones occurring in the marginally ischemic penumbra zone. Here, the problem is one of incipient pump failure, the threat being "spontaneous" depolarizations of the SD type, or microvascular failure, with a further compromise of ATP production or enhancement of the leak fluxes.

Calcium-related damage

The major events triggered by a rise in Ca_i^{2+} and the molecular havoc they give rise to, are illustrated in Fig. 1. Phospholipids and proteins are degraded by calcium-dependent enzymes, explaining why a rise in Ca_i^{2+} leads to rapid hydrolysis of phospholipids, with accumulation of lysophospholipids (LPLs), diacylglycerides (DAGs) and free fatty acids (FFAs), and to degradation of cellular proteins. Such events may be pathogenetically important since they alter membrane and cytoskeletal function. However, it now seems likely that changes in protein phosphorylation are equally important, and that an altered gene expression may contribute to the final damage incurred.

Protein phosphorylation

As discussed in detail by Wieloch et al. (this

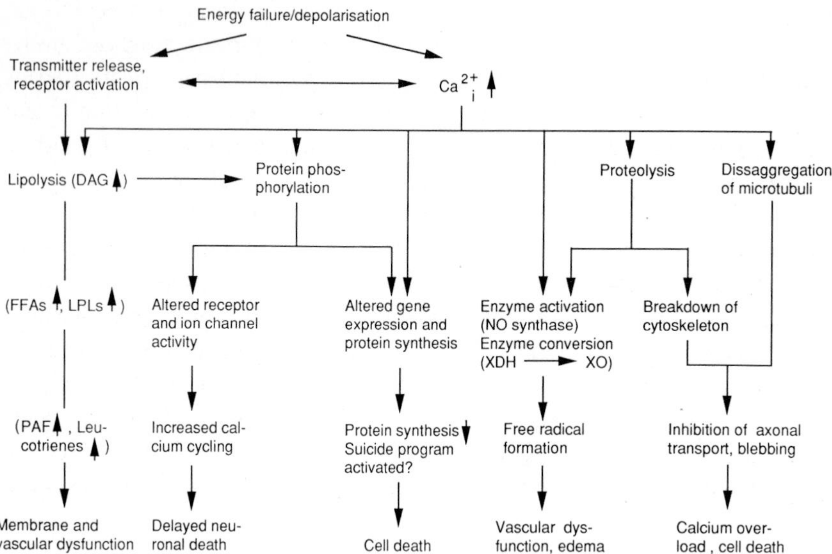

Fig. 1. Schematic diagram illustrating events which are secondary to depolarization, transmitter release, receptor activation and rise in cytosolic calcium concentration. (Modified after Siesjö, 1991.)

volume), the activity of many proteins depends on phosphorylation or dephosphorylation of important functional domains. Since such domains modulate the function of receptors, ion channels/translocators and enzymes, phosphorylation or dephosphorylation normally serves the purpose of altering membrane function and enzymatic activity to match the functional and metabolic needs.

Some of the protein kinases and phosphatases involved are directly activated by calcium or by calcium-calmodulin complexes. For example, both calcium-calmodulin-dependent kinase II (CaM kinase II) and protein kinase C (PKC) are activated by calcium; in the case of PKC calcium may be primarily involved in translocating the enzyme to the membrane where it is activated by DAG. Since DAG arises as a result of phospholipase C activity, and since the latter is modulated by calcium, a rise in Ca_i^{2+} plays a pivotal role in PKC activation (e.g., Nishizuka, 1986; Huang, 1989).

In this sequence of events, calcium and the calcium-dependent protein kinases and phosphatases can be regarded as second messengers which transform an external message into a purposeful response. This is usually considered to be brief (seconds to minutes). However, it has been recognized that a strong stimulus, or repeated calcium transients, can give rise to a long-lasting response, involving a sustained rise in Ca_i^{2+} due to PKC activation (Alkon and Rasmussen, 1988; Connor et al., 1988). Such findings have led to the proposal that a pathological calcium transient can lead to cell death which is secondary to sustained translocation/activation of PKC (Manev et al., 1989). Although the experimental results addressing this hypothesis are contradictory (Louis et al., 1988; Onodera et al., 1989; Wieloch et al., 1991; Domanska-Janik and Zalewska, 1992) we recognize the novelty of the concept: cell death is the result of an activation or a deactivation of second messengers which has gone out of control (Wieloch et al., this volume).

A sustained rise in Ca_i^{2+} and sustained activation or deactivation of protein kinases clearly represent a threat to the survival of cells since it could alter the functions of receptors and ion channels. It has been proposed (Alkon and Rasmussen, 1988) that an up-regulation of this type can serve to prolong the rise in Ca_i^{2+} by positive feedback. This could conceivably shift the balance between degradation and resynthesis of phospholipids and proteins in the direction of increased catabolism. It could also lead to a potentially detrimental inhibition of protein synthesis. Thus, as discussed by Wieloch et al. (this volume), studies on several experimental systems demonstrate that protein synthesis can be inhibited by an altered phosphorylation of the initiation factor 2 (eIF-2) (see also Nowak et al., 1984; Widmann et al., 1991).

Genome expression

It is now widely held that the expression of new genes represents a means for communication within the CNS. For example, repetitive stimulation or seizure activity leads to the expression of immediate early genes (IEGs), resulting in the production of gene products (proteins) which are triggering the expression of late response genes (Morgan and Curran, 1989; Sheng and Greenberg, 1990). This synthesis thus seems to be the third step in a communication sequence which starts with the depolarization and influx of calcium (millisecond time frame), which then leads to the activation of second messengers such as the protein kinases or phosphatases (seconds to minutes), and which ends with the expression of mRNAs for a variety of proteins (minutes to hours). The translocation of this message into protein synthesis may be a cornerstone in the adaptability of the organism to changing environmental demands; however, when the message is not a physiological one, the response may jeopardize the survival of the system.

Ischemia is now known to induce dramatic changes in genome expression since it induces the expression of IEGs such as *c-fos* and *c-jun* (Onodera et al., 1989; Uemura et al., 1991), as well as mRNAs for growth factors (Lindvall et al., 1992). Here, the expression of IEGs may represent a primary "upstream" effect, and the expression of genes for growth factors a secondary effect. Such downstream effects are indeed complex.

The genomic events encompass the synthesis of new proteins, such as the "heat shock" (hs) and "stress" proteins, known to be produced by a variety of cells in response to a variety of harmful stimuli (Dienel et al., 1986; Nowak et al., 1990; Gonzalez et al., 1991; for current overviews, see Brown, 1990; Nowak, 1990). Very probably, these proteins have important functions in the cellular defense against environmental threats, e.g., by handling denatured or otherwise altered, constitutive proteins. However, since such proteins are preferentially synthetized under conditions in which overall protein synthesis is suppressed one has to postulate that priorities of protein synthesis exist in the metabolically perturbed cell. The cause of such priorities and the consequences they may have are unknown (Wieloch et al., this volume).

The genomic events discussed are probably, at least in part, triggered by changes in Ca_i^{2+} (Morgan and Curran, 1989; Sheng and Greenberg, 1990). One can envisage, therefore, that an non-physiological rise in Ca_i^{2+} elicits a series of reactions encompassing activation of both second messengers (e.g., the protein kinases and phosphatases) and third messengers (the genomic events). The calcium transients discussed thus lead to exceedingly complex events which may have far-reaching implications for the ability of cells to survive such transients.

Free radical-mediated damage

The concept of free radical-mediated cell damage is an old one (Barber and Bernheim, 1967), and so is its application to ischemia research (Demopoulos et al., 1977). A decade ago, it seemed very likely that free radicals generated during incomplete ischemia or during recirculation following complete ischemia, significantly contributed to the final brain damage incurred (Siesjö, 1981). The case could also be made for free radical-mediated brain damage as a result of trauma (Kontos, 1985). However, it proved difficult to obtain definitive evidence of free radical-mediated damage, even though Watson et al. (1984) provided some evidence of diene conjugation, probably reflecting lipid peroxidation. In spite of that, the evidence which can be quoted in support of lipid peroxidation being an important pathogenetic event during or following ischemia is surprisingly weak (Watson, this volume).

At first sight, the negative results could be explained by the fact that lipid peroxidation is neither a prominent nor an early sign of free radical damage (Halliwell, 1987). In support of this assumption, evidence was recently reported that even short-lasting ischemia gives rise to oxidative damage to proteins, including enzymes such as glutamine synthetase (Floyd, 1990; Oliver et al., 1990). However, it has been difficult to reproduce these findings, obtained in gerbils, in other species such as the rat (Folbergrová et al., 1992). Thus, at present the best evidence for a free radical component of the ischemic brain damage is that the damage is ameliorated in animals treated with drugs whose best (or only known) effect is to scavenge free radicals (see Liu et al., 1989; Martz et al., 1989), or in transgenic mice in which the human Cu-Zn superoxide dismutase is overexpressed (Chan et al., this volume).

Free radical damage, if incurred, is likely triggered by events which are related to production of reduced compounds (such as NADH and NADPH), and to reoxygenation. Thus, formation of free radicals during reoxygenation should be related to both the accumulation of reduced compounds during ischemia, and to the post-ischemic burst of production of free radicals, e.g., during the metabolism of arachidonic acid. It has long been recognized that calcium enters as an important modulator of such reactions (Siesjö, 1981; Braughler et al., 1985). This is emphasized in Fig. 1 in which calcium is shown to trigger three important events: (1) accumulation of FFAs, including arachidonic acid; (2) modification of enzymes, exemplified by the conversion of xanthine dehydrogenase to xanthine oxidase; and (3) activation of nitric oxide synthethase.

Although these schemes are persuasive, it remains to be shown by what molecular mechanisms free radicals could contribute to ischemic brain damage. It also remains to be shown under what particular circumstances free radical production becomes prominent, and which are the primary targets. Available results only give hints. Thus, it is possible that the adverse effects of pre-ischemic hyperglycemia and of intra-ischemic, excessive acidosis are related to the effect of H^+ ions on equilibria determining the production of the pro-oxidant $H{\bullet}O_2$ from the "innocuous"$\bullet O_2^-$, or to the release of Fe^{3+}/Fe^{2+} from protein bindings in proteins such as transferrin (Siesjö, 1985; Siesjö et al., this volume).

It is possible that microvessels are the primary target of free radicals. Circumstantial evidence which can be quoted in support is the high concentration of xanthine dehydrogenase/xanthine oxidase and of nitric oxide synthetase (NOS) in the microvascular fraction (Beckman et al., 1990; Garthwaite, 1991). One can envisage that microvascular failure is related to the production of NO•, as a result of NOS activity and of $\bullet O_2^-$ (from xanthine oxidase), to the reaction of NO• and $\bullet O_2^-$ to yield peroxynitrate ($ONOO^-$) and to the decomposition of the latter to yield •OH, according to the reactions discussed by Beckman et al. (1990; see also Siesjö, 1992a,b). We recognize that this reaction sequence also emphasizes the possible participation of H^+ in the formation of injurious free radicals.

We can only speculate about the importance of these mechanisms for ischemic brain damage. It is conceivable that the coupling between loss of cell calcium homeostasis, acidosis and free radical damage is strong. In fact, one can argue that the primary effect of acidosis is to prolong and/or accentuate the calcium transient, e.g., by reducing the binding or sequestration of calcium (Siesjö, 1992a,b).

Summary and conclusions

The last 20–30 years of research has brought detailed information on the pathophysiology and the neurochemistry of anoxic/ischemic brain damage. On the basis of this information, impor-

Thorn, W., Scholl, H., Pfeiderer, G. and Mueldener, B. (1958) Stoffwechselvorgänge im Gehirn bei normaler und herabgesetzter Körpertemperatur unter ischämischer und anoxischer Belastung. *J. Neurochem.,* 2: 150 – 165.

Uemura, Y., Kowall, N.W. and Flint Beal, M. (1991) Global ischemia induces NMDA receptor-mediated *c-fos* expression in neurons resistant to injury in gerbil hippocampus. *Brain Res.,* 542: 343 – 347.

Watson, B.D., Busto, R., Goldberg, W.J., Santiso, M., Yoshida, S. and Ginsberg, M.D. (1984) Lipid peroxidation in vivo induced by reversible global ischemia in rat brain. *J. Neurochem.,* 42: 268 – 274.

Widmann, R., Kuroiwa, T., Bonnekoh, P. and Hossmann, K.-A. (1991) [^{14}C]Leucine incorporation into brain proteins in gerbils after transient ischemia: relationship to selective vulnerability of hippocampus. *J. Neurochem., 56,* 789 – 796.

Wieloch, T. (1985a) Hypoglycemia-induced neuronal damage prevented by an *N*-methyl-D-aspartate antagonist. *Science,* 230: 681 – 683.

Wieloch, T. (1985b) Neurochemical correlates to selective neuronal vulnerability. In: K.-A.H.K. Kogure, B. Siesjö and F. Welsh (Eds.), *Progress in Brain Research, Vol. 63,* Elsevier, Amsterdam, pp. 69 – 85.

Wieloch, T., Cardell, M., Bingren, H., Zivin, J. and Saitoh, T. (1991) Changes in the activity of protein kinase C and the differential subcellular redistribution of its isozymes in the rat striatum during and following transient forebrain ischemia. *J. Neurochem., 56,* 1227 – 1235.

SECTION I

Temperature, Acid – Base Homeostasis and Microcirculation

K. Kogure, K.-A. Hossmann and B.K. Siesjö (Eds.)
Progress in Brain Research, Vol. 96

CHAPTER 2

Temperature modulation of ischemic brain injury – a synthesis of recent advances

Myron D. Ginsberg, Mordecai Y.-T. Globus, W. Dalton Dietrich and Raul Busto

Cerebral Vascular Disease Research Center, Department of Neurology, University of Miami School of Medicine, Miami, FL 33101, U.S.A.

Introduction

Profound hypothermia has long been recognized as a potent means of lowering rates of organ metabolism and hence of protecting tissue during circulatory stasis. Thus, moderate-to-profound degrees of whole-body cooling have been used to confer organ protection during cardiovascular and neurosurgical procedures (Lougheed and Kahn, 1955; Little, 1959; Negrin, 1961; Connolly et al., 1962; Venugopal et al., 1973), and to protect against experimentally induced cerebral ischemia (Marshall et al., 1956; Rosomoff, 1957, 1959; Kramer et al., 1968; Michenfelder and Theye, 1970; Kopf et al., 1975; Berntman et al., 1981; Young et al., 1983). Hirsch and Müller (1962) described neurological and histological abnormalities in rabbits when complete brain ischemia was carried out at temperatures above 36°C but not at temperatures of 24 – 36°C. These studies will not be reviewed in detail here. Only in recent years has it become widely appreciated that mild-to-moderate degrees of brain cooling, even when induced selectively without whole-body temperature alterations, are capable of conferring dramatic cerebroprotection; and conversely, mild degrees of temperature elevation may be markedly deleterious to the injured brain. The present contribution synthesizes these recent advances, drawing upon a number of recent summaries of this subject from our own laboratory (Ginsberg, 1990, 1993; Dietrich, 1992; Ginsberg et al., 1992b; Globus et al., 1993).

Selective brain hypothermia during global ischemia

The issue initially arose in our laboratory as a result of unexplained and frustrating variability in the outcomes of apparently "standardized" animal models of global cerebral ischemia. It was anecdotally observed, for example, that reflection of the scalp tissues for EEG monitoring appeared to confer protection from ischemic injury in some studies (Vibulsresth et al., 1987). In retrospect, other laboratories had also been plagued by similar problems (e.g., Blomqvist et al., 1984; Smith et al., 1984), such that at times severe degrees of ischemic injury were observed with relatively minor insults, or unexplained side-to-side asymmetries of neuropathology were observed with bilaterally symmetrical insults – in retrospect, possibly due to asymmetric placement of heating lamps over the animal's head.

These observations led us to undertake a controlled study of the problem, in which *brain temperature* was directly monitored and regulated, and its effect on ischemic neuropathology ascertained. In our initial studies, we employed 20 min of four-vessel occlusion produced by the Pulsinelli-Brierley method (Pulsinelli and Brierley, 1979), in which

Wistar rats first received bilateral vertebral artery electrocauterization, and one day later were exposed to temporary bilateral common carotid artery occlusions with control of mean arterial blood pressure (MABP) (Busto et al., 1987). The temperature of the striatum was measured via an implanted thermocouple probe. We observed that, despite maintenance of rectal temperature at 37°C throughout the study, there occurred a steady, spontaneous decline in brain temperature of approximately 0.5°C/min over the first 10 min of the ischemic insult; and brain temperatures of 30 – 31°C were commonly achieved. Recirculation was followed by spontaneous brain warming to 35°C over 5 – 10 min. There was considerable inter-animal variability with respect to these observations, however.

The above findings prompted the use of a protocol in which, in different animal groups, the brain temperature was selectively modulated so as to be thermostated at fixed values of 30 – 36°C during the ischemic period but at normothermic levels (36°C) prior to and following ischemia. Histopathology performed following a three day animal survival revealed, in rats with normothermic ischemia, marked ischemic cell change in the central and dorsolateral striatum and in the CA1 sector of hippocampus (Busto et al., 1987). In contrast, when intra-ischemic temperature was 33 – 34°C, ischemic changes were reduced by approximately 75% in the dorsolateral and by 100% in the central zones of the striatum, and there was marked protection as well against CA1 cytopathology. With ischemia at 30 – 31°C, ischemic cell change was seen only in the hippocampal subiculum of some rats and only to a mild degree (Busto et al., 1987). This study thus showed that by carefully regulating brain temperature during ischemia, one could obtain vastly different neuropathological outcomes with intra-ischemic temperature variations of as little as 2°C, independent of body temperature maintenance (Busto et al., 1987, 1989b). A side result of this study was the demonstration that temporalis muscle temperature correlated well to intrastriatal temperature and could be used (via a computed regression line) to predict brain temperature, although it was necessary to establish a calibration curve for each experimental protocol.

Careful studies were performed to assure ourselves that the *severity* of ischemia was in fact the same at all temperature groups. This was established via autoradiographic measurements of CBF, revealing virtually absent flow at all ischemic temperatures (Busto et al., 1987, 1989c) and by enzymatic-fluorometric assays of high-energy metabolites, revealing severe energy metabolite depletion at the end of the ischemic insult to a similar degree in all groups. It should be noted, however, that other workers have shown that brains freeze-trapped after just 2 min of ischemia show intermediate degrees of ATP levels during mild intra-ischemic hypothermia but low levels with normothermic ischemia (Welsh et al., 1990). Thus, some initial retardation of ATP depletion appears to be conferred by mild hypothermia.

Measurements in our laboratory of individual free fatty acids released at the end of 20 min of four-vessel occlusion (Busto et al., 1989c) showed a paradoxical *increase* of free stearic and arachidonic acids in the striatum of hypothermic rats when compared to rats undergoing normothermic ischemia. This observation has no ready explanation inasmuch as free fatty acid release is now known to be a general concomitant of ischemia owing to phospholipase activation and breakdown of membrane phospholipids (Edgar et al., 1982; Ikeda et al., 1986; Yoshida et al., 1986) and to disturbed reacylation consequent to brain energy failure (Bazan, 1976).

As might be expected from the protective effect of hypothermia, local cerebral glucose utilization measured in the early post-ischemic period (2 h recirculation following 20 min ischemia at 30°C) was improved in various cortical and subcortical regions by approximately 45% compared to animals undergoing a comparable insult at normothermia (Ginsberg et al., 1989). A similar trend was observed in the CBF data.

In an extensive recent investigation of regional brain energy metabolites (Ginsberg et al., 1992a), rats received 20 min of global forebrain ischemia with maintenance of cranial temperature at either

30, 37 or 39°C; all three groups were normothermic prior to ischemia and during recirculation. Energy metabolites were assayed in the striatum, neocortex and hippocampus at either 30 min, 1 h or 4 h of recirculation in each of the three temperature groups. At all times, there was surprisingly complete recovery of brain energy metabolites in all three structures. However, an influence of altered intra-ischemic temperature was nonetheless evident in the somewhat less complete recovery of both ATP and Σ adenylates following ischemia at 39°C than at 30°C in all three structures, particularly at the 4 h recovery point. Although energy charge recovered to within 95% or more of control values in all structures by 30 min of recirculation, a significant reduction was nonetheless evident in the 39°C group compared to the other groups.

Other studies from our laboratory have documented important evidence of improved *functional* outcome following hypothermic ischemia (Dietrich et al., 1991a). Rats were subjected to 10 min of global forebrain ischemia under either normothermic (37°C) or hypothermic (30°C) brain temperatures. One day later, while awake, they received unilateral stimulation of the large whiskers (vibrissae) in an effort to activate the contralateral barrel-field somatosensory circuit. Control rats showed the expected robust activation of the barrel-field cortex. Animals recovering from normothermic ischemia had reduced resting levels of glucose utilization and a complete impairment of contralateral activation. By contrast, animals recovering from hypothermic ischemia showed more nearly normal levels of resting metabolic rate and significant degrees of metabolic activation in response to the stimulus. Correlative behavioral observations by our group (Green et al., 1992) have shown that histological protection is associated with improved performance on the water maze test – a measure of hippocampal memory function.

Other laboratories have provided data that amply support our own. Thus, Minamisawa et al. (Minamisawa et al., 1990b) confirmed that brain temperature declines during 15 min of forebrain ischemia despite maintenance of rectal temperature. These workers, by controlling both rectal and skull temperatures at levels of 33 – 38°C during 20 min of ischemia, noted that ischemic cell change in the caudate nucleus was severe in the 37 – 38°C groups but almost absent at 33 – 35°C, and that the neocortex showed histologic protection which increased with the degree of hypothermia. Partial protection of hippocampus was also seen at lower temperatures. This same group (Minamisawa et al., 1990c) later used a temperature-controlled high-humidity enclosure which ensured careful maintenance of whole body temperature. They confirmed that temperatures of even 35°C were associated with a protective effect in CA1 hippocampus. In further publications, this group has shown that the high-humidity box is capable of maintaining nearly constant brain temperature during ischemia (Minamisawa et al., 1990a).

Influence of brain temperature modulation on neurotransmitter release in ischemia

Our laboratory and others have previously documented marked release, into the extracellular space, of a variety of monoaminergic and amino acid neurotransmitters in ischemia (Benveniste et al., 1984; Hagberg et al., 1985; Globus et al., 1988a; Hillered et al., 1989; Benveniste, 1991). Decreased temperature may inhibit the biosynthesis, release and uptake of various neurotransmitters (Vanhoutte et al., 1981; Boels et al., 1985; Haikala et al., 1986; Okuda et al., 1986; Graf et al., 1992). Studies in our laboratory, employing a microdialysis probe implanted stereotaxically in the striatum of rats undergoing 20 min global ischemia, revealed a seven-fold release of glutamate during normothermic ischemia; in contrast, ischemia performed at either 30 or 33°C resulted in the complete suppression of glutamate release (Globus et al., 1988a,b; Busto et al., 1989c). Similarly, dopamine, which is massively released to the extent of over 500-fold with normothermic ischemia, rose more slowly during hypothermic ischemia, and its peak release was attenuated by approximately 60%.

The above observations take on pathogenetic

significance vis-a-vis a vast accumulating literature implicating neurotransmitter release in the pathogenesis of ischemic injury. Beginning with the observations of Lucas and Newhouse (1957) on glutamate-induced retinal neuronal destruction, and the observations of Olney and collaborators that blood-brain barrier-deficient brain regions could be injured by systemic glutamate (Olney, 1969; Rothman and Olney, 1986), observations in cell culture (Rothman, 1983) have clearly established that anoxic and dysmetabolic cell toxicity is dependent upon synaptic connections and can be blocked by prevention of synaptic acitivity or blockade of excitatory amino acids (Rothman, 1983, 1984). The development of selective excitatory amino acid antagonists (Watkins and Olverman, 1987) has permitted studies of pharmacoprotection to be carried out in a variety of systems. Extensive studies in in vitro systems have confirmed neurotoxicity mediated by the NMDA receptor/ionophore, and rapid and delayed forms of glutamate-induced neurotoxicity have been characterized (Rothman and Olney, 1986). Non-NMDA receptors have also been shown to mediate a more slowly occurring form of excitotoxicity (Meldrum and Garthwaite, 1990). A large number of studies involving deafferentation, local infusion of pharmacological antagonists and systemic administration of agents in animal ischemia models have permitted the conclusion that at least some forms of regional ischemic brain injury are convincingly mediated by excitatory neurotransmission (Simon et al., 1984; Swan et al., 1988; Albers, 1990; Buchan, 1990; Scatton et al., 1991).

A series of observations in our own laboratory has established with equal assurance that not only glutamatergic mechanisms are involved in ischemic brain injury, but other neurotransmitter systems are also participatory. Thus, a prior substantia nigra lesion in rats, which depletes striatal dopamine and prevents its rise when global forebrain ischemia is subsequently induced, has been shown in microdialysis/neuropathology studies to blunt the ischemia-induced release of dopamine and to protect the striatum from ischemic neuronal injury as well (Globus et al., 1988b). These studies, taken together with the microdialysis observations in hypothermic ischemia cited above, would suggest that both glutamate and dopamine are required to injure the striatum. Consistent with this are findings from our laboratory that the combined administration of an NMDA antagonist (MK-801) and a dopamine D1 antagonist (SCH-23390) confers synergistic protection in the hippocampus of rats subjected to 10 min of global ischemia (Globus et al., 1989). Thus by extension, the complete suppression of glutamate by hypothermia during ischemia, coupled with 60% suppression of dopamine release, may have a joint influence in the cerebroprotection conferred by intra-ischemic hypothermia.

Important work from other laboratories has shed additional light on intracellular mechanisms possibly mediating the protective effect of hypothermia. The enzyme calcium/calmodulin-dependent protein kinase II (CaM kinase II), which is responsible for signal transduction linking intracellular increases in free calcium ion to regulation of protein phosphorylation, has been shown to be permanently inhibited by forebrain ischemia of only 5 min (Taft et al., 1988). This phenomenon appears to be highly temperature-dependent, such that normothermic ischemia in gerbils leads to a 39% reduction in CaM kinase II activity in the forebrain at 2 h following forebrain ischemia, whereas the enzyme is unaffected following hypothermic ischemia; hyperthermic ischemia produces an even more severe depression. In correlative studies, loss of hippocampal CA1 neurons assessed at seven days parallels the loss of CaM kinase II activity. A post-translational modification of CaM kinase II is thought to be responsible for its ischemia-induced inactivation.

Efficacy of post-ischemic brain cooling

From the clinical perspective, it is important to determine the therapeutic window of efficacy for cooling initiated *following* an ischemic event. In our initial observations (Busto et al., 1987), a reduction in brain temperature to 33°C for the first hour of recirculation tended to confer partial protection on the striatum. In a subsequent study of 10 min of normothermic forebrain ischemia produced by bilateral carotid artery occlusions and hypotension, we compared the effects of hypothermic recirculation (30°C) either begun at 5 min following ischemia and maintained for 3 h, or begun at 30 min of recirculation and maintained for the same duration (Busto et al., 1989a). The former regimen led to approximately 50% protection of CA1 pyramidal neurons, while the latter regimen was ineffective. Others (Chopp et al., 1991) have established that the efficacy of post-ischemic cooling depends, as well, upon the duration of antecedent ischemia. In that study, whole body hypothermia to 34°C applied for 2 h following 8 min of normothermic ischemia was partially protective, but the same regimen following 12 min of ischemia was not.

Importantly, Kuroiwa et al. (Kuroiwa et al., 1990) have established the converse observation, namely, that subtle post-ischemic temperature elevations (of only approximately 1.5°C) are important in determining outcome. In that study, halothane was found to blunt the post-ischemic hyperthermic response and to confer protection as well; but the same degree of temperature blunting in the absence of halothane was equally protective. The above observations taken together would suggest that the first hour of post-ischemic recirculation is of particularly critical importance as a window of potential therapeutic opportunity.

Our group introduced the concept of the "excitotoxic index" as a descriptor reflecting the composite magnitude of excitatory/inhibitory amino acid neurotransmitter balance (Globus et al., 1991b,c). It was defined as [glutamate] × [glycine]/[GABA]. In rats subjected to 12.5 min of ischemia by bilateral carotid artery occlusions plus hypotension, and evaluated by intrastriatal microdialysis, animals maintained at 37°C throughout the study showed a significant increase in the excitotoxic index beginning at 1 – 2 h of recirculation and persisting at 3 – 4 h. The magnitude of increase in the excitotoxic index in these animals was 7 – 12-fold. By contrast, animals with post-ischemic hypothermia (30°C induced after 12 min of ischemia and maintained for 3 h) showed no significant changes in the excitotoxic index during the entire recirculation period (Globus et al., 1991a).

Pharmacoprotection and hypothermia

An important by-product of brain hypothermia research has been the realization that many "cerebroprotective" effects ascribed to pharmacotherapeutic agents might be explicable on the basis of inadvertent brain temperature modification. A particularly apposite example concerns the use of the non-competitive NMDA antagonist, MK-801 (dizocilpine). Although initially reported to be highly effective in preventing injury to CA1 hippocampus produced by global ischemia in gerbils (Gill et al., 1987, 1988) and rats (Rod and Auer, 1989), other studies failed to confirm cerebroprotection (Buchan, 1990). When a careful effort was made to repeat the earlier studies (Buchan and Pulsinelli, 1990), the initially described neuroprotective effect was reproduced, but prolonged hypothermia was also observed in treated animals. When normothermia was instead maintained, the protective effect was lost. In a subsequent, more extensive study, MK-801 in a variety of regimens was confirmed not to be effective in severe forebrain ischemia (Buchan et al., 1991).

In a recent study, we explored the potential of combining post-ischemic hypothermia with dextromethorphan, a non-competitive NMDA antagonist, in a rat model of 10 min bilateral carotid artery occlusions plus hypotension. Interestingly, combination therapy tended to be synergistically protective in the neocortex: ischemic cytopathology in layer 3 of the lateral frontoparietal cortex tended to be most marked in normothermic rats not receiving dextromethorphan; intermediate in rats given either hypothermia or dextromethorphan; and strikingly diminished in the combined therapy group. By contrast, there was no synergistic protection observed in the hippocampus, the major site of ischemic cell change in this model (Ginsberg et al., 1990).

The studies reviewed above have had the effect of making workers in experimental cerebral ischemia more broadly aware of the necessity of both controlling and monitoring brain temperature as a separate independent variable. No longer can this be disregarded, even in animals with rectal temperature control. An obvious effect of this change of experimental design has been increased reproducibility of experimental ischemia models. It can be debated, however, what level of brain temperature should be considered "normal" during ischemia. As noted earlier (Busto et al., 1987), brain temperature spontaneously declines with ongoing ischemia. Thus, in theory, one might thermostat brain temperature at a moderately hypothermic level so as to simulate the temperature "epicenter" of the spontaneous situation. A disadvantage of this approach, however, is that many pathomechanisms (including neurotransmitter release, CaM kinase II inactivation, etc.) would in fact not then be at play, and a degree of cerebroprotection would be conferred (as summarized above). Thus, we would argue in favor of the appropriateness of maintaining normothermic brain temperature during ischemia so as to summon the participation of relevant pathomechanisms, which may then be studied.

Deleterious effects of cerebral hyperthermia

In our initial studies (Busto et al., 1987), mild brain hyperthermia (at 39°C) during 20 min of global ischemia was associated with severe ischemic change to striatum, hippocampus, superficial layers of neocortex, and foci of thalamic injury. In a subsequent study (Dietrich et al., 1990b), brain temperature was held at either 37 or 39°C during 20 min of four-vessel occlusion, and pathologic outcome was assessed at one and three days. Although the non-ischemic brain warmed to 39°C showed no histopathology, hyperthermia during ischemia led to increased morbidity and mortality and to severe neuronal injury apparent even at one day survival, consisting of severe ischemic change throughout the striatum and the pyramidal layer of CA1, laminar necrosis in the somatosensory cortex and foci of infarction and ischemic change in ventrolateral thalamus. Cerebellum and pars reticulata of the substantia nigra were also affected, as were dentate granule cells of the hippocampus. This study (Dietrich et al., 1990b) thus concluded that hyperthermia both intensifies the pathologic change in those structures considered traditionally vulnerable to ischemia and, moreover, recruits additional areas of injury not present following normothermic ischemia. Finally, an *acceleration* of pathologic change is produced by hyperthermic ischemia.

Other laboratories have supported many of these findings. Thus, in rats undergoing 5 – 15 min of global forebrain ischemia at either 35, 37 or 39°C, hyperthermic ischemia of even 5 min significantly enhanced ischemic change in both neocortex and thalamus, while 15 min ischemia was associated with a high rate of infarction in neocortex and caudate (Minamisawa et al., 1990c). Studies in gerbil ischemia models have also tended to support these conclusions (Churn et al., 1990).

In a recent study (Sternau et al., 1992), rats received 20 min of forebrain ischemia by bilateral carotid occlusion and hypotension, while undergoing striatal microdialysis sampling. Intra-ischemic brain temperature was held at either 37 or 39°C, but normothermia was maintained before and following the insults. Interestingly, the magnitude of glutamate release during hyperthermic ischemia was significantly greater than was observed with normothermia (37-fold vs. 21-fold), and there was a tendency for higher persistent glutamate levels with recirculation. Extracellular GABA levels increased to a greater degree in the hyperthermic group as well. Glycine also attained higher levels in the hyperthermic group and remained high during a 4 h recirculation period. The excitotoxic index (Globus et al., 1991b,c) differed markedly in the two groups, showing only a two-fold rise in normothermia but a 20-fold increase during the recirculation period following hyperthermia (Sternau et al., 1992).

The blood-brain barrier has emerged from recent studies as being particularly susceptible to ischemia under hyperthermic conditions. Thus, in rats subjected to 20 min of four-vessel occlusion at brain temperatures ranging from 30 to 39°C, the blood-brain barrier remained intact to horseradish peroxidase in the early post-ischemic period following ischemia at 30 or 33°C, showed minor foci of neocortical protein extravasation following normothermic ischemia, but exhibited surprisingly widespread extravasation of protein tracer throughout cortical and subcortical structures following the 39°C insult (Dietrich et al., 1990a). In an extension of these studies, sites of blood-brain barrier disruption correlated well with foci of acute neuronal injury, suggesting that post-ischemic microvascular abnormalities might contribute to the process of neuronal cell death (Dietrich et al., 1991b). Others have noted that hyperthermic ischemia severely accentuates the ischemia-induced inhibition of calcium-calmodulin kinase II (Churn et al., 1990).

Brain temperature modulation in focal cerebral ischemia

In a recent study from our laboratory, three models of proximal middle cerebral artery (MCA) occlusion were used to assess the effects of both moderate hypothermia (30°C) and hyperthermia (39°C) on brain infarct volume. In permanent proximal MCA occlusion with an initial 30 min period of hypotension, large infarcts were demonstrated in both normo- and hypothermic animal groups. In permanent MCA occlusion without hypotension, statistical analysis revealed a hypothermia-induced alteration in the topographic pattern of the cortical infarct but no reduction in its volume compared to normothermia. By contrast, in a model of 2 h *reversible* MCA clip occlusion, infarct volume was lowest in animals with brain temperatures of 30°C during the occlusion period, intermediate in the normothermic group and largest in animals held at 39°C for 2 h. Infarct volume tended to be higher in animals with early post-ischemic hyperemia, as measured by laser Doppler flowmetry. Thus, manipulations of brain temperature in MCA occlusion appear to have a greater influence on cortical infarction in the setting of transient ischemia than in permanent occlusion (Morikawa et al., 1992).

Clinical directions

The demonstration that milder degrees of brain temperature reduction confer cerebroprotection has stimulated efforts to monitor and, eventually, to modulate the brain temperature of patients with ischemic and traumatic brain injury. By incorporating micro-thermistors into a standard ventriculostomy cannula used for the monitoring of intracranial pressure, it has become possible to record temperature simultaneously at ventricular and cortical sites and to correlate it with systemic temperature (Sternau et al., 1991). Pilot observations have suggested that human brain temperature is somewhat higher than core temperature. During febrile episodes in head-injured patients, brain temperatures of 39 – 40°C and above have been noted – levels known from the experimental work reviewed above to exacerbate ischemic injury. Other centers have also begun to monitor brain temperature (Mellergard et al., 1990; Mellergard and Nordström, 1991). Some neurosurgeons are now beginning more routinely to incorporate brain temperature measurements at epidural or subdural sites as a monitoring technique during intracranial operative procedures. We look forward, within the next several years, to controlled clinical trials of brain temperature modulation as a therapeutic tool in such contexts as acute stroke, head injury, post-resuscitation from cardiac arrest and in the setting of operations which pose a risk of brain injury.

Acknowledgements

We acknowledge the support of USPHS Grants NS05820 and NS22603. Dr. Ginsberg is the recipient of a Jacob Javits Neuroscience Investigator Award of the NIH. Dr. Globus is an Established Investigator of the American Heart Association. Ms. Helen Valkowitz helped to prepare the typescript.

References

Albers, G.W. (1990) Review. Potential therapeutic uses of *N*-methyl-D-aspartate antagonists in cerebral ischemia. *Clin. Neuropharmacol.*, 13: 177 – 197.

Bazan, N.G. (1976) Free arachidonic acid and other lipids in the nervous system during early ischemia and after electroshock. *Adv. Exp. Med. Biol.*, 72: 317 – 335.

Benveniste, H. (1991) The excitotoxin hypothesis in relation to cerebral ischemia. *Cerebrovasc. Brain Metab. Rev.*, 3: 213 – 245.

Benveniste, H., Drejer, J., Schousboe, A. and Diemer, N.H. (1984) Elevation of the extracellular concentrations of glutamate and aspartate in rat hippocampus during transient cerebral ischemia monitored by intracerebral microdialysis. *J. Neurochem.*, 43: 1369 – 1374.

Berntman, L., Welsh, F.A. and Harp, J.R. (1981) Cerebral protective effect of low-grade hypothermia. *Anesthesiology,* 55: 495 – 498.

Blomqvist, P., Mabe, H., Ingvar, M. and Siesjö, B.K. (1984) Models for studying long-term recovery following forebrain ischemia in the rat. 1. Circulatory and functional effects of 4-vessel occlusion. *Acta Neurol. Scand.*, 69: 376 – 384.

Boels, P.J., Verbeuren, T.J. and Vanhoutte, P.M. (1985) Moderate cooling depresses the accumulation and the release of newly synthesized catecholamines in isolated canine saphenous veins. *Experientia,* 41: 1374 – 1377.

Buchan, A. (1990) Do NMDA antagonists protect against cerebral ischemia: are clinical trials warranted? *Cerebrovasc. Brain Metab. Rev.*, 2: 1 – 26.

Buchan, A. and Pulsinelli, W.A. (1990) Hypothermia but not the *N*-methyl-D-aspartate antagonist MK-801 attenuates neuronal damage in gerbils subjected to transient global ischemia. *J. Neurosci.*, 10: 311 – 316.

Buchan, A., Li, H. and Pulsinelli, W.A. (1991) The *N*-methyl-D-aspartate antagonist, MK-801, fails to protect against neuronal damage caused by transient, severe forebrain ischemia in adult rats. *J. Neurosci.*, 11: 1049 – 1056.

Busto, R., Dietrich, W.D., Globus, M.Y.-T., Valdés, I., Scheinberg, P. and Ginsberg, M.D. (1987) Small differences in intraischemic brain temperature critically determine the extent of ischemic neuronal injury. *J. Cereb. Blood Flow Metab.*, 7: 729 – 738.

Busto, R., Dietrich, W.D., Globus, M.Y.-T. and Ginsberg, M.D. (1989a) Postischemic moderate hypothermia inhibits CA1 hippocampal ischemic neuronal injury. *Neurosci. Lett.*, 101: 299 – 304.

Busto, R., Dietrich, W.D., Globus, M.Y.-T. and Ginsberg, M.D. (1989b) The importance of brain temperature in cerebral ischemic injury. *Stroke,* 20: 1113 – 1114.

Busto, R., Globus, M.Y.-T., Dietrich, W.D., Martinez, E., Valdés, I. and Ginsberg, M.D. (1989c) Effect of mild hypothermia on ischemia-induced release of neurotransmitters and free fatty acids in rat brain. *Stroke,* 20: 904 – 910.

Chopp, M., Chen, H., Dereski, M.O. and Garcia, J.H. (1991) Mild hypothermic intervention after graded ischemic stress in rats. *Stroke,* 22: 37 – 43.

Churn, S.B., Taft, W.C., Billingsley, M.S., Blair, R.E. and DeLorenzo, R.J. (1990) Temperature modulation of ischemic neuronal death and inhibition of calcium/calmodulin-dependent protein kinase II in gerbils. *Stroke,* 21: 1715 – 1721.

Connolly, J.E., Boyd, R.J. and Calvin, J.W. (1962) The protective effect of hypothermia in cerebral ischemia: experimental and clinical application by selective brain cooling in the human. *Surgery,* 52: 15 – 24.

Dietrich, W.D. (1992) The importance of brain temperature in cerebral injury. *J. Neurotrauma,* 9 (Suppl. 2): S475 – S485.

Dietrich, W.D., Busto, R., Halley, M. and Valdés, I. (1990a) The importance of brain temperature in alterations of the blood-brain barrier following cerebral ischemia. *J. Neuropathol. Exp. Neurol.*, 49: 486 – 497.

Dietrich, W.D., Busto, R., Valdés, I. and Loor, Y. (1990b) Effects of normothermic versus mild hyperthermic forebrain ischemia in rats. *Stroke,* 21: 1318 – 1325.

Dietrich, W.D., Busto, R., Alonso, O., Pita-Loor, Y., Globus, M.Y.-T. and Ginsberg, M.D. (1991a) Intraischemic brain hypothermia promotes postischemic metabolic recovery and somatosensory circuit activation. *J. Cereb. Blood Flow Metab.*, 11 (Suppl. 2): S846.

Dietrich, W.D., Halley, M., Valdés, I. and Busto, R. (1991b) Interrelationships between increased vascular permeability and acute neuronal damage following temperature-controlled brain ischemia in rats. *Acta Neuropathol. (Berl.),* 81: 615 – 625.

Edgar, A.D., Strosznajder, J. and Horrocks, L.A. (1982) Activation of ethanolamine phospholipase A_2 in brain during ischemia. *J. Neurochem.*, 39: 1111 – 1116.

Gill, R., Foster, A.C. and Woodruff, G.N. (1987) Systemic administration of MK-801 protects against ischemia-induced hippocampal neurodegeneration in the gerbil. *J. Neurosci.*, 7: 3343 – 3349.

Gill, R., Foster, A.C. and Woodruff, G.N. (1988) MK-801 is neuroprotective in gerbils when administered during the post-ischaemic period. *Neuroscience,* 25: 847 – 855.

Ginsberg, M.D. (1990) Local metabolic responses to cerebral ischemia. *Cerebrovasc. Brain Metab. Rev.*, 2: 58 – 93.

Ginsberg, M.D. (1993) Emerging strategies for the treatment of ischemic brain injury. In: S.G. Waxman (Ed.), *Molecular and Cellular Approaches to the Treatment of Ischemic Brain Disease – ARNMD Research Publication Series, Vol. 71,* Raven Press, New York, pp. 207 – 237.

Ginsberg, M.D., Busto, R., Castella, Y., Valdés, I. and Loor, J. (1989) The protective effect of moderate intra-ischemic brain hypothermia is associated with improved postischemic glucose utilization and blood flow. *J. Cereb. Blood Flow Metab.*, 9 (Suppl. 1): S380.

Ginsberg, M.D., Globus, M.Y.-T., Busto, R. and Dietrich W.D. (1990) The potential of combination pharmacotherapy in cerebral ischemia. In: J. Krieglstein and H. Oberpichler (Eds.), *Pharmacology of Cerebral Ischemia, 1990,* Wissenschaftliches Verlagsgesellschaft, Stuttgart, pp. 499 – 510.

Ginsberg, M.D., Busto, R., Martinez, E., Globus, M.Y.-T., Valdés, I. and Loor, J.Y. (1992a) The effects of cerebral ischemia on energy metabolism. In: A. Schousboe, N.H. Diemer and H. Kofod (Eds.), *Drug Research Related to Neuroactive Amino Acids – Alfred Benzon Symposium 32,* Munksgaard, Copenhagen, pp. 207 – 224.

Ginsberg, M.D., Sternau, L.L., Busto, R., Dietrich, W.D. and Globus, M.Y.-T. (1992b) Brain temperature modulation – relevance to ischemic brain injury. *Cerebrovasc. Brain Metab. Rev.,* 4: 189 – 225.

Globus, M.Y.-T., Busto, R., Dietrich, W.D., Martinez, E., Valdés, I. and Ginsberg, M.D. (1988a) Effect of ischemia on the in vivo release of striatal dopamine, glutamate, and gamma-aminobutyric acid studied by intracerebral microdialysis. *J. Neurochem.,* 51: 1455 – 1464.

Globus, M.Y.-T., Busto, R., Dietrich, W.D., Martinez, E., Valdés, I. and Ginsberg, M.D. (1988b) Intra-ischemic extracellular release of dopamine and glutamate is associated with striatal vulnerability to ischemia. *Neurosci. Lett.,* 91: 36 – 40.

Globus, M.Y.-T., Dietrich, W.D., Busto, R., Valdés, I. and Ginsberg, M.D. (1989) The combined treatment with a dopamine D-1 antagonist (SCH-23390) and NMDA receptor blocker (MK-801) dramatically protects against ischemia-induced hippocampal damage. *J. Cereb. Blood Flow Metab.,* 9 (Suppl. 1): S5

Globus, M.Y.-T., Busto, R., Martinez, E., Valdés, I., Dietrich, W.D. and Ginsberg, M.D. (1991a) Early moderate postischemic hypothermia attenuates the rise in excitotoxic index in the hippocampus – a possible mechanism for the beneficial effects of early postischemic moderate cooling. *J. Cereb. Blood Flow Metab.,* 11 (Suppl. 2): S10.

Globus, M.Y.-T., Busto, R., Martinez, E., Valdés, I., Dietrich, W.D. and Ginsberg, M.D. (1991b) Comparative effect of transient global ischemia on extracellular levels of glutamate, glycine, and gamma-aminobutyric acid in vulnerable and nonvulnerable brain regions in the rat. *J. Neurochem.,* 57: 470 – 478.

Globus, M.Y.-T., Ginsberg, M.D. and Busto, R. (1991c) Excitotoxic index – a biochemical marker of selective vulnerability. *Neurosci. Lett.,* 127: 39 – 42.

Globus, M.Y.-T., Busto, R., Dietrich, W.D., Sternau, L., Morikawa, E. and Ginsberg, M.D. (1993) Temperature modulation of excitotoxic-induced ischemic damage. *J. Neurotrauma,* 2 (Suppl. 2): in press.

Graf, R., Matsumoto, K., Risse, F., Rosner, G. and Heiss, W.-D. (1992) Effect of mild hypothermia on glutamate accumulation in cat focal ischemia. *Stroke,* 23: 150.

Green, E.J., Dietrich, W.D., Van Dijk, F., Busto, R., Markgraf, C.G., McCabe, P.M., Ginsberg, M.D. and Schneiderman, N. (1992) Protective effects of brain hypothermia on histopathology and behavior following global cerebral ischemia in rats. *Brain Res.,* 580: 197 – 204.

Hagberg, H., Lehmann, A., Sandberg, M., Nyström, B., Jacobson, I. and Hamberger, A. (1985) Ischemia-induced shift of inhibitory and excitatory amino acids from intra- to extracellular compartments. *J. Cereb. Blood Flow Metab.,* 5: 413 – 419.

Haikala, H., Karmalahti, T. and Ahtee, L. (1986) The nicotine-induced changes in striatal dopamine metabolism of mice depend on body temperature. *Brain Res.,* 375: 313 – 319.

Hillered, L., Hallström, A., Segersvard, S., Persson, L. and Ungerstedt, U. (1989) Dynamics of extracellular metabolites in the striatum after middle cerebral artery occlusion in the rat monitored by intracerebral microdialysis. *J. Cereb. Blood Flow Metab.,* 9: 607 – 616.

Hirsch, H. and Müller, H.A. (1962) Funktionelle und histologische Veränderungen des Kaninchengehirns nach kompleter Gehirnischämie. *Pflügers Arch.,* 275: 277 – 291.

Ikeda, M., Yoshida, S., Busto, R., Santiso, M. and Ginsberg, M.D. (1986) Polyphosphoinositides as a probable source of brain free fatty acids accumulated at the onset of ischemia. *J. Neurochem.,* 47: 123 – 132.

Kopf, G.S., Mirvis, D.M. and Myers, R.E. (1975) Central nervous system tolerance to cardiac arrest during profound hypothermia. *J. Surg. Res.,* 18: 29 – 34.

Kramer, R.S., Sanders, A.P., Lesage, A.M., Woodhall, B. and Sealy, W.C. (1968) The effect of profound hypothermia on preservation of cerebral ATP content during circulatory arrest. *J. Thorac. Cardiovasc. Surg.,* 56: 699 – 709.

Kuroiwa, T., Bonnekoh, P. and Hossmann, K.-A. (1990) Prevention of postischemic hyperthermia prevents ischemic injury of CA1 neurons in gerbils. *J. Cereb. Blood Flow Metab.,* 10: 550 – 556.

Little, D.M. (1959) Hypothermia. *Anesthesiology,* 20: 942 – 977.

Lougheed, W.M. and Kahn, D.S. (1955) Circumvention of anoxia during arrest of cerebral circulation for intracranial surgery. *J. Neurosurg.,* 12: 226 – 239.

Lucas, D.R. and Newhouse, J.P. (1957) The toxic effect of sodium-L-glutamate on the inner layers of retina. *AMA Arch. Ophthalmol.,* 58: 193 – 201.

Marshall, S.B., Owens, J.C. and Swan, H. (1956) Temporary circulatory occlusion to the brain of the hypothermic dog. *Arch. Surg.,* 72: 98 – 106.

Meldrum, B. and Garthwaite, J. (1990) Excitatory amino acid neurotoxicity and neurodegenerative disease. *Trends Pharmacol. Sci.,* 11: 379 – 387.

Mellergard, P. and Nordström, C.-H. (1991) Intracerebral temperature in neurosurgical patients. *Neurosurgery,* 28: 709 – 713.

Mellergard, P., Nordström, C.-H. and Christensson, M. (1990) A method for monitoring intracerebral temperature in neurosurgical patients. *Neurosurgery,* 27: 654 – 657.

Michenfelder, J.D. and Theye, R.A. (1970) The effects of anesthesia and hypothermia on canine cerebral ATP and lactate during anoxia produced by decapitation. *Anesthesiology,* 33: 430 – 439.

Minamisawa, H., Mellergard, P., Smith, M.-L., Bengtsson, F., Theander, S., Boris-Moller, F. and Siesjö, B.K. (1990a)

Preservation of brain temperature during ischemia in rats. *Stroke,* 21: 758 – 764.

Minamisawa, H., Nordström, C.-H., Smith, M.-L. and Siesjö, B.K. (1990b) The influence of mild body and brain hypothermia on ischemic brain damage. *J. Cereb. Blood Flow Metab.,* 10: 365 – 374.

Minamisawa, H., Smith, M.-L. and Siesjö, B.K. (1990c) The effect of mild hyperthermia and hypothermia on brain damage following 5, 10 and 15 minutes of forebrain ischemia. *Ann. Neurol.,* 28: 26 – 33.

Morikawa, E., Ginsberg, M.D., Dietrich, W.D., Duncan, R.C., Kraydieh, S., Globus, M.Y.-T. and Busto, R. (1992) The significance of brain temperature in focal cerebral ischemia: histopathological consequences of middle cerebral artery occlusion in the rat. *J. Cereb. Blood Flow Metab.,* 12: 380 – 389.

Negrin, J. (1961) Selective local hypothermia in neurosurgery. *N. Y. State J. Med.,* 61: 2951 – 2965.

Okuda, C., Saito, A., Miyazaki, M. and Kuriyama, K. (1986) Alteration of the turnover of dopamine and 5-hydroxytryptamine in rat brain associated with hypothermia. *Pharmacol. Biochem. Behav.,* 25: 79 – 83.

Olney, J.W. (1969) Brain lesions, obesity and other disturbances in mice treated with monosodium glutamate. *Science,* 164: 719 – 721.

Pulsinelli, W.A. and Brierley, J.B. (1979) A new model of bilateral hemispheric ischemia in the unanesthetized rat. *Stroke,* 10: 267 – 272.

Rod, M.R. and Auer, R.N. (1989) Pre- and post-ischemic administration of dizocilpine (MK-801) reduces cerebral necrosis in the rat. *Can. J. Neurol. Sci.,* 16: 340 – 344.

Rosomoff, H.L. (1957) Hypothermia and cerebral vascular lesions. II. Experimental middle cerebral artery interruption followed by induction of hypothermia. *AMA Arch. Neurol. Psychiatry,* 78: 454 – 464.

Rosomoff, H.L. (1959) Experimental brain injury during hypothermia. *J. Neurosurg.,* 16: 177 – 187.

Rothman, S.M. (1983) Synaptic activity mediates death of hypoxic neurons. *Science,* 220: 536 – 537.

Rothman, S.M. (1984) Synaptic release of excitatory amino acid neurotransmitter mediates anoxic neuronal death. *J. Neurosci.,* 4: 1884 – 1891.

Rothman, S.M. and Olney, J.W. (1986) Glutamate and the pathophysiology of hypoxic-ischemic brain damage. *Ann. Neurol.,* 19: 105 – 111.

Scatton, B., Carter, C., Benavides, J. and Giroux, C. (1991) *N*-methyl-D-aspartate receptor antagonists: a novel therapeutic perspective for the treatment of ischemic brain injury. *Cerebrovasc. Dis.,* 1: 121 – 135.

Simon, R.P., Swan, J.H., Griffiths, T. and Meldrum, B.S. (1984) Blockade of *N*-methyl-D-aspartate receptors may protect against ischemic damage in the brain. *Science,* 226: 850 – 852.

Smith, M.-L., Auer, R.N. and Siesjö, B.K. (1984) The density and distribution of ischemic brain injury in the rat following 2 – 10 min of forebrain ischemia. *Acta Neuropathol. (Berl.),* 64: 319 – 332.

Sternau, L., Thompson, C., Dietrich, W.D., Busto, R., Globus, M.Y.-T. and Ginsberg, M.D. (1991) Intracranial temperature – observations in the human brain. *J. Cereb. Blood Flow Metab.,* 11 (Suppl. 2): S123.

Sternau, L.L., Globus, M.Y.-T., Dietrich, W.D., Martinez, E., Busto, R. and Ginsberg, M.D. (1992) Ischemia-induced neurotransmitter release: effects of mild intraischemic hyperthermia. In: M.Y.-T. Globus and W.D. Dietrich (Eds.), *Role of Neurotransmitters in Brain Injury,* Plenum Press, New York, pp. 33 – 38.

Swan, J.H., Evans, M.C. and Meldrum, B.S. (1988) Long-term development of selective neuronal loss and the mechanism of protection by 2-amino-7-phosphonoheptanoate in a rat model of incomplete forebrain ischaemia. *J. Cereb. Blood Flow Metab.,* 8: 64 – 78.

Taft, W.C., Tennes-Rees, K.A., Blair, R.E., Clifton, G.L. and DeLorenzo, R.J. (1988) Cerebral ischemia decreases endogenous calcium-dependent protein phosphorylation in gerbil brain. *Brain Res.,* 447: 159 – 163.

Vanhoutte, P.M., Verbeuren, T.J. and Webb, R.C. (1981) Local cerebral modulation of the adrenergic neuroeffector interaction in the blood vessel wall. *Physiol. Rev.,* 61: 151 – 247.

Venugopal, P., Olszowka, J., Wagner, H., Vlad, P., Lambert, E. and Subramanian, S. (1973) Early correction of congenital heart disease with surface-induced deep hypothermia and circulatory arrest. *J. Thorac. Cardiovasc. Surg.,* 66: 375 – 386.

Vibulsresth, S., Dietrich, W.D., Busto, R. and Ginsberg, M.D. (1987) Failure of nimodipine to prevent ischemic neuronal damage in rats. *Stroke,* 18: 210 – 216.

Watkins, J.C. and Olverman, H.J. (1987) Agonists and antagonists for excitatory amino acid receptors. *Trends Neurosci.,* 10: 265 – 272.

Welsh, F.A., Sims, R.E. and Harris, V.A. (1990) Mild hypothermia prevents ischemic injury in gerbil hippocampus. *J. Cereb. Blood Flow Metab.,* 10: 557 – 563.

Yoshida, S., Ikeda, M., Busto, R., Santiso, M., Martinez, E. and Ginsberg, M.D. (1986) Cerebral phosphoinositide, triacylglycerol, and energy metabolism in reversible ischemia: origin and fate of free fatty acids. *J. Neurochem.,* 47: 744 – 757.

Young, R.S., Olenginski, T.P., Yagel, S.K. and Towfighi, J. (1983) The effect of graded hypothermia on hypoxic-ischemic brain damage: a neuropathologic study in the neonatal rat. *Stroke,* 14: 929 – 934.

K. Kogure, K.-A. Hossmann and B.K. Siesjö (Eds.)
Progress in Brain Research, Vol. 96

CHAPTER 3

Acidosis-related brain damage

Bo K. Siesjö, Ken-ichiro Katsura, Pekka Mellergård, Anders Ekholm, Johan Lundgren and Maj-Lis Smith

Laboratory for Experimental Brain Research, Experimental Research Center, Lund University Hospital, S-221 85 Lund, Sweden

Introduction

As discussed in two recent review articles (Siesjö, 1985, 1988a) pre-ischemic or intra-ischemic hyperglycemia aggravates damage due to transient ischemia, probably because the increased tissue glucose concentration or the continued/accelerated glucose delivery to the energy-depleted tissue enhances accumulation of lactate$^-$ plus H^+. It is then tacitly assumed that cell damage is secondary to a reduction in intra- or extracellular pH (pH_i and pH_e, respectively). The presumed coupling between acidosis and aggravated brain damage is not unique to the brain, nor is it observed exclusively in ischemia. For example, it has been proposed that flooding intolerance in plants is, at least in part, caused by acidosis (Roberts et al., 1984). Furthermore, cells in culture are so readily killed by intracellular acidification that the procedure can be used to select mutants underexpressing or overexpressing membrane transporters responsible for H^+ extrusion (Pouysségur et al., 1984; Pouysségur, 1985). It is also known from studies on tissue slices (Patel et al., 1973) and cultured astrocytes (Norenberg et al., 1987; Goldman et al., 1989) that a reduction of pH_e, particularly if severe, leads to cell necrosis.

In spite of the evidence in favor of acidosis being a mediator of cell death, discrepant results have been published. These results, most of which were obtained in models of hypoxia or permanent middle cerebral artery (MCA) occlusion, have failed to confirm the relationship between hyperglycemia and aggravated damage. However, as will be discussed below the results could reflect the fact that plasma glucose concentration or glucose delivery are not the sole determinants of intra- and extracellular acidosis in the models studied. Thus, the results may not provide evidence against the proposed coupling between acidosis and cell damage.

The objective of this article is to update information on the coupling among hyperglycemia, intra- and extracellular acidosis and brain damage due to ischemia or hypoxia, and to discuss cellular and molecular mechanisms which may be involved. Since new information has been gained on several basic aspects of the subject, and since controversies have arisen around some others, we will begin by discussing a few key issues.

Sources of H^+ in normal and ischemic tissue

As discussed by Krebs et al. (1975) H^+ ions are produced in large quantities in a multitude of metabolic reactions. Since cerebral metabolism is dominated by the oxidation of glucose, our immediate concern is H^+ generated by glycolysis and during pyruvate oxidation. In general, H^+ is produced in reactions in which ATP is used or NAD^+ is reduced (see Krebs et al., 1975; Alberti and Cuthbert, 1982). We may take as examples the phosphorylation of glucose to glucose-6-phosphate (G-6-P) and the oxidation of glyceraldehyde 3-phosphate (GAP) to 1,3-diphosphoglycerate (DPG):

$$\text{glucose} + \text{ATP}^{4-} \rightarrow \text{G-6-P}^{2-} + \text{ADP}^{3-} + \text{H}^+ \quad (1)$$

$$\text{GAP} + \text{NAD}^+ + \text{HPO}_4^{2-} \rightarrow \text{DPG} + \text{NADH} + \text{H}^+ \quad (2)$$

However, this net acid production is balanced by a corresponding consumption of H^+. The reactions involved encompass those leading to synthesis of ATP or oxidation of NADH (and NADPH). As examples, we may take the final two reactions in the glycolytic sequence, i.e., those which lead to conversion of phosphoenolpyruvate (PEP) to pyruvate, and to reduction of pyruvate to lactate:

$$\text{PEP}^{5-} + \text{ADP}^{3-} + \text{H}^+ \rightarrow \text{pyruvate}^- + \text{ATP}^{4-} + \text{HPO}_4^{2-} \quad (3)$$

$$\text{pyruvate}^- + \text{NADH} + \text{H}^+ \rightarrow \text{lactate}^- + \text{NAD}^+ \quad (4)$$

The net result of glycolysis, i.e., the anaerobic conversion of one mol of glucose to two moles of lactate can be described by two reactions (see Krebs et al., 1975):

$$\text{glucose} + 2\,\text{HPO}_4^{2-} + 2\,\text{ADP}^{3-} \rightarrow 2\,\text{lactate}^- + 2\,\text{ATP}^{4-} \quad (5)$$

$$\text{glucose} + 2\,\text{H}_2\text{PO}_4^- + 2\,\text{ADP}^{3-} \rightarrow 2\,\text{lactate}^- + 2\,\text{ATP}^{4-} + 2\,\text{H}^+ \quad (6)$$

Since Eqn. 5 predominates over Eqn. 6 glycolysis would seem to lead to little production of H^+. However, the ATP formed does not accumulate but is used as soon as it is formed. Hydrolysis of ATP can be described by two reactions:

$$\text{ATP}^{4-} + \text{H}_2\text{O} \rightarrow \text{ADP}^{3-} + \text{HPO}_4^{2-} + \text{H}^+ \quad (7)$$

$$\text{ATP}^{4-} + \text{H}_2\text{O} \rightarrow \text{ADP}^{3-} + \text{H}_2\text{PO}_4^- \quad (8)$$

We note that Eqn. 5 is coupled to Eqn. 7 and Eqn. 6 to Eqn. 8. Thus, although the lactate dehydrogenase reaction (Eqn. 4) *consumes* H^+ when catalyzing lactate formation, glycolysis occurring at constant ATP concentration is always associated with the production of equal amounts of lactate$^-$ and H^+ (see Hochachka and Mommsen, 1983).

This fact has sometimes been overlooked, as has the production of H^+ in the reaction exemplified by Eqn. 6. That equation, and the preceding one (Eqn. 5), represent oversimplifications. In reality, the relative proportions between Eqns. 5 and 6, and between Eqns. 7 and 8 depend on both pH and on the free Mg^{2+} concentration (Gevers, 1977, 1979; Wilkie, 1979; Hochachka and Mommsen, 1983; Nioka et al., 1987). However, the fact remains that, at constant ATP, glycolysis yields equal amounts of lactate$^-$ and H^+.

It is clear that if ischemia/hypoxia leads to hydrolysis of the pre-existing ATP stores some extra H^+ will be released (Gevers, 1977, 1979; Hochachka and Mommsen, 1983). The ATP available is both that stored in the tissue (about 3 mmol/kg) and that formed by the creatine kinase reaction (about 5 mmol/kg). However, the hydrolysis of these 8 mmol/kg of ATP would not lead to the release of 8 mmol/kg of H^+ because less than 1 mmol of H^+ will appear for each ATP hydrolyzed and because the creatine kinase reaction *consumes* H^+. We thus obtain:

$$\text{ATP} + \text{HOH} \rightarrow \text{ADP} + \text{P}_i + n' \cdot \text{H}^+ \quad (9)$$

$$\text{PCr} + \text{ADP} + n'' \cdot \text{H}^+ \rightarrow \text{Cr} + \text{ATP} \quad (10)$$

where n' and n'' vary with pH and Mg^{2+} concentration (Lawson and Veech, 1979; Vink et al., 1988). Probably, hydrolysis of all PCr and ATP during ischemia yields 2–4 mmol/kg of H^+. The exact figure cannot be stated since n' and n'' depend on pH, and thereby on the amount of lactate accumulated. Furthermore, ischemia also leads to breakdown of other nucleoside triphosphates, such as UTP, CTP and GTP (Kleihues et al., 1974; for corresponding data on hypoglycemia, see Chapman et al., 1981).

What additional sources of H^+ generation exist, which could contribute to the acidosis of ischemia/hypoxia? Breakdown of triglycerides and phospholipids to free fatty acids (FFAs) would be expected to release H^+. However, the breakdown is quantitatively small, compared to glycolysis. Another source of H^+ is the electron transport chain. Thus, as pointed out by Krebs et al. (1975) oxidation of substrate-bound hydrogen atoms must lead to H^+ release according to the general reaction:

$$2\,Fe^{3+} + 2\,H \rightarrow 2\,Fe^{2+} + 2\,H^+ \qquad (11)$$

However, there is probably no net release of H^+ from the mitochondria because the reactions are reversed when the reduced respiratory carriers are reoxidized. Furthermore, although H^+ should be absorbed when electron transport yields ATP, these H^+ ions are probably released when the ATP is hydrolyzed. In general, therefore, the mitochondria probably do not generate H^+ under normal steady state conditions, but they could do so if they are marginally uncoupled in disease states (Radda, 1982).

One can tentatively conclude that the amount of H^+ generated in anoxia corresponds to the amount of lactate$^-$ accumulated plus the H^+ released when the pre-ischemic ATP stores are hydrolyzed. If little ATP has been hydrolyzed but PCr has been extensively broken down, as occurs during the first 30 sec of anoxia (Folbergrová et al., 1990; Ekholm et al., 1992), the total amount of H^+ released will be less than the lactate$^-$ accumulated. This is because the creatine kinase reaction consumes H^+ (see above, and because n'' in Eqn. 10 exceeds n' in Eqn. 9). Two findings strongly support these general conclusions. First, although hypoglycemic coma leads to extensive ATP hydrolysis and lipolysis, pH_i is either unchanged or slightly increased, as would be expected from the consumption of metabolic acids, exemplified by the *decreased* lactate levels (Siesjö, 1988b). Second, when complete ischemia is induced in rats whose pre-ischemic plasma and tissue glucose concentrations are varied over wide limits, extrapolation of the pH_i/lactate curve to normal tissue lactate content yields a moderately reduced pH_i value, suggesting that 3 – 5 mmol/kg of the H^+ accumulated is derived from other sources than glycolysis (Katsura et al., 1992b).

Regulation of pH_i

It has been known for many decades that pH_i in nerve and muscle cells is maintained at about 7.0, i.e., 0.3 – 0.4 units more acid than pH_e (Roos and Boron, 1981). Since the membrane potential (Ψ) of nerve, glial and muscle cells is maintained at negative values of at least 60 mV, passive distribution of H^+ would require a pH_i of 6.3 or lower. As suggested by Hill already in 1955, the inescapable conclusion is that metabolic energy is used to extrude H^+ or accumulate HCO_3^-.

The molecular mechanisms have been extensively studied, and at least in part defined (Roos and Boron, 1981; Boron, 1983; Thomas, 1984; Mahnen-

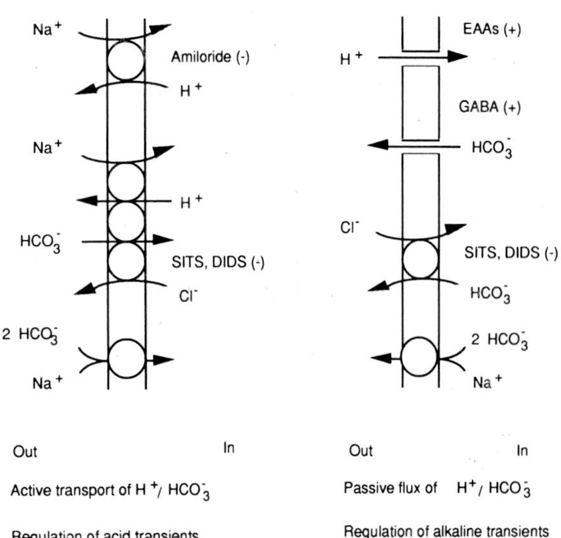

Fig. 1. Schematic diagram, illustrating energy-dependent mechanisms for H^+ extrusion (left panel), and passive mechanisms for accumulation of H^+ or loss of HCO_3^- (right panel).

smith and Aronson, 1985; Grinstein and Rothstein, 1986; Frelin et al., 1988; Chesler, 1990). Many cells, particularly of vertebrate origin, contain a Na^+/H^+ exchanger which extrudes H^+ in exchange for Na^+ (Fig. 1). This extrusion requires the presence of external Na^+ (or Li^+), and is usually inhibited by amiloride or its derivatives. Energetically, the exchanger is driven by the Na^+ gradient. Since the extra- to intracellular Na^+ gradient is about 10:1, the exchanger could theoretically set the H^+ gradient to 1:10, and maintain pH_i at a value of > 8.0. Since this is not the case, regulation of pH_i by the exchanger is assumed to be kinetic, rather than thermodynamic. It is now commonly assumed that, apart from containing an internal substrate site (for H^+), the exchanger also has a pH-sensing modulatory site which activates the exchanger when pH_i falls below the "set point", which is usually around 7.0 (Boron et al., 1979; Grinstein et al., 1983; Jean et al., 1986). The result is that the rate of H^+ efflux (and Na^+ influx) increases with falling pH_i to a maximal value which is usually around 10 mmol/l per minute (see, e.g., Grinstein et al., 1983). However, the rate also depends on pH_e, suggesting that H^+ competes with Na^+ for an external site of the exchanger, or that it decreases the affinity of the external site for Na^+. As a result of this interaction the rate of H^+ extrusion of two studied cell types decreased towards zero when pH_e fell to values approaching 6.0, even though pH_i was low enough to markedly activate the exchanger (Grinstein et al., 1983; Jean et al., 1986). As will be discussed below, the actual regulation of pH_i shows an even larger dependence on pH_e and $[HCO_3^-]_e$).

Many invertebrate and some vertebrate cells contain another H^+ extruding device, one which translocates HCO_3^- inwards in exchange for Cl^- (see Roos and Boron, 1981; Boron, 1983; Thomas, 1984). The presence of this exchanger allows H^+ extrusion to proceed faster in HCO_3^-/CO_2^- containing media, even though pH_i and pH_e are similar. The energy source of this exchange is not obvious since an "isolated" HCO_3^-/Cl^- exchanger would translocate HCO_3^- outwards, acidifying the cell. This is because the extra- to intracellular Cl^- gradient (10:1) is usually much larger than the HCO_3^- gradient (2:1), favoring influx of Cl^- in exchange for HCO_3^-.

It seems likely that an "active" HCO_3^-/Cl^- exchanger, i.e., one translocating HCO_3^- inwards, is somehow coupled to (and driven by) the Na^+ gradient. Thomas (1984) proposed several alternative models, one of which involves influx of Na^+ and HCO_3^- in exchange for H^+ and Cl^- (Fig. 1, left panel). More recently, Boron and his colleagues (Boron and Knakal, 1989) have suggested that net acid extrusion occurs by the influx of the $NaCO_3^-$ pair in exchange for internal Cl^-. We have tentatively assumed that the two acid-extruding exchangers (Na^+/H^+ and HCO_3^-/Cl^-) coexist in the membranes of many cells.

A third pH_i-regulating mechanism, originally proposed to explain HCO_3^--dependent pH_i regulation in kidney cells (see Boron, 1983), seems to exist in glial cells of the leach and the mudpuppy optic nerve (Deitmer and Schlue, 1987; Astion and Orkand, 1988). It is an electrogenic Na^+/HCO_3^- symporter, probably shuttling 1 Na^+ and 2 HCO_3^- across the membrane. Its presence is revealed by a rise in pH_i, and an increase in Ψ, when Hepes buffer is replaced by HCO_3^-/CO_2 (at the same pH_e). It is not unlikely that such a translocase is reversible and poised close to equilibrium. Since it is electrogenic it could then translocate HCO_3^- inwards in response to depolarization of the membrane (see below). By the same token, though, it should translocate HCO_3^- outwards when the membrane hyperpolarizes. The potential importance of such a HCO_3^--transporting mechanism is that it couples changes in membrane potential to transmembrane fluxes of HCO_3^- (and thereby of H^+).

The H^+ extrusion mechanisms discussed must work against a constant leak, involving entry of H^+ and egress of HCO_3^- (Fig. 1, right panel). This leak consists of Na^+-independent ("passive") HCO_3^-/Cl^- exchangers and of conductance channels for H^+ and HCO_3^-; if present, a reversible $Na^+/2\ HCO_3^-$ cotransporter could also catalyze loss of HCO_3^-, and notably when the membrane hyperpolarizes, $[HCO_3^-]_i$ increases or $[HCO_3^-]_e$ decreases. Many, if not most, cells contain a Na^+-independent HCO_3^-/Cl^- exchanger which may function both to transport Cl^- inwards, and to regulate pH_i during alkaline transients (reviewed by Boron, 1983; Olsnes et al., 1987; Frelin et al., 1988). Many years ago, it was generally assumed that leak fluxes were small. In particular, transmembrane fluxes of H^+ were considered almost negligible at the existing intra- and extracellular concentrations. It has been less certain that HCO_3^- fluxes can be neglected since HCO_3^- concentrations are about 10^4 times the H^+ concentrations. It is now recognized that fluxes of H^+ and HCO_3^- may be appreciable. As discussed previously (Siesjö, 1988a), likely pathways for H^+ encompass the non-specific cation channels gated by glutamate receptors (see also Obrenovitch et al., 1990), and for HCO_3^- encompass the Cl^- channels regulated by GABA receptors (Kaila and Voipio, 1987, 1990).

An additional and important mechanism for translocation of H^+ across membranes is provided by permeation of organic acids, like lactic acid. This can either occur by non-ionic diffusion of the acid across the lipid bilayer or by the facilitated transport of lactate$^-$ plus H^+ (see below). Such mechanisms are probably important in reducing differences in pH between different compartments when acid is produced within one of them; however, the mechanism cannot be an important one in causing acid-loading of cells under normal conditions.

It is generally taken for granted that, at steady state or following an acid transient, the extrusion of H^+ is adjusted so that a pH_i of close to 7.0 is maintained. Clearly, though, regulation of pH_i can only occur if the rate of H^+ extrusion matches the downhill leakage of H^+ or HCO_3^- via conductive or ion exchange pathways. This was recognized by Roos and Boron (1981) who emphasized that although an acid transient is usually followed by regulation of pH_i back to normal if pH_e is kept constant, regulation is incomplete or absent if pH_e is appreciably lowered. Theoretically, this follows from the postulate that a lowering of pH_e (or $[HCO_3^-]_e$) decreases the rate of pumping, and increases the leak for H^+ and HCO_3^-; at some point, the leak is equal to the (reduced) rate of pumping.

Boron (1983; see also Roos and Boron, 1981) considered the case in which a cell is exposed to a weak acid (Ha) and its conjugate weak base (a^-), discussing the factors which determine the behavior of pH_i following the initial acidification due to entrance of Ha. Since this case is applicable to the weak acid H_2CO_3 and its conjugate base HCO_3^-, we have redrawn Boron's figure so that it covers acidification due to a rise in PCO_2 (Fig. 2). The figure shows three examples of acid-base response: pH_i regulates back to normal, it initially falls to a value which is then maintained, and it continues to drift in the acid direction. The examples were considered to represent cells which are essentially impermanent to the anion (a^-), those which allowed a^- to leave at a rate which matches the capacity of the pump, and those having such a high permeability to a^- that cycling of Ha and a^- continues to acidify the cell.

This is a useful model and analysis. However, re-

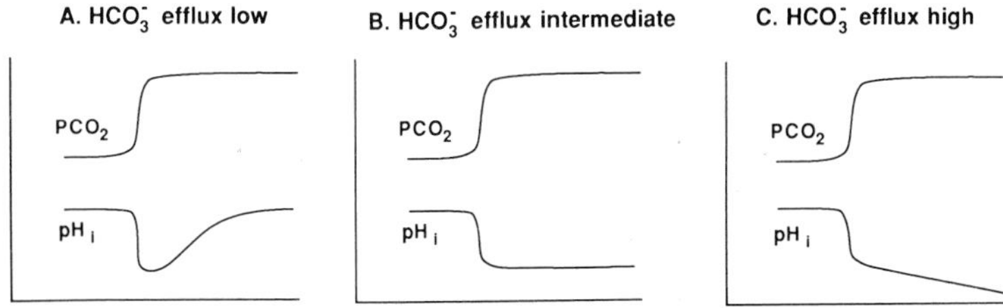

Fig. 2. Schematic diagram illustrating three different responses of pH_i to a rise in PCO_2. The responses are assumed to represent the case when membrane permeability to HCO_3^- is very low (*A*), when it is intermediate (*B*) and when it is high (*C*). (Modified after Boron, 1983.)

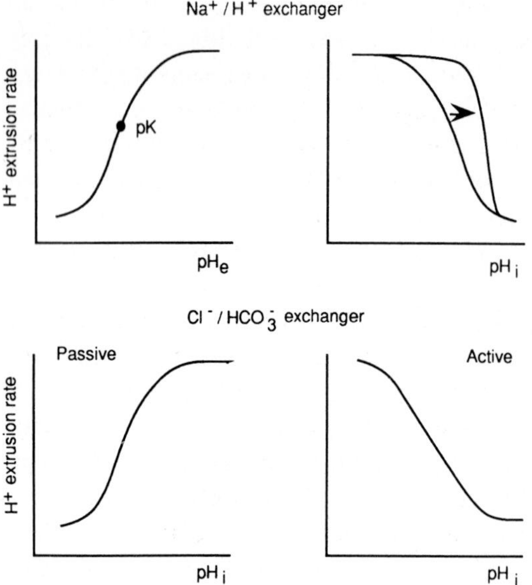

Fig. 3. Schematic diagram, illustrating factors regulating H^+ extrusion by a Na^+/H^+ antiporter (upper two panels) and those regulating Na^+-dependent and Na^+-independent Cl^-/HCO_3^- exchangers (lower two panels). For further explanation, see text.

cent data suggest that additional factors should be taken into account when regulation of pH_i is considered (Fig. 3). One of this is the influence of pH_e and pH_i on the rate of H^+ extrusion (see Grinstein and Rothstein, 1986; Frelin et al., 1988). Although H^+ extrusion is modulated by pH_e as shown in Fig. 3 (upper left panel), the pK values probably vary from one cell to the other and, at least in one glioma cell line studied, the position of the curve was influenced by pH_i, suggesting that the dependence of H^+ extrusion on pH_e is not necessarily fixed (Jean et al., 1986). As shown in the upper right panel of Fig. 3 the dependence of this extrusion on pH_i is described by a curve which can be shifted along the pH_i axis and vary in slope. A rightward shift of the curve – and thus in the pH_i dependence of acid extrusion – is typically observed upon addition of various growth factors and hormones which act by stimulating protein kinase C or other kinases (Grinstein and Rothstein, 1986; Frelin et al., 1988). Even under unstimulated conditions, the slope suggests cooperativity in the interaction of H^+ with the modulatory site, with a Hill coefficient exceeding unity. An up-regulation of the exchanger by phosphorylation may lead to both a rightward shift of the curve and increased cooperativity. Two conclusions can be drawn from these facts: (1) there is no fixed set point but pH_i can be regulated to a value which is higher than normal; and (2) the slope of the curve can be so steep that pH_i is very tightly regulated.

Although information on the modulation of HCO_3^-/Cl^- exchange is limited, certain important facts have emerged (see Olsnes et al., 1987; Frelin et al., 1988). Thus, as shown in the lower panels of Fig. 3, also the Na^+-dependent HCO_3^-/Cl^- exchanger varies with pH_i in a purposeful way. In contrast, the passive HCO_3^-/Cl^- exchanger is inhibited at low pH_i. This would make the exchanger suited to aid in the regulation of pH_i following alkaline transients and prevent simultaneous activation of Na^+/H^+ and Cl^-/HCO_3^- antiporters. Such activation could otherwise lead to a wasteful cycling of ions across the membrane and to loading of the cell with Na^+ and Cl^- (see below). However, since regulation of HCO_3^-/Cl^- exchange is probably also controlled by phosphorylation/dephosphorylation, i.e., by kinases and phosphatases, regulation could be upset in disease.

As illustrated in Fig. 1 (see above), most cells exposed to CO_2/HCO_3^--containing fluids have one, two or three molecular mechanisms for extruding H^+, and several leak pathways most of which allow HCO_3^- to leave. Furthermore, both the extrusion mechanisms and the leak pathways are subject to control by mechanisms which probably encompass conformational changes due to titration of protein groups and phosphorylation/dephosphorylation. Our present concern is the balance of pump and leak pathways in neurons and glial cells.

As extensively discussed by Chesler (1990), nerve and glial cells from vertebrate sources use H^+ extrusion mechanisms similar to those described for other vertebrate (and many invertebrate) cells. The relative importance of Na^+/H^+ and HCO_3^-/Cl^- exchangers in regulating pH_i during acid transients varies between cells; very probably, similar variations exist in the role played by $Na^+:2\,HCO_3^-$ symporters, and by Na^+-independent HCO_3^-/Cl^- antiporters in catalyzing influx or efflux of HCO_3^-. Hippocampal neurons in culture seem to rely on a Na^+/H^+ exchanger for regulation of pH_i during acid transients; however, this was reported as a pharmacologically distinct variant of the ubiquitous Na^+/H^+ antiporter, and the participation of Na^+-dependent HCO_3^-/Cl^- exchange seemed obvious (Raley-Susman et al., 1991). The results of these authors suggest that hippocampal cells in culture have an appreciable leak to H^+ or HCO_3^- and that the "resting" pH_i represents the balance between passive influx of H^+ (or efflux of HCO_3^-) and active efflux of H^+ by any of the mechanisms discussed.

Recent results obtained on primary cultures of cortical astrocytes give comparable information on the relative importance of H^+-extruding mechanisms. However, the results hint to an unorthodox relationship between pH_i and H^+ extrusion (Mellergård and Siesjö, 1991; Mellergård et al., 1992). When suspended in a HCO_3^-/Cl^--containing buffer the cells behaved as those depicted in Fig. 2*A*, i.e., they regulated pH_i back to normal (Mellergård et al., in preparation). However, this behavior was only observed at constant pH_e (7.35); regulation was attenuated when pH_e was reduced to 7.0 – 7.1 and absent at a pH_e of about 6.8 (Mellergård et al., 1992, in preparation). Results were similar if acidification was induced with an ammonia prepulse, i.e., regulation of pH_i to "normal" occurred if pH_e was kept constant, but not if it was reduced to values below normal. At first sight, this suggests that glial cells maintain a normally high rate of HCO_3^- efflux. However, similar results were obtained in the nominal absence of HCO_3^-/CO_2. Furthermore, whether the cells were suspended in Hepes buffer or in HCO_3^-/CO_2 buffer, a lowering of pH_e induced a rapid decrease in pH_i, giving a $\Delta pH_i/\Delta pH_e$ relationship of about 0.7.

These results raise the question whether cultured cells have an unfavorable pump/leak relationship for H^+ (or HCO_3^-), or whether regulation of pH_i is modulated by pH_e in a manner which is not clarified by the experiments. As a third alternative, one may speculate that the rate of extrusion does not vary with pH_i as expected, i.e., that the extrusion rate is relatively constant when $\Delta\mu_{H^+}$ and $\Delta\mu_{HCO_3^-}$ vary over wide ranges. Information on membrane potentials is needed to settle this issue. What is clear is that cultured astrocytes have both a high rate of H^+ extrusion (at normal or reduced pH) and high leak fluxes for H^+ and HCO_3^-. This makes it imperative to study how uphill and downhill fluxes of H^+/HCO_3^- are regulated.

The importance of these in vitro findings is not known at present, and further data are required to assess if neurons and glia cells are capable of regulating pH_i when pH_e is appreciably reduced. Some experiments suggest that although regulation of pH_i occurs during hypercapnia in vivo, it is slower and probably less complete than what is usually observed in vitro at constant pH_e (Messeter and Siesjö, 1971a). It is tempting to speculate that an appreciable part of the acute regulation of pH_i occurs by consumption of metabolic acids (Siesjö, 1973) and that regulation of pH_i by H^+ extrusion heavily depends on mechanisms which regulate pH_e (see Messeter and Siesjö, 1971b). This speculation is supported by recent data reported by Cohen et al. (1990), demonstrating absence of regulation of pH_i in animals exposed to very high CO_2 concentrations (50%) for 75 min. We submit that this is because pH_e falls to such low values that H^+ extrusion can no longer match the passive leak of H^+ (or HCO_3^-).

Although these in vitro and in vivo data suggest that pH_i cannot be fully regulated by H^+ extrusion if pH_e is low, other results demonstrate that this is feasible. As Fig. 4 shows, recovery from 20 min of status epilepticus is followed by a rapid increase of pH_i to values exceeding control, although pH_e remains low for a prolonged period (Siesjö et al., 1985). The results are compatible with enhanced Na^+/H^+ exchange, acidifying the extracellular and alkalinizing the intracellular fluids. We also have to explain why pH_i can be regulated back towards normal when flow is reinstated in hyperglycemic animals subjected to 15 min of ischemia, although pH_e remains below 7.0 in that period (Smith et al., 1986). It could be argued that

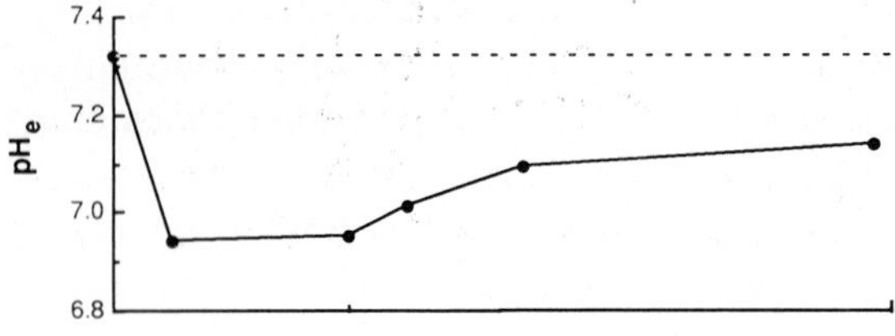

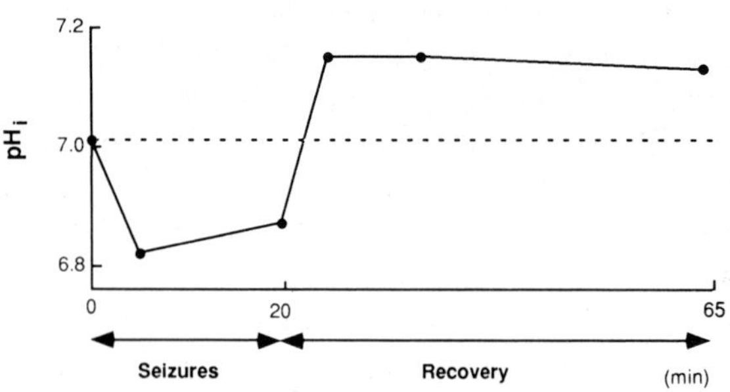

Fig. 4. Changes in pH_e and pH_i during and following drug-induced status epilepticus in rats (data from Siesjö et al., 1985). Changes in pH_e were measured by a microelectrode while the pH_i data were obtained by calculation from total CO_2, $PtCO_2$ and pH_e. Note "overregulation" of pH_i during recovery in spite of persistence of extracellular acidosis.

pH_i is regulated by consumption of metabolic acids (chiefly lactic acid) when the insults are terminated. What speaks against this possibility is that "clearance" of lactate is slow following these transient insults (Hillered et al., 1985). Furthermore, we have seen a similar dissociation between extra- and intracellular pH following hypoglycemic coma, an insult which is followed by *production* of acids consumed during the insult (Bengtsson et al., 1990; and unpublished results).

Very likely, these results reflect variations in the pump/leak relationship for H^+ and HCO_3^-. Conceivably, certain insults (or conditions) reduce the leaks or increase the pump rates. It is perhaps most likely that the set point for the influence of internal H^+ on the Na^+/H^+ exchanger is shifted in the alkaline direction, or that the curve describing the H^+ extrusion rate as a function of pH_e is shifted towards more acid values. The first possibility is compatible with the known effect of growth factors and protein kinase C (PKC) activators in up-regulating the Na^+/H^+ antiporter, i.e., in changing the set point for the antiporter (Grinstein and Rothstein, 1986; Moolenaar, 1986; Frelin et al., 1988; Saldet et al., 1991). As already remarked, the second possibility has some precedence since Jean et al. (1986) reported that, at least in one glia-derived cell line, the influence of pH_e on the H^+ extrusion rate seemed to vary with pH_i.

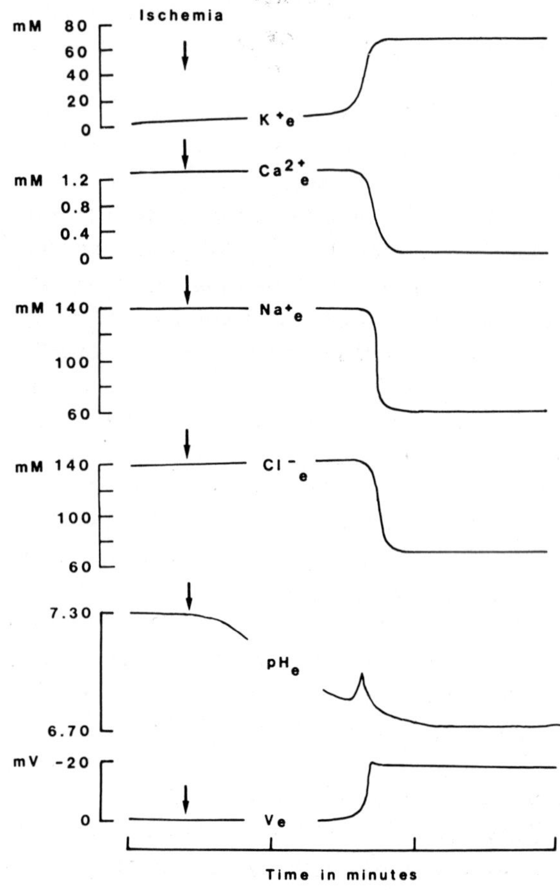

Fig. 5. Schematic diagram illustrating transmembrane fluxes of H^+ (or HCO_3^-) in relationship to the ionic fluxes and to the DC potential change accompanying ischemia. (Reproduced with permission from Siesjö et al., 1989b.)

Compartmentation of H^+

Compartmentation of H^+ exists on several levels. First, the extracellular fluid usually has a pH which is about 0.3 units more alkaline than "average" pH_i. Second, although the cytoplasmic pH_i measured under control conditions in cortical astrocytes is very close to this average pH_i, stimulation of neuronal activity with a rise in K_e^+ triggers dynamic changes of pH_i which differ between neurons and glia, as well as changes in pH_e which may be in the opposite direction to those in pH_i (Chesler, 1990). Third, compartmentation of H^+ within cells is obvious since mitochondria maintain a higher, and lysosomes as well as transmitter-containing granulae/vesicles a lower pH than the cytosol (see Roos and Boron, 1981). In fact, gradients of pH_i can be created between different parts of the same cell. To take only two examples, activation of receptors gating H^+- or HCO_3^--permeable channels must lead to local changes in pH_i (and pH_e), and growth cones have been reported to have a higher pH_i than the rest of the cell.

Compartmentation of H^+ between and within cells is thus a fact, and further data on the complex functional responses of neuronal networks and the various forms of glia may well reveal even larger differences in pH responses. Our present concern is a different one: do cells respond differently to ischemia and are H^+ gradients maintained in the energy-deprived and grossly acidotic tissue of an ischemic subject? Before discussing this question, we will briefly recall compartmentation of H^+ during functional activation.

Synaptic activity may cause two types of transients in which extra- and intracellular pH change in opposite directions (Chesler, 1990). One is the alkaline shift of pH_e observed during electrical stimulation (e.g., Kraig et al., 1983; Sykova and Svoboda, 1990). Typically, such stimulation leads to an alkaline followed by an acid shift. However, results obtained during spreading depression (SD) or in ischemia showed that an initial acid shift was followed by a transient alkaline shift (Kraig et al., 1983; Mutch and Hansen, 1984). Since this alkaline shift occurred at the time when K^+ was rapidly released from cells and Ca^{2+} and Na^+ was taken up together with Cl^- (Fig. 5), it could be speculated that the alkalosis was caused by influx of H^+ through unspecific cation channels, e.g., those gated by glutamate receptors, or by efflux of HCO_3^- through GABA-activated Cl^--channels (Siesjö, 1988a). The transient nature of the alkalosis would then follow from the fact that, once the membranes depolarize, the electrochemical gradients for passive flux of H^+ or HCO_3^- reverse. Experimental support for this hypothesis has been reported (Obrenovitch et al., 1990), and recent studies of activity-dependent pH_e shifts promise to clarify the mechanisms involved (Chen and Chesler, 1991, 1992).

The other activity-dependent transient is that in which pH_i in glial cells increases in response to electrical stimulation or SD, at a time when pH_e and neuronal pH seem to decrease (Chesler and Kraig, 1987, 1989). The results raise the question about the mechanisms involved (see Chesler, 1990). In theory, influx of HCO_3^- could occur via an electrogenic Na^+/HCO_3^- cotransporter and be driven by the depolarization of the glial cell membrane; however, we recognize that stimulation of Na^+/H^+ exchange would lead to the same result. Such stimulation of the exchanger could conceivably be caused by activation of kinases, triggered as a result of the depolarization. It is highly justified that the mechanisms are clarified.

It was proposed by Kraig et al. (1986) that compartmentation of H^+ between glia cells, neurons and ECF occurs also during ischemia. These authors based their analyses on the fact that pre-ischemic hyperglycemia aggravates damage due to transient ischemia, and set out to correlate $PtCO_2$, pH_e, TCO_2 and tissue lactate content in animals whose pre-ischemic tissue glucose concentration varied over wide limits. Their results suggested that marked shifts of H^+ and HCO_3^- occur in the tissue lactate range of 15 – 20 mmol/kg, i.e., in the range over which ischemic damage is aggravated in hyperglycemic animals (Siesjö, 1981, 1984). Such shifts were reflected in both the pH_e and the $PtCO_2$

records. Thus, over the lactate range of 9–40 mmol/kg, pH_e showed two plateau values with ΔpH of about 0.5 and 1.1, respectively, and a transition zone at lactate values of 15–20 mmol/kg. In this zone the $PtCO_2$ increased abruptly but remained constant at higher lactate values. The results hinted to the formation of lactic acid in a compartment whose HCO_3^- content was close to zero (explaining the constancy of PCO_2 at high lactate contents). The authors suggested that, at high tissue glucose contents, lactate is preferentially formed in glia cells which suffer damage from the lactic acidosis. In other words, compartmentation of H^+ was invoked to explain the pannecrotic lesions of hyperglycemic subjects.

Although the direct pH_i measurements reported by Kraig and Chesler (1990) suggest that the ischemic tissue of grossly hyperglycemic animals contains compartments with pH values of about 5.3, the concept of marked compartmentation of H^+ in ischemic tissue has not received additional support. Boris-Möller et al. (1988) did not detect a splitting of the P_i peak in ^{31}P-NMR studies on ischemic tissue, and pointed out that non-ionic diffusion of lactic acid must be expected to attenuate or obliterate any H^+ gradients. This issue was directly addressed by Walz and Mukerji (1990) who failed to find evidence that cultured astrocytes, loaded with lactic acid, could trap the acid; on the contrary, lactic acid rapidly equilibrated between glia, neurons and extracellular fluid (see also Walz and Mukerji, 1988). We also wish to recall that the pH_i of cultured astrocytes changes rapidly when pH_e is reduced, suggesting a high membrane conductance to H^+ (see above). In view of this it seems unlikely that appreciable H^+ gradients can be maintained across the glial cell membranes.

Additional data on this controversy have recently been collected. Thus, in the hands of our own group the relationship between lactate and either PCO_2 or pH_e in ischemic tissue is linear (Fig. 6, data from Katsura et al., 1992a,b). Such a relationship does not support the notion of compartmentation of H^+, but suggests that pH_e and pH_i of a lumped intracellular space change in parallel when increasing amounts of lactate accumulate in the ischemic tissue (Katsura et al., 1992a).

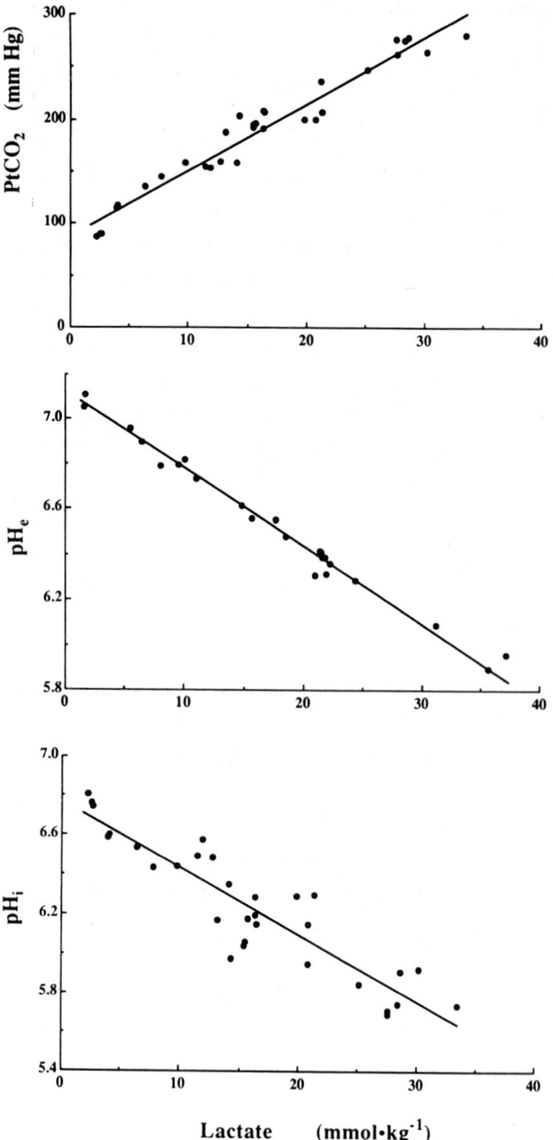

Fig. 6. Relationship between tissue lactate and $PtCO_2$ (upper), pH_e (middle) or pH_i (lower) in normocapnic rats. The correlation coefficients (*r*) of the linear fitting were 0.975 (upper), 0.991 (middle) and 0.912 (lower), respectively. (Data from Katsura et al., 1992a,b.)

In summary, considerable interest is at present directed towards two aspects of the acid-base metabolism of the brain. One is the well-known sensitivity of neurons and glial cells to excessive acidosis, which is most dramatically observed in the exaggeration of brain damage in hyperglycemic animals subjected to transient ischemia. The other aspect concerns changes in extracellular pH (pH_e) and in intracellular pH (pH_i) of neurons and glial cells during functional alterations (see Chesler, 1990). Such changes, and those observed during SD, demonstrate that pH_e and pH_i can move in opposite directions, and furthermore that glial cells can show an alkaline shift when neurons and extracellular fluid are acidified. Although compartmentation of H^+, with glial cells becoming excessively acid, has been assumed to arise during complete ischemia, this hypothesis has been refuted.

Brain damage in hyperglycemic subjects: mediators and modulators

As discussed in a recent review article (Siesjö, 1988a), hyperglycemia, whether caused by stress in fed subjects or by the intentional pre-ischemic administration of glucose, aggravates brain damage due to transient ischemia. Typical features of such aggravation are extensive neuronal damage, glial swelling and destruction, gross edema and post-ischemic seizures. Usually, the damage appears after a delay which varies between minutes and many hours. Short "maturation" periods are observed after long ischemic periods in grossly hyperglycemic subjects (see Ginsberg et al., 1980; Welsh et al., 1980; Kalimo et al., 1981; Rehncrona et al., 1981). For example, although reperfusion occurs after 30 min of incomplete ischemia in such subjects, a secondary compromise of microcirculation with deterioration of energy metabolism may be observed already during the first 1 – 2 h of recovery. In contrast, if ischemia is of short duration (e.g., 10 min) and hyperglycemia is less severe, the cell damage matures over hours (Smith et al., 1988) and the characteristic audiogenic seizures ("running fits") may be delayed by up to 24 h (Warner et al., 1987; Voll and Auer, 1988). However, this long delay is at least in part due to a seizure-suppressing effect of the anesthetic used. Thus many animals anesthetized with isoflurane showed clinical seizure activity during the first 1 – 4 h (Lundgren et al., 1990a,b).

In starved, normoglycemic subjects short periods of ischemia typically lead to damage which is confined to selectively vulnerable neurons and which appears after a delay which varies depending on the region affected (Kirino, 1982; Pulsinelli et al., 1982a; Smith et al., 1984a,b). Hyperglycemia alters this pattern in three ways: the evolution of the damage is faster; glial cells become involved yielding pannecrotic lesions; and new areas are affected (Pulsinelli et al., 1982b; Smith et al., 1988). Prominent among the latter are cingulate cortex, some thalamic nuclei and substantia nigra pars reticulata (SNPR) (Inamura et al., 1987; Smith et al., 1988; Lundgren et al., 1991a, 1992). The frequent damage to the SNPR is noticeable since the nucleus is only moderately ischemic, at least in the forebrain model used for induction of ischemia in our laboratory.

The sequence of events described has been so extensively documented that little doubt exists of a causal relationship between hyperglycemia and exaggerated brain damage. Nonetheless, some published findings are seemingly at variance with the concept, and the coupling among hyperglycemia, acidosis and brain damage is not as straightforward as a cursory analysis would suggest. We will discuss some of the problems, identifying each of them by a question.

Is a trickle of flow detrimental because it allows delivery of additional glucose?

The original en passant observation that incomplete ischemia, allowing a trickle of flow, had a worse outcome than complete ischemia, was assumed to reflect the adverse vascular effects of blood stagnating in the tissue (Hossmann and Kleihues, 1973). Although our own group could verify the finding as such, we favored another explanation, i.e., that the continued delivery of oxygen or glucose triggered oxygen-dependent or acidosis-dependent damage (Nordström et al., 1976, 1978). Subsequent experiments showed that the speculation about a detrimental effect of excessive acidosis was correct (for early reviews, see Myers, 1979; Siesjö, 1981, 1984). However, conflicting results were reported on the importance of a trickle of flow (e.g., Steen et al., 1979).

It can be speculated that incomplete ischemia carries a worse outcome in hyperglycemic subjects in which a remaining flow can cause excessive accumulation of lactate$^-$ plus H^+ (see Siesjö, 1984, 1988a). Furthermore, in starved and normoglycemic subjects a trickle of flow may have a survival value and improve recovery. This may be due to two factors. First, in the absence of acidosis, the delivery of some oxygen could support energy production. Second, continued perfusion of the microvessels may prevent an excessive increase in the relative viscosity and reduce detrimental interaction between platelets or neutrophils and endothelial cells. By the same token, complete ischemia is harmful because it increases relative viscosity and hinders reperfusion so that perfusion defects appear (Kågström et al., 1983a,b; Dietrich et al., 1987). One can also speculate that the remarkable recovery of brain function after 60 min of complete ischemia, reported by Hossmann and colleagues (see Hossmann and Kleihues, 1973; Hossmann, 1982, 1985), was possible only because these workers took precautions to promote reperfusion by reducing blood osmolarity and viscosity, to prevent intravascular coagulation and to increase perfusion pressure.

If this speculation is valid, we may conclude that two different factors are potentially detrimental: complete cessation of flow and excessive acidosis. Conceivably, they both exert adverse effects which are at least in part exerted on the microcirculation. This possibility justifies efforts to explore how excessive acidosis influences capillary and arteriolar function. However, as pointed out by Hossmann (1991), the results reported in the literature are equivocal and further data are required before the issue is settled.

Is hyperglycemia always detrimental?

If hyperglycemia exaggerates damage by increasing production of lactate$^-$ plus H^+, one would expect such exaggeration only in situations where glucose supply for glycolysis is limited. Vannucci et al. (1988; see also Voorhies et al., 1986), inducing hypoxia/ischemia in immature rats, failed to find worse damage in subjects injected with enough glucose to raise the blood glucose concentration almost three-fold. However, although tissue glucose concentrations were also raised by this treatment, the tissue lactate concentrations varied only to a limited extent between normo- and hyperglycemic rats. Furthermore, since information on pH_i was lacking it was not possible to state whether or not hyperglycemia aggravated the acidosis.

The failure of hyperglycemia to raise tissue lactate content in models of hypoxia/ischemia is not unexpected. Thus, previous results have shown that, unless flow decreases to low values, the increase in tissue lactate content correlates with the fall in adenylate energy charge (or ATP concentration) and not with plasma glucose concentration (Salford and Siesjö, 1974; Gardiner et al., 1982). Obviously, when flow is normal or increased glycolysis is not limited by glucose supply but is determined by the degree of deterioration of cerebral energy state. It follows from this that hyperglycemia is only harmful if it exaggerates production of lactate$^-$ plus H^+.

Another situation in which hyperglycemia does not invariably aggravate ischemic damage is focal ischemia due to middle cerebral artery (MCA) occlusion. Thus, although hyperglycemia aggravates damage incurred as a result of *transient* MCA occlusion (Venables et al., 1985; Nedergaard, 1987; De Courten-Myers et al., 1989), results differ in experiments with *permanent* occlusion. One group found that hyperglycemia in cats subjected to permanent MCA occlusion increased the size of infarct and caused fatal brain swelling in some animals (De Courten-Myers et al., 1988); however, divergent results were obtained by other workers (Zasslow et al., 1989). The results obtained in rats are equally variable. Thus, although acute hyperglycemia increased infarct size in one study (Duverger and MacKenzie, 1988) and chronic hyperglycemia caused by streptozotocin-induced diabetes had a similar effect in another study (Nedergaard and Diemer, 1987), other results showed no such effect (Ginsberg et al., 1987); in fact, in at least one study hyperglycemic animals had smaller infarcts (Ginsberg et al., 1987). By comparing three different models for inducing focal ischemia due to MCA occlusion, Prado et al. (1988) came to the conclusion that hyperglycemia increased infarct size in collaterally perfused areas, usually neocortical, but not in end-arterial vascular territories, such as the caudo-putamen.

This is a reasonable mechanistic explanation but it is only applicable to permanent MCA occlusion; besides, it does not address the issue whether or not hyperglycemia aggravates local acidosis in focal or penumbral tissues. This is a crucial issue which we will discuss below. In the present context, we wish to recall the intriguing findings of Nedergaard and Diemer (1987) who induced permanent MCA occlusion in hypo-, normo- and hyperglycemic rats, assessing infarct size and density of perifocal neuronal necrosis. Hypoglycemic subjects had reduced infarct size but increased density of neuronal necrosis, mainly localized to layers 2 and 3 of the neocortex. Such perifocal neuronal injury was also observed in normoglycemic subjects, but to a lesser extent. Animals made acutely hyperglycemic before MCA occlusion failed to show an increased infarct size or perifocal neuronal necrosis; however, they showed lesions with total destruction of all cellular elements including glia and microvessels. Thus, hyperglycemia prevented perifocal neuronal lesions but reinforced the pannecrotic character of the focal lesion.

Is hyperglycemia detrimental because it exaggerates lactic acidosis?

As reviewed in a previous article (Siesjö, 1988a) substantial evidence exists that the exaggeration of ischemic lesions by pre-ischemic hyperglycemia is related to enhanced production of lactate$^-$ plus H^+. However, some findings question this coupling. These findings pertain to the surprisingly small changes in plasma glucose (or tissue lactate) concentration required to dramatically worsen the damage and to paradoxical results on the role of hyperglycemia in focal ischemia.

Even moderate hyperglycemia triggers events leading to grossly exaggerated brain damage (Siesjö, 1981; Pulsinelli et al., 1982b). On analysis of available data, it appears that a change in tissue lactate from 15 to 20 mmol/kg is enough to precipitate the cascade of events described above. Such a pronounced threshold effect could possibly be explained by a threshold change in pH_i or pH_e (Kraig et al., 1985). However, since the data supporting this contention have been refuted we are faced with the problem of explaining why an increase in tissue lactate content by 5 mmol/kg or less can dramatically change the outcome of transient ischemia. Since pH_i and pH_e change hardly over this range of lactate concentration (Katsura et al., 1992a), one has to postulate that either this narrow pH threshold reflects the titration of functionally critical protein groups, or that a raised glucose concentration per se is essential for the same functions. This will remain an open question until further data are available.

The problems at stake are highlighted by the results reported by Welsh et al. (1983), who induced hypoxia in animals with a unilateral carotid artery occlusion, varied the pre-ischemic plasma glucose concentration and recorded short-term metabolic recovery. These authors found a narrow range of plasma glucose concentrations over which recovery was adversely affected; however, the corresponding range of tissue lactate concentrations was so narrow that the question had to be posed whether lactate was the critical variable. The potential objection against any conclusion drawn from such data is that since the model used represents an open system, allowing exchange of ions between tissue and blood, it is not known if lactate content correlates with the severity of acidosis. Nonetheless, the possibility must be kept in mind that hyperglycemia is detrimental, not because it aggravates acidosis but because it triggers other adverse reactions. Thus, the glucose molecule per se may be important, e.g., by influencing glucosylation of essential molecules. As a very speculative possibility, one has to consider the possibility that hyperglycemia inhibits oxidative phosphorylation, referred to as the Crabtree effect (Crabtree, 1929). As suggested by Krebs (1972), cells with a high glycolytic capacity may show this effect which may lead to a competition between glycolysis and the respiratory chain for ADP and P_i. In support of this possibility, Siemkowicz et al. (1982) found that hyperglycemia caused increased post-ischemic glucose phosphorylation and decreased oxygen consumption. However, there is no indication that pre-ischemic hyperglycemia affects post-ischemic phosphorylation state (Hillered et al., 1985); besides, post-ischemic administration of glucose has been claimed not to enhance ischemic brain damage (Rehncrona et al., 1981; Pulsinelli et al., 1982b). For these reasons, we will adopt the working assumption that hyperglycemia is detrimental because it causes a further decrease in pH. This conclusion receives support from in vitro data on astrocytes in primary culture, demonstrating that high glucose treatment (30 min) for 24 h before hypoxia did not affect cell viability to a hypoxic insult (Tombaugh and Sapolsky, 1990a). Such treatment is unlikely to alter pH_i.

The variable effect of hyperglycemia on the severity of a focal ischemic lesion remains to be clarified. In discussing this crucial issue we can assume, on good grounds, that hyperglycemia does not aggravate damage to the focus caused by permanent occlusion, simply because focal blood flow is low enough to yield an infarct, irrespective of the plasma glucose concentration. The problem thus revolves around events in the penumbra. Two questions arise. First, does pH fall to values low enough to trigger acidosis-related damage? Second, is acidosis exaggerated by hyperglycemia?

The answer to the first question is far from straightforward since perifocal flow rates may differ from one species to another, and also depend on the models employed. As discussed elsewhere (Siesjö, 1992b), MCA occlusion may be accompanied by surprisingly moderate reductions in extra- or intracellular pH. Additional data, attesting to this fact, have recently appeared (Nedergaard et al., 1991). However, two recent studies in the rat (Nakai et al., 1988) and the baboon (Obrenovitch et al., 1988) clearly demonstrate that the reduction in pH_i

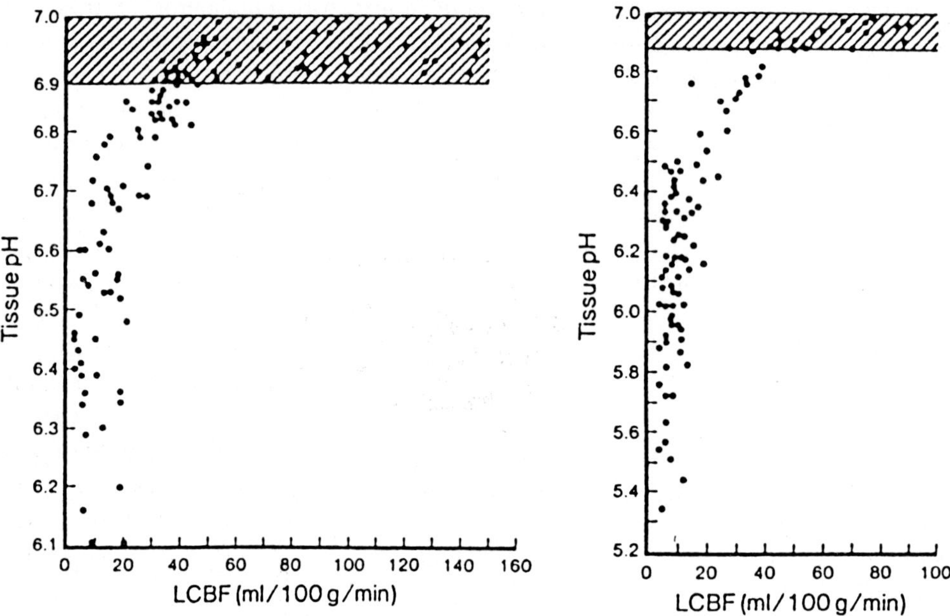

Fig. 7. Relationship between local CBF and tissue pH during focal ischemia in normo- and hyperglycemic rats. The values were obtained with autoradiographic techniques (4-^{18}F-fluoroantipyrine and ^{14}C-dimethyloxazolidine-2,5-dione, respectively). (Reproduced with permission from Nakai et al., 1988.)

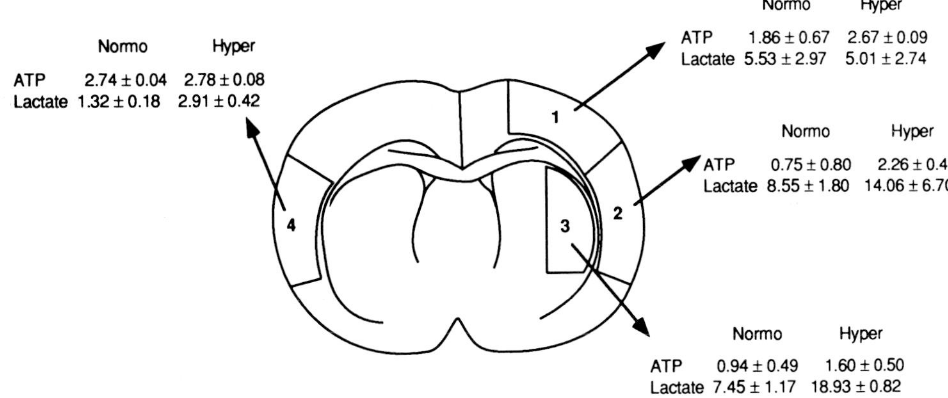

Fig. 8. Focal and perifocal changes in labile tissue metabolites in a rat model of middle cerebral artery (MCA) occlusion. Normal values for ATP and lactate are those obtained on neocortical samples from the contralateral side (area 4). On the side ipsilateral to the MCA occlusion, the lateral caudo-putamen (area 3) and the overlying neocortex (area 2) constitute the focus, while the upper part of the neocortex (area 1, bordering to the area irrigated by the anterior cerebral artery) represents penumbral tissue in the sense that it is potentially salvageable by drugs or reperfusion. The terms "Normo" and "Hyper" denote normoglycemia and hyperglycemia, respectively.

is tightly correlated with the fall in CBF, and also that pH values fall to or even below 6.0 at the lowest flow rates recorded. As shown in Fig. 7 one of these studies also clearly documents the aggravation of acidosis by hyperglycemia (Nakai et al., 1988). However, the results do not clarify the role of acidosis in aggravating damage to penumbral tissues; neither do they give clues to why hyperglycemia in some models *reduce* infarct size.

A recent study from our own group provides information on the influence of hyperglycemia on cellular energy state in focal and perifocal tissues following a 30 min period of MCA occlusion in rats (Fig. 8, data from Folbergrová et al., 1991). The results demonstrate that hyperglycemia aggravates lactate accumulation in the densely ischemic focal tissues, but not in the less densely ischemic penumbra. Two additional findings are noteworthy. First, although focal tissues have low ATP, glucose and glycogen concentrations, the lactate contents are lower than expected, considering the pre-ischemic substrate stores and the potential for delivery of additional glucose during ischemia. This suggests that some of the lactate formed during ischemia leaves the tissue by the circulation. Nonetheless, hyperglycemia causes a massive accumulation of lactate, demonstrating that glycolysis is at least in part substrate-limited. Second, increased glucose delivery in the hyperglycemic animals does not only raise the lactate but also the ATP contents. This suggests that limitation of substrate supply may contribute to the decrease in ATP concentration.

Clearly, the influence of hyperglycemia on marginally ischemic tissue cannot be predicted with certainty. This is because glycolytic lactate production in moderately ischemic tissues may not be substrate-limited; furthermore, in more densely ischemic tissues both lactate and ATP production may be limited by substrate supply. In addition, a lowering of pH, at least if moderate, may inhibit potentially detrimental reactions. Thus, a reduction in pH to the range of 6.4 – 6.6 reduces membrane currents mediated by NMDA receptors (Morad et al., 1988; Tang et al., 1989; Giffard et al., 1990b) and decreases glutamate-induced toxicity in cortical and hippocampal cultures (Giffard et al., 1990a,b; Tombaugh and Sapolsky, 1990a,b). Such results suggest that moderate acidosis can protect neurons from ischemic injury: however, if the acidosis is sustained, glial damage may develop (Giffard et al., 1990a; however, see also Tombaugh and Sapolsky, 1990a). Clearly, if hyperglycemia reduces pH to these tolerable levels and at the same time enhances ATP production, the short-term effect could well be an amelioration of the ischemic lesion.

Are there any important modulatory factors in the hyperglycemia-related damage?

At least in rats, pre-ischemic hyperglycemia triggers a series of post-ischemic events which are dominated by pannecrotic tissue lesions and by seizures. The question arises whether the seizures contribute to the gross tissue lesions. Experiments on perinatal animals suggest that the effect is small (Williams et al., 1990). Furthermore, whereas halothane anesthesia postpones seizure discharge in mature animals (Warner et al., 1987; Lundgren et al., 1991a, 1992), it does not prevent the evolution of tissue lesions (Smith et al., 1988).

Extensive brain damage must enhance the tendency to seizure discharge. However, it seems likely that seizures can occur in the absence of gross tissue lesions. In support of this, when large amounts of insulin were administered after the ischemic insult to reduce post-ischemic blood glucose concentration all animals died from seizures although brain damage was markedly curtailed (Voll and Auer, 1988). This study was later followed up, and it was shown that insulin plus glucose (to maintain normal plasma levels) ameliorated the lesions and suppressed the seizures (Voll and Auer, 1991; Auer and Voll, 1991). This suggests that insulin in high doses ameliorates the ischemic lesion.

It has been discussed for some time whether the difference in outcome following ischemia in starved and glucose-infused animals is related to another factor than blood (and tissue) glucose concentrations. Evidence exists that ketone bodies play a role. Thus 1,3-butanediol, an ethanol dimer which is a precursor to β-hydroxybutyrate, has been reported to ameliorate brain damage due to hypoxia/ischemia and transient forebrain ischemia, an effect which may have been secondary to suppression of tissue lactate production (Marie et al., 1987). A study, designed to unravel differences in plasma concentrations of substrates and hormones in starved and glucose-infused animals subjected to ischemia, also suggested plasma ketone body concentrations as an additional modulator of hyperglycemia-related damage (Lundgren et al., 1990b). However, a subsequent attempt to ameliorate the lesions with administration of 1,3-butanediol gave negative results (Lundgren et al., 1992). Thus, of all conceivable modulatory factors insulin is emerging as the potentially most important one.

Cellular and molecular mechanisms involved

A previous review article of acidosis-related damage discusses mechanisms which may be responsible for both the rapidly evolving damage seen after protracted ischemic periods and the delayed type seen after brief periods of transient ischemia (Siesjö, 1988a). In the following paragraphs we will summarize the mechanisms discussed in that article, update information on selected issues and speculate about the molecular basis of acidosis-related damage. Any discussion of such mechanisms should be based on established facts pertaining to the evolution of this type of damage and its characteristics; specifically, attention should be focused on the pannecrotic type of lesions incurred, on the profuse edema, and on the association between pre-ischemic ischemia and post-ischemic seizures.

Although it is tempting to state that excessive acidosis leads to cell damage, this statement must be qualified. Thus, although cell damage is readily induced in vitro by a reduction of external pH (Pouysségur et al., 1984; Norenberg et al., 1987; Goldman et al., 1989), in vivo results demonstrate that rats can be exposed to 50% CO_2 for 75 min, with a reduction of pH_i to about 6.6, without signs of cell damage (Cohen et al., 1990). There are several possible explanations for these seemingly discrepant results. For example, in order to kill astrocytes in primary culture, Norenberg et al. (1987) had to reduce pH_e to 6.0 for 60 min. In most published reports the critical pH_e is even lower (Goldman et al., 1989; Staub et al., 1990) and, if the exposure period is limited to 10 min, the critical pH is close to or below 5.0 (Goldman et al., 1989). A reduction of pH_i to 6.6 may thus not be enough to kill cells by acidosis alone; alternatively, acidosis due to an increase in PCO_2 is less damaging than that caused by accumulation of non-volatile acids (Siesjö, 1988a; Rehncrona et al., 1989). Furthermore, experiments involving a reduction of pH_i/pH_e in vitro or in vivo cannot reproduce conditions prevailing during ischemia and recirculation, since the latter encompasses an anaerobic/aerobic transition favoring production of partially reduced oxygen species. Besides, since ischemia leads to energy failure and activation of degradative enzymes, the impact of acidosis may be a different one in the absence of such perturbation.

At the very outset of this discussion of cellular and molecular mechanisms responsible for the acidosis-related damage, we wish to direct attention to the fact that pannecrotic lesions and post-ischemic seizures occur under other circumstances than hyperglycemia and exaggerated acidosis. Thus, if starved animals are subjected to ischemia of increasing duration, pannecrotic lesions appear, edema becomes a more conspicuous feature and post-ischemic seizures develop (Pulsinelli and Brierley, 1979; Smith et al., 1984a,b). Furthermore, even if ischemic duration is not increased, an increase in brain temperature can elicit pannecrotic lesions (Minamisawa et al., 1990). However, if ischemic duration is the same and temperature is constant, pH changes seem to play a very critical role. Thus, normoglycemic and very moderately hyperglycemic subjects differ dramatically with respect to the outcome of ischemia.

It was proposed by Kraig et al. (1987) that the critical pH_e may be below 6.0, and that such pH values are obtained in ischemic animals, not during ischemia but after reperfusion had started (see also Nemoto and Frinak, 1981). Although such a secondary, additional decrease in pH_e may occur, the observations cannot form the basis of a generalized concept. This is because typical acidosis-related damage can occur in animals in which such secondary acidosis is not observed (Smith et al., 1986). In moderately hyperglycemic animals with typical acidosis-induced damage, pH_e does not fall below 6.2 (Smith et al., 1986; see also Katsura et al., 1992a); since much lower pH values were required to kill astrocytes and neurons in vitro (Norenberg et al., 1987; Goldman et al., 1989; Staub et al., 1990) the relevance of the in vitro studies for the in vivo events is not immediately obvious.

With these considerations as a background, we can proceed to discuss mechanisms which conceivably contribute to acidosis-related brain damage. It seems justified to discuss mechanisms of acidosis-related damage in relationship to the three cardinal features of this damage: pannecrosis, edema and seizures, and to end by discussing molecular mechanisms in both rapidly evolving and slowly maturing lesions.

Pannecrotic lesions and their pathophysiology

Lesions affecting both neurons and glial cells, sometimes also endothelial cells, typically occur following ischemia of long duration and ischemia which is either complicated by hyperthermia or by excessive acidosis. The lesions are often circumscribed, e.g., affecting parts of the neocortex or subcortical nuclei; however, they seem to reflect a "community disease" in the sense that all or most cells in a particular neighborhood are affected. This neighborhood may be constituted by cells nourished by a compromised arteriole branch, or drained by a compressed venule. However, since there is probably only a transitional state between laminar neuronal necrosis and total necrosis, one can envisage that if many neighboring neurons die they "infect" the neighbors by releasing toxins (such as excitatory amino acids, free radical precursors or initiators (e.g., H_2O_2, Fe^{3+}/Fe^{2+}) or free radicals) that will reach other cells by diffusion and convection.

As outlined elsewhere, it can be speculated that pannecrosis arises because conditions favor production of free radicals (Siesjö et al., 1989a). It can be further speculated that the primary target of attack of such radicals are the microvessels (Siesjö et al., 1991; Siesjö, 1992a,b; Siesjö and Katsura, 1992). This view thus favors the suggestion of Nedergaard and Diemer (1987) that microvessels are the target in severely acidotic tissue, rather than that of Plum

(1983) and Kraig et al. (1986) who focus the attention on glial cells.

There are two major reasons why enhanced free radical production can be linked to acidosis (Siesjö, 1985, 1988a; Siesjö and Katsura, 1992). One is that a lowering of pH releases pro-oxidant iron from protein bindings in transferrin and ferritin, favoring chelation of iron to low-molecular weight compounds which are pro-oxidant. We still lack definitive proof that this hypothesis is valid. The other link between acidosis and free radical reaction is provided by the sequences leading to the production of nitric oxide (NO•), and its decomposition in the presence of $\bullet O_2^-$, i.e., superoxide anions (see Beckman et al., 1990; Garthwaite, 1991). If a source of $\bullet O_2^-$ exists, e.g., the xanthine oxidase reaction, we can write the following three reactions for the production of NO• by NO• synthetase (NOS), the reaction between NO• and $\bullet O_2^-$ to yield peroxynitrate and the decomposition of the latter to yield hydroxyl radicals and NO_2:

$$\text{arginine} + O_2 + \text{NADPH} \xrightarrow{\text{NOS}} \text{citrulline} + \text{NO}\bullet + \text{NADPH} \quad (12)$$

$$\text{NO}\bullet + \bullet O_2^- \rightarrow \text{ONOO}^- + H^+ \rightarrow \text{ONOOH} \quad (13)$$

$$\text{ONOOH} \rightarrow \bullet\text{OH} + NO_2 \quad (14)$$

Since xanthine oxidase is concentrated to the microvessels the reaction between NO• and $\bullet O_2^-$, normally a physiological event, can attain pathological significance and cause microvascular damage if the production of both NO• and $\bullet O_2^-$ is enhanced. In this sequence of events, acidosis could have the dual function of increasing decompartmentalization of pro-oxidant iron and accelerating decomposition of ONOOH to yield the extremely toxic •OH species.

We thus envisage that pannecrotic lesions are favored in situations which are prone to accelerate decompartmentalization of iron, production of free radicals and formation and decomposition of peroxynitric acid, and furthermore that the primary target of attack are the microvessels of the tissue.

Edema

As discussed in the preceding review article (Siesjö, 1988a), cell edema arises either because endogenous osmoles are formed in excessive amounts (e.g., lactate$^-$ plus H^+) or because exogenous osmoles enter the cells; these osmoles essentially comprise Na^+ and Cl^- (see Hossmann and Takagi, 1976; Schuier and Hossmann, 1980). Although a mere inhibition of Na^+/K^+ pumping by energy-driven ATPase is supposed to cause tissue swelling (MacKnight and Leaf, 1977), anoxia per se leads to little swelling, at least in vitro (Kempski et al., 1987, 1988). This suggests that the establishment of a leak pathway for Na^+ (and Cl^-) is even more important or at least a prerequisite for edema to develop. In fact, one can envisage that the most "explosive" cell swelling could occur if the leak pathways are activated and the pumps still operative (see below).

It has been discussed whether hyperglycemia causes tissue damage by increasing cellular osmolarity, thereby causing post-ischemic water influx, distension and perhaps even rupture of cell membranes, blebbing and abnormal membrane permeability (see Siesjö, 1988a; Kempski et al., 1988; Staub et al., 1990). No support for this possibility was provided when edema formation was assessed in normo- and hyperglycemic rats subjected to 10 min of ischemia (Gisselsson et al., 1992). Somewhat surprisingly, hyperglycemic subjects did not develop more severe edema. This could have been due to a maintained osmolarity gradient between tissue and plasma, simply because hyperglycemic animals had a higher plasma osmolarity. The possibility remains that cell swelling and membrane rupture contribute to the rapid deterioration of circulation and energy metabolism when hyperglycemic animals are subjected to long periods of ischemia (see Kalimo et al., 1981). In the absence of more substantial evidence it is difficult to argue, however, that the exaggerated brain damage in hyperglycemic subjects is due to excessive cellular accumulation of endogenous osmoles.

It seems likely that cellular edema arises because leak pathways are created for Na^+ and Cl^-. This could either occur by activation of a co-transport mechanism, shuttling Na^+, K^+ and Cl^- into the cell at the energetic expense of the Na^+ gradient, or by the simultaneous activation of Na^+/H^+ and Cl^-/HCO_3^- antiporters (Siesjö, 1988a). As discussed in a previous section of this article, the Na^+/H^+ and the Cl^-/HCO_3^- antiporters are independently regulated, probably by phosphorylation/dephosphorylation, so that the Na^+/H^+ antiporter is activated in acidotic states and the Cl^-/HCO_3^- antiporter in alkalotic ones. We envisage that in disease both antiporters could be simultaneously activated, catalyzing the accumulation of Na^+ and Cl^- with osmotically obliged water. We recognize that this mechanism is especially detrimental in states where the Na^+/K^+-activated pump is operative, and regenerates the Na^+ gradient. Thus, since the normal extra- to intracellular Na^+ gradient is far in excess of that required to drive Na^+/H^+ exchange, the coupled mechanisms could achieve substantial cellular accumulation of Na^+ and Cl^-.

Seizures

It is not unlikely that post-ischemic seizures arise because ischemia in hyperglycemic subjects inflicts damage upon cell systems operative in seizure control, or upon cell structures which maintain an inhibitory tone. Control of activity of burst-firing neurons, or other neurons which can participate in seizure discharge, is at least in part subserved by GABAergic neurons which hyperpolarize neuronal membranes or reduce dendritic calcium influx. It was suggested by Sloper et al. (1980) that damage to GABAergic cells due to hypoxia could explain the occurrence of post-hypoxic seizures.

One group of GABAergic neurons, obviously serving the function of a gating system in control of seizure activity, is that organized in SNPR (Gale, 1985, 1986). This is the system which is frequently damaged in hyperglycemic animals subjected to transient ischemia (see above). Such damage may, at least in part, reflect dysinhibition by necrosis of GABAergic cells in the caudo-putamen. At the local level, gross acidosis undoubtedly contributes (Inamura et al., 1988).

Damage to GABAergic neurons due to ischemia is not a general phenomenon; for example, in the CA1 sector of the hippocampus GABAergic neurons are resistant to ischemic damage (Johansen et al., 1983; Nitsch et al., 1989a,b). However, a GABAergic nucleus such as the lateral reticular nucleus of the thalamus is frequently involved (Smith et al., 1984), and the affectation of SNPR in hyperglycemic subjects could reflect a more general involvement of GABAergic neurons. Francis and Pulsinelli (1982) documented a reduction of glutamate decarboxylase (GAD) activity in the caudo-putamen following 40 min of normoglycemic ischemia. In our own studies, 10 min of ischemia in hyperglycemic subjects was enough to significantly reduce GAD activity in caudo-putamen and SNPR (Fig. 9, data from Folbergrová et al., 1989). It seems highly justified that the possibility is explored that hyperglycemia and/or excessive acidosis affect GABAergic systems of key importance for the control of seizure activity (see below). However, it is equally justified to study effects of hyperglycemia/acidosis on receptors and ion channels which subserve inhibitory functions in seizure-prone neurons.

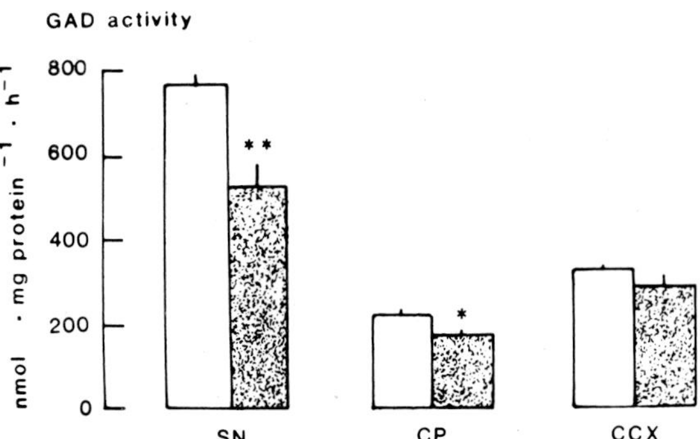

Fig. 9. Glutamate decarboxylase (GAD) activity in substantia nigra (SN), caudo-putamen (CP), and cerebral cortex (CCX), as measured one day after either sham operation (open bars) or 10 min of hyperglycemic ischemia (shaded bars). Values are means ± S.E.M.; $n = 6$ in each group. * $P < 0.05$; ** $P < 0.01$, by Student's *t*-test.

Rapidly developing and slowly evolving lesions

As discussed elsewhere (Siesjö et al., 1990; Siesjö, 1992b), marked acidosis during prolonged ischemia may prevent or retard recovery by at least four different mechanisms. First, the hyperglycemia-induced acidosis causes swelling of vascular cells and predisposes to sludge and other phenomena, decreasing the quality of reperfusion and promoting inflammatory reactions in the microvasculature. Second, extracellular acidosis will slow down Na^+-coupled H^+ extrusion, preventing or delaying normalization of pH_i. Third, since intracellular acidosis retards oxidative phosphorylation, ATP production is reduced. This leads to a precarious situation in which too little energy is formed by the acidotic cell which, in the absence of an energy source to build up a Na^+ gradient, cannot correct the acidosis. Fourth, what could contribute to this vicious circle is that the oxidase part of the lactate dehydrogenase complex is inhibited because an essential substrate group has been titrated; if this is so, the H^+ ion cannot be removed by oxidation of lactate$^-$. We envisage that all these factors could come into play when transient ischemia of long duration is followed by rapidly evolving cell swelling and tissue destruction.

Although the borderline is not too distinct, other hyperglycemic lesions are conspicuously delayed with a free interval during which metabolism and function are resumed. The mechanisms have not been defined but two possible mediators have been identified. One is the iron-catalyzed or NO•-coupled production of free radicals which possibly could cause cell death, albeit after a delay. The other mechanism is an even more speculative one. Experiments on ischemic animals with pre-ischemic hyperglycemia have demonstrated marked chromatin clumping (Kalimo et al., 1981), and acidosis in vitro has similar effects on astrocytic nuclei (Norenberg et al., 1987). It may be assumed, therefore, that hyperglycemia and/or acidosis causes activation of endonucleases and that this secondarily gives rise to cell death similar to that described for extraneuronal cells (Orrenius et al., 1988). It seems highly justified that the possiblity is explored that such "programmed" cell death is initiated by the enhanced acidosis.

An unifying hypothesis

On the basis of available information in the literature an unifying hypothesis can be set up, which purportedly explains both why hyperglycemic animals show more extensive and more rapidly developing lesions, and why they show a propensity to develop seizures. The hypothesis is based on the following findings.

(1) Animals subjected to ischemia under hyperglycemic conditions show a more pronounced decrease in pH_i and pH_e during ischemia and, when recirculation is instituted, the duration of the acid transients is longer in hyper- than in normoglycemic animals (Smith et al., 1986, see also Chopp et al., 1988). This means that when cellular ATP production is restituted, and ion pumps are re-energized, pH_i and pH_e differ between normo- and hyperglycemic animals.

(2) Although recordings of Ca_e^{2+} show relatively small differences during recovery following ischemia in hyper- and normoglycemic animals (Siemkowicz and Hansen, 1981), there are reasons to believe that Ca_i^{2+} is higher in hyperglycemic than in normoglycemic subjects in the period before pH_i has normalized (Smith et al., 1986). One reason why this could be so is that H^+ outcompetes Ca^{2+} for intracellular binding sites; the other that enhanced regulation of pH_i by Na^+/H^+ exchange sets the stage for reversed 3 Na^+/Ca^{2+} exchange, i.e., influx of Ca^{2+}. This suggestion is supported by two findings. First, hyperglycemic animals have higher active fractions of the pyruvate dehydrogenase complex (PDHC) during the first 15 min of recovery, suggesting a high Ca_i^{2+}, transmittance of calcium into the mitochondria and relative activation of PDHC phosphatase (Lundgren et al., 1990a). Second, Araki et al. (1990), using a fluorometric technique, recently showed that Ca_i^{2+} recovery from transient ischemia was slower in hyper- than in normoglycemic subjects.

(3) Previous (Sloper et al., 1980) as well as more recent results (Romijn et al., 1988) suggest that

hypoxia/ischemia and other adverse conditions cause damage to GABAergic cells, which may form key elements in the control of seizure activity. Many of these metabolically highly active cells contain parvalbumin, a calcium-binding protein (Kosaka et al., 1987). This suggests that the cells use calcium as a first and second messenger; hence, they may require a high concentration of a calcium-binding protein to prevent untoward rises in Ca_i^{2+}. Conceivably, calcium binding to parvalbumin is pH-sensitive.

Based on these three basic findings we suggest the following.

(1) The damage incurred by cells in hyperglycemic subjects is related to the more pronounced and more sustained fall in pH_i, which gives rise to a correspondingly accentuated and delayed rise in Ca_i^{2+}. This is the detrimental factor. Thus, since a rise in Ca_i^{2+} triggers enhanced lipolytic, proteolytic and endonucleic activity and since some of these degradative enzymes only work in the presence of ATP, their activation may give rise to post-ischemic damage. Since some of these events, involving proteolytic or lipolytic activities, give rise to production of free radicals, it is to be expected that free radicals are components of the final damage. Essentially therefore, excessive and prolonged acidosis prolongs the calcium transient into the recovery period, triggering calcium-induced damage by mechanisms which probably encompass free radical formation.

(2) Cells handling calcium transients as part of their stimulus-response coupling, and thus requiring a high concentration of calcium-binding proteins, may be particularly prone to damage caused by acidosis since an increase in $[H^+]$, by competing with $[Ca^{2+}]$ for the binding sites, could cause Ca_i^{2+} to rise to toxic levels. If this is the scenario with GABAergic cells, their destruction could set the stage for the post-ischemic seizures.

In summary, when ischemia is complicated by excessive acidosis the ischemic damage encompasses post-ischemic seizures, edema and pannecrosis. The cellular and molecular mechanisms responsible for these alterations have not been adequately defined. However, it seems likely that the acidosis causes damage to inhibitory GABAergic cells by raising Ca_i^{2+} to levels which will overload the buffering systems and cause cell death, thereby explaining the proclivity to post-ischemic seizure discharge. Furthermore, the rapidly evolving damage following long periods of ischemia is probably caused by several adverse effects of a raised H^+ activity: inhibition of Na^+/H^+ exchange and lactate$^-$ oxidation, inhibition of mitochondrial respiration, and acceleration of coupled Na^+/H^+ and Cl^-/HCO_3^- exchange. However, an important factor may be a lingering rise in Ca_i^{2+} in cells whose pH_i is reduced over a longer period, predisposing to Ca^{2+}-related damage. Finally, the molecular mechanisms underlying delayed acidosis-related damage probably comprise Fe^{2+} and NO•-related production of free radicals which have the microvessels as their main target. We also speculate that such damage could be programmed, being triggered by an activation of Ca^{2+}-activated endonucleases, fragmenting DNA.

References

Alberti, K.G.M.M. and Cuthbert, C. (1982) The hydrogen ion in normal metabolism: a review. In: R. Porter and G. Lawrenson (Eds.), *Metabolic Acidosis – CIBA Foundation Symposium, Vol. 87,* Pitman, London, pp. 1–19.

Araki, N., Uematsu, D., Greenberg, J.H. and Reivich,M. (1990) The effect of hyperglycemia on intracellular calcium in stroke. *Neurology,* 40 (Suppl. 1): 383.

Astion, M. and Orkand, R. (1988) Electrogenic Na^+/HCO_3^- cotransport in neuroglia. *Glia,* 1(5): 355–357.

Auer, R.N. and Voll, C.L. (1991) Insulin reduces ischemic brain damage by a direct CNS effect. *J. Cereb. Blood Flow Metab.,* 11 (Suppl. 2): S760.

Beckman, J., Beckman, T., Chen, J., Marshall, P. and Freeman, B. (1990) Apparent hydroxyl radical production by peroxynitrite: implications for endothelial injury from nitric oxide and superoxide. *Proc. Natl. Acad. Sci. U.S.A.,* 87: 1620–1624.

Bengtsson, F., Boris-Möller, F., Hansen, A.J. and Siesjö, B.K. (1990) Extracellular pH in the rat brain during hypoglycemic coma and recovery. *J. Cereb. Blood Flow Metab.,* 10: 262–269.

Boris-Möller, F., Drakenberg, T., Elmdén, K., Forsén, S. and Siesjö, B.K. (1988) Evidence against major compartmentalization of H^+ in ischemic rat brain tissue. *Neurosci. Lett.,* 85: 113–118.

Boron, W. (1983) Topical review: transport of H^+ and ionic weak acids and bases. *J. Membr. Biol.,* 72: 1 – 16.

Boron, W. and Knakal, R. (1989) Intracellular pH-regulating mechanism of the squid axon. Interaction between DNDS and extracellular Na^+ and HCO_3^-. *J. Gen. Physiol.,* 93: 123 – 150.

Boron, W., McCormick, W. and Roos, A. (1979) pH regulation in barnacle muscle fibers: dependence on intracellular and extracellular pH. *Am. J. Physiol.,* 237: C185 – C193.

Chapman, A., Westerberg, E. and Siesjö, B. (1981) The metabolism of purine and pyrimidine nucleotides in rat cortex during insulin-induced hypoglycemia and recovery. *J. Neurochem.,* 36: 179 – 189.

Chen, J.C.T. and Chesler, M. (1991) Extracellular alkalinization evoked by GABA and its relationship to activity-dependent pH shifts in turtle cerebellum. *J. Physiol. (Lond.),* 442: 431 – 446.

Chen, J.C.T. and Chesler, M. (1992) Modulation of extracellular pH by glutamate and GABA in rat hippocampal slices. *J. Neurophysiol.,* 67: 29 – 36.

Chesler, M. (1990) The regulation and modulation of pH in the nervous system. *Prog. Neurobiol.,* 34: 401 – 427.

Chesler, M. and Kraig, R. (1987) Intracellular pH of astrocytes increases rapidly with cortical stimulation. *Neuroscience,* 253: R666 – R670.

Chesler, M. and Kraig, R. (1989) Intracellular pH transients of mammalian astrocytes. *J. Neurosci.,* 9(6): 2011 – 2019.

Chopp, M., Welch, K.M.A., Tidwell, C.D. and Helpern, J.A. (1988) Global cerebral ischemia and intracellular pH during hyperglycemia and hypoglycemia in cats. *Stroke,* 19: 1383 – 1387.

Cohen, Y., Chang, L.-H., Litt, L., Kim, F., Severinghaus, J.W., Weinstein, P.R., Davis, R.L., Germano, I. and James, T.L. (1990) Stability of brain intracellular lactate and ^{31}P-metabolite levels at reduced intracellular pH during prolonged hypercapnia in rats. *J. Cereb. Blood Flow Metab.,* 10: 277 – 284.

Crabtree, H.G. (1929) Observations on the carbohydrate metabolism of tumours. *Biochem. J.,* 23: 536 – 545.

De Courten – Myers, G., Myers, R.E. and Schoolfield, L. (1988) Hyperglycemia enlarges infarct size in cerebrovascular occlusion in cats. *Stroke,* 19: 623 – 630.

De Courten-Myers, G., Kleinholz, M., Wagner, K. and Myers, R. (1989) Fatal strokes in hyperglycemic cats. *Stroke,* 20: 1707 – 1715.

Deitmer, J. and Schlue, W.-R. (1987) The regulation of intracellular pH by identified glial cells and neurones in the central nervous system of the leech. *J. Physiol. (Lond.),* 388: 261 – 283.

Dietrich, W., Busto, R., Yoshida, S. and Ginsberg, M. (1987) Histopathological and hemodynamic consequences of complete versus incomplete ischemia in the rat. *J. Cereb. Blood Flow Metab.,* 7: 300 – 308.

Duverger, D. and MacKenzie, E. (1988) The quantification of cerebral infarction following focal ischemia in the rat: influence of strain, arterial pressure, blood glucose concentration and age. *J. Cereb. Blood Flow Metab.,* 4: 449 – 463.

Ekholm, A., Asplund, B. and Siesjö, B.K. (1992) Perturbation of cellular energy in complete ischemia: relationship to dissipative ion fluxes. *Exp. Brain Res.,* 90: 47 – 53.

Folbergrová, J., Smith, M.-L., Inamura, K. and Siesjö, B.K. (1989) Decrease of glutamate decarboxylase activity in substantia nigra and caudoputamen following transient hyperglycemic ischemia in the rat. *J. Cereb. Blood Flow Metab.,* 9: 897 – 901.

Folbergrová, J., Minamisawa, H., Ekholm, A. and Siesjö, B.K. (1990) Phosphorylase *a* and labile metabolites during anoxia: correlation to membrane fluxes of K^+ and Ca^{2+}. *J. Neurochem.,* 55: 1690 – 1696.

Folbergrová, J., Memezawa, H., Smith, M.-L. and Siesjö, B. (1991) Focal and perifocal changes in tissue energy state during middle cerebral artery occlusion in normo- and hyperglycemic rats. *J. Cereb. Blood Flow Metab.,* in press.

Francis, A. and Pulsinelli, W. (1982) The response of GABAergic and cholinergic neurons to transient cerebral ischemia. *Brain Res.,* 243: 271 – 278.

Frelin, C., Vigne, P., Ladoux, A. and Lazdunski, M. (1988) The regulation of the intracellular pH in cells from vertebrates. *Eur. J. Biochem.,* 174: 3 – 14.

Gale, K. (1985) Mechanisms of seizure control mediated by *g*-aminobutyric acid: role of the substantia nigra. *Fed. Proc.,* 44: 2414 – 2424.

Gale, K. (1986) Role of the substantia nigra in GABA-mediated anticonvulsant action. *Adv. Neurol.,* 44: 343 – 364.

Gardiner, M., Smith, M.-L., Kågström, E., Shohami, E. and Siesjö, B.K. (1982) Influence of blood glucose concentration on brain lactate accumulation during severe hypoxia and subsequent recovery of brain energy metabolism. *J. Cereb. Blood Flow Metab.,* 2: 429 – 438.

Garthwaite, J. (1991) Glutamate, nitric oxide and cell-cell signalling in the nervous system. *Trends Neurosci.,* 14: 60 – 67.

Gevers, W. (1977) Generation of protons by metabolic process in heart cell. *J. Mol. Cell. Cardiol.,* 9: 867 – 874.

Gevers, W. (1979) Reply to Wilkie 1979. *J. Mol. Cell. Cardiol.,* 11: 328 – 330.

Giffard, R.G., Monyer, H. and Choi, D.W. (1990a) Selective vulnerability of cultured cortical glia to injury by extracellular acidosis. *Brain Res.,* 530: 138 – 141.

Giffard, R.G., Monyer, H., Christine, C.W. and Choi, D.W. (1990b) Acidosis reduces NMDA receptor activation, glutamate neurotoxicity, and oxygen-glucose deprivation neuronal injury in cortical cultures. *Brain Res.,* 506: 339 – 342.

Ginsberg, M.D., Welsh, F.A. and Budd, W.W. (1980) Deleterious effect of glucose pretreatment on recovery from diffuse cerebral ischemia in the cat. I. Local cerebral blood flow and glucose utilization. *Stroke,* 11: 347 – 354.

Ginsberg, M.D., Prado, R., Dietrich, W., Busto, R. and Watson, B. (1987) Hyperglycemia reduces the extent of cerebral infarction in rats. *Stroke,* 18: 570 – 574.

Gisselsson, L., Smith, M.-L. and Siesjö, B. (1992) Influence of preischemic hyperglycemia on osmolality and early postischemic edema in the rat brain. *J. Cereb. Blood Flow Metab.,* 12: 809 – 816.

Goldman, S.A., Pulsinelli, W.A., Clarke, W.Y., Kraig, R.P. and Plum, F. (1989) The effects of extracellular acidosis on neurons and glia in vitro. *J. Cereb. Blood Flow Metab.,* 9: 471 – 477.

Grinstein, S. and Rothstein, A. (1986) Mechanisms of regulation of the Na^+/H^+ exchanger: topical review. *J. Membr. Biol.,* 90: 1 – 12.

Grinstein, S., Clarke, C. and Rothstein, A. (1983) Activation of Na^+/H^+ exchange in lymphocytes by osmotically induced volume changes and by cytoplasmatic acidification. *J. Gen. Physiol.,* 82: 619 – 638.

Hill, A.V. (1955) The influence of the external medium on the internal pH of muscle. *Proc. R. Soc. B.,* 144: 1 – 22.

Hillered, L., Smith, M.-L. and Siesjö, B.K. (1985) Lactic acidosis and recovery of mitochondrial function following forebrain ischemia in the rat. *J. Cereb. Blood Flow Metab.,* 5: 259 – 266.

Hochachka, P. and Mommsen, T. (1983) Protons and anaerobiosis. *Science,* 219: 1391 – 1397.

Hossmann, K.A. (1982) Treatment of experimental cerebral ischemia. *J. Cereb. Blood Flow Metab.,* 2: 275 – 297.

Hossmann, K.A. (1985) Post-ischemic resuscitation of the brain: selective vulnerability versus global resistance. *Progr. Brain Res.,* 63: 3 – 17.

Hossmann, K.A. (1991) Tolerance of the brain to complete and incomplete ischemia. *Neuropathology (Suppl.),* 4: 445 – 449.

Hossmann, K.A. and Kleihues, P. (1973) Reversibility of ischemic brain damage. *Arch. Neurol.,* 29: 375 – 382.

Hossmann, K.A. and Takagi, S. (1976) Osmolality of brain in cerebral ischemia. *Exp. Neurol.,* 51: 124 – 131.

Inamura, K., Olsson, Y. and Siesjö, B.K. (1987) Substantia nigra damage induced by ischemia in hyperglycemic rats. A light and electron microscopic study. *Acta Neuropathol. (Berl.),* 75: 131 – 139.

Inamura, K., Smith, M.-L., Olsson, Y. and Siesjö, B.K. (1988) Pathogenesis of substantia nigra lesions following hyperglycemic ischemia. *J. Cereb. Blood Flow Metab.,* 8: 375 – 384.

Jean, T., Frelin, C., Vigne, P. and Lazdunski, M. (1986) The Na^+/H^+ exchange system in glial cell lines. Properties and activation by an hyperosmotic shock. *Eur. J. Biochem.,* 160: 211 – 219.

Johansen, F.F., Jørgensen, M.B. and Diemer, N.H. (1983) Resistance of hippocampal CA1 interneurons to 20 min transient cerebral ischemia in the rat. *Acta Neuropathol. (Berl.),* 61: 135 – 140.

Jørgensen, M., Deckert, J., Wright, D. and Gehlert, D. (1989) Delayed *c-fos* proto-oncogene expression in the rat hippocampus induced by transient global cerebral ischemia: an in situ hybridization study. *Brain Res.,* 484: 393 – 398.

Kågström, E., Smith, M.-L. and Siesjö, B.K. (1983a) Recirculation in the rat brain following incomplete ischemia. *J. Cereb. Blood Flow Metab.,* 3: 183 – 192.

Kågström, E., Smith, M.-L. and Siesjö, B.K. (1983b) Local cerebral blood flow in the recovery period following complete cerebral ischemia in the rat. *J. Cereb. Blood Flow Metab.,* 3: 170 – 182.

Kaila, K. and Voipio, J. (1987) Postsynaptic fall in intracellular pH induced by GABA-activated bicarbonate conductance. *Nature,* 330: 163 – 165.

Kaila, K. and Voipio, J. (1990) GABA-activated bicarbonate conductance. Influence on E_{GABA} and on postsynaptic pH regulation. In: F. Alvarez-Leefmans and J. Russell (Eds.), *Chloride Channels and Carriers in Nerve, Muscle and Glial Cells,* Plenum, New York, pp. 331 – 352.

Kalimo, H., Rehncrona, S., Söderfeldt, B., Olsson, Y. and Siesjö, B.K. (1981) Brain lactic acidosis and ischemic cell damage: 2. Histopathology. *J. Cereb. Blood Flow Metab.,* 1: 313 – 327.

Katsura, K., Asplund, B., Ekholm, A. and Siesjö, B.K. (1992a) Extra- and intracellular pH in the brain during ischemia, related to tissue lactate content in normo- and hypercapnic rats. *Eur. J. Neurosci.,* 4: 166 – 176.

Katsura, K., Ekholm, A. and Siesjö, B.K. (1992b) Tissue PCO_2 in brain ischemia related to lactate content in normo- and hypercapnic rats. *J. Cereb. Blood Flow Metab.,* 12: 270 – 280.

Kempski, O., Zimmer, M., Neu, A., von Rosen, F., Fansen, M. and Baethmann, A. (1987) Control of glial cell volume in anoxia. In vitro studies on ischemic cell swelling. *Stroke,* 18: 623 – 628.

Kempski, O., Staub, F., Jansen, M., Schödel, F. and Baethmann, A. (1988) Glial swelling during extracellular acidosis in vitro. *Stroke,* 19: 385 – 392.

Kirino, T. (1982) Delayed neuronal death in the gerbil hippocampus following transient ischemia. *Brain Res.,* 239: 57 – 69.

Kleihues, P., Kobayashi, K. and Hossman, K.-A. (1974) Purine nucleotide metabolism in the cat brain after one hour of complete ischemia. *J. Neurochem.,* 23: 417 – 425.

Kosaka, T., Heizmann, C.W., Tateishi, K., Hamaoka, Y. and Hama, K. (1987) An aspect of the organizational principle of the γ-aminobutyric acid-ergic system in the cerebral cortex. *Brain Res.,* 412: 403 – 408.

Kraig, R. and Chesler, M. (1990) Astrocytic acidosis in hyperglycemic and complete ischemia. *J. Cereb. Blood Flow Metab.,* 10: 104 – 114.

Kraig, R., Ferreira-Filho, C. and Nicholson, C. (1983) Alkaline and acid transients in the cerebellar microenvironment. *J. Neurophysiol.,* 49: 831 – 849.

Kraig, R.P., Pulsinelli, W.A. and Plum, F. (1985) Hydrogen ion buffering during complete brain ischemia. *Brain Res.,* 342: 281 – 290.

Kraig, R.P., Pulsinelli, W.A. and Plum, F. (1986) Carbonic acid buffer changes during complete brain ischemia. *Am. J. Physiol.*, 250: R348 – R357.

Kraig, R.P., Petito, C.K., Plum, F. and Pulsinelli, W.A. (1987) Hydrogen ions kill brain at concentrations reached in ischemia. *J. Cereb. Blood Flow Metab.*, 7: 379 – 386.

Krebs, H.A. (1972) The Pasteur effect and the relations between respiration and fermentation. *Essays Biochem.*, 8: 1 – 34.

Krebs, H., Woods, H. and Alberti, K. (1975) Hyperlactataemia and lactic acidosis. *Essays Med. Biochem.*, 1: 81 – 103.

Lawson, J.W. and Veech, R.L. (1979) Effects of pH and free Mg^{2+} on the Keq of the creatine kinase reaction and other phosphate hydrolyses and phosphate transfer reactions. *J. Biol. Chem.*, 254: 6528 – 6537.

Lundgren, J., Cardell, M., Wieloch, T. and Siesjö, B.K. (1990a) Preischemic hyperglycemia and postischemic alteration of rat brain pyruvate dehydrogenase activity. *J. Cereb. Blood Flow Metab.*, 10: 536 – 541.

Lundgren, J., Mans, A. and Siesjö, B.K. (1990b) Ischemia in normo- and hyperglycemic rats: plasma energy substrates and hormones. *Am. J. Physiol.*, 258: E767 – E774.

Lundgren, J., Smith, M. and Siesjö, B.K. (1991a) Influence of moderate hypothermia on ischemic brain damage incurred under hyperglycemic conditions. *Exp. Brain Res.*, 84: 91 – 101.

Lundgren, J., Zhang, H., Agardh, C.-D., Smith, M.-L., Evans, P., Halliwell, B. and Siesjö, B. (1991b) Acidosis-induced ischemic brain damage: are free radicals involved? *J. Cereb. Blood Flow Metab.*, 11: 587 – 596.

Lundgren, J., Smith, M.-L., Mans, A. and Siesjö, B.K. (1992) Ischemic brain damage is not ameliorated by 1,3-butanediol in hyperglycemic rats. *Stroke*, 23: 719 – 724.

MacKnight, A. and Leaf, A. (1977) Regulation of cellular volume. *Physiol. Rev.*, 57: 510 – 573.

Mahnensmith, R. and Aronson, P. (1985) The plasma membrane sodium-hydrogen exchanger and its role in physiological and pathophysiological processes. *Circ. Res.*, 56: 773 – 788.

Marie, C., Bralet, A. and Bralet, J. (1987) Protective action of 1,3-butanediol in cerebral ischemia. A neurologic, histologic and metabolic study. *J. Cereb. Blood Flow Metab.*, 7: 794 – 800.

Mellergård, P. and Siesjö, B.K. (1991) Astrocytes fail to regulate intracellular pH at moderately reduced extracellular pH. *Neuroreport*, 2: 695 – 698.

Mellergård, P., Ou Yang, Y. and Siesjö, B.K. (1992) Regulation of intracellular pH in cultured astrocytes and neuroblastoma cells: dependence on extracellular pH. *Can. J. Physiol.*, in press.

Messeter, K. and Siesjö, B.K. (1971a) The intracellular pH in the brain in acute and sustained hypercapnia. *Acta Physiol. Scand.*, 83: 210 – 219.

Messeter, K. and Siesjö, B.K. (1971b) Regulation of the CSF pH in acute and sustained respiratory acidosis. *Acta Physiol. Scand.*, 83: 21 – 30.

Minamisawa, H., Smith, M.-L. and Siesjö, B.K. (1990) The effect of mild hyperthermia (39°C) and hypothermia (35°C) on brain damage following 5, 10 and 15 min of forebrain ischemia. *Ann. Neurol.*, 28: 26 – 33.

Moolenaar, W. (1986) Regulation of cytoplasmic pH by Na^+/H^+ exchange. *Trends Biochem. Sci.*, 11: 141 – 143.

Morad, M., Dichter, M. and Tang, C.M. (1988) The NMDA activated current in hippocampal neurons is highly sensitive to $[H^+]_o$. *Soc. Neurosci. Abstr.*, 14: 791.

Mutch, W.A. and Hansen, A.J. (1984) Extracellular pH changes during spreading depression and cerebral ischemia: mechanisms of brain pH regulation. *J. Cereb. Blood Flow Metab.*, 4: 17 – 27.

Myers, R.E. (1979) Lactic acid accumulation as a cause of brain edema and cerebral necrosis resulting from oxygen deprivation. In: R.K. and G. Guilleminault (Eds.), *Advances in Perinatal Neurology*, Spectrum, New York, pp. 85 – 114.

Nakai, H., Yamamoto, Y., Diksic, M., Worsley, K. and Takara, E. (1988) Triple-tracer autoradiography demonstrates effects of hyperglycemia on cerebral blood flow, pH, and glucose utilization in cerebral ischemia of rats. *Stroke*, 19: 764 – 772.

Nedergaard, M. (1987) Transient focal ischemia in hyperglycemic rats is associated with increased cerebral infarction. *Brain Res.*, 408: 79 – 85.

Nedergaard, M. and Diemer, N. (1987) Focal ischemia of the rat brain, with special reference to the influence of plasma glucose concentration. *Acta Neuropathol. (Berl.)*, 73: 131 – 137.

Nedergaard, M., Kraig, R., Tanabe, J. and Pulsinelli, W. (1991) Dynamics of interstitial and intracellular pH in evolving brain infarct. *Am. J. Physiol.*, 260: R581 – R588.

Nemoto, E. and Frinak, S. (1981) Brain tissue pH after global brain ischemia and barbiturate loading in rats. *Stroke*, 6: 77 – 82.

Nioka, S., Chance, B., Hilberman, M., Subramanian, H.V., Leigh Jr., J.S., Veech, R.L. and Forster, R.E. (1987) Relationship between intracellular pH and energy metabolism in dog brain as measured by ^{31}P-NMR. *J. Appl. Physiol.*, 62: 2094 – 2102.

Nitsch, C., Goping, G. and Klatzo, I. (1989a) Preservation of GABAergic perikarya and boutons after transient ischemia in the gerbil hippocampal CA1 field. *Brain Res.*, 495: 243 – 252.

Nitsch, C., Scotti, A., Sommacal, A. and Kalt, G. (1989b) GABAergic hippocampal neurons resistant to ischemia-induced neuronal death contain the CA^{2+}-binding protein parvalbumin. *Neurosci. Lett.*, 105: 263 – 268.

Nordström, C.-H., Rehncrona, S. and Siesjö, B.K. (1976) Restitution of cerebral energy after complete and incomplete ischemia of 30 min duration. *Acta Physiol. Scand.*, 97: 270 – 272,.

Nordström, C.-H., Rehncrona, S. and Siesjö, B.K. (1978) Restitution of cerebral energy state, as well as of glycolytic metabolites, citric acid cycle intermediates and associated amino acids after 30 min of complete ischemia in rats anaesthetized with nitrous oxide or phenobarbital. *J. Neurochem.*, 30: 479 – 486.

Norenberg, M., Mozes, L., Gregorios, J. and Norenberg, L.-O. (1987) Effects of lactic acid on astrocytes in primary culture. *J. Neuropathol. Exp. Neurol.,* 46: 154 – 166.

Obrenovitch, T.P., Garofalo, O., Harris, R.J., Bordi, L., Ono, M., Momma, F., Bachelard, H.S. and Symon, L. (1988) Brain tissue concentration of ATP, phosphocreatine, lactate and tissue pH in relation to reduced cerebral blood flow following experimental acute middle cerebral artery occlusion. *J. Cereb. Blood Flow Metab.,* 8: 866 – 874.

Obrenovitch, T.P., Scheller, D., Matsumoto, T., Tegtmeier, F., Höller, M. and Symon, L. (1990) A rapid redistribution of hydrogen ions is associated with depolarization and repolarization subsequent to cerebral ischemia reperfusion. *J. Neurophysiol.,* 64: 1125 – 1133.

Olsnes, S., Ludt, J., Tonnessen, T. and Sandvig, K. (1987) Bicarbonate/chloride antiport in vero cells: II. Mechanisms for bicarbonate-dependent regulation of intracellular pH. *J. Cell. Physiol.,* 132: 192 – 202.

Orrenius, S., McConkey, D., Jones, D. and Nicotera, P. (1988) Ca^{2+}-activated mechanisms in toxicity and programmed cell death. *ISI Atlas Sci: Pharmacology,* 2: 319 – 324.

Patel, K., Hartmann, J. and Cohen, M. (1973) Effect of pH on metabolism and ultrastructure of guinea pig cerebral cortex slices. *Stroke,* 4: 221 – 231.

Plum, F. (1983) What causes infarction in ischemic brain?: the Robert Wartenburg lecture. *Neurology,* 33: 222 – 233.

Pouysségur, J. (1985) The growth factor-activable Na^+/H^+ exchange system: a genetic approach. *Trends Neurosci.,* 8: 453 – 455.

Pouysségur, J., Sardet, C., Franchi, A., L'Allemain, G. and Paris, S. (1984) *Proc. Natl. Acad. Sci. U.S.A.,* 81: 4833 – 4837.

Prado, R., Ginsberg, M., Dietrich, W., Watson, B. and Busto, R. (1988) Hyperglycemia increases infarct size in collaterally perfused but not end-arterial vascular territories. *J. Cereb. Blood Flow Metab.,* 8: 186 – 192.

Pulsinelli, W.A. and Brierley, J.B. (1979) A new model of bilateral hemispheric ischemia in the unanesthetized rat. *Stroke,* 10: 267 – 272.

Pulsinelli, W.A., Brierley, J.B. and Plum, F. (1982a) Temporal profile of neuronal damage in a model of transient forebrain ischemia. *Ann. Neurol.,* 11: 491 – 498.

Pulsinelli, W.A., Waldman, S., Rawlinson, D. and Plum, F. (1982b) Moderate hyperglycemia augments ischemic brain damage: a neuropathological study in the rat. *Neurology,* 32: 1239 – 1246.

Radda, G. (1982) Discussion: H^+ in normal metabolism. In: R. Porter and G. Lawrenson (Eds.), *Metabolic Acidosis,* Pitman, Bath, p. 18.

Raley-Susman, K., Cragoe, E., Sapolsky, R. and Kopito, R. (1991) Regulation of intracellular pH in cultured hippocampal neurons by an amiloride-insensitive Na^+/H^+ exchanger. *J. Biol. Chem.,* 266: 2739 – 2745.

Rehncrona, S., Rosén, I. and Siesjö, B.K. (1981) Brain lactic acidosis and ischemic cell damage: 1. Biochemistry and neurophysiology. *J. Cereb. Blood Flow Metab.,* 1: 297 – 311.

Rehncrona, S., Hauge, H.N. and Siesjö, B.K. (1989) Enhancement of iron-catalyzed free radical formation by acidosis in brain homogenates: difference in effect by lactic acid and CO_2. *J. Cereb. Blood Flow Metab.,* 9: 65 – 70.

Roberts, J., Callis, J., Jardetzky, O., Walbot, V. and Freeling, M. (1984) Cytoplasmic acidosis as a determinant of flooding intolerance. *Proc. Natl. Acad. Sci. U.S.A.,* 81: 6029 – 6033.

Romijn, H.J., Ruijter, J.M. and Wolters, P.S. (1988) Hypoxia preferentially destroys GABAergic neurons in developing rat neocortex explants in culture. *Exp. Neurol.,* 100: 332 – 340.

Roos, A. and Boron, W. (1981) Intracellular pH. *Physiol. Rev.,* 61: 296 – 434.

Saldet, C., Counillon, L., Franchi, A. and Pouysségur, J. (1991) Growth factors induce phosphorylation of the Na^+/H^+ antiporter, a glycoprotein of 110 kD. *Science,* 247: 723 – 726.

Salford, L.G. and Siesjö, B. (1974) The influence of arterial hypoxia and unilateral carotid artery occlusion upon regional blood flow and metabolism. *Acta Physiol. Scand.,* 92: 130 – 141.

Schuier, F.J. and Hossmann, K.A. (1980) Experimental brain infarcts in cats. II. Ischemic brain edema. *Stroke,* 11: 593 – 601.

Siemkowicz, E. and Hansen, A.J. (1981) Brain extracellular ion composition and EEG activity folllowing 10 min ischemia in normo- and hyperglycemic rats. *Stroke,* 12: 236 – 240.

Siemkowicz, E., Hansen, A.J. and Gjedde, A. (1982) Hyperglycemic ischemia of rat brain: the effect of post-ischemic insulin on metabolic rate. *Brain Res.,* 243: 386 – 390.

Siesjö, B.K. (1973) Metabolic control of intracellular pH. (Editorial). *Scand. J. Clin. Lab. Invest.,* 32: 97 – 104.

Siesjö, B.K. (1981) Cell damage in the brain: a speculative synthesis. *J. Cereb. Blood Flow Metab.,* 1: 155 – 185.

Siesjö, B.K. (1984) Cerebral circulation and metabolism (review article). *J. Neurosurg.,* 60: 883 – 908.

Siesjö, B.K. (1985) Acid-base homeostasis in the brain: physiology, chemistry, and neurochemical pathology. In: K.-A.H.K. Kogure, B. Siesjö and F. Welsh (Eds.), *Progress in Brain Research, Vol. 63,* Elsevier Science Publishers, Amsterdam, pp. 121 – 154.

Siesjö, B.K. (1988a) Acidosis and ischemic brain damage. *Neurochem. Pathol.,* 9: 31 – 88.

Siesjö, B.K. (1988b) Hypoglycemia, brain metabolism, and brain damage. *Diabetes Metab. Rev.,* 4(2): 113 – 144.

Siesjö, B.K. (1992a) The role of calcium in cell death. In: D. Price, A. Aguayo and H. Thoenen (Eds.), *Neurodegenerative Disorders: Mechanisms and Prospects for Therapy,* Wiley, New York, pp. 35 – 59.

Siesjö, B.K. (1992b) Pathophysiology and treatment of focal cerebral ischemia. *J. Neurosurg.,* 77: 169 – 184, 337 – 354.

Siesjö, B.K. and Katsura, K. (1992) Ischemic brain damage: focus on lipids and lipid mediators. In: N. Bazan (Ed.), *Neurobiology of Essential Fatty Acids,* pp. 41 – 56.

Siesjö, B.K., von Hanwehr, R., Nergelius, G., Nevander, G. and

Ingvar, M. (1985) Extra- and intracellular pH in the brain during seizures and in the recovery period following the arrest of seizure activity. *J. Cereb. Blood Flow Metab.*, 5: 47 – 57.

Siesjö, B.K., Agardh, C.-D. and Bengtsson, F. (1989a) Free radicals and brain damage. *Cerebrovasc. Brain Metab. Rev.*, 1: 165 – 211.

Siesjö, B.K., Bengtsson, F., Grampp, W. and Theander, S. (1989b) Calcium, excitotoxins, and neuronal death in the brain. *Ann. N.Y. Acad. Sci.*, 568: 234 – 251.

Siesjö, B.K., Ekholm, A., Katsura, K. and Theander, S. (1990) Acid-base changes during complete brain ischemia. *Stroke*, 21: 194 – 199.

Siesjö, B.K., Memezawa, H. and Smith, M.-L. (1991) Neurocytotoxicity: pharmacological implications. *Fundam. Clin. Pharmacol.*, 5: 755 – 767.

Sloper, J.J., Johnson, P. and Powell, T.P.S. (1980) Selective degeneration of interneurons in the motor cortex of infant monkeys following controlled hypoxia: a possible cause of epilepsy. *Brain Res.*, 198: 204 – 209.

Smith, M.-L., Auer, R.N. and Siesjö, B.K. (1984a) The density and distribution of ischemic brain injury in the rat following 2 – 10 min of forebrain ischemia. *Acta Neuropathol. (Berl.)*, 64: 319 – 332.

Smith, M.-L., Bendek, G., Dahlgren, N., Rosén, I., Wieloch, T. and Siesjö, B.K. (1984b) Models for studying long-term recovery following forebrain ischemia in the rat. 2. A 2-vessel occlusion model. *Acta Neurol. Scand.*, 69: 385 – 401.

Smith, M.-L., von Hanwehr, R. and Siesjö, B.K. (1986) Changes in extra- and intracellular pH in the brain during and following ischemia in hyperglycemic and in moderately hypoglycemic rats. *J. Cereb. Blood Flow Metab.*, 6: 574 – 583.

Smith, M.-L., Kalimo, H., Warner, D.S. and Siesjö, B.K. (1988) Morphological lesions in the brain preceding the development of postischemic seizures. *Acta Neuropathol. (Berl.)*, 76: 253 – 264.

Staub, F., Baethmann, A., Peters, J., Weigt, H. and Kempski, O. (1990) Effects of lactacidosis on glial cell volume and viability. *J. Cereb. Blood Flow Metab.*, 10: 866 – 876.

Steen, P., Michenfelder, J. and Milde, J. (1979) Incomplete versus complete cerebral ischemia: improved outcome with a minimal blood flow. *Ann. Neurol.*, 6: 389 – 398.

Sykova, E. and Svoboda, J. (1990) Extracellular alkaline-acid-alkaline transients in the rat spinal cord evoked by peripheral stimulation. *Brain Res.*, 512: 181 – 189.

Tang, C.M., Dichter, M. and Morad, M. (1989) Mechanism of NMDA channel modulation by H^+ at near physiologic pH. *Soc. Neurosci. Abstr.*, 15: 325.

Thomas, R. (1984) Experimental displacement of intracellular pH and the mechanisms of its subsequent recovery. *J. Physiol. (Lond.)*, 354: 3 – 22.

Tombaugh, G.C. and Sapolsky, R.M. (1990a) Mechanistic distinctions between excitotoxic and acidotic hippocampal damage in an in vitro model of ischemia. *J. Cereb. Blood Flow Metab.*, 10: 527 – 535.

Tombaugh, G.C. and Sapolsky, R.M. (1990b) Mild acidosis protects hippocampal neurons from injury induced by oxygen and glucose deprivation. *Brain Res.*, 506: 343 – 345.

Vannucci, R., Lyons, D. and Vasta, F. (1988) Regional cerebral blood flow during hypoxia-ischemia in immature rats. *Stroke*, 19: 245 – 250.

Venables, G., Miller, S., Gibson, G., Hardy, J. and Strong, A. (1985) The effects of hyperglycaemia on changes during reperfusion following focal cerebral ischaemia in the cat. *J. Neurol. Neurosurg. Psychiatry*, 48: 663 – 669.

Vink, R., Faden, A.I. and Mcintosh, T.K. (1988) Changes in cellular bioenergetic state following graded traumatic brain injury in rats: determination by phophorus 31 magnetic resonance spectroscopy. *J. Neurotrauma*, 5: 315 – 330.

Voll, C.L. and Auer, N.R. (1988) The effect of postischemic blood glucose levels on ischemic brain damage in the rat. *Ann. Neurol.*, 24: 638 – 646.

Voll, C.L. and Auer, N.R. (1991) Postischemic seizures and necrotizing ischemic brain damage: neuroprotective effect of postischemic diazepam and insulin. *Neurology*, 41: 423 – 428.

Voorhies, T., Rawlinson, D. and Vannucci, R. (1986) Glucose and perinatal hypoxic-ischemic brain damage in the rat. *Neurology*, 36: 1115 – 1118.

Walz, W. and Mukerji, S. (1988) Lactate production and release in cultured astrocytes. *Neurosci. Lett.*, 86: 296 – 300.

Walz, W. and Mukerji, S. (1990) Simulation of aspects of ischemia in cell culture: changes in lactate compartmentation. *Glia*, 3: 522 – 528.

Warner, D.S., Smith, M.-L. and Siesjö, B.K. (1987) Ischemia in normo- and hyperglycemic rats: effects on brain water and electrolytes. *Stroke*, 18: 464 – 471.

Welsh, F.A., Ginsberg, M.D. and Budd, W.W. (1980) Deleterious effect of glucose pretreatment on recovery from diffuse cerebral ischemia in the cat. II. Regional metabolite levels. *Stroke*, 11: 355 – 363.

Welsh, F.A., Sims, R. and McKee, A. (1983) Effect of glucose on recovery of energy metabolism following hypoxia-oligemia in mouse brain: dose dependence and carbohydrate specificity. *J. Cereb. Blood Flow Metab.*, 3: 486 – 492.

Wilkie, D. (1979) Generations of protons by metabolic processes other than glycolysis in muscle cells: a critical view. *J. Mol. Cell. Cardiol.*, 11: 325 – 330.

Williams, C.E., Gunn, A.J., Synek, B. and Gluckman, P.D. (1990) Delayed seizures occurring with hypoxic-ischemic encephalopathy in the fetal sheep. *Pediatr. Res.*, 27: 561 – 565.

Zasslow, M., Pearl, R., Shuer, L., Steinberg, G., Lieberson, R. and Larson Jr., C. (1989) Hyperglycemia decreases acute neuronal ischemic changes after middle cerebral artery occlusion in cats. *Stroke*, 20: 519 – 523.

K. Kogure, K.-A. Hossmann and B.K. Siesjö (Eds.)
Progress in Brain Research, Vol. 96

CHAPTER 4

Cerebral ischemia: the microcirculation as trigger and target

Ulrich Dirnagl

Department of Neurology, University of Munich, 8000 Munich 70, Germany

Introduction

During the last decade, great advances have been made in the understanding of the pathophysiology of cerebral ischemia. Particularly at the molecular level, an array of mechanisms and mediators of ischemic damage to nerve cells and glia has been identified: hydrogen ions, excitatory amino acids, Ca_i^{2+}, disturbed protein synthesis, oxygen free radicals, nitric oxide, etc. Each of those mechanisms has been reviewed extensively (see below), and in this volume excellent updates on the current progress in the understanding of each mechanism can be found. It is therefore not the purpose of this communication to review mechanisms in isolation, but rather to relate them to our knowledge of the pathophysiology of the ischemic cerebral microcirculation. Since it is a disturbance of the microcirculation that triggers the cascade that eventually leads to ischemic cell death, since the microcirculation itself is a target of mediators of ischemic damage, and since re-establishment of microcirculatory flow has to be a prime goal of therapy, understanding of the interaction of ischemic brain tissue and the cerebral microcirculation may prove essential for successful stroke therapy.

In the course of this article, I will review some of the current knowledge on the pathophysiology of ischemic cell death, discuss the potential contribution of the cerebral microcirculation in this process, and emphasize some technological advances which may help to promote our understanding of the underlying pathophysiology.

Cerebral ischemia: the microcirculation as trigger

Cerebral ischemia is caused by reduced blood supply to the brain tissue, which results in reduced substrate supply and waste removal at the microcirculatory level. It is important to discriminate at least two different types of cerebral ischemia, namely focal and global cerebral ischemia (Siesjö et al., 1990a). Although both may share a final common pathway of cell death, the sequence of events that triggers damage to the tissue may be completely different.

Before I discuss specific mechanisms of cellular and microcirculatory mechanisms of ischemic tissue damage, I therefore would like to briefly review those major types of cerebral ischemia. Focal ischemia is localized to a part of the brain, may be of long duration or even permanent and the reduction in perfusion is not complete. Global cerebral ischemia has the following key features: it affects the entire forebrain, it is severe and of short duration. The most important clinical correlates of focal and global cerebral ischemia are ischemic stroke and circulatory arrest, respectively.

The histopathological correlate of the difference between focal and global cerebral ischemia is infarction (Tyson et al., 1984) and selective neuronal necrosis (Pulsinelli, 1985). Infarction irreversibly strikes all cell types, including neurons, glia and endothelial cells, whereas selective neuronal necrosis only affects highly vulnerable neurons in specific brain regions. These cell changes are correlated to two different blood flow patterns to the cerebral cells.

(i) In the first hours after onset of focal cerebral ischemia, even in the core of the perfusion defect, a trickle of blood flow is preserved (< 20%). The ischemic core is surrounded by an area of compromised blood flow (25 – 50%), where neuronal excitability is suppressed but the cellular energy state is normal or only slightly abnormal (Astrup, 1982; Strong et al., 1983). In this area, the so called ischemic penumbra, CBF changes dynamically, with a potential of restoration to normal, hence salvage of the tissue, or of further decrease in perfusion with infarction. It is particularly this area where microcirculatory changes may prevent or augment tissue destruction. When reperfusion is allowed within 1 – 4 h, hyperperfusion develops even in the core of the infarct; then moderate hypoperfusion develops or even normal CBF prevails (Nagasawa and Kogure, 1989; Kaplan et al., 1991; Buchan et al., 1992a). Especially in higher mammals, flow patterns in the reperfusion phase become increasingly complex, with the coexistence of areas of local hyperperfusion adjacent to hypoperfusion (Hossmann et al., 1985).

(ii) In models of global cerebral ischemia, forebrain CBF is temporarily (usually 5 – 30 min) reduced to below 10% of normal. Lower brain-stem perfusion remains greater than 30%, which is critical for survival (Pulsinelli et al., 1982b). Immediately with reperfusion, hyperperfusion develops with CBF reaching 2 – 3 times baseline values. After this hyperemic response, which lasts approximately as long as the ischemic period, hypoperfusion develops with CBF values around 50% of baseline (Fig. 1), with a wide variability between different anatomical structures (20 – 80%; Kagström et al., 1983) and models of ischemia. CBF in the reperfusion phase may be heterogeneous, with hyperperfusion close to hypoperfusion areas (Dietrich et al., 1987). With prolonged ischemic periods, some perfusion defects may result (areas of "no-reflow"; Kagström et al., 1983). In regions which later develop neuronal injury, CBF (and ATP levels) may return to nearly normal (Suzuki et al., 1983) and even rise above normal as the cells begin to die (Pulsinelli et al., 1982a).

I will return to the distinction between focal and global ischemia after I have reviewed general principles of ischemic cell death and ischemia effects on the microcirculation.

Putative mechanisms of ischemic cell death

In Fig. 2, putative mechanisms of ischemic cell death are summarized. Regardless the mechanism of CBF reduction, when microcirculatory blood flow to the cerebral tissue is dramatically reduced, substrate supply to the brain and metabolic waste product removal ceases, energy-dependent ionic pumps fail, and sodium, chloride and calcium influx occurs (Siesjö, 1981; Siesjö and Bengtsson, 1989; Meyer, 1989; Choi, 1990). Reversal of the direction of the electrogenic 3 Na/Ca-antiporter (Nachsen et al., 1986; Barcenas-Ruiz et al., 1987) may follow, with a further rise in $[Ca_i^{2+}]$. Energy-dependent reuptake of excitatory amino acids (particularly gluta-

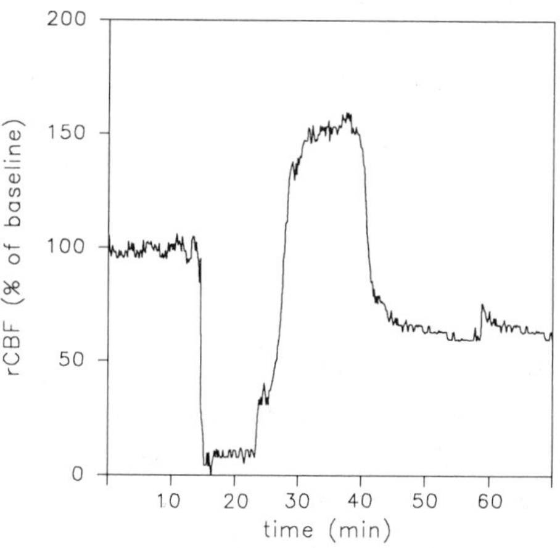

Fig. 1. Effect of 10 min of global forebrain ischemia (Dirnagl et al., 1992b) on cortical rCBF measured with laser-Doppler flowmetry. During ischemia, rCBF drops to below 10% of baseline. Immediately upon reperfusion, hyperfusion develops, and plateaus for 10 min at 150% of baseline. Within less than 25 sec, hypoperfusion (approx. 65% of baseline) develops.

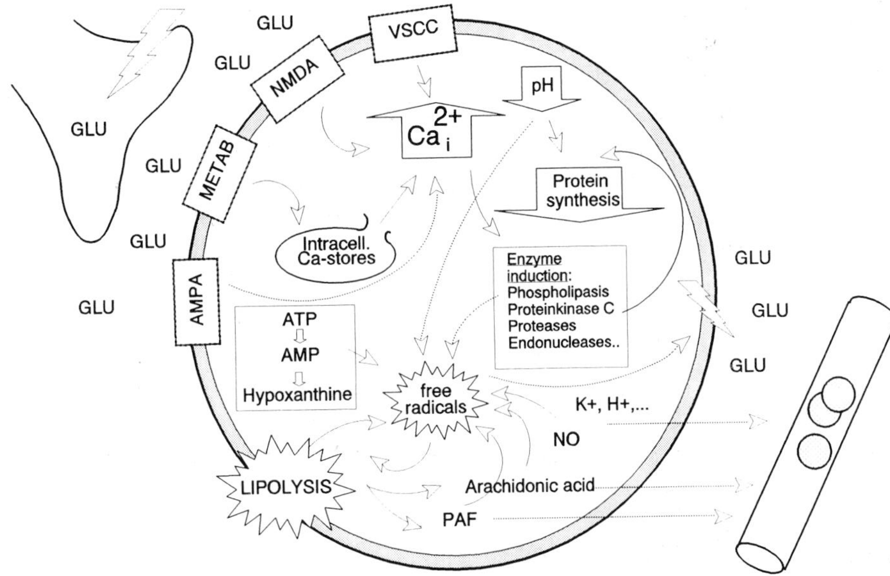

Fig. 2. Putative mechanisms of cell death in cerebral ischemia (for details see text).

mate) is impaired, and with anoxic depolarization further quanta of excitatory amino acids are released into the extracellular space (Benveniste, 1991). Here they activate receptor-operated ion channels, resulting in direct (NMDA receptor) or indirect (via Na^+/K^+ fluxes, AMPA and kainate receptors) increases in intracellular Ca^{2+} (Choi, 1988; Farooqui and Horrocks, 1991). In addition, metabotropic receptors are activated, resulting in massive mobilization of Ca^{2+} from intracellular stores via phospholipase C (PLC) and inositol-triphosphate (IP3) (Nahorski, 1988; Berridge and Irvine, 1989).

At this point, intracellular Ca^{2+} levels are sufficiently high to trigger the induction of a variety of enzymes, resulting in protein phosphorylation (protein kinase C; Huang, 1989), proteolysis (proteases; Melloni and Pontremoli, 1989), DNA fragmentation (endonucleases; Nicotera et al., 1989) and lipolysis (phospholipase A2; Farooqui and Horrocks, 1991).

As a consequence of lipolysis (Yamasaki and Kogure, 1990), platelet activating factor (PAF; Goracci, 1990; Lindsberg et al., 1991), and arachidonic acid (AA) and its metabolites are formed (Abe et al., 1988). Increased PAF and AA metabolism leads to the formation of oxygen free radicals (Siesjö et al., 1990b). Nitric oxide (NO) generation, particularly in nitric oxide synthetase/NADPH diaphorase co-localizing neurons (Koh and Choi, 1988; Dawson et al., 1991a,b), is triggered by NMDA receptor activation (Garthwaite et al., 1988) and forms the reactive peroxinitrites in the presence of superoxide anion (Beckman et al., 1990; Nowicki et al., 1991). Oxygen free radicals, especially the hydroxyl radical, react at very high rate constants with almost any type of molecule found in brain cells: sugars, amino acids, phospholipids, DNA bases and organic acids (Halliwell and Gutteridge, 1984). By causing lipolysis (Hall and Braughler, 1989; Braughler and Hall, 1989) and release of glutamate (Pellegrini-Giampietro et al., 1988, 1990), oxygen free radicals initiate vicious circles. Oxygen free radical formation as potential mechanism of damage has to be considered primarily when oxygen becomes available again (reperfusion) or when some oxygen tension within the tissue is preserved to some degree (e.g., incomplete ischemia around the core; Halliwell and Gutteridge, 1985; Ernster, 1988; Traystman et al., 1991). In addition to the oxygen free radicals derived from lipolysis and NO, the degradation products of adenosine phosphates via xanthine oxidase (Betz, 1985) and the iron-catalyzed Haber-Weiss reaction (mobilization of iron when pH is low) may contribute to reactive oxygen species formation (Watson and Ginsberg, 1989; Ikeda and Long, 1990; but see also Lundgren et al., 1991).

In the absence of oxygen or with very low tensions of oxygen, the metabolism of glucose, stored in tissue or supplied by residual perfusion, leads to an accumulation of lactate and protons. Low pH, at levels reached during cerebral ischemia, was shown to kill neurons (Plum, 1983; Petito et al., 1987; Kraig et al., 1987; Goldman et al., 1989; Nedergaard et al., 1991). The deleterious effect of protons, by which excessive cellular acidity destroys brain cells is unknown. The acidic reduction of ferric to ferrous iron and the release of iron from organic stores may catalyze free radical production (see above), and acidosis may impair cellular protein synthesis (see below). Recently, the concept of extracellular acidosis as "foe" in ischemia has been challenged, and it was speculated that extracellular acidity may in fact be a "friend" having a specific, favorable effect on ischemic tissue by reducing NMDA receptor-mediated toxicity (Tang et al., 1990; Choi et al., 1990).

Protein synthesis of the ischemic tissue may be reduced due to an array of mechanisms: the shortage of energy-rich phosphates (Mies et al., 1991), a decreased tissue pH (Morimoto et al., 1978), polysome disaggregation (Kleinhues and Hossmann, 1971) and a disturbed phosphorylation initiation factor as a consequence of the phosphorylation of subunits of the polypeptide chain initiation factor (Schatzman et al., 1983; Duncan and Hershey, 1989) by protein kinase C.

The ischemic cerebral microcirculation as target

As outlined above, tissue ischemia, which starts as a disturbance of the cerebral circulation, leads to a derangement of the intra- and extracellular ion homeostasis and the generation of a variety of effectors, which may act on the parenchymal and pial vasculature, changing the trigger into a target.

Focal cerebral ischemia

In focal cerebral ischemia, there is evidence for a reduction of the number of perfused capillaries in the affected area (Mchedlishvili et al., 1987; Buchweitz-Milton and Weiss, 1988; Anwar et al., 1988; Anwar and Weiss, 1989; Ennis et al., 1990), indicating a disturbance of the microcirculation. However, at least during the early stages of focal ischemia and reperfusion, the capillary bed is probably not completely obstructed. This has been demonstrated by labeled plasma, which does reach all ischemic and post-ischemic capillaries (although delayed; Little et al., 1981; Anwar and Weiss, 1989), and the finding of isolated plasma flow in the penumbra (Kogure et al., 1987). Isolated plasma flow, which has been described under physiological conditions in a number of vascular beds of different organs (Mchedlishvili, 1986), including brain (Mchedlishvili et al., 1987; Yoshimine et al., 1989; Villringer et al., 1991b), may remove waste and secure osmotic homeostasis under conditions of compromised flow, but has not been studied in detail so far. Nevertheless, quantitative CBF methods measuring plasma flow, like ^{14}C-iodoantipyrine autoradiography, correlate well under normal and ischemic conditions with methods measuring corpuscular perfusion (laser-Doppler flowmetry: Dirnagl et al., 1989; microspheres: Marcus et al., 1976); it is therefore unlikely that there is a significant mismatch between plasma and red cell perfusion under ischemic conditions.

At later stages of ischemia, there may be a failure of the microcirculation to reperfusion, the so called "no reflow" phenomenon (Ames, 1968; Crowell and Olsson, 1972; Fisher, 1973).

What are the potential mechanisms accounting for the microcirculatory disturbance in focal cerebral ischemia (Fig. 3)?

As outlined above, the ischemic cerebral tissue is capable of producing a variety of vasoactive substances, capable of both vasodilatation and vasoconstriction. The resulting net effect may de-

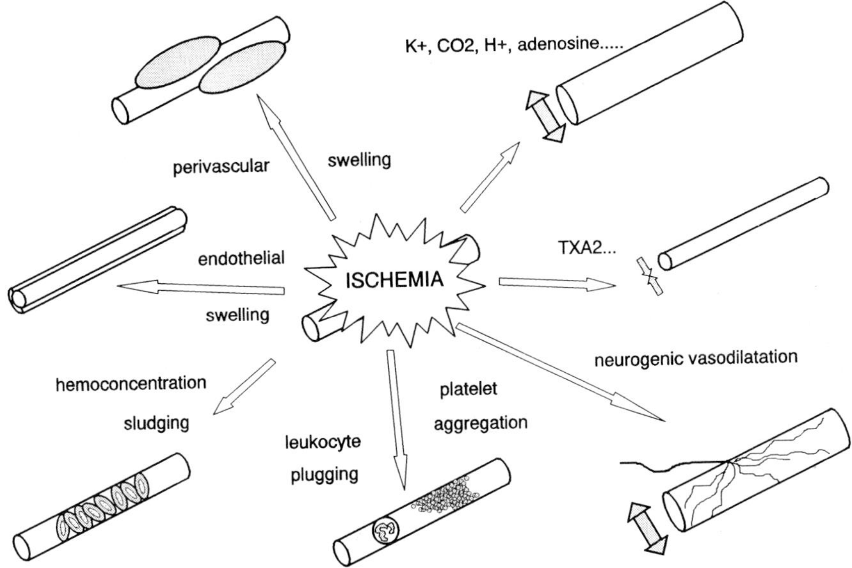

Fig. 3. Ischemia effects on the microcirculation (for details see text).

pend on the severity of ischemia, degree of reperfusion, etc. The following ischemic and post-ischemic changes in the ECF will lead to precapillary vasodilatation: increases in the concentrations of potassium, protons, CO_2, adenosine (Berne et al., 1974; Hagberg et al., 1987; Rudolphi et al., 1990), prostaglandines (PGG2, PGE2, PGH2, PGI2) and NO, and a decrease in the ECF-Ca^{2+} concentration. The ensuing vasodilatation may serve to increase flow to areas critically impaired in perfusion. However, other substances, like the ischemia-induced lipolysis product thromboxane A2, will constrict cerebral vessels.

In response to the drop in local perfusion, flow to the ischemic area may be promoted by conducted vasodilatation (Segal and Duling, 1986; Segal, 1991) or by neurogenic vasodilatation (Lembeck et al., 1982; Moskowitz et al., 1989a).

An array of mechanical factors may compromise capillary flow in the penumbra:

– Neuronal, glial and pericytal swelling causing pericapillary edema (Leaf, 1973; Ito et al., 1979).

– As a consequence of endothelial energy depletion, exposure to toxic substances diffusing from the ischemic tissue or from intravasal blood cells (oxygen free radicals, proteases, etc.), the blood-brain barrier may be disturbed, allowing the extravasation of plasma proteins and increasing the interstitial edema (Schuier and Hossmann, 1980; Sage et al., 1984; Shigeno et al., 1985).

– Disturbed autoregulation (Dirnagl and Pulsinelli, 1990), possibly augmenting interstitial edema (Kogure et al., 1981).

– Endothelial swelling (Leaf, 1973; Dietrich et al., 1984).

– Intracapillary hemoconcentration and sludging (Wood and Kee, 1985).

– Leukocytes and platelets plugging the capillary microcirculation and the venous vascular bed (Fig. 4; Del Zoppo et al., 1991).

Recently, leukocytes have received increasing attention in ischemia research. Polymorphonuclear leukocytes (PMLs) may be activated during ischemia/reperfusion via substances generated by the ischemic tissue (see above). Leukotrienes (Lindström et al., 1990) and superoxide (Suzuki et al., 1989) will up-regulate leukocytic β_2-integrins (leukocyte adhesive glycoprotein complex CD11/CD18) on the surface of PMLs. Superoxide will also up-regulate the leukocyte adhesion molecule GMP-

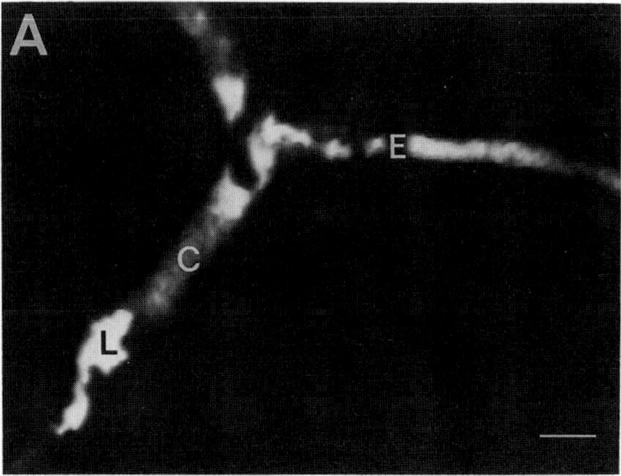

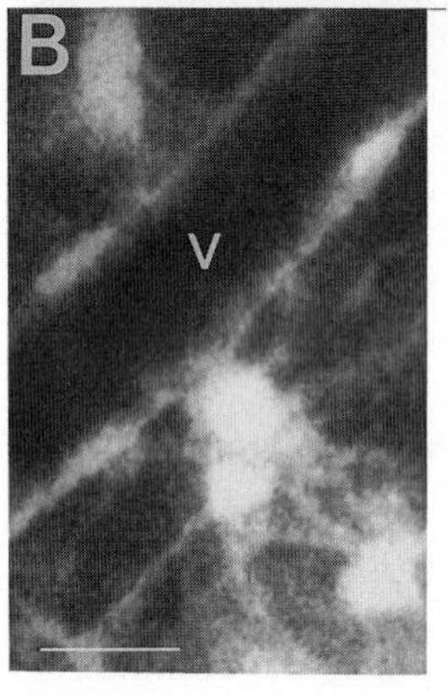

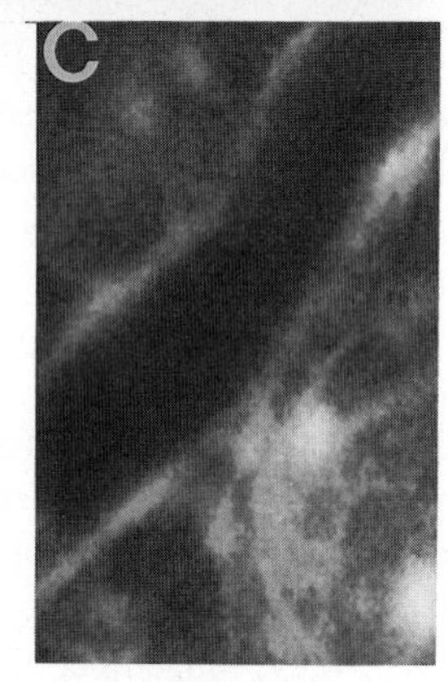

Fig. 4. *A*. Leukocyte (L) plugging capillary (C) during hypoperfusion after 10 min of global forebrain ischemia. Erythrocytes (E) in negative contrast. Focal plane 150 μm beneath the surface of the brain. Epifluorescence confocal microscopy in vivo, leukocytes stained with rhodamine 6G, plasma stained with fluorescein sodium (for details, see Villringer et al., 1991a and Dirnagl et al., 1992c). Scale bar is 5 μm. *B*. Brain cells close to an intraparenchymal vessel (V). Cells loaded with the [H^+]-sensitive dye BCECF. *C*. Same cells immediately after 10 min of global forebrain ischemia. Note the drop in fluorescence, indicating a drop in pH. Vasodilatation during hyperemia (for details, see Dirnagl et al., 1991b). Scale bar is 20 μm.

140 at the endothelial surface (Patel et al., 1991). TNF and interleukin-1, both of which are products of PAF-stimulated monocytes/macrophages (Pignol et al., 1987; Valone et al., 1988), up-regulate other endothelium-confined leukocyte adhesion receptor molecules (e.g., ICAM; Pober and Cotran, 1990). This may lead to adhesion of the leukocytes to the endothelial wall with damage to the endothelium (Harlan, 1985; Fein et al., 1991), microvascular occlusion, release of toxic (e.g., oxygen free radicals; Fantone and Ward, 1982) and proaggregatory (e.g., PAF; Uchiyama et al., 1991) leukocytic products, and migration of the leukocytes into the brain tissue (Weiss, 1989; Villringer et al., 1991a), creating vicious circles.

There are several lines of evidence supporting a role of leukocytes in the pathophysiology of cerebral ischemia. Animals rendered leukopenic or with impaired leukocyte function (CD18 antibody treatment) show less damage and improved outcome in a variety of focal ischemia models when compared to controls (Clark et al., 1991; Bednar et al., 1991; Heinel et al., 1991). Accumulation of leukocytes in capillaries in focal cerebral ischemia has been shown histologically and with autoradiography (Hallenbeck et al., 1986; Del Zoppo et al., 1986, 1991) in the early reperfusion phase. In humans, the leukocyte count after ischemic stroke correlates with the severity of the neurologic impairment and infarct size (Pozilli et al., 1985), and granulocyte adhesion (Grau et al., 1992), filterability (Mercuri et al., 1989) and aggregability (Uchiyama et al., 1991) of leukocytes is enhanced in patients with ischemic stroke. Leukocyte activation and endothelial damage, together with the release of proaggregatory substances from the ischemic tissue (e.g., PAF, ADP and thromboxane A2), may also trigger platelet aggregation, which has been demonstrated in focal ischemic cerebral tissue (Obrenovitch and Hallenbeck, 1985; Figols et al., 1987).

However, the hypothesis that leukocytes play a key role in ischemia and reperfusion damage has been challenged (Aspey et al., 1987; Schürer et al., 1991; Steimle et al., 1992; Takeshima et al., 1992). The interpretation of the above cited studies is hampered by methodological problems, especially the confounding effects of experimentally induced leukopenia and the artifacts caused by fixation of the brain tissue when looking for leukocyte plugging. In vivo studies are needed to demonstrate the involvement of leukocytes (see below) and the functional significance of this phenomenon has to be proven.

It is noteworthy that there is a puzzling similarity in the extent of protection afforded by very different experimental treatment strategies in models of focal ischemia. Free radical scavengers (Martz et al., 1989; Liu et al., 1989; Imaizumi et al., 1990; Pereira et al., 1990; Matsumiya et al., 1991; Lin and Phillis, 1991; Kinouchi et al., 1991), NMDA receptor antagonists (Park et al., 1988; Ozyurt et al., 1988; Dirnagl et al., 1990), AMPA receptor antagonists (Gill and Lodge, 1991; Nowicki et al., 1991), dihydropyridine antagonists (Mohamed et al., 1985; Sauter and Rudin, 1986; Jacewicz et al., 1990), gangliosides (Karpiak et al., 1990; Mazzari et al., 1990), PAF antagonists (Bielenberg and Wagener, 1988) etc. are capable of protecting 25 – 50% of the tissue that otherwise would undergo infarction. A compatible degree of protection was demonstrated by electrical stimulation of the cerebellar fastigial nucleus (Reis et al., 1991), a measure to increase rCBF via a cholinergic mechanism (Nakai et al., 1982). Some of the experimental treatment strategies mentioned above have been shown to increase ischemic CBF, particularly in moderately ischemic tissue (Takizawa et al., 1991; Steinberg et al., 1991; Buchan et al., 1992b; Dirnagl et al., 1992a). Hence, at least some of the protection attributed to specific mechanisms may in fact be due to a rather unspecific effect of those substances on the microcirculation in the penumbra.

In summary, in focal cerebral ischemia with its preservation of a trickle of blood flow to the tissue over extended periods of time, humoral and mechanical factors may lead to a variety of dynamic microcirculatory changes, which may have the potential of improving flow above the threshold of infarction (vasodilatation), or lead to a further decrease in perfusion with subsequent infarction. Most of those detrimental effects, particularly the activation of leukocytes, may be self-sustaining and even self-exacerbating.

Global cerebral ischemia

Most of the factors causing microcirculatory derangement cited above have also been implied as contributors to damage in global cerebral ischemia/reperfusion. It is generally accepted that the hyperemic response after global ischemia is due to a maximal vasodilatation caused by the accumulation of vasoactive metabolic products (see above), such as protons, CO_2, K^+, adenosine, etc. (Siesjö, 1981; Crumrine and LaManna, 1991). Since trigeminal gangliectomy was shown to attenuate the post-ischemic hyperemic response (Moskowitz et al., 1989b), a contribution of axonal reflex-like mechanisms, leading to the release of vasodilator neuropeptides (substance P, neurokinin A, calcitonin gene-related peptide; Moskowitz et al., 1989a) from unmyelinated C-fibers surrounding cerebral vessels, has to be considered as an additional mechanism responsible for post-ischemic hyperperfusion.

Reperfusion hyperemia, which is very intense but of short duration after global cerebral ischemia as compared to focal ischemia, may have beneficial as well as detrimental effects. Obviously, hyperemia delivers substrate to the tissue and removes waste accumulated during ischemia. On the other hand, the blood-brain barrier may be disrupted during hyperperfusion (Ito et al., 1979; Kuroiwa et al., 1985), causing extravasation of plasma proteins and brain edema. More importantly, with reperfusion there is delivery of excess O_2 to the tissue which is at this time biochemically ready to produce a burst of oxygen free radicals (see above; Ernster, 1988; Ikeda and Long, 1990; Traystman et al., 1991). Nevertheless, treatment with a free radical scavenger did not affect the hyperemic response after global ischemia (Helfaer et al., 1991).

It is less clear what causes the hypoperfusion that follows hyperperfusion, and what the pathophysiological significance of this phenomenon is. The involvement of mechanical obstruction of the microcirculatory bed, particularly by leukocytes and platelets, is controversial. Obstruction of capillaries in the post-ischemic phase has been demonstrated after global ischemia in a number of tissues (heart: Engler et al., 1986; skeletal muscle: Quinones-Baldrich et al., 1991) including the brain (Mchedlishvili et al., 1987; Del Zoppo et al., 1991). Induction of leukopenia ameliorates post-ischemic hypoperfusion (Grögaard et al., 1989) and improves functional outcome (Vasthare et al., 1990). Hossman et al. (1980) found accumulation of platelets in the post-ischemic brain, and artificial reduction of blood platelets alleviates post-ischemic brain edema (Turcani et al., 1988). Imdahl and Hossmann (1986) found a reduced density of perfused capillaries seven days after global cerebral ischemia in areas particularly vulnerable to this type of ischemia. They speculated that there may be a link between a local microcirculatory disturbance and selective neuronal vulnerability in those areas. However, others found no morphological abnormality in cerebrovascular endothelial cells and no aggregates occluding the vascular lumen (Petito et al., 1982; Pulsinelli et al., 1982a). Although Grögaard et al. (1989) reported an improvement of post-ischemic hypoperfusion with experimental neutrophil depletion, in the same model no neuroprotection could be demonstrated (Schürer et al., 1991).

It is interesting that the onset of hypoperfusion is precipitous (Frerichs et al., 1991; Dirnagl et al., 1992b; Fig. 1), and that selective neuronal depletion does not abolish the hyperemic phase but prevents the abrupt onset of hypoperfusion (Frerichs et al., 1991). From this it can be speculated that a local neurogenic mechanism triggers the microvascular collapse of post-ischemic hypoperfusion.

To assess the significance of post-ischemic hypoperfusion, it is critical to know whether there is a metabolic CBF mismatch during hypoperfusion. Hypoperfusion may create areas of local ischemia (Levy et al., 1979; Siesjö, 1981; Hossmann, 1982), or on the other hand be an epiphenomenon caused by a decreased CBF demand. More recent work did not find a CBF metabolic mismatch during hypoperfusion (Blomqvist and Wieloch, 1985; Michenfelder and Milde, 1990; Crumrine and LaManna, 1991) and no correlation was found between the degree and duration of hypoperfusion following total cerebral ischemia (LaManna et al., 1988). Hence, hypoperfusion per se may have little effect on the death or survival of cerebral tissue. Instead, global ischemia itself may have triggered events that, within days, lead to neuronal death despite adequate perfusion. This process may be totally independent of the microvascular perfusion, involving only neurons. The vasculature or blood components may play a role in this process by fueling vicious circles with neurotoxic substances, rather than in further restricting substrate supply to the post-ischemic tissue.

The contribution of the microcirculation to the pathophysiology of ischemia: a hypothesis

Weighing the above reviewed data on the mechanisms of ischemic cell damage, its induction by the ischemic microcirculation and the possible contribution of the microcirculation in either alleviating or worsening the consequences of the initial ischemic event, the following hypothesis is proposed:

In focal cerebral ischemia, a plethora of mechanisms, humoral as well as mechanical, may further compromise microvascular flow to the core of the perfusion defect and the surrounding penumbra. A permanent supply of oxygen enables the production of toxic active oxygen species, but may be insufficient for aerobic glycolysis, with the resultant production of lactic acid and protons. Leukocytes and platelets are activated, leading to vascular occlusion and enhanced production of oxygen free radicals and vasoactive substances, driving vicious circles. At the same time, various factors promote a restoration of blood flow above the threshold of infarction, particularly vasodilators like K^+, CO_2, H^+, adenosine, etc. The resulting dynamic process, which is mainly localized within the penumbra, can be successfully reinforced towards normalization of flow and metabolism by a number of strategies aimed at cellular and vascular effectors, but only when started early after onset of ischemia.

In global cerebral ischemia, the initital ischemic event may trigger neuronal events (Ca-cycling

TABLE I

Selection of methods potentially useful for the investigation of microcirculation and tissue biochemistry in vivo and in situ

Method	Evaluation of:	Spatial resolution	Advantage	Disadvantage	Literature
PET	Glucose metabolism, oxygen consumption, blood volume flow, receptor imaging	Several mm^3	Imaging capabilities, genuinely non-invasive, quantitative	Very expensive, low time resolution	Phelps and Mazziotta (1985)
NMR	Energy-rich phosphates and pH_i (P^{31}NMR), lactate, *N*-acetyl-aspartate, glutame (H^1-NMR) rCBF and plasma volume (“capillary perfusion”, Gd(DTPA)-NMR), diffusion	Spectroscopy: 1 cm^3; rCBF imaging: several mm^3	Imaging capabilities, genuinely non-invasive, quantitative	Expensive, low time resolution, repeated rCBF measurements only every 30 min	Petroff et al. (1985), Rudin and Sauter (1991), Moonen et al. (1990)
Near infrared spectroscopy	Cytochrome a/a3 redox state, Hb/HbO_2, blood volume and flow	Several cm^3	Genuinely non-invasive, non-ionizing radiation, relatively inexpensive, high temporal resolution	Low spatial resolution	Jöbsis (1977), Chance (1991), Villringer et al. (1992)
Microfluorimetry	NADH, blood volume, blood flow, pH_i (umbelliferone clearance), $[Ca^{2+}]$ (indo-1)	Several 100 mm^3	Simultaneous measurements of flow and metabolism, high temporal resolution	Cranial window, only relative measurements, U.V.-light (damage), unknown sample volume, brain cortex only	Sundt and Andersson (1980), Meyer et al. (1986), Uematsu et al. (1988)
Confocal laser scanning microscopy	Brain cortex microcirculatory morphology, erythrocyte, leukocyte and plasma perfusion, $[Ca_i^{2+}]$, $[H_i^+]$	Single cells, $< 1\ \mu m$ (depending on depth)	Imaging, high spatial resolution, simultaneous (?) imaging of capillary perfusion and tissue biochemistry	Cranial window, biochemistry, only relative measurements, brain cortex only	Villringer et al. (1989, 1991a), Dirnagl et al. (1991a, 1992c)
Laser Doppler flowmetry	Microcirculatory rCBF	1 mm^3	High temporal resolution, simple and inexpensive	Cranial window, quantitation of relative changes only	Stern (1975), Haberl et al. (1989), Dirnagl et al. (1989)
Ion-selective microelectrodes	Extra and intracellular $[Ca^{2+}]$, $[H^+]$, $[K^+]$ etc.	Single cells	Quantitative, high temporal resolution	Invasive, difficult (especially intracellular ISM)	Ammann et al. (1981), Chesler and Kraig (1989)
Microdialysis	Almost any substance in the ECF (e.g., excitatory amino acids)			Invasive	Benveniste (1989)

across the neuronal membrane (Siesjö and Bengtsson, 1989); production of NO by "killer cells" (Dawson et al., 1991a,b); changes in the regulation of AMPA receptor splice variants (Sommer et al., 1990; Monyer et al., 1991)), which are sufficient to explain delayed neuronal necrosis. Only very long periods of the ischemic interval may involve an additional microvascular contribution (including "no reflow"), particularly via the production of oxygen free radicals.

Instrumentation for the simultaneous investigation of the microcirculation and tissue biochemistry in vivo

Many questions regarding the interrelationship of microcirculation and cellular mechanisms in cerebral ischemia remain unanswered. Methodological difficulties hamper the progress of understanding: the study of the cerebral microcirculation, which resists scrutiny by lying within the cortex, covered by the meninges, bone and skin, is possible only in vivo and in situ. In vitro models have promoted understanding of molecular mechanisms of ischemic cell death, but it is not possible to bridge the link to the microcirculation in those models. It is therefore necessary to develop techniques that allow the simultaneous investigation of the microcirculation and the surrounding environment (neurons, glia, ECF, etc.) in vivo. It is desirable that those methods are capable of in situ investigation and that they have a high spatial and temporal resolution. Table I presents a selection of such methods, with their inherent advantages and disadvantages. Combinations of methods (e.g., laser-Doppler flowmetry and ion-selective microelectrodes) have been applied, broadening their potential. The temporal and spatial resolution of those methods will probably greatly increase in the near future.

The only method currently available providing a resolution high enough to resolve intracortical capillaries and cells is confocal laser scanning microscopy. The method allows the quantification of capillary perfusion (erythrocyte- and leukocyte-flux rates and velocities) within the outer layers of the cortex (Fig. 4*A*; Dirnagl et al., 1991a, 1992c; Villringer et al., 1991a; Sixt et al., 1992). With the use of ion-sensitive fluorescent dyes (BCECF, Fluo-3 etc.), simple intracellular biochemistry ([Ca^{2+}], [H^+], [Na^+], etc.) of the brain tissue is feasible (Dirnagl et al., 1991b,c; Them et al., 1992; Them, 1993; Fig. 4*B,C*). Due to technical limitations, quantitation (i.e., ratioing; Tsien, 1989) of ion concentrations is not feasible so far, but new microsopes, light sources and dyes will enable quantitation. New dyes for the imaging of second messengers (Adams et al., 1991) and cellular hypoxia (Hodgkiss et al., 1991) are being developed. This method, which has been successfully used to investigate capillary recruitment in normal brain (Villringer et al., 1991b), has yet to prove its usefulness for ischemia research.

Conclusions

Because cerebral ischemia is a disturbance of blood flow to areas of the brain, early research into the pathophysiology of this disease has mainly focused on blood flow-related topics. With the advent of sophisticated methods of molecular neurobiology, the interest has shifted towards understanding the molecular mechanism of damage to brain cells as a consequence of cerebral ischemia. Indeed, in this area great progress has been made during the last decade. It was the purpose of this review to relate our new understanding of molecular mechanisms to some of the "old fashioned" as well as recent data on the microvascular changes during and after cerebral ischemia. It was emphasized that the disturbance of the flow to the microcirculation may not only trigger changes at the neuronal/glial level, but also be a target for ischemic damage itself, thereby participating in vicious circles boosting the damage to the brain tissue. The hypothesis was forwarded that this is true particularly in focal cerebral ischemia, whereas in global cerebral ischemia mechanisms independent of the microcirculation lead to neuronal death. If ischemic microcirculation is an active part of the process of focal cerebral ischemia, microcirculation is a prime target for therapy.

Acknowledgements

Supported by the Deutsche Forschungsgemeinschaft (Di 454/4-1). I thank Dr. Arno Villringer and Dr. Andreas Them for their helpful suggestions during the preparation of this article.

References

Abe, K., Yuki, S. and Kogure, K. (1988) Strong attenuation of ischemic and postischemic brain edema in rats by a novel free radical scavenger. *Stroke,* 19: 480 – 485.

Adams, S.R., Harootunian, A.T., Buechler, Y.J., Taylor, S.S. and Tsien, R.Y. (1991) Fluorescence ratio imaging of cyclic AMP in single cells. *Nature,* 349: 694 – 697.

Ames, A. (1968) Cerebral ischemia II: The no reflow phenomenon. *Am. J. Pathol.,* 52: 437 – 453.

Ammann, D., Lanter, F., Steiner, R.A., Schulthero, P., Shijo, Y. and Simon, W. (1982) Neutral carrier based hydrogen in a selective microelectrode for extra and intracellular studies. *Anal. Chem.,* 53: 2267 – 2269.

Anwar, M. and Weiss, H.R. (1989) Adenosine and cerebral capillary perfusion and blood flow during middle cerebral artery occlusion. *Am. J. Physiol.,* 257: H1656 – H1662.

Anwar, M., Buchweitz-Milton, E. and Weiss, H.R. (1988) Effect of prazosin on microvascular perfusion during middle cerebral artery ligation in the rat. *Circ. Res.,* 63: 27 – 34.

Aspey, B.S., Ehteshami, S., Hurst, C.M., McCoy, A.L. and Harrison, M.J.G. (1987) The effect of increased blood pressure on hemispheric lactate and water content during acute cerebral ischemia in the rat and gerbil. *J. Neurol. Neurosurg. Psychiatry,* 50: 1493 – 1498.

Astrup, J. (1982) Energy-requiring cell functions in the ischemic brain. *J. Neurosurg.,* 56: 482 – 497.

Barcenas-Ruiz, L., Beukelmann, D.J. and Wier, W.G. (1987) Sodium-calcium exchange in heart: membrane currents and changes in Ca_i^{2+}. *Science,* 238: 1720 – 1722.

Beckman, J.S., Beckman, T.W., Chen, J., Marshall, P.A. and Freeman, B.A. (1990) Apparent hydroxyl radical production by peroxinitrite: implications for endothelial injury from nitric oxide and superoxide. *Proc. Natl. Acad. Sci. U.S.A.,* 87: 1620 – 1624.

Bednar, M.M., Raymond, S., McAuliffe, T., Lodge, P.A. and Gross, C.E. (1991) The role of neutrophils and platelets in a rabbit model of thromboembolic stroke. *Stroke,* 22: 44 – 50.

Benveniste, H. (1989) Brain microdialysis. *J. Neurochem.,* 52: 1667 – 1679.

Benveniste, H. (1991) The excitotoxin hypothesis in relation to cerebral ischemia. *Cerebrovasc. Brain Metab. Rev.,* 3: 213 – 245.

Berne, R.M., Rubio, R. and Curnish, R.R. (1974) Release of adenosine from ischemic brain. Effect on cerebral vascular resistance and incorporation into cerebral adenine nucleotides. *Circ. Res.,* 35: 262 – 271.

Berridge, M.J. and Irvine, R.F. (1989) Inositol phosphates and cell signalling. *Nature,* 341: 197 – 205.

Betz, A.L. (1985) Identification of hypoxanthine transport and xanthine oxidase activity in brain capillaries. *J. Neurochem.,* 44: 574 – 579.

Bielenberg, G.W. and Wagener, G. (1988) PAF antagonists reduce infarct size in focal cerebral ischemia in the rat brain. In: J. Krieglstein (Ed.), *Pharmacology of Cerebral Ischemia,* Wissenschaftliche Verlagsgesellschaft, Stuttgart, pp. 281 – 284.

Blomqvist, P. and Wieloch, T. (1985) Ischemic brain damage in rats following cardiac arrest using a long-term recovery model. *J. Cereb. Blood Flow Metab.,* 5: 420 – 431.

Braughler, J.M. and Hall, E.D. (1989) Central nervous system trauma and stroke, I. Biochemical considerations for oxygen radical formation and lipid peroxidation. *Free Radicals Biol. Med.,* 6: 289 – 301.

Buchan, A.M., Xue, D. and Slivka, A. (1992a) A new model of temporary focal neocortical ischemia in the rat. *Stroke,* 23: 273 – 279.

Buchan, A., Slivka, A. and Xue, D. (1992b) The effect of the NMDA receptor antagonist MK-801 on cerebral blood flow and infarct volume in experimental focal stroke. *Brain Res.,* 574: 171 – 177.

Buchweitz-Milton, E. and Weiss, H.R. (1988) Perfused microvascular morphometry during middle cerebral artery occlusion. *Am. J. Physiol.,* 255: H623 – H628.

Chance, B. (1991) Optical method. *Annu. Rev. Biophys. Chem.,* 20: 1 – 28.

Chesler, M. and Kraig, R.P. (1989) Intracellular pH of mammalian astrocytes. *J. Neurosci.,* 9: 2011 – 2019.

Choi, D. (1988) Calcium-mediated neurotoxicity: relationship to specific channel types and role in ischemic damage. *Trends Neurosci.,* 11: 465 – 469.

Choi, D.W. (1990) Cerebral hypoxia: some new approaches and unanswered questions. *J. Neurosci.,* 10: 2493 – 2501.

Choi, D., Giffard, R.G., Monyer, H. and Goldberg, M.P. (1990) Modification of "ischemic" injury in cortical cell culture by extracellular acidity. In: J. Krieglstein and H. Oberpichler (Eds.), *Pharmacology of Cerebral Ischemia,* Wissenschaftliche Verlagsgesellschaft, Stuttgart, pp. 177 – 181.

Clark, W.M., Madden, K.P., Rothlein, R. and Zivin, J.A. (1991) Reduction of central nervous system ischemic injury by monoclonal antibody to intercellular adhesion molecule. *J. Neurosurg.,* 75: 623 – 627.

Crowell, R.M. and Olsson, Y. (1972) Impaired microvascular filling after focal cerebral ischemia in the monkey. *Neurology,* 22: 500 – 504.

Crumrine, R.C. and LaManna, J.C. (1991) Regional cerebral metabolites, blood flow, plasma volume, and mean transit time in total cerebral ischemia in the rat. *J. Cereb. Blood Flow Metab.,* 11: 272 – 282.

Dawson, T.M., Dawson, V.L., Bredt, D.S., Fotuhi, M., Hwang, P.M., Uhl, G.R. and Snyder, S.H. (1991a) Nitric oxide synthetase/NADPH diaphorase neurons: role in neurotoxicity. *Soc. Neurosci. Abstr.,* 17: 784.

Dawson, V.L., Dawson, T.M., London, E.D., Bredt, D.S. and Snyder, S.H. (1991b) Glutamate neurotoxicity is mediated by nitric oxide. *Soc. Neurosci. Abstr.,* 17: 783.

Del Zoppo, G.J., Copeland, B.R., Harker, L.A., Waltz, T.A., Zyroff, J., Hanson, S.R. and Battenberg, E. (1986) Experimental acute thrombotic stroke in baboons. *Stroke,* 17: 1254 – 1265.

Del Zoppo, G.J., Schmid-Schönbein, G.W., Mori, E., Copeland, B.R. and Chang, C.-M. (1991) Polymorphonuclear leukocytes occlude capillaries following middle cerebral artery occlusion and reperfusion in baboons. *Stroke,* 22: 1276 – 1283.

Dietrich, W.D., Busto, R. and Ginsberg, M.D. (1984) Cerebral endothelial microvilli: formation following global forebrain ischemia. *J. Neuropathol. Exp. Neurol.,* 43: 72 – 83.

Dietrich, W.D., Busto, R., Yoshida, S. and Ginsberg, M.D. (1987) Histopathological and hemodynamic consequences of complete versus incomplete ischemia in the rat. *J. Cereb. Blood Flow Metab.,* 7: 300 – 308.

Dirnagl, U. and Pulsinelli, W. (1990) Autoregulation of cerebral blood flow in experimental focal brain ischemia. *J. Cereb. Blood Flow Metab.,* 10: 327 – 336.

Dirnagl, U., Kaplan, B., Jacewicz, M. and Pulsinelli, W. (1989) Continuous measurement of cerebral cortical blood flow by laser-Doppler flowmetry in a rat stroke model. *J. Cereb. Blood Flow Metab.,* 9: 589 – 596.

Dirnagl, U., Tanabe, J. and Pulsinelli, W. (1990) Pre- and post-treatment with MK-801 but not pretreatment alone reduces neocortical damage after focal cerebral ischemia in the rat. *Brain Res.,* 527: 62 – 68.

Dirnagl, U., Villringer, A., Gebhardt, R., Haberl, R.L. and Einhäupl, K.M. (1991a) Three-dimensional reconstruction of the rat brain cortical microcirculation in vivo. *J. Cereb. Blood Flow Metab.,* 11: 353 – 360.

Dirnagl, U., Villringer, A. and Einhäupl, K.M. (1991b) Imaging of intracellular pH in normal and ischemic rat brain neocortex using confocal laser scanning microscopy in vivo. *J. Cereb. Blood Flow Metab.,* 11 (Suppl. 2): S206.

Dirnagl, U., Villringer, A., Them, A., Sixt, G. and Einhäupl, K.M. (1991c) In vivo imaging of intracellular ion concentrations in rat brain neocortex: a feasibility study. *Soc. Neurosci. Abstr.,* 17: 1480.

Dirnagl, U., Jacewicz, M. and Pulsinelli, W. (1992a) The effect of MK-801 on cerebral blood flow in spontaneously hypertensive rats subjected to focal cerebral ischemia. *J. Cereb. Blood Flow Metab.,* submitted.

Dirnagl, U., Thoren, P., Villringer, A., Sixt, G., Them, A. and Einhäupl, K.M. (1992b) Global forebrain ischemia in the rat: controlled reduction of cerebral blood flow by hypobaric hypotension and two vessel occlusion. *Neurol. Res.,* in press.

Dirnagl, U., Villringer, A. and Einhäupl, K.M. (1992c) In-vivo confocal laser scanning-microscopy of the cerebral microcirculation. *J. Microsc.,* 165: 147 – 158.

Duncan, R.F. and Hershey, J.W.B. (1989) Protein synthesis and protein phosphorylation during heat stress, recovery, and adaptation. *J. Cell Biol.,* 109: 1467 – 1481.

Engler, R.L., Dahlgren, M.D., Morris, D.D., Peterson, M.A. and Schmid-Schönbein, G.W. (1986) Role of leukocytes in response to acute myocardial ischemia and reflow in dogs. *Am. J. Physiol.,* 251: H314 – H322.

Ennis, S.R., Keep, R.F., Schielke, G.P. and Betz, A.L. (1990) Decrease in perfusion of cerebral capillaries during incomplete ischemia and reperfusion. *J. Cereb. Blood Flow Metab.,* 10: 213 – 230.

Ernster, L. (1988) Biochemistry of reoxygenation injury. *Crit. Care Med.,* 16: 947 – 953.

Fantone, J.C. and Ward, P.A. (1982) Role of oxygen-derived free radicals and metabolites in leukocyte-dependent inflammatory reactions. *Am. J. Pathol.,* 107: 397 – 418.

Farooqui, A.A. and Horrocks, L.A. (1991) Excitatory amino acid receptors, neural membrane phospholipid metabolism and neurological disorders. *Brain Res. Rev.,* 16: 171 – 191.

Fein, A.M., Grant, M.M., Niederman, M.S. and Kantrowitz, N. (1991) Neutrophil-endothelial cell interaction in critical illness. *Chest,* 99: 1456 – 1462.

Figols, J., Cervos-Navarro, J., Solo, S. and Ferszt, R. (1987) Microthrombi in the development of ischemic irreversible brain infarct. In: J. Cervos-Navarro and R. Ferszt (Eds.), *Stroke and Microcirculation,* Raven Press, New York, pp. 69 – 74.

Fisher, E.G. (1973) Impaired perfusion following cerebrovascular stasis. *Arch. Neurol.,* 29: 361 – 366.

Frerichs, K.U., Siren, A.-L. and Hallenbeck, J.M. (1991) The onset of cortical hypoperfusion after forebrain ischemia is precipitous and may be triggered neuronally. *J. Cereb. Blood Flow Metab.,* 11 (Suppl. 2): S856.

Garthwaite, J., Charles, S.L. and Chess-Williams, R. (1988) Endothelium derived relaxing factor release on activation of NMDA receptors suggests role as intracellular messenger in the brain. *Nature,* 336: 385 – 388.

Gill, R. and Lodge, D. (1991) The neuroprotective action of 2,3-dihydroxy-6-nitro-7-sulfamoylbenzo(f)quinoxaline (NBQX) in a rat focal ischemia model. *J. Cereb. Blood Flow Metab.,* 11 (Suppl.2): S303.

Goldman, S.A., Pulsinelli, W.A., Clarke, W.Y., Kraig, R.P. and Plum, F. (1989) The effects of extracellular acidosis on neurons and glia in vitro. *J. Cereb. Blood Flow Metab.,* 9: 471 – 477.

Goracci, G. (1990) PAF in the nervous system: biochemistry and pathophysiology. In: J. Krieglstein and H. Oberpichler (Eds.),

Pharmacology of Cerebral Ischemia, Wissenschaftliche Verlagsgesellschaft, Stuttgart, pp. 377 – 390.

Grau, A.J., Berger, E., Sung, K.-L.P. and Schmid-Schönbein, G.W. (1992) Granulocyte adhesion deformability, and superoxide formation in acute stroke. *Stroke,* 23: 33 – 39.

Grögaard, B., Schürer, L., Gerdin, B. and Arfors, K.E. (1989) Delayed hypoperfusion after incomplete forebrain ischemia in the rat. The role of polymorphonuclear leukocytes. *J. Cereb. Blood Flow Metab.,* 9: 500 – 505.

Haberl, R.L., Heizer, M.L., Marmarou, A. and Ellis, E.F. (1989) Laser Doppler assessment of the brain microcirculation. *Am. J. Physiol.,* 256: H1247 – H1254.

Hagberg, H., Andersson, P., Lacarewicz, J., Jacobson, I., Butcher, S. and Sandberg, M. (1987) Extracellular adenosine, inosine, hypoxanthine, and xanthine in relation to tissue nucleotides and purines in rat striatum during transient ischemia. *J. Neurochem.,* 49: 227 – 231.

Hall, E.D. and Braughler, J.M. (1989) Central nervous system trauma and stroke, II. Physiological and pharmacological evidence for involvement of oxygen radicals and lipid peroxidation. *Free Radicals Biol. Med.,* 6: 303 – 313.

Hallenbeck, J.M., Dutka, A.J., Tanishima, T., Kochanek, P.M., Kumaroo, K.K., Thompson, C.B., Obrenovitch, T.P. and Contreras, T.J. (1986) Polymorphonuclear leukocyte accumulation in brain regions with low blood flow during the early postischemic period. *Stroke,* 17: 246 – 253.

Halliwell, B. and Gutteridge, J.M.C. (1984) Oxygen toxicity, oxygen radicals, transition metals and disease. *Biochem. J.,* 219: 1 – 14.

Halliwell, B. and Gutteridge, J.M.C. (1985) Oxygen radicals and the nervous system. *Trends Neurosci.,* 8: 22 – 26.

Harlan, J.M. (1985) Leukocyte-endothelial interactions. *Blood,* 65: 513 – 525.

Heinel, L.A., Rubin, S., Vasthare, U.S., Rosenwasser, R.H. and Tuma, R.F. (1991) WBC involvement in infarct generation following cerebral ischemia and reperfusion injury. *FASEB J.,* 5: A1279.

Helfaer, M.A., Kirsch, J.R., Haun, S.E., Moore, L.E. and Traystman, R.J. (1991) Polyethylene glycol-conjugated superoxide dismutase fails to blunt postischemic reactive hyperemia. *Am. J. Physiol.,* 261: H548 – H553.

Hodgkiss, R.J., Jones, G.W., Long, A., Middleton, R.W., Parrick, J., Stratford, M.R.L., Wardman, P. and Wilson, G.D. (1991) Fluorescent markers for hypoxic cells: a study of nitroaromatic compounds, with fluorescent heterocyclic side chains, that undergo bioreductive binding. *J. Med. Chem.,* 34: 2268 – 2274.

Hossmann, K.A. (1982) Treatment of experimental cerebral ischemia. *J. Cereb. Blood Flow Metab.,* 2: 275 – 297.

Hossmann, K.A., Mies, G., Paschen, W., Csiba, L., Bodsch, W., Rapin, J.R., Le Poncin-Lafitte, M. and Takahashi, K. (1985) Multiparametric imaging of blood flow and metabolism after middle cerebral artery occlusion in cats. *J. Cereb. Blood Flow Metab.,* 5: 97 – 107.

Hossmann, V., Hossmann, K.A. and Tagaki, S. (1980) Effect of intravascular platelet aggregation on blood recirculation following prolonged ischemia of the cat brain. *J. Neurol.,* 222: 159 – 170.

Huang, K.P. (1989) The mechanism of protein kinase C activation. *Trends Neurosci.,* 12: 425 – 432.

Ikeda, Y.L. and Long, D.M. (1990) The molecular basis of brain injury and brain edema: the role of oxygen free radicals. *Neurosurgery,* 27: 1 – 11.

Imaizumi, S., Woolworth, V., Fishman, R.A. and Chan, P.H. (1990) Liposome-entrapped superoxide dismutase reduces cerebral infarction in cerebral ischemia in rats. *Stroke,* 21: 1312 – 1317.

Imdahl, A. and Hossmann, K.A. (1986) Morphometric evaluation of post-ischemic capillary perfusion in selectively vulnerable areas of gerbil brain. *Acta Neuropathol. (Berl.),* 69: 267 – 271.

Ito, U., Ohno, K., Nakamura, R., Suganuma, F. and Inaba, Y. (1979) Brain edema during ischemia and after restoration of blood flow. Measurement of water, sodium, potassium content and plasma protein permeability. *Stroke,* 10: 542 – 547.

Jacewicz, M., Brint, S., Tanabe, J., Wang, X.J. and Pulsinelli, W.A. (1990) Continuous nimodipine treatment attenuates cortical infarction in rats subjected to 24 hours of focal cerebral ischemia. *J. Cereb. Blood Flow Metab.,* 10: 89 – 96.

Jöbsis, F.F. (1977) Noninvasive, infrared monitoring of cerebral and myocardial oxygen sufficiency and circulatory parameters. *Science,* 198: 1264 – 1267.

Kagström, E., Smith, M.L. and Siesjö, B.K. (1983) Local cerebral blood flow in the recovery period following complete cerebral ischemia in the rat. *J. Cereb. Blood Flow Metab.,* 3: 170 – 182.

Kaplan, B., Brint, S., Tanabe, J., Jacewicz, M., Wang, X.J. and Pulsinelli, W. (1991) Temporal thresholds for neocortical infarction in rats subjected to reversible focal cerebral ischemia. *Stroke,* 22: 1032 – 1039.

Karpiak, S.E., Mahadik, S.P. and Wakade, C.G. (1990) Ganglioside reduction of ischemic injury. *CRC Crit. Rev. Neurobiol.,* 5: 221 – 237.

Kinouchi, H., Epstein, C.J., Mizui, T., Carlson, E., Chen, S.F. and Chan, P.H. (1991) Attenuation of focal cerebral ischemic injury in transgenic mice overexpressing CuZn superoxide dismutase. *Proc. Natl. Acad. Sci. U.S.A.,* 88: 11158 – 11162.

Kleinhues, P. and Hossmann, K.A. (1971) Protein synthesis in the cat brain after prolonged cerebral ischemia. *Brain Res.,* 35: 409 – 418.

Kogure, K., Busto, R. and Scheinberg, P. (1981) The role of hydrostatic pressure in ischemic brain edema. *Ann. Neurol.,* 9: 273 – 282.

Kogure, K., Izumiyama, M., Tanaka, J., Tobita, M. and Ido, T. (1987) An autoradiographic study of plasma skimming in cerebral ischemia. In: A. Hartmann and W. Kuschinsky (Eds.), *Cerebral Ischemia and Hemorheology,* Springer, Heidelberg, pp. 342 – 348.

Koh, J. and Choi, D. (1988) Vulnerability of cultured cortical neurons to damage by excitotoxins: differential susceptibility of neurons containing NADPH diaporase. *J. Neurosci.*, 8: 2153 – 2163.

Kraig, R.P., Petito, C.K., Plum, F. and Pulsinelli, W.A. (1987) Hydrogen ions kill brain at concentrations reached in ischemia. *J. Cereb. Blood Flow Metab.*, 7: 379 – 386.

Kuroiwa, T., Ting, P., Martinez, H. and Klatzo, I. (1985) The biphasic opening of the blood brain barrier to proteins following temporary middle cerebral artery occlusion. *Acta Neuropathol. (Berl.)*, 68: 122 – 129.

LaManna, J.C., Crumrine, R.C. and Jackson, D.L. (1988) No correlation between cerebral blood flow and neurologic recovery after total cerebral ischemia in the dog. *Exp. Neurol.*, 101: 234 – 247.

Leaf, A. (1973) Cell swelling; a factor in ischemic tissue injury. *Circulation*, 48: 455 – 458.

Lembeck, F., Donnerer, J. and Bartho, L. (1982) Inhibition of neurogenic vasodilation and plasma extravasation by substance P antagonists, somatostatin and d-Met2(Pro5)enkephalinamide. *Eur. J. Pharmacol.*, 85: 171 – 176.

Levy, D.E., Van Uitert, R.L. and Pike, C.L. (1979) Delayed postischemic hypoperfusion: a potentially damaging consequence of stroke. *Neurology*, 29: 1245 – 1252.

Lin, Y. and Phillis, J.W. (1991) Oxypurinol reduces focal ischemic brain injury in the rat. *Neurosci. Lett.*, 126: 187 – 190.

Lindsberg, P.J., Hallenbeck, J.M. and Feuerstein, G. (1991) Platelet-activating factor in stroke and brain injury. *Ann. Neurol.*, 30: 117 – 129.

Lindström, P., Lerner, R., Palmblad, J. and Patarroyo, M. (1990) Rapid adhesive responses of endothelial cells and of neutrophils induced by leukotriene B4 are mediated by leukocytic adhesion protein CD18. *Scand. J. Immunol.*, 31: 737 – 744.

Little, J.R., Cook, A., Cook, S.A. and MacIntyre, W.J. (1981) Microcirculatory obstruction in focal cerebral ischemia: albumin and erythrocyte transit. *Stroke*, 12: 218 – 223.

Liu, T.H., Beckman, J.S., Freeman, B.A., Hogan, E.L. and Hsu, C.Y. (1989) Polyethylene glycol conjugated superoxide dismutase and catalase reduce ischemic brain injury. *Am. J. Physiol.*, 256: H589 – H593.

Lundgren, J., Zhang, H., Agardh, C.D., Smith, M.L., Evans, P.J., Halliwell, B. and Siesjö, B.K. (1991) Acidosis-induced ischemic brain damage: are free radicals involved? *J. Cereb. Blood Flow Metab.*, 11: 587 – 596.

Marcus, M.L., Heistad, D.D., Ehrhardt, J.C. and Abboud, F.M. (1976) Total and regional cerebral blood flow measurement with 7-, 10-, 15-, 25-, and 50-μm microspheres. *J. Appl. Physiol.*, 40: 501 – 507.

Martz, D., Rayos, G., Schielke, G.P. and Betz, L.A. (1989) Allpurinol and dimethylurea reduce brain infarction following middle cerebral occlusion in rats. *Stroke*, 20: 488 – 494.

Matsumiya, N., Koehler, R.C., Kirsch, J.R. and Traystman, R.J. (1991) Conjugated superoxide dismutase reduces extent of caudate injury after transient focal ischemia in cats. *Stroke*, 22: 1193 – 1200.

Mazzari, S., Lipartiti, M., Seren, S., Fadda, E., Koga, T., Lazzaro, A., Leon, A. and Toffano, G. (1990) Monoganglioside GM1 neuroprotective effects on ischemic brain injury models. In: J. Krieglstein and H. Oberpichler (Eds.), *Pharmacology of Cerebral Ischemia*, Wissenschaftliche Verlagsgesellschaft, Stuttgart, pp. 513 – 527.

Mchedlishvili, G. (1986) *Arterial Behaviour and Blood Circulation in the Brain*, Plenum Press, New York.

Mchedlishvili, G., Varazahvili, M. and Sikharulidze, N. (1987) Microcirculatory disturbances in brain cortex during postischemic edema. In: J. Cervos-Navarro and R. Ferszt (Eds.), *Stroke and Microcirculation*, Raven Press, New York, pp. 63 – 69.

Melloni, E. and Pontremoli, S. (1989) The calpains. *Trends Neurosci.*, 12: 438 – 444.

Mercuri, M., Ciuffetti, G., Robinson, M. and Toole, J. (1989) Blood cell rheology in acute cerebral infarction. *Stroke*, 20: 959 – 962.

Meyer, F.B. (1989) Calcium, neuronal hyperexcitability, and ischemic injury. *Brain Res. Rev.*, 14: 227 – 243.

Meyer, F.B., Anderson, R.E., Sundt, T.M. and Yaksh, T.L. (1986) Intracellular brain pH, indicator tissue perfusion, electroencephalography, and histology in severe and moderate focal cortical ischemia in the rabbit. *J. Cereb. Blood Flow Metab.*, 6: 71 – 78.

Michenfelder, J.D. and Milde, J.A. (1990) Postischemic canine cerebral blood flow appears to be determined by cerebral metabolic needs. *J. Cereb. Blood Flow Metab.*, 10: 71 – 76.

Mies, G., Ishimaru, S., Xie, Y., Seo, K. and Hossmann, K.A. (1991) Ischemic thresholds of cerebral protein synthesis and energy state following middle cerebral artery occlusion in rat. *J. Cereb. Blood Flow Metab.*, 11: 753 – 761.

Mohamed, A.A., Gotoh, O., Graham, D.I., Osborne, K.A., McCulloch, J., Mendelow, A.D., Teasdale, G.M. and Harper, A.M. (1985) Effect of pretreatment with the calcium antagonist nimodipine on local cerebral blood flow and histopathology after middle cerebral artery occlusion. *Ann. Neurol.*, 18: 705 – 711.

Monyer, H., Nellgard, B., Seeburg, P.H. and Wieloch, T. (1991) Differential regulation of AMPA-receptor splice variants in the CA1 region following ischemia. *Soc. Neurosci. Abstr.*, 17: 184.

Moonen, C.T.W., Van Zijl, P.C.M., Frank, J.A., Le Bihan, D. and Becker, E.D. (1990) Functional magnetic resonance imaging in medicine and physiology. *Science*, 250: 53 – 61.

Morimoto, K., Brengman, J. and Yanagihara, T. (1978) Further evaluation of polypeptide synthesis in cerebral anoxia, hypoxia and recovery. *J. Neurochem.*, 31: 1277 – 1282.

Moskowitz, M.A., Buzzi, M.G., Dakas, D.E. and Linnik, M.D. (1989a) Pain mechanisms underlying vascular headaches. *Rev. Neurol. (Paris)*, 145: 181 – 193.

Moskowitz, M.A., Sakas, D.E., Wei, E.P., Kano, M., Buzzi, M.G., Ogilvy, C. and Kontos, H.A. (1989b) Postocclusive cerebral hyperemia is markedly attenuated by chronic trigeminal ganglionectomy. *Am. J. Physiol.,* 257: H1736 – H1739.

Nachsen, D.A., Sanchez-Armass, S. and Weinstein, A.M. (1986) The regulation of cytosolic calcium in rat brain synaptosomes by sodium-dependent calcium efflux. *J. Physiol. (Lond.),* 381: 17 – 28.

Nagasawa, H. and Kogure, K. (1989) Correlation between cerebral blood flow and histologic changes in a new rat model of cerebral artery occlusion. *Stroke,* 20: 1037 – 1043.

Nahorski, S.R. (1988) Inositol polyphosphates and neuronal calcium homeostasis. *Trends Neurosci.,* 11: 444 – 448.

Nakai, M., Iadecola, C. and Reis, D.J. (1982) Global cerebral vasodilation by stimulation of rat fastigial cerebellar nucleus. *Am. J. Physiol.,* 243: H226 – H235.

Nedergaard, M., Goldman, S.A., Desai, S. and Pulsinelli, W.A. (1991) Acid-induced death in neurons and glia. *J. Neurosci.,* 11: 2487 – 2489.

Nicotera, P., McConkey, D.J., Dypbukt, J.M., Jones, D.P. and Orrenius, S. (1989) Ca^{2+}-activated mechanisms in cell killing. *Drug Metab. Rev.,* 20: 193 – 201.

Nishigaya, K., Yoshida, Y., Sagusa, M., Nukui, H. and Ooneda, G. (1991) Effect of recirculation on exacerbation of ischemic vascular lesions in rat brain. *Stroke,* 22: 635 – 642.

Nowicki, J.P., Duval, D., Poignet, H. and Scatton, B. (1991) Nitric oxide mediates neuronal death after focal cerebral ischemia in the mouse. *Eur. J. Pharmacol.,* 204: 339 – 340.

Obrenovitch, T.P. and Hallenbeck, J.M. (1985) Platelet accumulation in regions of low blood flow during the postischemic period. *Stroke,* 16: 224 – 234.

Ozyurt, E., Graham, D.I., Woodruff, G.N. and McCulloch, J. (1988) Protective effect of the glutamate antagonist, MK-801 in focal cerebral ischemia in the cat. *J. Cereb. Blood Flow Metab.,* 8: 138 – 143.

Park, C.K., Nehls, D.G., Graham, D.I., Teasdale, G.M. and McCulloch, J. (1988) The glutamate antagonist MK-801 reduces focal ischemic brain damage in the rat. *Ann. Neurol.,* 24: 543 – 551.

Patel, K.D., Zimmerman, G.A., Prescott, S.M., McEver, R.P. and McIntyre, T.M. (1991) Oxygen radicals induce human endothelial cells to express GMP140 and bind neutrophils. *J. Cell Biol.,* 112: 749 – 760.

Pellegrini-Giampietro, D.E., Cherici, G., Alesiana, M., Carla, V. and Moroni, F. (1988) Excitatory amino acid release from rat hippocampal slices as a consequence of free radical formation. *J. Neurochem.,* 51: 1960 – 1963.

Pellegrini-Giampietro, D.E., Cherici, G., Alesiana, M., Carla, V. and Moroni, F. (1990) Excitatory amino acid release and free radical formation may cooperate in the genesis of ischemia-induced neuronal damage. *J. Neurosci.,* 10: 1035 – 1041.

Pereira, B.M., Chan, P.H., Weinstein, P.R. and Fishman, R.A. (1990) Cerebral protection during reperfusion with superoxide dismutase in focal cerebral ischemia. *Adv. Neurol.,* 52: 97 – 103.

Petito, C.K., Pulsinelli, W.A., Jacobson, G. and Plum, F. (1982) Edema and vascular permeability on cerebral ischemia: comparison between ischemic neuronal damage and infarction. *J. Neuropathol. Exp. Neurol.,* 41: 423 – 436.

Petito, C.K., Kraig, R.P. and Pulsinelli, W.A. (1987) Light and electron-microscopic evaluation of hydrogen induced brain necrosis. *J. Cereb. Blood Flow Metab.,* 6: 625 – 632.

Petroff, O.A.C., Prichard, J.W., Behar, K.L., Alger, J.R., Den Hollander, J.A. and Shulman, R.G. (1985) Cerebral intracellular pH by ^{31}P nuclear magnetic resonance spectroscopy. *Neurology,* 35: 781 – 788.

Phelps, M.E. and Maziotta, J.C. (1985) Positron emission tomography: human brain function and biochemistry. *Science,* 228: 799 – 809.

Pignol, P., Silvie, H., Mencia-Huerta, J.M. and Rola Plesczynski (1987) Effect of platelet-activating factor (PAF-acether) and its specific receptor antagonist, BN 52021, on interleukin-1 (IL1) release and synthesis by rat spleen adherent monocytes. *Prostaglandins,* 33: 931 – 939.

Plum, F. (1983) What causes infarction in ischemic brain?: the Robert Wartenberg lecture. *Neurology,* 33: 222 – 233.

Pober, J.S. and Cotran, R.S. (1990) The role of endothelial cells in inflammation. *Transplantation,* 50: 537 – 544.

Pozilli, C., Lenzi, G.L., Argentino, C., Bozzoa, L., Raisura, M., Giubilei, F. and Fieschi, C. (1985) Peripheral white blood cell count in cerebral ischemic infarction. *Acta Neurol. Scand.,* 71: 396 – 400.

Pulsinelli, W.A. (1985) Selective neuronal vulnerability: morphological and molecular characteristics. *Prog. Brain Res.,* 63: 29 – 37.

Pulsinelli, W.A., Brierley, J. and Plum, F. (1982a) Temporal profile of bilateral hemispheric ischemia in a model of transient forebrain ischemia. *Ann. Neurol.,* 11: 491 – 498.

Pulsinelli, W.A., Levy, D.E. and Duffy, T.E. (1982b) Regional cerebral blood flow and glucose metabolism following transient forebrain ischemia. *Ann. Neurol.,* 11: 499 – 509.

Quinones-Baldrich, W.J., Chervu, A., Hernandez, J.J., Colburn, M. and Moore, W.S. (1991) Skeletal muscle function after ischemia: "no reflow" versus reperfusion injury. *J. Surg. Res.,* 51: 5 – 12.

Reis, D.J., Berger, S.B., Underwood, M.D. and Khayata, M. (1991) Electrical stimulation of cerebellar fastigial nucleus induces ischemic infarction elicited by middle cerebral artery occlusion in rat. *J. Cereb. Blood Flow Metab.,* 11: 810 – 818.

Rudin, M. and Sauter, A. (1991) Noninvasive determination of regional cerebral blood flow in rats using dynamic imaging with Gd(DTPA). *Magn. Reson. Med.,* 22: 32 – 46.

Rudolphi, K.A., Keil, M. and Grome, J.J. (1990) Adenosine – a pharmacological concept for the treatment of cerebral ischemia? In: J. Krieglstein and H. Oberpichler (Eds.), *Pharmacology of Cerebral Ischemia,* Wissenschaftliche

Verlagsgesellschaft, Stuttgart, pp. 439 – 449.

Sage, E., Van Uitert, R.L. and Duffy, T.E. (1984) Early changes in blood-brain barrier permeability to small molecules after transient cerebral ischemia. *Stroke,* 15: 46 – 50.

Sauter, A. and Rudin, M. (1986) Calcium antagonists reduce the extent of infarction in rat middle cerebral artery occlusion model as determined by quantitative magnetic resonance imaging. *Stroke,* 17: 1228 – 1234.

Schatzman, R.C., Grifo, J.A., Merrick, W.C. and Kuo, J.F. (1983) Phospholipid sensitive Ca^{2+}-dependent protein kinase phosphorylates the beta unit eukaryotic initiation factor 2 (eIF-2). *FEBS Lett.,* 159: 167 – 170.

Schuier, F.J. and Hossmann, K.A. (1980) Experimental brain infarcts in cats II. Ischemic brain edema. *Stroke,* 11: 593 – 600.

Schürer, L., Grögaard, B., Gerdin, B., Kempski, O. and Arfors, K.E. (1991) Leucocyte depletion does not affect post-ischaemic nerve cell damage in the rat. *Acta Neurochir. (Wien),* 111: 54 – 60.

Segal, S.S. (1991) Microvascular recruitment in hamster striated muscle: role for conducted vasodilation. *Am. J. Physiol.,* 261: H181 – H189.

Segal, S.S. and Duling, B.R. (1986) Flow control among microvessels coordinated by intercellular conduction. *Science,* 234: 868 – 870.

Shigeno, T., Teasdale, G.M., McCulloch, J. and Graham, D.I. (1985) Recirculation model following MCA occlusion in rats. *J. Neurosurg.,* 63: 272 – 277.

Siesjö, B.K. (1981) Cell damage in the brain: a speculative synthesis. *J. Cereb. Blood Flow Metab.,* 1: 155 – 185.

Siesjö, B.K. and Bengtsson, F. (1989) Calcium fluxes, calcium antagonists, and calcium-related pathology in brain ischemia, hypoglycemia, and spreading depression: a unifying hypothesis. *J. Cereb. Blood Flow Metab.,* 9: 127 – 140.

Siesjö , B.K., Ekholm, A., Katsura, K., Memezawa, H., Ohta, S. and Smith, M.L. (1990a) The type of ischemia determines the pathophysiology of brain lesions and the therapeutic response to calcium channel blockade. In: J. Krieglstein and H. Oberpichler (Eds.), *Pharmacology of Cerebral Ischemia,* Wissenschaftliche Verlagsgesellschaft, Stuttgart, pp. 79 – 88.

Siesjö, B.K., Lundgren, J. and Pahlmark, K. (1990b) The role of free radicals in ischemic brain damage: a hypothesis. In: J. Krieglstein and H. Oberpichler (Eds.), *Pharmacology of Cerebral Ischemia,* Wissenschaftliche Verlagsgesellschaft, Stuttgart, pp. 319 – 323.

Sixt, G., Villringer, A. and Dirnagl, U. (1992) Leukocyte behavior during acute reperfusion after global cerebral ischemia in the rat brain microcirculation. *Soc. Neurosci. Abstr.,* 18(2): 1262.

Sommer, B., Keinänen, K., Verdoorn, T.A., Wisden, W., Burnashev, N., Herb, A., Köhler, M., Takagi, T., Sakmann, B. and Seeburg, P.H. (1990) Flip and flop: a cell-specific functional switch in glutamate-operated channels of the CNS. *Science,* 249: 1580 – 1585.

Steimle, C.N., Guynn, T.P., Morganroth, M.L., Bolling, S.F., Carr, K. and Deeb, G.M. (1992) Neutrophils are not necessary for ischemia-reperfusion lung injury. *Ann. Thorac. Surg.,* 53: 64 – 73.

Steinberg, G.K., Lo, E.H., Kunis, D.M., Grant, G.A., Poljak, A. and DeLaPaz, R. (1991) Dextromethorphan alters cerebral blood flow and protects against cerebral injury following focal ischemia. *Neurosci. Lett.,* 133: 225 – 228.

Stern, M.D. (1975) In vivo evaluation of microcirculation by coherent light scattering. *Nature,* 254: 56 – 58.

Strong, A.J., Venables, G.S. and Gibson, G. (1983) The cortical ischaemic penumbra associated with occlusion of the middle cerebral artery in the cat: 1. Topography of changes in blood flow, potassium ion activity and EEG. *J. Cereb. Blood Flow Metab.,* 3: 86 – 96.

Sundt, T.M. and Anderson, R.E. (1980) Umbelliferone as an intracellular pH-sensitive fluorescent indicator and blood brain barrier probe. *J. Neurophys.,* 44: 60 – 75.

Suzuki, M., Inauen, W., Kvietys, P.R., Grisham, M.B., Meininger, C., Schelling, M.E., Granger, H.J. and Granger, D.N. (1989) Superoxide dismutase mediates reperfusion-induced leukocyte endothelial cell interactions. *Am. J. Physiol.,* 257: H1740 – H1745.

Suzuki, R., Yamaguchi, T., Kirino, T., Orzi, F. and Klatzo, I. (1983) The effects of 5-minute ischemia in mongolian gerbils: I. Blood-brain barrier, cerebral blood flow, and local cerebral glucose utilization changes. *Acta Neuropathol. (Berl.),* 60: 207 – 216.

Takeshima, R., Kirsch, J.R., Koehler, R.C., Gomoll, A.W. and Traystman, R.J. (1992) Monoclonal leukocyte antibody does not decrease the injury of transient focal cerebral ischemia in cats. *Stroke,* 23: 247 – 252.

Takizawa, S., Hogan, M. and Hakim, A. (1991) The effects of a competitive NMDA receptor antagonist (CGS-19755) on cerebral blood flow and pH in focal ischemia. *J. Cereb. Blood Flow Metab.,* 11: 786 – 793.

Tang, C.M., Dichter, M. and Morad, M. (1990) Modulation of the *N*-methyl-D-aspartate channel by extracellular H^+. *Proc. Natl. Acad. Sci. U.S.A.,* 87: 6445 – 6449.

Them, A., (1993) Brain cortex pH/Ca^{2+} imaging in situ. *Adv. Exp. Med. Biol.,* in press.

Them, A., Villringer, A., Büttner, U.R. and Dirnagl, U. (1992) Confocal fluorescence imaging of Ca_i^{2+}-transients in acute rat brain slices using Fluo-3-AM and a small volume merged chamber system. *Soc. Neurosci. Abstr.,* 18(2): 967.

Traystman, R.J., Kirsch, J.R. and Koehler, R.C. (1991) Oxygen radical mechanisms of brain injury following ischemia and reperfusion. *J. Appl. Physiol.,* 71(4): 1185 – 1195.

Tsien, Y. (1989) Fluorescent indicators of ion concentrations. *Methods Cell Biol.,* 30: 127 – 156.

Turcani, P., Gotoh, F., Ishihara, N., Tanaka, K., Gomi, S., Takashima, S. and Mihara, B. (1988) Are blood platelets involved in the pathogenesis of ischemic brain edema in gerbils? *Stroke,* 19: 486 – 489.

Tyson, G.W., Teasdale, G.M., Graham, D.I. and McCulloch, J.

(1984) Focal cerebral ischemia in the rat: topography of hemodynamic and histopathological changes. *Ann. Neurol.,* 15: 559 – 567.

Uchiyama, S., Yamazaki, M. and Maruyama, S. (1991) Role of platelet-activating factor in aggregation of leukocytes and platelets in cerebral ischemia. *Lipids,* 26: 1247 – 1249.

Uematsu, D., Greenberg, J.H., Reivich, M., Kobayashi, S. and Karp, A. (1988) In vivo fluorometric measurement of changes in cytosolic free calcium from the cat cortex during anoxia. *J. Cereb. Blood Flow Metab.,* 8: 367 – 374.

Valone, Fh., Philip, R. and Debs, R.J. (1988) Enhanced human monocyte toxicity by platelet-activating factor. *Immunology,* 166: 715 – 718.

Vasthare, U.S., Heinel, L.A., Rosenwasser, R.H. and Tuma, R.F. (1990) Leukocyte involvement in cerebral ischemia and reperfusion injury. *Surg. Neurol.,* 33: 261 – 265.

Villringer, A., Haberl, R.L., Dirnagl, U., Anneser, F., Verst, M. and Einhäupl, K.M. (1989) Confocal laser microscopy to study microcirculation on the rat brain surface in vivo. *Brain Res.,* 504: 159 – 160.

Villringer, A., Dirnagl, U., Them, A., Schürer, L., Krombach, F. and Einhäupl, K.M. (1991a) Imaging of leukocytes within the rat brain cortex in vivo. *Microvasc. Res.,* 42: 305 – 315.

Villringer, A., Dirnagl, U., Gebhardt, R. and Einhäupl, K.M. (1991b) An in vivo approach to assess the capillary recruitment hypothesis in the brain microcirculation using confocal laser scanning microscopy. *J. Cereb. Blood Flow Metab.,* 11 (Suppl. 2): S441.

Villringer, A., Bötzel, K., Hock, C., Schleinkofer, L. and Dirnagl, U. (1992) Noninvasive monitoring of local cerebral blood volume and tissue oxygenation during cognitive tasks in man using near infrared spectoscopy. *Soc. Neurosci. Abstr.,* 18(1): 864.

Watson, B.D. and Ginsberg, M.D. (1989) Ischemic injury in the brain – role of oxygen radical-mediated processes. *Ann. N.Y. Acad. Sci.,* 559: 269 – 275.

Weiss, S.J. (1989) Tissue destruction by neurophils. *N. Engl. J. Med.,* 320: 365 – 376.

Wood, J.H. and Kee, D.B. (1985) Hemorheology of the cerebral circulation in stroke. *Stroke,* 16: 765 – 772.

Yamasaki, Y. and Kogure, K. (1990) The involvement of free radical formation and lipid peroxidation on the post-ischemic neuronal damage. In: J. Krieglstein and H. Oberpichler (Eds.), *Pharmacology of Cerebral Ischemia,* Wissenschaftliche Verlagsgesellschaft, Stuttgart, pp. 325 – 333.

Yoshimine, T., Nakajima, S., Hayakawa, T., Kato, A. and Mushiroi, T. (1989) rCBF versus microvascular plasma circulation in focal cerebral ischemia. *J. Cereb. Blood Flow Metab.,* 9 (Suppl. 1): S170.

SECTION II

Free Radicals and Excitatory Amino Acids

K. Kogure, K.-A. Hossmann and B.K. Siesjö (Eds.)
Progress in Brain Research, Vol. 96

CHAPTER 5

Evaluation of the concomitance of lipid peroxidation in experimental models of cerebral ischemia and stroke

Brant D. Watson

Cerebral Vascular Disease Research Center, Department of Neurology, University of Miami School of Medicine, Miami, FL 33101, U.S.A.

Introduction: lipid peroxidation and its significance to cell injury

Early, aggressive clinical treatment intended to limit the extent and severity of brain injury caused by stroke is uncommon. A clinician first must determine if indeed a stroke has occurred, whether it is hemorrhagic, thrombotic or embolic, and then whether to intercede by means of attempts to restore blood flow to the afflicted zones of the brain. Direct intercession with a thrombolytic enzyme is initiated only with great caution, inasmuch as the problem of induced hemorrhage leading to excessive morbidity and mortality, formerly seen with streptokinase treatment, still occurs but to a much less lethal degree with human tissue plasminogen activator (Del Zoppo, 1990). This candidate for a widely accepted, available method for mitigating stroke-in-evolution is still in development.

Recirculation of ischemic tissue may not reinstitute normal metabolism and complete recovery, however. Instead, attempts to resuscitate tissue from an ischemic state may damage it irreversibly. This undesirable outcome, known as reperfusion injury, is now thought to be mediated by free radical forms of molecular oxygen (Braunwald and Kloner, 1985). Free radicals contain one or more "unpaired" electrons, and are chemically reactive because in order to regain thermodynamic stability (all electrons paired) they tend to strip electrons or hydrogen atoms from neighboring molecules, thus radicalizing these molecules in turn. The oxygen radicals, also referred to as "active oxygens", arise in sequential fashion from molecular oxygen by successive single-electron reduction reactions (Halliwell and Gutteridge, 1985a,b). They are respectively identified as the superoxide anion radical (O_2^-), its protonated form the perhydroxyl radical ($HO_2^\bullet$), hydrogen peroxide and the hydroxyl radical ($OH^\bullet$). These active oxygen species comprise the oxygen radical cascade, of which the superoxide anion radical is the precursor; its presence is taken as strongly indicating that the other species are also being produced. Acute ischemic injury potentiates oxygen radical formation during reperfusion, owing to the interaction of molecular oxygen with an excess of reduced species (e.g., mitochondrial ubisemiquinone radical) accumulated during the period of metabolic suppression.

An important consequence of oxygen radical formation is the subject of this article: lipid peroxidation (reviewed by Tappel, 1973; Siesjo, 1981; Sevanian and Hochstein, 1985; Halliwell and Gutteridge, 1985a; Watson and Ginsberg, 1988, 1989; Braughler and Hall, 1989; Hall and Braughler, 1989; Watson, 1990a,b). Lipid peroxidation arises during and following disruption of membrane structure via oxygen-consuming rancidity reactions. Membrane viscosity and rigidity are increased (Dobretsov et al., 1977) and microscopically visible fissures or holes are formed in the membrane lipid bilayer (Anderson et al., 1976; Pasquali-Ronchetti et al., 1980; Yagi et al., 1981; Noronha-Dutra and Steen, 1982; Thaw et al., 1983; Dietrich et al., 1987). Consistent with these defects are reports of enhanced permeability (Smolen and Shohet, 1974; Hicks and Gebicki, 1978) and the development of edema (Thaw et al., 1983; Burton et al., 1984). Lipid peroxidation can inhibit the function of important membrane-bound enzymes as well. For example, the hydroperoxide formed from arachidonic acid inhibits endothelial prostacyclin synthase (Bunting et al., 1983; Warso and Lands, 1983), thereby inactivating an important response of endothelium to aggregating platelets. Lipid peroxides are chemically unstable and can continue to degrade into many other products which are also chemically reactive. Such decomposition reactions are encompassed by the term "lipid peroxidation" also. In particular, reactive species such as aldehydes can be produced; these can also induce changes in membrane structure and function by cross-linking amino groups of proteins (Chio and Tappel, 1969; Fletcher and Tappel, 1971) or polar head groups of phospholipid molecules (Bidlack and Tappel, 1973). Owing to these deleterious effects, monitoring the development of lipid peroxidation is believed to provide an index of tissue injury on the molecular scale.

Lipid peroxidation is damaging to tissues principally because it is a chain process; a single initiating free radical can precipitate the destruction of many adjacent molecules in a cellular structure and thus compromise its function. Peroxidation of a susceptible molecule such as an unsaturated fatty acid is initiated by abstraction of a methylene hydrogen atom; the resultant carbon-centered fatty acid radical transforms structurally to yield a conjugated diene moiety. This molecular fragment is quickly peroxidized by direct addition of O_2 to yield a peroxy radical. The peroxy free radical can then reinitiate a new reaction cycle, by repeating the hydrogen atom abstraction step at the expense of another susceptible molecule. This final step of a typical cycle thus yields another lipid free radical, and also a lipid (hydro)peroxide molecule – the product of lipid peroxy radical neutralization. These reactions thus form a regenerative chain process driven by oxygen. Such a reaction sequence may well proceed until the propagating radical is neutralized by an organic scavenger compound. (More information on these processes appears in the Appendix.)

The identity of the chain-initiating oxygen free radical is generally presumed to be the hydroxyl radical ($OH^\bullet$), or at low pH, the perhydroxyl radical ($HO_2^\bullet$). The hydroxyl radical arises from decomposition of hydrogen peroxide or lipid hydroperoxides by metal ions (Fenton reaction; cf. Appendix). Convincing evidence for the initiating role of hydroxyl (or perhydroxyl) radical is derived from radiochemical experiments performed on aqueous suspensions of unsaturated fatty acids (Hasegawa and Patterson, 1978; Bielski et al., 1983). However, its initiating role in biological systems is less convincingly established. Chain peroxidation of lipids to observable amounts may instead be initiated by metal-ion-induced decomposition of the small quantity of lipid hydroperoxides already present. The peroxy and alkoxy lipid radicals resulting from such decomposition are able to sustain the chain process and, in the presence of iron ions, are more likely to be produced than the hydroxyl radical (Gutteridge, 1988). The role of ferrous or ferric ion in hydroperoxide decomposition is also less clear; complexes of ionic iron and oxygen have been invoked but not identified unequivocally.

The question of just what initial conditions are minimally sufficient to initiate processes leading to cell death by any means, let alone free radical processes, is still open, however. The answer to this question will likely involve assessment of the functional capacity of the enzymic defense system against peroxidation reactions (cf. Appendix). Briefly, enzymic reduction of lipid hydroperoxides and hydrogen peroxide by glutathione peroxidase prevents their degradation to hydroxyl, peroxy or alkoxy radicals or to other reactive products such as aldehydes. A complementary function of the defense system is to generate the hydrogen peroxide, by enzymic dismutation of the superoxide anion radical by superoxide dismutase (SOD). Ultimately, however, this system is dependent on maintenance of sufficient metabolic potential via glucose utilization (cf. Appendix), not only for the purpose of cellular defense but also for its own sake: superoxide anion inactivates catalase and glutathione peroxidase while hydrogen peroxide inactivates superoxide dismutase (reviewed by Kontos, 1989a), hence these enzymes also exhibit mutual protection. Nonetheless, tissue injury by any means leading to metabolic dysfunction may result in exacerbation of conditions for generation of free radicals and hydroperoxides. To illustrate, trauma in the form of focal ischemia elicits a secondary inflammatory response (McCord, 1987), in which infiltrating neutrophils release a cascade of secretions including oxygen radicals (Clifford and Repine, 1982) of such intensity that the defense system is unable to mitigate its effects focally. The resultant damage done to adjacent tissues can then accentuate the severity and expand the volume of the ischemic zone, in concert with the development of edema facilitated by peroxidative damage to membranes (McCord, 1987).

However, the location, character and magnitude of free radical-induced alterations at the earliest stages of cell injury are not yet known, nor are their presumed contributions to the development of edema of sufficient severity and persistence to cause cell death. For example, it is possible that the contribution of edema to cellular morbidity is a function of pores formed by oxygen radical-induced lipid peroxidative injury to the surface membrane, but that the levels of oxygen radicals or their product lipid peroxides are too low to detect by existing methods. On the other hand, a completely different mechanism may lead to similarly lethal effects: the non-peroxidative formation of pores by protein (perforin) aggregates, followed by development of lethal edema in target cells, has recently been revealed as at least one strategy employed by cytotoxic T (killer) cells (Young and Cohn, 1988). In nucleated cells such pores may be absorbed by endocytosis, so long as metabolism remains intact (Carney et al., 1985), but apparently this has not yet been investigated as a potential response to lipid peroxidative damage to the plasma membrane. As membrane breakdown proceeds, however, concomitant with a profusion of events such as excessive calcium ion influx (Cheung et al., 1986) and free fatty acid release (Bazan, 1970), the chain process of lipid peroxidation may proceed to detectable levels concomitant with the development of frank cellular rancidity, provided that the interacting components are not diluted. However, at this point the cell is probably in a quiescent state and may well be dying or already dead. The disorder engendered by primary (but undetected) oxygen radical processes is sufficient in this scenario to sever any directly observable connection of lipid peroxides derived from these radicals to *primary induction* of cell death, and further suggests that the transition from developing cell morbidity to frank mortality is not distinct. Therefore, if lipid peroxidation is rendered observable only by the compoundment of such degenerative processes, it cannot be proven that lipid peroxidation is not an epiphenomenon – a sequel of cell death rather than its precedent (Halliwell and Gutteridge, 1984). It thus seems necessary to develop means to detect lipid peroxides at very early times after compromise of tissue metabolism, but before structural disruption is pervasive.

Mechanisms for in vivo production and detection of oxygen radicals

The hypothesis that lipid peroxidation mediates cell rancidity and death arose about forty years ago, but the connection of lipid peroxidation with oxygen radicals was not widely appreciated until considerably later. Mechanisms for production of the precursor radical, superoxide anion, during ordinary or compromised metabolic processes in vivo have been discovered only within the past 25 years (Fridovich, 1978). In that time, awareness among bioscientists (and the general public) of the putative involvement of free radicals in degenerative diseases of all types has increased markedly. This is due largely to the marketing efforts of companies selling antioxidants (such as vitamin E) as nutritional supplements, as well as to popular accounts of scientific literature describing biological effects attributed to free radical reactions, e.g., aging.

In the contexts of cerebral ischemia and stroke, several mechanisms of superoxide radical production are considered to be of significant or likely relevance (Kontos, 1989a,b; Ikeda and Long, 1990; Schmidley, 1990).

(1) Purine catabolism. Ischemia triggers two parallel transformations, one being conversion of ATP into its metabolites AMP, adenosine, inosine, hypoxanthine and xanthine, and the other being transformation of xanthine dehydrogenase to xanthine oxidase. During reperfusion (reoxygenation), xanthine oxidase successively catabolizes hypoxanthine to xanthine and xanthine to urea, releasing superoxide anion (O_2^-) at each step (McCord, 1985).

(2) Respiration. Oxidation of ubisemiquinone radical, the diffusible electron transfer agent in the mitochondrial respiratory chain, yields O_2^- (Turrens et al., 1985). This pathway operates during normal metabolism but its enhancement (following reoxygenation) is potentiated by the reducing conditions present during ischemia.

(3) Prostaglandin (PG) synthesis. After conversion of free arachidonic acid to PGG_2, the conversion of PGG_2 to PGH_2 by prostaglandin synthase is accomplished by the enzyme operating as a classical (hydro)peroxidase; i.e., the enzyme itself assumes free radical character through compounds I and II. In a concomitant reaction, the enzyme radicals can abstract hydrogen atoms from pyridine nucleotides (NAD(P)H), and their resultant radical forms (NAD(P)•) can be oxidized by molecular oxygen to yield O_2^- (Kukreja et al., 1986). Although this process occurs normally, it is presently conjectured that any type of tissue trauma (including ischemia) leading to arachidonic acid release can amplify this pathway. Ischemia further potentiates this reaction via enhanced accumulation of reduced pyridine nucleotides, which then facilitates O_2^- production during reperfusion.

(4) Excitatory amino acid release. Another consequence of ischemia currently receiving much attention is the release of excitatory amino acids (EAA) such as glutamate. Because this further stimulates arachidonic acid release (Dumuis et al., 1988), tissue toxicity may be expressed via superoxide-dependent reactions according to mechanism (3). The interconnectedness of these toxic responses is further illustrated by the stimulated release of EAA from tissue by oxygen radicals (Pellegrini-Giampietro et al., 1990).

(5) Neutrophil activation. Phagocytosis stimulates O_2^- synthesis by NADPH oxidase during the respiratory burst. Neutrophils responding to tissue injury (as signaled chemotactically by O_2^- release) may inappropriately enhance local, or possibly remote, destruction of tissue by releasing a flood of toxic free radicals (McCord, 1987). The resultant secondary tissue damage (Weiss, 1989) may further confuse assessments of the contribution of lipid peroxidation to primary tissue injury.

Discovering pathways that produce superoxide anion is important because superoxide is the radical from which more potently reactive oxygen radicals are derived, prior to initiating lipid peroxidation. Hydroxyl radical is commonly believed to arise from the iron-catalyzed, superoxide-driven Haber-Weiss reaction (cf. Appendix for reaction equations). In this coupled reaction scheme, superoxide anion interacts with iron-binding proteins to release ferrous iron derived from the bound ferric form (Thomas et al., 1985), while in parallel, superoxide anions are converted into hydrogen peroxide and oxygen by superoxide dismutase. Hydroxyl radical then arises and ferric iron is regenerated via the well-known ferrous iron-catalyzed Fenton reaction. By recycling the redox state of iron ions, the superoxide anion thus facilitates the continuous generation of hydroxyl radical and subsequent initiation of the chain process of lipid peroxidation. Conversion and release of bound iron to its elemental, reactive form is also enhanced by protease activation upon tissue disruption (Halliwell and Gutteridge, 1986) and by tissue acidosis (Barber and Bernheim, 1967). By means of these latter processes, lipid peroxidation is amplified and likely extended from microfocal sites to outlying regions, thereby expanding the zone of damaged tissue and facilitating still more oxygen radical-mediated reactions. Such a generalized tissue response, comprised of regenerative events leading to tissue destruction, is reminiscent of the cyclic nature of oxygen radical-mediated processes and is generally thought to result from the concatenation of these processes on a greatly expanded scale (Watson, 1990b). This illustrates the importance of maintaining intact membrane barriers, in order to prevent spurious admixture of reactive substances by means of molecular or cellular *decompartmentation.*

Much current research involves collecting evidence for the existence, and appearance in time, of one or more of these superoxide-producing schemes after the onset of tissue injury in a particular context. The supporting evidence is mainly indirect, however; it is usually based on detection of a (presumably) specific product formed by reaction of a quencher compound with superoxide anion or hydroxyl radical, or on attenuation of the development of tissue deterioration by compounds which scavenge oxygen radicals. For example, superoxide anion is often detected by its reaction with nitroblue tetrazolium to yield an insoluble formazan precipitate. Inhibition by allopurinol of superoxide radical formation from xanthine oxidase or scavenging of superoxide by superoxide dismutase are utilized to test indirectly for the involvement of superoxide in the process under examination. Molecular scavengers of hydroxyl radical, such as mannitol, dimethylsulfoxide or dimethylthiourea, have also been used to protect membranes from the initial assault of hydrogen atom abstraction.

Direct in vivo detection of oxygen radicals is very uncommon and to this point dependent on the technique of electron paramagnetic resonance (EPR) to detect the unpaired electron of a specific radical. This requires optimization of the conditions for producing a sufficient number of electron "spins", which is difficult unless the free radicals can be produced in a highly concentrated burst. This condition is more likely to occur in the intravascular space, at the point of transition between high-grade ischemia and reperfusion, instead of at a focus of non-reperfusible traumatic tissue injury. More recently, EPR spectra attributed to peroxidation-induced radical intermediates were detected by infusion of the spin trap PBN within the first 5 min following reperfusion of ischemic dog heart in vivo (Bolli et al., 1989). These spectral intensities were suppressed, and recovery of contractile function observed, by administering the potent hydroxyl radical scavenger N-(2-mercaptopropionyl)-glycine (MPG) just before reperfusion. Infusion of MPG at 1 min after the start of reperfusion did not restore contractile function, presumably owing to the propagation of lipid peroxidation reactions initiated during the first minute of reperfusion. Hydroxyl radical production in vivo following reperfusion of ischemic gerbil brain (Cao et al., 1988) or during microdialysis of rat striatum (Boisvert, 1991) has also been assayed by high-performance liquid chromatography (hplc) in terms of 2,5-dihydroxybenzoate, assumed to result from hydroxylation of infused salicylate. Increased production of this salicylate adduct was enhanced by infusion of ferrous sulfate (Boisvert, 1991). However, because 2,5-hydroxybenzoate is also produced by activation of the microsomal cytochrome P-450 system, it has been suggested that detection of 2,3-dihydroxybenzoate should be utilized as a more rigorous indicator of hydroxyl radical formation (Halliwell et al., 1991). Lastly, free radicals were detected by EPR with phenyl-N-tert-butyl nitrone (PBN) as spin probe in the brains of pigs subjected to global ischemia/reperfusion (Kirsch et al., 1991). The signal, identified as originating from carbon-centered radicals, became apparent during ischemia while during the reperfusion period the signal decayed. This may reflect the ischemia-induced accumulation of normally occurring mitochondrial radicals (e.g., ubisemiquinone) in the parenchyma and their dissipation during reperfusion. On the other hand, the loss of radical signal during reperfusion may simply indicate dilution of the (unidentified) radicals in the intravascular space, or progressive neutralization by antioxidants in the blood. Such evidence may be insufficient to implicate free radicals as primary inducers of tissue damage, however.

Determining whether the appearance of oxygen radicals is concomitant with ischemic brain injury is another active approach. Behavioral abnormalities and cerebral edema were significantly attenuated by allopurinol administration to spontaneously hypertensive rats subjected to global cerebral ischemia and recirculation (Itoh et al., 1986). In a similar but specifically conditioned rat model leading to infarcts of reproducible volume, infarct size was reduced by pretreatment with Cu,Zn superoxide dismutase (Beckman et al., 1987). The xanthine dehydrogenase-to-oxidase transition was also observed and quantitated; summed activities of both enzymes remained constant during ischemia and reperfusion. In similar work, the summed brain activities of these enzymes were progressively decreased (in contrast to allopurinol-dosed animals), as were hydrogen peroxide levels and the severity of edema, in gerbils maintained on a tungsten-rich diet or administered dimethylthiourea (DMTU) and then subjected to 1 h of unilateral carotid artery occlusion followed by 6 h of reperfusion (Patt et al., 1988). For animals exhibiting neurologic deficits, survival at 48 h after treatment with either tungsten or DMTU was complete, as opposed to less than 40% after treatment with saline or allopurinol. In a rat model of focal ischemia induced by permanent occlusions of the middle cerebral (MCA) and both common carotid (CCA) arteries, preadministered liposome-entrapped SOD reduced regional infarct volumes by up to 33% (Imaizumi et al., 1990). The development of vasogenic edema following cold-induced focal ischemic injury was mitigated by pre- and post-administration of liposomes containing SOD, while the concomitance of superoxide anion production was confirmed by NBT staining (Chan et al., 1987). Polyethylene glycol (PEG)-conjugated SOD has recently become available; this has the advantages of much longer persistence of circulating activity as well as enhanced uptake by endothelium. In combination with preadministered PEG-conjugated catalase (a complementary scavenger of hydrogen peroxide), PEG SOD reduced infarct volume at 24 h by 24% in rats subjected to permanent MCA occlusion and 90 min bilateral CCA occlusion (Liu et al., 1989). Given such evidence of the efficacy of SOD in mitigating ischemic brain injury, the protective effect of enhancing intrinsic SOD activity by transgenically implanting the gene coding for human SOD was recently studied in mice (Kinouchi et al., 1991). Animals expressing a 2.6-fold increase in Cu,Zn SOD activity, and subjected to permanent MCA and left CCA occlusion and 1 h of right CCA occlusion, displayed a 37% reduction in infarct volume at 24 h.

These experiments offer strong support for the association of the superoxide anion radical and (by inference or observation) the derivative forms of active oxygen, with progression of brain tissue degeneration following traumatic or ischemic injury. Convincing evidence for the *initiating* role of the oxyradical cascade in expression of tissue damage requires *acute* detection of oxygen radicals, however. Experiments based on suppression of the tissue-degrading effects of oxygen radical-induced reactions (exemplified by lipid peroxidation) are less likely to yield information about initiation because lipid peroxidation, once started, may be occurring in cellular regions inaccessible to specific oxygen radical scavengers and therefore resists quenching by them. To illustrate, hepatocytes permeabilized by electroporation generated lipid peroxides at the same rate (normalized to protein content) as did similarly stimulated preparations of liver microsomes (Hallinan et al., 1991); peroxidation was initiated by incubation with decompartmentalized ferrous iron in the form of an EDTA chelate. Nonetheless, the concentration of Fenton reaction-generated hydroxyl radical detected by scavenger molecules, including dimethylsulfoxide, was much greater in the microsomal system than in the permeabilized hepatocytes. The difference was attributed to the competitive capability of cytosolic antioxidant proteins (such as glutathione peroxidase) remaining in the hepatocytes to eliminate hydrogen peroxide, the precursor of hydroxyl radical; the data also suggest, however, that membrane lipid peroxidation can be initiated and sustained with very small amounts of hydroxyl radical.

In further examples, the effectiveness of superoxide dismutase in preventing death mediated by starvation in neuronal cell cultures (Saez et al., 1987), or mediated by exposure to hydrogen peroxide or activated neutrophils in endothelial cell cultures (Markey et al., 1990) was greatly enhanced by artificially increasing the cellular content of SOD. Markey et al. (1990) attributed these protective effects to inhibition of the superoxide-mediated reduction of ferric iron to ferrous iron, a necessary step in recycling the Fenton reaction.

Experiments of this type, however, cannot yield information on the biomolecular structural changes that are presumably concomitant with tissue degeneration. That is to say, the structurally damaging process of lipid peroxidation cannot be inferred rigorously from evidence of the presence of oxygen radicals derived either from EPR spectra or from quenching experiments. As an example of the difficulty inherent in assuring such a connection, a transgenic mouse model overexpressing human Cu,Zn SOD activity (and therefore increased hydrogen peroxide concentration) was invented originally in the hope that tissue-damaging processes (including lipid peroxidation) presumed to occur in Down syndrome would be facilitated (Epstein et al., 1987). However, these authors also predicted that the deleterious effects of conditions thought to involve exogenous attack by oxygen radicals might be avoided in this model (cf. Kinouchi et al., 1991).

Detection methods for lipid peroxidation reactions

To be convincingly implicated in the expression of acute tissue injury, lipid peroxides or their reaction products must be detected directly, and very early in time after the onset of injury. This has not yet been attempted, however, owing to disagreement about what consitutes a direct method as well as to insensitivity and absence of rigorous specificity of existing methods of assay. Inasmuch as lipid peroxidation is a consequence of oxygen radical attack it will likely require some time to become manifest, at least to detectable levels by current techniques. To this point, it has not been possible to attain overlap of the complementary methodologies of direct oxygen radical detection or of lipid peroxidation in either time or space (i.e., in specific tissue regions). Another complicating factor is that generation of superoxide anion may continue for a considerable time after the original insult (Kontos, 1987); as suggested by the above schemes for superoxide production, only schemes (1) and (2) are acutely expressed, while schemes (3) through (5) are based on secondary responses (see pp. 72, 84). Further, because the detection of lipid peroxides in vivo has yet to precede or predict foci of ischemic damage, the initiating role of lipid peroxidation in engendering irreversible neuronal damage and infarction has not been established.

Nearly all the commonly used assays for lipid peroxidation were developed in the context of in vitro studies in which the tissues were placed under untoward oxidative stress; i.e., tissue degradation was often induced by means which do not reflect accurately the initial conditions leading to oxygen radical-induced processes. For example, the combination of ferrous iron and ascorbic acid has long been used to stimulate indicators of lipid peroxidation such as thiobarbituric acid-reactive substances (TBARS), and losses of GSH, vitamin E and unsaturated fatty acids. This type of experiment should now be regarded as outmoded, however, and the results obvious, because the membrane breakdown sensitized is so fulminant that the observed lipid peroxides likely arise as a result of cell death, rather than vice versa. It must be re-emphasized that *compartmentation* of cells and cellular organelles by membranes must be preserved in order to prevent adventitious mixture of susceptible substrates with reactive agents such as ferrous iron (Halliwell and Gutteridge, 1986); the results are likely to have little to do with the natural processes of *initial* tissue degradation. This would appear to be true also in recent experiments in which several assays (TBA reactants, diene conjugation, fatty acid loss) of lipid peroxidative damage by free radical intermediates during the metabolism of bromobenzene in liver tissue were linearly related (Pompella et al., 1987).

On the other hand, brain homogenates incubated with ferrous iron and ascorbate were found to generate TBA-reactive material at a pH optimum of 6.0 – 6.5 (Siesjo et al., 1985). It was proposed that this increase in putative peroxidation products was facilitated by the intracellular decompartmentation of iron to the ferrous form and also to increased concentration of the chain-initiating perhydroxyl radical, both conditions being favored during ischemia-induced tissue acidosis.

The TBA test (Dahle et al., 1962), in particular, is still widely employed despite a great profusion of inherent difficulties which render the TBA test inappropriate for assessing the contribution of lipid peroxidation to the early stages of irreversible brain damage. As originally envisioned, the test is intended to detect the small amount of malonaldehyde arising from decomposition of intrinsic tissue lipid hydroperoxides by the acid-heating conditions of the test. However, these conditions also create new lipid hydroperoxides, whose decomposition in kind yields the vast bulk of malonaldehyde detected; the final concentration of malonaldehyde so generated is assumed to be proportional to the amount intrinsic to the tissue sample. The reaction product of thiobarbituric acid with malonaldehyde yields a TBARS chromophore which can be detected either spectrophotometrically (by absorbance at 532 nm) or by fluorometry (by emission at 550 nm; Yagi, 1976). However, TBARS are not specific indicators of lipid peroxidation inasmuch as they include many substances, such as sialic acid, prostaglandins, deoxyribose and aldehydes other than malonaldehyde (Gutteridge, 1986, 1988). Also, the intensity of the color reaction is inconsistent, because its amplification from initial small amounts of reactive products is accelerated by ferrous iron (which decomposes lipid hydroperoxides) and mitigated by antioxidant compounds (such as vitamin E). Quantitation is not comparable among laboratories owing to variations in technical procedure intended to impose reproducibility, such as extrinsic manipulation of iron or antioxidant content.

More seriously, owing to its incubation of pulverized tissue at high temperature, the TBA test creates adventitious products which are likely not representative of peroxidic mediators of membrane destabilization hypothesized to form during the development of ischemic tissue damage. Such use of the TBA test to obtain information about tissue-degrading processes even before membrane damage is microscopically detectable does not recognize that the test was originally invented only to measure intrinsic tissue rancidity (i.e., liquefaction) over much longer time scales than presently desired. Of course, in the case of traumatic injury to tissue, the TBA test could be expected more accurately to detect lipid peroxide formation owing to acceleration of rancidity reactions in the crushed, decompartmentalized tissue. Finally, one might conclude justifiably that the TBA test is inherently flawed, from perusing the many publications on how to modify it to analyze tissue samples properly (Asakawa and Matsushita, 1979, 1980; Gutteridge, 1986, 1988), and that its alleged connection with meaningful assessments of early intrinsic peroxidative damage to tissue should be viewed quite skeptically.

Unequivocal evidence for the existence of intrinsic (not derivatized) lipid peroxides – the purported membrane molecular damage products of free radical reactions – is very uncommon in ischemia/reperfusion injury, but is of much interest. Inasmuch as diene conjugation in unsaturated fatty acids is generally accepted as the first structural manifestation of free radical damage, a method was developed (Watson et al., 1984) which represents an attempt to rigorously define the spectroscopic conditions under which the conjugated diene structure can be observed and quantified unarguably. In this method, the tissue total lipid fraction is isolated by the Bligh/Dyer technique (1959); an aliquot from the pure chloroform lower layer containing the lipid fraction is dried under nitrogen gas and then taken up in heptane for absorption spectroscopic analysis. By scanning from 350 nm down to about 310 nm, a steadily increasing but featureless background absorption is seen. In most cases this can be accounted for by the Rayleigh scattering formula. When this correction is made over the entire spectral range, the resulting spectrum may be attributed entirely to light absorption. Continuing the scan, absorbance inflections corresponding to higher-order structures such as conjugated trienes are seen in the 260 – 280 nm range, while the conjugated diene itself appears in the vicinity of 232 – 240 nm. Continuing farther into the ultraviolet, the absorbance increases rapidly and reaches a peak at approximately 190 – 194 nm, which represents light absorption by non-conjugated (i.e., non-transformed) double bonds.

The main feature of this technique is to derive a true difference spectrum between spectra obtained under (presumably) peroxidizing and control conditions. This is done by matching the amplitudes of the control spectrum and the peroxidized sample spectrum at the peak of the latter (approximately 193 nm), and then adjusting the remainder of the control spectrum according to the 193 nm amplitude ratio (Watson et al., 1984). From the absorbance difference at the conjugated diene peak, the conjugated diene concentration can be calculated to a first approximation. This concentration is proportional to the concentration of isolated double bonds lost during diene conjugation. Adding the equivalent absorbance to the absorbance of the control spectrum at 193 nm, and then renormalizing, yields a spectrum which is intended to simulate the sample spectrum before it was submitted to peroxidizing conditions. The difference between this final control spectrum and the peroxidized sample spectrum reveals a difference spectrum which not only displays the conjugated diene peak prominently, but also indicates the conversion of isolated double bonds into the diene structure as shown by negative absorbance in the 190 – 210 nm region (Watson et al., 1984). These spectral features are illustrated in Figs. 1 and 2, which display spectra derived from sampling plasma lipids of nominally healthy and chronically diseased humans.

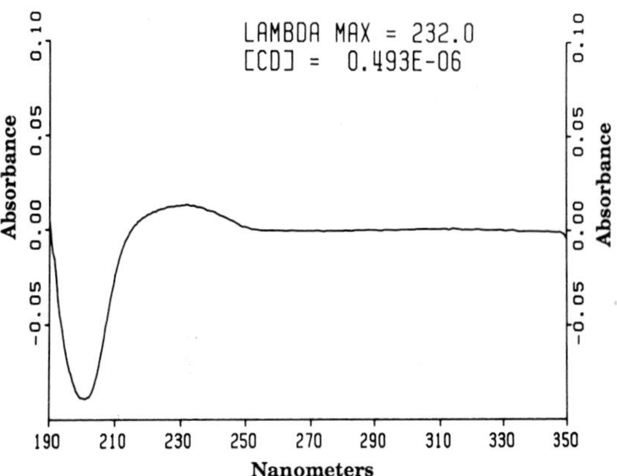

Fig. 2. Difference spectrum obtained by subtracting spectrum (C) from spectrum (P). The negative absorbance seen in the 190 – 210 nm region represents relative loss of isolated double bonds (i.e., relative decrease in fatty acid unsaturation index) and their conversion into the conjugated diene structure (Holman and Burr, 1946), as shown by the clearly resolved spectrum peaking at 232 nm. The absorbance difference corresponds to a 300 μM excess of plasma conjugated diene, concomitant with the chronically ill state of the anephric patient.

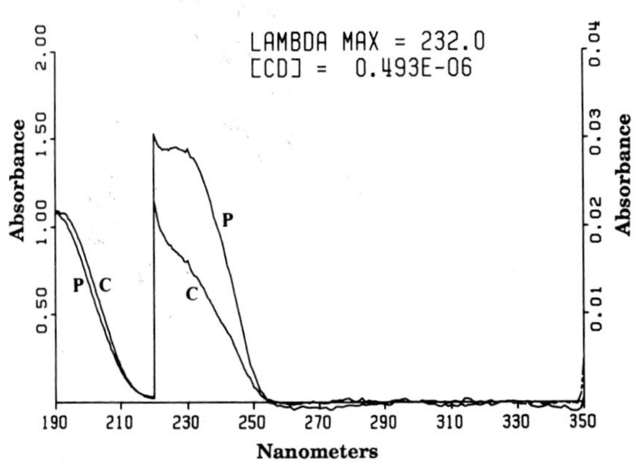

Fig. 1. Ultraviolet absorption spectra, Rayleigh-corrected for background scattering, of heptane-solubilized total lipid extracts from human plasma (note the expanded absorbance scale from 220 to 350 nm). The spectrum labeled (P) was derived from a chronically diseased anephric patient on dialysis (sample obtained by courtesy of G. Zilluerelo and J. Strauss). The spectrum labeled (C) was derived from a nominally healthy person. The control spectrum (C) was equivalenced to the patient spectrum (P) by the procedure given in the text. Both spectra display positive inflections in the 230 – 240 nm range suggestive of conjugated diene, although the inflection corresponding to the anephric patient is much larger. The spectral peaks in the 190 nm region are due to absorption by isolated double bonds (Rusoff et al., 1945).

Specific evidence for CNS tissue damage attributed to lipid peroxidation

Evidence for lipid peroxidation in the context of

brain ischemia/reperfusion has appeared in many forms, in the main adapted from previous in vitro methods. The most commonly used techniques include observation of vitamin E consumption (Yoshida et al., 1982; Hall et al., 1991); disappearance of ascorbyl radical (Demopoulos et al., 1980) or of unsaturated fatty acid content (Rehncrona et al., 1982; Yoshida et al., 1982); increases in content of oxidized glutathione (GSSG) at the expense of reduced glutathione (GSH) (Cooper et al., 1980; Rehncrona et al., 1980); changes in oxidized and reduced ubiquinones (Kinuta et al., 1989); detection of pentane (Mickel et al., 1987) from lipid peroxide decomposition or of chemiluminescence emitted from (presumably) peroxidizing tissue (Kogure et al., 1985); and spectroscopic assay for TBARS (Rehncrona et al., 1980; MacMillan, 1982). Reviews of this work have been pervasive and ubiquitous to the point of self-perpetuation (Ginsberg et al., 1988; Watson and Ginsberg, 1988, 1989; Watson, 1989, 1990a,b; Braughler and Hall, 1989; Hall and Braughler, 1989). Rather than comprehensively recycling this material yet again, only selected works will be discussed here in order to illustrate important conceptual aspects.

Although use of such indirect methods continues unabated, it is unlikely that the associated results will provide information on whether or how lipid peroxidation contributes fundamentally to the initiation of irreversible tissue degradation. One reason is that accurate regional assessment of peroxidation reactions generally cannot be done with these assays owing to the large volume of tissue required for sampling, thus obviating any correlation with the development of regional pathology. Another reason is that indirect assays, such as those cited, can yield results from in vivo experiments that are difficult to explain by reference to the (presumably) analogous in vitro results. This indicates that the conditions underlying the development of peroxidic markers in vitro simply do not mimic accurately the supposedly similar events occurring in real time in vivo.

Several examples will illustrate this point. In the setting of reversible global ischemia in the rat, Rehncrona et al. (1980) and Cooper et al. (1980) observed loss of reduced glutathione in cortical tissue with no correspondent increase in oxidized glutathione. This lack of evidence for in vivo lipid peroxidation was also observed by MacMillan (1982) who, in a similar in vivo system, found no changes in TBA reactants during ischemia or recirculation. In addition, Rehncrona et al. (1980) found that both aerobic and anaerobic incubation of homogenized cortical tissue in vitro with ferrous iron and ascorbic acid induced loss of reduced glutathione, which was stoichiometrically balanced by an increased content of oxidized glutathione only under aerobic conditions; also, TBA-reactive material was generated aerobically but not anaerobically. Kogure et al. (1982), while incubating a ''minced'' brain preparation (in which tissue is disintegrated but not homogenized) under *both* aerobic and anaerobic conditions, also observed loss of reduced glutathione without a compensating increase in oxidized glutathione content. Losses of vitamin E were similar and indistinguishable under both types of incubation. However, conjugated dienes were also clearly observed in total lipid extracts from the aerobically (but not anaerobically) incubated minces, and also ipsilaterally (but not contralaterally) in vivo in brains of rats 24 h after induction of embolic stroke. These observations by Kogure et al. (1982) of conjugated diene production must be acknowledged as accurately indicating lipid peroxidation, despite the lack of correlation with results obtained from indirect methods (especially the vitamin E results).

The explanation for the supposedly negative results of Rehncrona et al. (1980), Cooper et al. (1980) and Kogure et al. (1982) may lie within the response, as observed in cultured cells, of the glutathione redox cycle to an oxidative insult. Le et al. (1992) found that cultured myocytes, supplemented with glucose and exposed to cumene hydroperoxide, exhibited the same glutathione responses as reported by the above authors: loss of cellular reduced glutathione, maintenance of cellular oxidized glutathione, and no extracellular release of the latter (analogous to its observed lack in the CNS; Rehncrona et al., 1980). In the absence of glucose, reduced glutathione again decreased, while the levels of intracellular and especially extracellular oxidized glutathione increased almost linearly in time. Glucose supplementation also inhibited myocyte lysis and the development of TBA reactants. In contrast, inhibition of the latter presumed index of lipid peroxidation by incubation with oxidized glutathione or Trolox C (a water-soluble analog of vitamin E) did not entirely mitigate the onset of cell death, thereby suggesting the possible involvement of alternate pathways. Similarly, the level of oxidized glutathione in tumor cell cultures exposed to high concentrations of hydrogen peroxide increased slowly over 60 min, but increased immediately to 70% of the total glutathione fraction upon addition of a second bolus of hydrogen peroxide (Schraufstatter et al., 1985); deprivation of glucose yielded similar results. Depletion of cellular glutathione (reduced form) enhanced the rate of cell lysis upon exposure to hydrogen peroxide. Schraufstatter et al. (1985) concluded that the role of the hexose monophosphate shunt (cf. Appendix) in generating reducing equivalents was most critically evidenced by the maintenance of low cellular levels of oxidized glutathione. This in turn requires capability to maintain high turnover of the hexose monophosphate shunt, as measured by release of labeled CO_2. Therefore, as interpreted with the help of these data, the results of Rehncrona et al. (1980), Cooper et al. (1980) and Kogure et al. (1982) actually indicate that the glutathione redox cycle was indeed responding to the presumed oxidative insult of reperfusion (or to incubation with oxygen). The protective capacity of this pathway is remarkable, inasmuch as its saturation requires an extreme oxidative insult. This behavior is suggested by the production of appreciable oxidized glutathione in homogenized brain tissue incubated with a peroxidizing mixture of ferrous iron and ascorbic acid (Rehncrona et al., 1980), whereas the in vivo results did not reflect this response. The validity of determining the presence of oxidative damage by means of glutathione measurements per se is thus called into question. It would appear that direct measurements of hexose monophosphate shunt turnover are more useful for this purpose.

Finally, in oxygenated or nitrogenated brain homogenates derived from Wistar rats maintained at deficient, normal or supplemented brain levels of vitamin E derived from the diet, the levels of TBA reactants and conjugated dienes were inversely related to tissue vitamin E concentration (Yoshida et al., 1985), as expected, but were not significantly different between vitamin E-normal and vitamin E-supplemented homogenates. However, in vivo analysis of brains from these same rats grouped according to vitamin E status and subjected to 45 min of two-vessel ischemia (Nordstrom et al., 1976) and either 45 min or 4 h recirculation did not reveal differences in TBA reactants among any of these groups (R. Busto, unpublished results). Again, lipid peroxidation in the in vitro homogenates likely arose due to decompartmentation in the preparation of shattered tissue, leading to admixture of intrinsic reactive substances (such as ferrous iron) across broken membrane barriers (Halliwell and Gutteridge, 1986). This situation clearly is much less likely to occur during or after ischemia induced by properly performed mechanical occlusion of cerebral arteries.

Despite some positive evidence accumulated with indirect methods in vitro, the lack of direct evidence for lipid peroxidation in vivo following recirculation of globally ischemic brain was unexpected and quite disconcerting. The common perception was that the schemes for oxygen radical production should be applicable to brain ischemia/reperfusion, but without directly observing lipid peroxides intrinsically formed in the compromised tissue, there was still no proof that these modes actually participated in post-ischemic tissue degeneration. A contribution to understanding this problem was made by deciding to monitor conjugated diene content in small (less than 1 mg) tissue samples taken from brain coronal sections of rats subjected to 30 min of global ischemia (Pulsinelli and Brierley, 1979) and recirculation times of 30 min to 4 h (Watson et al., 1984). The fundamental idea was that the brain, be-

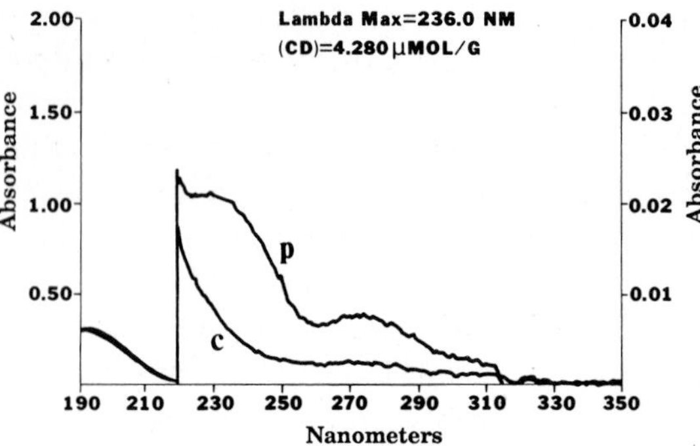

Fig. 3. Ultraviolet absorption spectra, Rayleigh-corrected for background scattering, of heptane-solubilized total lipid extracts from rat brains. The spectrum labeled (P) was derived from a 0.63 mg sample of lateral cerebral cortex of a rat subjected to photothrombotic occlusion of the middle cerebral artery (MCA) with 1 h bilateral common carotid artery ligation, and recirculated for 15 min following release of the ligatures. The spectrum labeled (C) is from a control tissue sample. The isolated double bond content of the control spectrum is equivalenced to that of the "peroxidized" spectrum (P), as described in the text. (Adapted from Ginsberg et al., 1988, with permission from the publisher.)

ing quite heterogeneous in structure and function, should not be assayed by methods (e.g., the TBA test, glutathiones) which required large amounts of tissue. The conjugated diene assay (in the modified form described above and shown in Figs. 3 – 6) met this criterion, because sufficient lipid can be extracted from 0.5 – 1 mg samples to facilitate spectroscopic analysis of particular brain regions (striatum, hippocampus, and dorsolateral, lateral and medial cortex). Approximately 15% of the total lipid extracts analyzed from these samples exhibited resolvable difference spectra indicative of the conjugated diene structure (Watson et al., 1984). No specificity in recirculation time or in regional susceptibility could be discerned, however. The reason that previous work in vivo had not succeeded became clear when all the regional spectra for each rat were computer-averaged, thus simulating the large amounts of tissue used for those assays. When this was done the small-scale positive effect was diluted so as to be indistinguishable from control samples. From this example, the difficulty of extrapolating methods which yield expected results in vitro to assessment of in vivo lipid peroxidation is made clear from a geometrical standpoint.

Further such work was continued with several models of photochemically induced thrombotic stroke of the middle cerebral artery (MCA) territory (Watson and Ginsberg, 1988; Ginsberg et al., 1988). A single occlusive thrombus was induced in the MCA trunk by means of an endothelial-damaging photochemical reaction, mediated by the interaction of a photosensitizing dye and a laser beam. In the first model, a thrombus resulting from rose bengal dye and helium-neon laser irradiation could be eroded by topical application of nimodipine, thus facilitating reperfusion of the ischemic MCA territory (Nakayama et al., 1988). In the second, rose bengal dye and argon laser irradiation created a permanent thrombus, which together with bilateral common carotid artery ligation, induced MCA territory ischemia which could be relieved by release of the carotid ligatures (Prado et al., 1988). In the third, an occlusive thrombus formed by the photochemical interaction of flavin mononucleotide and argon laser light at 457.9 nm could be recanalized by human tissue-type plasminogen ac-

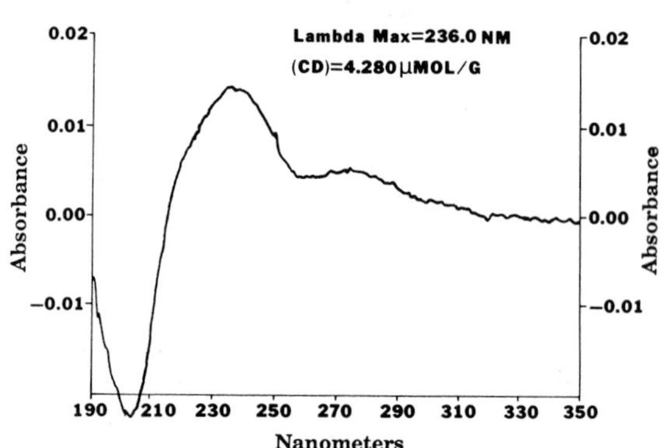

Fig. 4. Difference spectrum obtained by subtracting spectrum (C) from spectrum (P). Note again, that negative absorbance in the 190 – 210 nm region is counterbalanced by conversion of isolated double bonds into spectral peaks corresponding to the conjugated diene structure (maximum at 236 nm) and to higher order degradation products (maximum at 274 nm). The conjugated diene maximum is red-shifted compared to the plasma spectra (Figs. 1 and 2) owing to the greatly increased content of polyunsaturated fatty acids in brain compared to plasma. (Adapted from Ginsberg et al., 1988, with permission from the publisher.)

tivator after the desired period of MCA territory ischemia. Following 1 h of MCA territory ischemia in each model and the establishment of recirculation for times up to 15 min, punch biopsies of the MCA territory were taken and their total lipid extracts analyzed for conjugated dienes. An example of an ideally resolved spectrum selected from this series appears in Figs. 3 and 4. In our analysis a conjugated diene spectrum is evaluated only after it is identified positively by means of a difference spectrum; thus this method of analysis is very stringent. However, by far the most common appearance of the regional spectra is shown in Figs. 5 and 6. The featureless continuum of absorbance in the 210 – 330 nm range cannot be attributed to conjugated diene formation. If, however, the measurements were taken at just one wavelength (nominally 232 nm) as is usually the case in the literature, it is clear that the positive absorbances seen at that wavelength could be reported erroneously as due to conjugated diene absorption. Resolvable diene spectra observed during the recirculation periods (< 5% of samples) were thus rare and inconsistently located (even in contralateral hemisphere samples) despite the fact that the volume of MCA territory infarction at 24 h in these

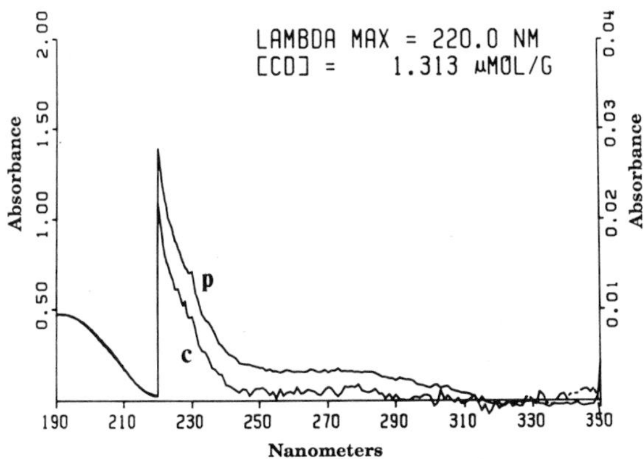

Fig. 5. Spectrum (P), derived from the lateral cortex of another rat treated similarly to the subject of Fig. 3 and compared to its control analog (C). The similarity of experimental spectra (P) to control spectra (C) was observed quite commonly following recirculation of rats subjected to focal ischemia induced by photothrombotic occlusion of the MCA; spectra similar to (P) of Fig. 3 were observed much less frequently.

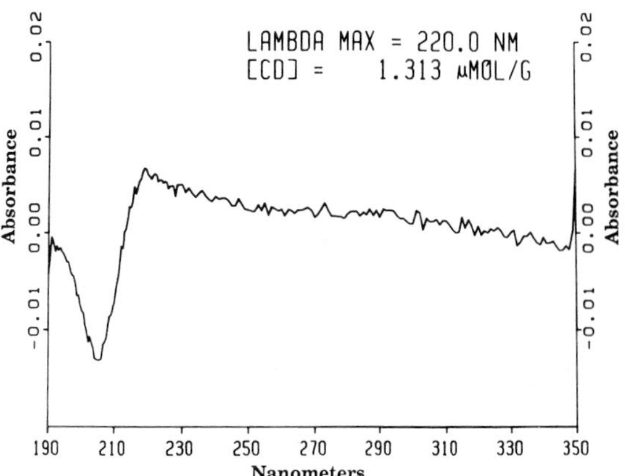

Fig. 6. Difference spectrum obtained by subtracting spectrum (C) from spectrum (P). This is by far the most common appearance of the difference spectra observed in the recirculated focal ischemia series. The featureless continuum of absorbance in the 210 – 330 nm range cannot be attributed to conjugated diene formation, despite the relative diminishment of absorbance due to isolated double bonds. It is clear that assessment of conjugated diene absorbance at one wavelength (e.g., 232 nm, as is still commonly done) would lead to a false positive report of "conjugated diene absorption".

models, although variable, still comprises much more than the 5% of tissue volume susceptible to diene formation. The focal character of conjugated diene concentration seen in these experiments was also observed histochemically in the livers of bromobenzene-poisoned mice (Pompella et al., 1987). Inasmuch as the regions exhibiting peroxidation cannot be localized beforehand with existing markers, lipid peroxidation in terms of conjugated diene biochemical analyses cannot yet be correlated with early morphologic changes.

The inconsistency of conjugated diene formation among these models of focal and global ischemia and reperfusion provides little correlation of this presumed marker of reperfusion injury with infarct development and certainly not with initiation of such injury. This leads us to conclude that spectroscopically measurable conjugated dienes are likely to develop in metabolically quiescent tissue regions; i.e., the tissues are already fatally compromised in microfocal, poorly collateralized regions. The existence of lipid peroxidation as a chain process, truncated by dilution after a small number of cycles and thus resulting in undetectable conjugated diene levels, cannot be ruled out. On the other hand, the existence of protective effects of free radical scavengers (in the absence of direct product detection) implies that a very low level of radical activity leading to peroxidation may contribute to the observed deleterious effects. These conjectured radical chain processes may be occurring in the small volume of the microvasculature rather than in the parenchyma.

Whether lipid peroxidation is involved in the earliest expression of tissue damage still remains an important and unanswered question. A very sensitive and specific test is needed to determine the existence of lipid peroxidation at much lower levels than currently can be detected. Given that the detection threshold for fluorescence is far more sensitive than that for absorption in appropriate compounds, we investigated whether diene bond conjugates in fatty acids exhibited autofluorescence (apparently there is no literature on this topic). We then observed that peroxidized fatty acid standards displayed characteristic fluorescence excitation and emission bands at room temperature for both the diene and triene structures (Watson and Busto, 1989). Eicosadieneoic acid containing a fraction of singly peroxidized molecules (by conjugated diene assay) and arachidonic acid peroxidizing in air both developed fluorescence excitation/emission (EX/EM) peaks at 228/330 nm. (These spectra are not corrected, however; these wavelengths are only approximate). In time the arachidonic acid sample developed a new pair of EX/EM maxima at 260/290 nm. A sample of 15-hydroperoxy arachidonic acid was then examined and found to exhibit both pairs of EX/EM spectra, thus lending credence to our qualitative peak assignments. This fluorometric technique appears to provide an enormous increase in sensitivity. For example, if one defines the sensitivity enhancement by relating the minimum observable concentrations (signal-to-noise ratio equal to 1) by the respective techniques of absorption and fluorescence, we found that the threshold for detection of the conjugated triene structure (region of 270 nm in Figs. 3 and 4) was at least 500 times lower by fluorescence. We have not yet determined the enhancement factor for dienes but it appears to be substantial.

Because detection of underivatized lipid peroxides in vivo is so difficult in the context of brain ischemia/reperfusion, it has been left fallow in recent years. Instead, much current activity has involved the synthesis of new drugs as putative inhibitors of lipid peroxidation, and characterization of their effects in vivo. The recently developed lazaroids, for example, were designed to incorporate several properties of compounds (e.g., vitamin E, methylprednisolone) known or strongly believed to exhibit antioxidant capacity (Braughler et al., 1987). The lazaroid U74006F (tirilazad mesylate), a 21-aminosteroid compound, has attenuated cerebral hypoperfusion after global cerebral ischemia (Hall and Yonkers, 1988) or subarachnoid hemorrhage (SAH) (Hall and Travis, 1988a), enhanced recovery of mean arterial blood pressure after hemorrhagic shock (Hall et al., 1988a), and mitigated the development of spinal cord ischemia after contusion injury (Hall, 1988), all in the cat. U74006F has also been used to enhance neurologic recovery following head injury in the mouse (Hall et al., 1988b). In the rat, blood-brain barrier permeability was decreased following SAH or injection of ferrous iron or arachidonic acid (Zucarello and Anderson, 1989), or injection of arachidonic acid (Hall and Travis, 1988b), and regional edema development after MCA occlusion was attenuated as well (Young et al., 1988). More recently, in the brains of gerbils subjected to focal cerebral ischemia/reperfusion and treated with U74006F, decreases in the post-ischemic tissue concentrations of vitamin E and extracellular calcium were mitigated (Hall et al., 1991); in the same model the extracellular calcium concentration as well as the neuronal density were partially conserved by the non-steroidal 2-methylaminochroman lazaroid U78517F, a compound designed with the intent to combine the properties of vitamin E with those of the amino moiety of U74006F (Hall et al., 1990). Recently, U74006F was found to reduce infarct volume at 24 h, independent of regional CBF, in transient (2 h) but not permanent MCA territory ischemia in Wistar and in SHR rats (Xue et al., 1992).

The mechanism of tissue protection afforded by the lazaroids is likely multifactorial, but these compounds are most often described as "potent inhibitors of iron-dependent lipid peroxidation". The evidence for this contention is based almost entirely upon the inhibition of color development in TBA test assessments of brain homogenates in vitro to which ferrous ion is added. In this respect U78517F is far more effective than vitamin E; its activity (as well as those of U74500A and U74006F) is attributed to its capacity to chelate iron (Hall et al., 1990). However, as outlined above the difficulties of interpretation of in vivo events from results obtained with indirect tests in vitro still remain; positive results obtained with such a test can only be considered suggestive so long as their meaning is not embellished beyond the limitations of the test. For example, U74006F has inhibited linoleic acid peroxidation by reaction with the peroxy radical intermediate, but curiously is much less active for this function than is vitamin E (Braughler and Pregenzer, 1989). Interestingly, the lazaroid U74500A inhibited the production of hydrogen peroxide by stimulated leukocytes and monocytes in vitro and also the associated chemiluminescence of leukocytes; from these data it was presumed that formation of lipid peroxides secondary to granulocyte activation would be inhibited in vivo (Fisher et al., 1990).

Despite such suggestions, there is still no evidence in terms of observations with a direct test, for lazaroid suppression of primary lipid peroxidation in vivo nor, accordingly, is there an inverse correlation of therapeutic effects with tissue lipid peroxide levels. From the in vivo work it appears that the lazaroids are most effective in mitigating damage to mechanically traumatized tissue. In such an environment, free radical mechanisms of tissue degeneration are amplified due to membrane damage, decompartmentation of reactants such as ferrous iron, and propagation of adventitious lipid peroxidation reactions. Thus, lazaroids evidently inhibit important but secondary mechanisms of tissue injury. Supporting this perception is the fact that their protective effects in the context of post-ischemic cerebral reperfusion typically have been examined at sufficiently long times (2 h at minimum) following the ictus to facilitate the development of such secondary processes. This notion is further supported by a report that U74006F decreases the malonaldehyde content of subarachnoid clot examined at seven days following emplacement; the correlation was better established when malonaldehyde was assayed directly by hplc rather than by the TBA test (Kanamaru et al., 1991). This is in contrast with the results of an acute ischemia/reperfusion experiment in which malonaldehyde as assessed by hplc did not increase in a rabbit heart preparation subjected to 60 min ischemia and 30 min reperfusion (Ceconi et al., 1991). Concurrently obtained TBA test results were positive but, because they were not correlated with the hplc determinations and were three orders of magnitude greater, were considered not to represent "lipid peroxidation" reliably. In summary, the lazaroids have displayed important protective properties in vivo despite the fact that their purported mechanism of action as "potent inhibitors of lipid peroxidation", as cast in terms of the TBA test, lacks direct biochemical proof. From current evidence it is likely more accurate to propose that these compounds may be "potent inhibitors of lipid peroxidation reactions arising secondary to destruction of tissue compartments in vitro and perhaps in vivo".

Deferoxamine, a chelator of ferric iron, has been utilized frequently to inhibit iron-catalyzed biochemical damage (Halliwell, 1989). In dogs subjected to cerebral ischemia induced by cardiac arrest of 7 min duration followed by cardiopulmonary resuscitation, deferoxamine in combination with superoxide dismutase facilitated recovery of somatosensory evoked potentials and normalization of cerebral blood flow profiles (Cerchiari et al., 1987). In a similar model employing 15 min of cardiac arrest examined at 2 h following resuscitation, the release of iron from cerebral stores was detected concomitant with the formation of TBA reactants and conjugated dienes; these indicators of lipid peroxidation were rendered indistinguishable from control levels by deferoxamine treatment (Komara et al., 1986). Subsequently these investigators found, at times of up to 8 h resuscitation, that either deferoxamine or superoxide dismutase administration partially inhibited the production of TBARS, but only deferoxamine preserved the degree of fatty acid unsaturation and the ionic ratio of potassium to sodium (White et al., 1988). This level of protection was still insufficient to prevent behavioral and morphological signs of reperfusion injury, however. The hypothesis that brain nuclear DNA is the critical site of oxygen radical reaction damage was then investigated. Genomic DNA was extracted from the brains of dogs subjected to 20 min cardiac arrest and recirculated for 2 or 8 h, but electrophoretic analysis revealed that the distribution pattern of DNA fragments presumably resulting from oxygen radical attack was not significantly different from control (White et al., 1991). To this point, resuscitation strategies based on current knowledge of post-ischemic reactions injurious to tissue are not yet capable of mitigating the high incidence of central nervous system injury observed clinically following resuscitation (Babbs, 1985).

It seems clear that a remarkable array of progressive and interactive complications, apparently based on oxygen radical potentiation and activity, can arise during and following cerebral ischemia. In recognition of this situation the developing consensus regarding treatment is to apply multifactorial strategies which can operate at different cellular levels and inhibit the development of deleterious events at different time scales. For example, reperfusing-isolated, 14 min ischemic dog brains with a combination of ginkgolide platelet-activating factor antagonist and dimethylsulfoxide (DMSO) restored relevant metabolic parameters and physiological responses to normal or near-normal levels at 60 min, while in brains treated with either DMSO alone or with the drug combination the level of TBARS (in contrast to untreated brains) did not rise above the control level (Gilboe et al., 1991). An additional benefit of using DMSO was likely enhanced dissolution of the ginkgolide into the brain tissue at risk. Recently, rats subjected to 30 min global forebrain ischemia (Pulsinelli and Brierley, 1979) were pretreated orally with the 4-thiazolidinone compound LY178002, a drug displaying multiple functionalities including inhibition of arachidonic acid cascade enzymes as well as apparent iron-scavenging capability (Clemens et al., 1991). Examination at three days of the striatum and CA1 hippocampus in treated brains revealed significant neuronal preservation, and also inhibition of TBARS formation in brain homogenates incubated with ferrous iron and LY178002. In rats subjected to focal cerebral ischemia induced by 30 min MCA occlusion, brain edema was reduced significantly by treatment with either dimethylthiourea (a hydroxyl radical scavenger) or by the excitotoxin antagonist MK-801, suggesting a connection between oxygen radical activity and excitotoxin production (Oh and Betz, 1991). This presumption is buttressed by comparatively less glutamate-induced toxicity in transgenically altered cultured neurons to overexpress Cu,Zn superoxide dismutase activity, compared to normal unaltered neurons (Chan et al., 1990). It therefore appears from these indirect tests that significant protection of brain tissue can be achieved by preventing oxygen radical-dependent events from escalating to irreversibility, even at delayed times from the onset of ischemia or reperfusion. Lipid peroxidation may be involved intimately in the progression of tissue-damaging events, but it is not at all known whether lipid peroxidation actually precipitates the onset of irreversible damage long before it is morphologically apparent. Nonetheless, drugs evidently exhibiting useful activity have been developed despite a lack of firm knowledge of their actual modes of action in vivo.

In addition, it has been realized recently that oxidative damage to other cellular components such as DNA or protein may be comparable in importance to the long-invoked lipid peroxidation process. It is believed that such damage is mediated by hydroxyl radical derived from hydrogen peroxide via Fenton reactions induced by low-molecular weight iron complexes (Imlay and Linn, 1988; Stadtman, 1990); these complexes arise from reduction of bound iron by superoxide anion produced during reperfusion (White et al., 1991). Exposure of calf thymus DNA to hydrogen peroxide from stimulated neutrophils yielded several damage products (e.g., following hydrolysis, 8-hydroxyguanine and thymine glycol) believed to arise during attack by Fenton-derived hydroxyl radicals (Jackson et al., 1989). This was evidenced by enhanced product formation in the presence of ferrous iron, and its inhibition by SOD, catalase, deferoxamine and dimethylsulfoxide. The hydroxyl radical damage product, 8-hydroxy-2′-deoxyguanosine, can be detected electrochemically in the ten femtomole range (Floyd et al., 1986), but has yet to be monitored during brain ischemia/reperfusion. Single strand breaks in DNA have been observed following exposure to hydrogen peroxide (transformed to hydroxyl radical by DNA-bound iron) even though the glutathione redox cycle is fully operational (Schraufstatter et al., 1985, 1986). This in turn activates NAD-dependent poly(ADP ribose) synthase in an attempted protective response, but results in loss of energy stores (ATP) and reducing power (NAD(P)H) (Schraufstatter et al., 1986). Continuation of such a response will lead to metabolic insufficiency, loss of protection against oxygen radical processes and finally disintegration of the plasma membrane resulting in cell death. In complementary fashion, Carney and Floyd (1991) have reported that the content of oxidized protein in the brain increases for recirculation times of up to 2 h, following a 10 min period of cerebral ischemia induced in gerbils. Interestingly, administration of the oxygen radical spin probe PBN (also cf. Kirsch et al., 1991) to these animals significantly inhibited protein oxidation and in particular largely preserved the activity of glutamine synthase, an enzyme believed to be sensitive to oxidative damage.

Future research must determine the initial modes of oxygen radical-dependent damage processes, their cellular and molecular locations and time dependencies and their distribution between vascular and parenchymal compartments. Further, can significant brain injury be induced by oxygen radicals themselves or does it require expression of lipid peroxidation initiated by oxygen radicals? The necessary experiments may be within the reach of modern techniques, such as confocal microscopy in conjunction with a tunable ultraviolet-visible laser system. If these devices were interfaced, it may become feasible to utilize fluorescence-based methods to locate and identify oxygen radicals and their products within cells. In this connection, the production of superoxide anion and hydrogen peroxide in stimulated phagocytes was analyzed by laser-activated flow cytometry. During the phagocytic respiratory burst, superoxide anion and hydrogen peroxide (in association with cellular peroxidase) were found to oxidize, respectively, the non-fluorescent dyes hydroethidine and dihydrorhodamine 123 to their fluorescent derivatives ethidium bromide (Rothe and Valet, 1990a) and rhodamine 123 (Rothe and Valet, 1990b). Chemiluminescent probes for superoxide anion (Hayashi et al., 1990) may also find utility, but their rates of light emission may be insufficient in comparison to laser-activated fluorescence. Further, the apparent autofluorescence (Watson and Busto, 1989) of the lipid-conjugated diene and triene moieties, if verified, may facilitate cellular mapping of damage due to lipid peroxidation. Finally, it may be possible to observe similarly the evolution of oxidative damage to DNA, inasmuch as the oxyradical product, 8-hydroxy-2′-deoxyguanosine, was found to be autofluorescent with excitation/emission maxima at 297/415 nm (B.D. Watson, unpublished data). Given the profusion of investigations in tissue damage based on oxygen radical schemes and the relative dearth of molecular evidence for lipid peroxidation-induced damage in vivo resulting from oxygen radical reactions, it seems quite timely and indeed necessary to resolve these issues as directly and unequivocally as possible.

Acknowledgements

The author wishes to thank Professor Bo K. Siesjö for the very stimulating questions provoked by his careful reading of the manuscript. This work was supported by USPHS Grant RO1 23244 from the National Institute of Neurological Diseases and Stroke. The author is a recipient of a Jacob Javits Neuroscience Investigator Award from this institute.

Appendix: chemical reactions associated with lipid peroxidation

The relationship between lipid peroxidation and free radicals

Electron orbitals in organic molecules each contain two electrons of opposite quantum-mechanical spin. If an electron pair is broken, leaving one electron in the corresponding orbital, a transient species known as a free radical results. Because this molecular fragment is no longer in a minimum energy configuration, it displays a strong tendency to attain thermodynamic stability by attracting an electron from another molecule. Two molecules are thus immediately transformed, owing to an initial alteration in one. Because the donor molecule is transformed into a new free radical, the process can be repeated at the expense of yet another molecule. This illustrates an important feature of free radical chemistry: that of propagation of chemical change from one molecule to many other molecules by means of a chain reaction.

This process of molecular radicalization followed by neutralization, usually by hydrogen atom abstraction from another molecule, is the basis of non-enzymatic lipid peroxidation. Unsaturated fatty acids are quite susceptible because they are easily radicalized by removal of a hydrogen atom from the methylene bridge linking two double bonds. Given a particular unsaturated fatty acid, ^1LH (see Eqn. 1) from which a methylene hydrogen atom is abstracted (by an initial free radical, discussed below), a fatty acid radical ($^1L_c\bullet$) results. (The symbol "•" denotes the unpaired electron associated with the free radical.) A bond shift occurs immediately (Eqn. 2), converting two double bonds isolated by the methylene bridge into the conjugated form (conjugated diene). Then, in the presence of oxygen, this fatty acid (or lipid) radical combines avidly with an oxygen molecule (Eqn. 3) to form a peroxy radical ($^1L_cO_2^\bullet$). Such a process of spontaneous combination with an oxygen molecule is also known as autoxidation. At this point the peroxy radical is liable to neutralize itself by abstracting a hydrogen atom from a neighboring lipid molecule (^2LH) yielding a new product hydroperoxide molecule (^1LOOH) and a new free radical ($^2L\bullet$), shown in Eqn. 4. Formation of this new free radical constitutes the basis of the regenerative chain process, also known as lipid autoxidation; the chain process can continue until the propagating free radical is quenched by a molecule such as vitamin E (tocopherol) which, although transformed into a free radical, does not fuel the chain process further. These reactions are listed below:

$$^1LH \xrightarrow{\text{Initiation}} {}^1L\bullet + H\bullet \quad (1)$$

$$^1L\bullet \xrightarrow{\text{Diene conjugation}} {}^1L_c^\bullet \quad (2)$$

$$^1L_c^\bullet + O_2 \xrightarrow{\text{Peroxy radical formation}} {}^1L_cO_2\bullet \quad (3)$$

$$^1L_cO_2\bullet + {}^2LH \xrightarrow{\text{Formation of lipid hydroperoxide and reinitiation of the chain process of Eqn. 1}} {}^1L_c\,OOH + {}^2L\bullet \quad (4)$$

An unusual exception to the general rule that molecules with unpaired electrons are chemically reactive is that of molecular oxygen. The most stable (ground state) configuration of molecular oxygen consists of two orbital electrons each having spin quantum numbers of the same sign, but in different orbitals. With this electronic configuration, direct addition of an oxygen molecule (peroxidation) to a target molecule is very unlikely under ordinary thermodynamic conditions. Filling the outer oxygen orbitals would require that two orbital electrons having the same spin direction be transferred simultaneously from the target molecule to oxygen; this necessitates breakage of two electron pairs, which is unfeasible at thermal energies. However, oxygen can react with a lipid radical due to the 50% probability that its orbital spins are opposite in sign to that of the lipid radical's; in effect, this reaction behaves as if two different free radicals were being combined. Owing to its two unpaired electrons, molecular oxygen is often referred to as a "diradical", but this character is exhibited only in single-sided fashion with another free radical, not a neutral molecule such as an unsaturated lipid.

The reactions of oxygen leading to initiation of lipid autoxidation are considered next.

Initiating radical species

Although it is agreed that the chain process of lipid autoxidation must be initiated by a free radical, the identity of the initiating radical (or radicals) and the process by which it is formed were for many years the source of controversy. A great deal of evidence for lipid peroxidation was accumulated in vitro and in vivo but the mechanisms of initiation were simply unknown. Although the controversy continues, it is now mostly abated in view of recent discoveries implicating the production in vivo of reactive species derived from oxygen molecules. These species, also known as "active oxygens", "reactive oxygen metabolites" or "oxygen radicals", are now thought to be formed in the mitochondrial respiratory chain during reperfusion of tissue compromised by ischemia. To a much lesser extent, they are formed similarly during normal mitochondrial respiration in healthy tissue and appear to be involved in other critical metabolic processes as well, such as phagocytosis and prostaglandin synthesis. The concept of "active oxygens" rests on the capability of the oxygen molecule to receive into its outer orbitals one electron at a time. Such single-electron reduction reactions comprise the following sequence:

$$O_2 + e^- \longrightarrow O_2^- \text{ (superoxide radical)} \quad (5a)$$

$$O_2^- + H^+ \longrightarrow HO_2^{\bullet} \quad \text{(perhydroxyl radical)} \quad (5b)$$

$$HO_2^{\bullet} + e^- + H^+ \longrightarrow H_2O_2 \quad \text{(hydrogen peroxide)} \quad (6)$$

$$H_2O_2 + e^- + H^+ \longrightarrow H_2O + OH^{\bullet} \quad \text{(hydroxyl radical)} \quad (7)$$

In eqns. 6 and [illegible] H^+ is equivalent to a hydrogen [illegible]

Eqns [illegible] indicate that the superoxide radic[illegible] form of its conjugate acid, the perhyd[illegible]cal, as well. At the physiological pH of 7.[illegible] concentration ratio of perhydroxyl radical to superoxide anion is a seemingly insignificant 1%, given a $pK(HO_2)$ of 4.7.

Although reports of alleged toxicity due to the superoxide anion and hydrogen peroxide are many and continuing, the most common interpretation of the evidence indicates that the hydroxyl radical, and quite possibly the perhydroxyl radical, are the principal agents of the initiation reaction (hydrogen atom abstraction) of lipid peroxidation referred to in Eqn. 1. This reaction, explicitly stated, has as products a lipid radical and either water (HOH) or hydrogen peroxide (HOOH) according to H atom abstraction by hydroxyl or perhydroxyl radical, respectively:

$$LH + HO(O)^{\bullet} \longrightarrow L^{\bullet} + HO(O)H \quad (8)$$

Eqn. 8 is equivalent to Eqn. 1 with the addition of the hydroxyl or perhydroxyl radical to both sides.

The hydroxyl radical is the most reactive free radical known. As a feature of its extreme avidity for organic molecules, the hydroxyl radical abstracts hydrogen atoms non-selectively and at short range from the site of its production; thus not only lipids but also proteins may be damaged, by subsequent cross-linking (polymerization) reactions. On the other hand, the less reactive (but still potent) perhydroxyl radical has been shown to selectively abstract methylene hydrogens from unsaturated fatty acids (Bielski et al., 1983). The potential of the hydroxyl and perhydroxyl radicals to induce damage in membranes is augmented by their electrical neutrality. To the extent their reactivities allow, these uncharged species may diffuse into plasma membranes toward their most vulnerable substrates. Further, the potential for perhydroxyl radical formation increases as the pH is lowered. This may be enhanced during metabolic dysfunctional states such as ischemia-induced lactic acidosis.

The origin of the controversy concerning the reactivity of superoxide anion and hydrogen peroxide apparently lies in reactions catalyzed by metal ion impurities, even in trace amounts in the preparations examined. Oxidation/reduction reactions mediated by single-electron transfer are easily facilitated by ferrous (Fe^{2+}) and ferric (Fe^{3+}) ions. Other ion pairs include cuprous (Cu^{+}) and cupric (Cu^{2+}) ions. Under the influence of metal ion catalysis a reaction similar to Eqn. 7 can be expressed:

$$Fe^{2+} + H_2O_2 \longrightarrow Fe^{3+} + OH^- + OH\bullet \qquad (9)$$

This reaction, known as the Fenton reaction, thus converts hydrogen peroxide into the hydroxyl radical. Because iron is bound in the ferric form in vivo, however, a complementary reaction is needed to generate ferrous ion, and this is mediated by superoxide anion:

$$Fe^{3+} + O_2^- \longrightarrow Fe^{2+} + O_2 \qquad (10)$$

The sum of eqns. 9 and 10 is known as the iron-catalyzed, superoxide-driven Haber-Weiss reaction. The summed reaction is facilitated more efficiently when the iron ions are chelated in proteins such as hemoglobin and ferritin. The "toxicities" of superoxide anion and hydrogen peroxide are therefore explained by their capability to potentiate the production of species which are able to abstract hydrogen atoms.

Another important source of propagating radicals is believed to arise from the small quantity of lipid hydroperoxides already existing in tissues. In the presence of iron ions these compounds can undergo scission according to:

$$Fe^{2+} + LOOH \longrightarrow Fe^{3+} + OH^- + LO\bullet \qquad (11)$$

$$Fe^{3+} + LOOH \longrightarrow Fe^{2+} + H^+ + LOO\bullet \qquad (12)$$

The lipid alkoxy (LO•) and peroxy (LOO•) radicals are themselves capable of initiating chain propagation processes (Borg and Schaich, 1988).

Natural means of protection against lipid peroxidation: enzyme-dependent mechanisms

It is an elegant paradox that the fundamental physical reason for the existence of lipid peroxidation is the very diffusibility of oxygen that makes life possible. The interaction of oxygen with ubiquinone (the only diffusible component of the respiratory chain) in its singly reduced form produces superoxide anion under normal conditions of metabolism. Thus, as the mechanism of respiration evolved to be based on single-electron reduction reactions of electron transport chain components, it became critically important to deter the non-enzymatic cascade of undesirable reactions initiated by superoxide anion. Fortunately, an enzyme was evolved for this purpose. Because it catalyzes the oxidation of one superoxide radical and the reduction of another, this enzyme is called superoxide dismutase. The reaction is shown below.

$$O_2^- + O_2^- + 2H^+ \xrightarrow{\text{superoxide dismutase}} H_2O_2 + O_2 \qquad (13)$$

Superoxide dismutase is ubiquitous in oxygen-dependent organisms. The rate constant for the reaction it catalyzes is remarkably high at $10^{11}\ M^{-1}$. Superoxide dismutase enzyme exists in two forms. The copper-zinc (Cu^{2+},Zn^{2+}) form is located in the cellular cytosol, while the manganese-containing form (Mn^{2+}) resides in the mitochondria.

However, hydrogen peroxide in vivo is highly labile itself and is likely to be a major source of hydroxyl radical (cf. Eqn. 9). This possibility is largely mitigated by another remarkable enzyme, glutathione peroxidase. This enzyme contains four covalently bound selenium atoms per molecule and is located in the mitochondrial matrix and cytosol. While converting reduced glutathione (GSH) into oxidized glutathione (GSSG), it is able to catalyze the reduction of hydrogen peroxide or fatty acid hydroperoxides (LOOH) to water or hydroxy fatty acids (LOH), respectively, according to the reactions:

$$2GSH + H_2O_2 \xrightarrow{\text{glutathione peroxidase}} 2H_2O + GSSG \quad (14a)$$

$$2GSH + LOOH \longrightarrow H_2O + GSSG + LOH \quad (14b)$$

Glutathione peroxidase lies at the end of a string of coupled enzymatic reactions which serve to keep the required substrates in intricate balance. The neighboring enzyme, glutathione reductase, recycles oxidized glutathione (GSSG) back into the reduced form (GSH):

$$GSSG + NADPH + H^+ \xrightarrow{\text{glutathione reductase}} 2GSH + NADP^+ \quad (15)$$

Recycling of NADPH is facilitated by the pentose phosphate pathway, also known as the phosphogluconate pathway or the hexose monophosphate shunt. This reaction, catalyzed by glucose 6-phosphate dehydrogenase, utilizes glucose 6-phosphate according to:

$$\text{glucose 6-phosphate} + NADP^+ \xrightarrow{\text{glucose 6-phosphate dehydrogenase}} \text{6-phosphogluconate} + NADPH + H^+ \quad (16)$$

Glucose 6-phosphate is produced by a phosphorylation reaction catalyzed by hexokinase:

$$\text{glucose} + ATP \xrightarrow{\text{hexokinase}} \text{glucose 6-phosphate} + ADP \quad (17)$$

The implication of eqns. 14 – 17 is that enzymic protection from lipid hydroperoxides depends fundamentally on the capability of tissue to conduct normal metabolic processes. Although much attention has been given to the protective role of superoxide dismutase in extinguishing the superoxide anion, sufficient protection is not obtained by transforming superoxide anion into hydrogen peroxide; an operating glutathione peroxidase system must be intact also (Schraufstatter et al., 1985). Catalase, although known for many years to decompose hydrogen peroxide to water and oxygen, is no longer regarded as the chief scavenger of hydrogen peroxide produced by superoxide dismutase. This function is attributed to glutathione peroxidase owing to its widespread subcellular distribution (especially in the mitochondrial matrix), whereas catalase is localized to the peroxisomal microbodies.

Identifying the synergism of superoxide dismutase with glutathione peroxidase instead of with catalase (in the face of classical bias) illustrates the important concept of *compartmentation.* Lipid peroxidation reactions are very much affected by membrane barriers, which serve to localize the effects of these reactions or their initiators. For this reason, a great amount of misinformation with respect to purported reaction schemes involving lipid peroxidation in vivo has been collected during in vitro experiments in which tissue homogenization was employed. Such experiments are conducted commonly by using compounds thought to be protective against lipid peroxidation, actually to initiate free radical processes. In the next section this apparently paradoxical activity will be discussed, together with non-enzymatic means of quenching lipid peroxidation.

Non-enzymatic protective mechanisms

By hydrogen atom donation, natural antioxidant compounds inhibit initiation or propagation of chain processes induced by free radicals. The usual products of this reaction are an organic (hydro) peroxide derived from the free radical and an organic radical formed from the quenching compound. The antioxidant radical, however, normally does not sustain the chain process because the half-filled orbital radical is delocalized; owing to this dilution of charge, the antioxidant radical is incapable of abstracting a hydrogen atom from a neighboring molecule. Instead, they often combine with each other, as illustrated in the following list of common antioxidant molecule reactions.

Reactions of alpha-tocopherol (TH).

$$O_2^- + TH \xrightarrow{H^+} \text{8a-hydroxy-alpha-tocopherone} + OH^-$$

$$\text{9a-hydroxy-alpha-tocopherone} \xrightarrow{H^+} \text{alpha-tocopheryl quinone}$$

Peroxy (LOO•), hydroperoxy ($HO_2^{\bullet}$) or hydroxyl (•OH) radical quenching:

$$TH + LO(O)\bullet \longrightarrow T\bullet + LO(O)H$$

Disproportionation of tocopherol radicals:

$$H^+ + T\bullet + T\bullet \longrightarrow T^+ + TH$$

Reactions of ascorbic acid (AH_2). Regeneration by ascorbic acid of alpha-tocopherol from its radical:

$$T\bullet + AH_2 \longrightarrow TH + AH\bullet$$

Peroxy (LOO•), hydroperoxy ($HO_2^{\bullet}$) or hydroxyl (•OH) radical quenching:

$$AH_2 + LO(O)\bullet \longrightarrow AH\bullet + LO(O)H$$

Reactions with superoxide anion:

$$O_2^- + AH_2 + H^+ \longrightarrow H_2O_2 + AH\bullet$$

$$O_2^- + AH\bullet + H^+ \longrightarrow H_2O_2 + A$$

Disproportionation of ascorbyl radical:

$$2AH\bullet \longrightarrow A + AH_2$$

Thus ascorbic acid regenerates alpha-tocopherol and scavenges superoxide anion as well. A major function in vivo may be prevention of superoxide-induced release of ferrous iron from ferritin. On the other hand, for exogenously added ferrous iron in vitro:

$$[Fe^{2+}] + LOOH \longrightarrow [Fe^{3+}] + OH^- + LO\bullet$$

$$Fe^{3+} + AH_2 \longrightarrow Fe^{2+} + AH\bullet$$

These reactions explain the propagation of lipid peroxidation by the ferrous iron-ascorbate (or ferrous iron-glutathione) combination in vitro and indicate the necessity of tightly binding iron in the ferric form in tissues.

References

Anderson, W.R., Tan, W.C., Takatori, T. and Privett, O.S. (1976) Toxic effects of hydroperoxide injections on rat lung. *Arch. Pathol. Lab. Med.*, 100: 154 – 162.

Asakawa, T. and Matsushita, S. (1979) Thiobarbituric acid test for detecting lipid peroxides. *Lipids*, 14: 401 – 406.

Asakawa, T. and Matsushita, S. (1980) Coloring conditions of thiobarbituric acid test for detecting lipid peroxides. *Lipids*, 15: 137 – 140.

Babbs, C.F. (1985) Role of iron ions in the genesis of reperfusion injury following successful cardipulmonary resuscitation. *Ann. Emerg. Med.*, 14: 777 – 783.

Barber, A.A. and Bernheim, F. (1967) Lipid peroxidation: its measurement, occurrence, and significance in animal tissues. *Adv. Gerontol. Res.*, 2: 355 – 403.

Bazan, N.G. (1970) Effects of ischemia and electroconvulsive shock on the free fatty acid pool in the brain. *Biochim. Biophys. Acta*, 218: 1 – 10.

Beckman, J.S., Liu, T.H., Hogan, E.L., Freeman, B.A. and Hsu, C.Y. (1987) Oxygen free radicals and xanthine oxidase in cerebral ischemic injury in the rat. *Soc. Neurosci. Abstr.*, 13 (Part 2): 1498.

Bidlack, W.R. and Tappel, A.L. (1973) Fluorescent products of phospholipids during lipid peroxidation. *Lipids*, 8: 203 – 207.

Bielski, B.H.J., Arudi, R.L. and Sutherland, M.W. (1983) A study of the reactivity of HO_2/O_2^- with unsaturated fatty acids. *J. Biol. Chem.*, 258: 4759 – 4761.

Bligh, E.G. and Dyer, W.J. (1959) A rapid method of lipid extraction and purification. *Can. J. Biophys. Biochem.*, 37: 911 – 917.

Boisvert, D.P. (1991) In vivo assessment of hydroxyl free radical production in the brain. *J. Cereb. Blood Flow Metab.,* 11: S637.

Bolli, R., Jeroudi, M.O., Patel, B.S., Aruoma, O.I., Halliwell, B., Lai, E.K. and McCay, P.B. (1989) Marked reduction of free radical generation and contractile dysfunction by antioxidant therapy begun at the time of reperfusion. *Circ. Res.,* 65: 607 – 622.

Borg, D.C. and Schaich, K.M. (1988) Iron and iron-derived radicals. In: B. Halliwell (Ed.), *Oxygen Radicals and Tissue Injury Symposium (Proceedings),* Federation of American Society for Experimental Biology, Bethesda, MD, pp. 20 – 26.

Braughler, J.M. and Hall, E.D. (1989) Central nervous system trauma and stroke. 1. Biochemical considerations for oxygen radical formation and lipid peroxidation. *Free Radical Biol. Med.,* 6: 289 – 301.

Braughler, J.M., Pregenzer, J.F., Chase, R., Duncan, L.A., Jacobsen, E.J. and McCall, J.M. (1987) Novel 21-amino steroids as potent inhibitors of iron-dependent lipid peroxidation. *J. Biol. Chem.,* 262: 10438 – 10440.

Braughler, J.M. and Pregenzer, J.F. (1989) The 21-aminosteroid inhibitors of lipid peroxidation: reactions with lipid peroxyl and phenoxy radicals. *Free Radical Biol. Med.,* 7: 125 – 130.

Braunwald, E. and Kloner, R.A. (1985) Myocardial reperfusion: a double-edge sword? *J. Clin. Invest.,* 76: 1713 – 1719.

Bunting, S., Moncada, S. and Vane, J.R. (1983) The prostacyclin-thromboxane A_2 balance: pathophysiological and therapeutic implications. *Br. Med. Bull.,* 39: 271 – 276.

Burton, K.P., McCord, J.M. and Ghai, G. (1984) Myocardial alterations due to free-radical generation. *Am. J. Physiol.,* 246: H776 – H783.

Cao, W., Carney, J.M., Duchon, A., Floyd, R.A. and Chevion, M. (1988) Oxygen free radical involvement in ischemia and reperfusion injury to brain. *Neurosci. Lett.,* 88: 233 – 238.

Carney, D.F., Koski, C.L. and Shin, M.L. (1985) Elimination of terminal complement intermediates from the plasma membrane of nucleated cells. *J. Immunol.,* 134: 1804 – 1809.

Carney, J.M. and Floyd, R.A. (1991) Protection against oxidative damage to CNS by α-phenyl-tert-butyl nitrone (PBN) and other spin-trapping agents: a novel series of nonlipid free radical scavengers. *J. Mol. Neurosci.,* 3: 47 – 57.

Ceconi, C., Cargnoni, A., Pasini, E., Condorelli, E., Curello, S. and Ferrari, R. (1991) Evaluation of phospholipid peroxidation as malonaldehyde during myocardial ischemia and reperfusion injury. *Am. J. Physiol.,* 260: H1057 – 1061.

Cerchiari, E.L., Hoel, T.M., Safar, P. and Sclabassi, R.J. (1987) Protective effects of combined superoxide dismutase and deferoxamine on recovery of cerebral blood flow and function after cardiac arrest in dogs. *Stroke,* 18: 869 – 878.

Chan, P.H., Longar, S. and Fishman, R.A. (1987) Protective effects of liposome-entrapped superoxide dismutase on posttraumatic brain edema. *Ann. Neurol.,* 21: 540 – 547.

Chan, P.H., Chu, L., Chen, S.F., Carlson, E.J. and Epstein, C.J. (1990) Reduced neurotoxicity in transgenic mice overexpressing human copper-zinc-superoxide dismutase. *Stroke,* 21 (Suppl. III): III-80 – III-82.

Cheung, J.Y., Bonventre, J.V., Malis, C.D. and Leaf, A. (1986) Calcium and ischemic injury. *N. Engl. J. Med.,* 314: 1670 – 1676.

Chio, K.S. and Tappel, A.L. (1969) Synthesis and characterization of fluorescent products derived from malonaldehyde and amino acids. *Biochem. J.,* 8: 2821 – 2832.

Clemens, J.A., Ho, P.P.K. and Panetta, J.A. (1991) LY178002 reduces rat brain damage after transient global forebrain ischemia. *Stroke,* 22: 1048 – 1052.

Clifford, D.E. and Repine, J.E. (1982) Hydrogen peroxide mediated killing of bacteria. *Mol. Cell. Biochem.,* 49: 143 – 149.

Cooper, A.J.L., Pulsinelli, W.A. and Duffy, T.E. (1980) Glutathione and ascorbate during ischemia and postischemic reperfusion in rat brain. *J. Neurochem.,* 35: 1242 – 1245.

Dahle, L.K., Hill, E.G. and Holman, R.T. (1962) The thiobarbituric acid reaction and the autoxidations of polyunsaturated fatty acid methyl esters. *Arch. Biochem. Biophys.,* 98: 253 – 261.

Del Zoppo, G.J. and the rt-PA Acute Stroke Study Group (1990) Open, multicenter trial of recombinant tissue plasminogen activator in acute stroke. A progress report. *Stroke,* 21: IV-174 – IV-175.

Demopoulos, H.D., Flamm, E.S., Pietronigro, D.D. and Seligman, M.L. (1980) The free radical pathology and the microcirculation in the major central nervous system disorders. *Acta Physiol. Scand. (Suppl.),* 492: 91 – 119.

Dietrich, W.D., Watson, B.D., Busto, R., Ginsberg, M.D. and Bethea, J.R. (1987) Photochemically induced cerebral infarction: 2. Edema and blood-brain barrier disruption. *Acta Neuropathol. (Berl.),* 72: 315 – 325.

Dobretsov, G.E., Borschevskaya, T.A., Petrov, V.A. and Vladimirov, Yu.A. (1977) The increase of phospholipid bilayer rigidity after lipid peroxidation. *FEBS Lett.,* 84: 125 – 128.

Dumuis, A., Sebben, M., Haynes, L., Pin, J.P. and Bockart, J. (1988) NMDA receptors activate the arachidonic acid cascade system in striatal neurons. *Nature,* 336: 68 – 73.

Epstein, C.J., Avraham, K.B., Lovett, M., Smith, S., Elroy-Stein, O., Rotman, G., Bry, C. and Groner, Y. (1987) Transgenic mice with increased Cu/Zn-superoxide dismutase activity: animal model of dosage effects in Down syndrome. *Proc. Natl. Acad. Sci. U.S.A.,* 84: 8044 – 8048.

Fisher, M., Levine, P.H. and Cohen, R.A. (1990) A 21-aminosteroid reduces hydrogen peroxide generation by and chemiluminescence of stimulated human leukocytes. *Stroke,* 21: 1435 – 1438.

Fletcher, B.L. and Tappel, A.L. (1971) Fluorescent modification of serum albumin by lipid peroxidation. *Lipids,* 6: 172 – 175.

Floyd, R.A., Watson, J.J., Wong, P.K., Altmiller, D.H. and Richard, R.C. (1986) Hydroxyl free radical adduct of deoxyguanosine: sensitive detection and mechanisms of formation.

Free Radical Res. Commun., 1: 163 – 172.

Fridovich, I. (1978) The biology of oxygen radicals. *Science*, 201: 875 – 880.

Gilboe, D.D., Kintner, D., Fitzpatrick, J.H., Emoto, S.E., Esanu, A., Braquet, P.G. and Bazan, N.G. (1991) Recovery of postischemic brain metabolism and function following treatment with a free radical scavenger and platelet-activating factor antagonists. *J. Neurochem.*, 56: 311 – 319.

Ginsberg, M.D., Watson, B.D., Busto, R., Yoshida, S., Prado, R., Nakayama, H., Ikeda, M., Dietrich, W.D. and Globus, M.Y-T. (1988) Peroxidative damage to cell membranes following cerebral ischemia. A cause of ischemic brain injury? *Neurochem. Pathol.*, 9: 171 – 193.

Gutteridge, J.M.C. (1986) Aspects to consider when detecting and measuring lipid peroxidation. *Free Radical Res. Commun.*, 1: 173 – 184.

Gutteridge, J.M.C. (1988) Lipid peroxidation: some problems and concepts. In: B. Halliwell (Ed.), *Oxygen Radicals and Tissue Injury Symposium (Proceedings)*, Federation of American Society for Experimental Biology, Bethesda, MD, pp. 9 – 19.

Hall, E.D. (1988) Effects of the 21-aminosteroid U74006F on post-traumatic spinal cord injury in cats. *J. Neurosurg.*, 68: 462 – 465.

Hall, E.D. and Braughler, J.M. (1989) Central nervous system trauma and stroke. II. Physiological and pharmacological evidence for involvement of oxygen radicals and lipid peroxidation. *Free Radical Biol. Med.*, 6: 303 – 313.

Hall, E.D. and Travis, M.A. (1988a) Effects of the nonglucocorticoid 21-aminosteroid U74006F on acute cerebral hypoperfusion following experimental subarachnoid hemorrhage. *Exp. Neurol.*, 102: 244 – 248.

Hall, E.D. and Travis, M.A. (1988b) Inhibition of arachidonic acid-induced brain vasogenic brain edema by the non-glucocorticoid 21-aminosteroid U74006F. *Brain Res.*, 451: 350 – 352.

Hall, E.D. and Yonkers, P.A. (1988) Attenuation of postischemic cerebral hypoperfusion by the 21-aminosteroid U74006F. *Stroke*, 19: 340 – 344.

Hall, E.D., Yonkers, P.A. and McCall, J.M. (1988a) Attentuation of hemorrhagic shock by the non-glucocorticoid 21-aminosteroid U74006F. *Eur. J. Pharmacol.*, 147: 299 – 303.

Hall, E.D., Yonkers, P.A., McCall, J.M. and Braughler, J.M. (1988b) Effects of the 21-aminosteroid U74006F on experimental head injury in mice. *J. Neurosurg.*, 68: 456 – 461.

Hall, E.D., Pazara, K.E., Braughler, J.M., Linseman, K.L. and Jacobsen, E.J. (1990) Nonsteroidal lazaroid U78517F in models of focal and global ischemia. *Stroke*, 21: III-83 – III-87.

Hall, E.D., Pazara, K.E. and Braughler, J.M. (1991) Effects of tirilazad mesylate on postischemic brain lipid peroxidation and recovery of extracellular calcium in gerbils. *Stroke*, 22: 361 – 366.

Hallinan, T., Gor, J., Rice-Evans, C.A., Stanley, R., O'Reilly, R. and Brown, D. (1991) Lipid peroxidation in electroporated hepatocytes occurs much more readily than does hydroxyl-radical formation. *Biochem. J.*, 277: 767 – 771.

Halliwell, B. (1989) Protection against tissue damage in vivo by desferrioxamine: what is its mechanism of action? *Free Radical Biol. Med.*, 7: 645 – 651.

Halliwell, B. and Gutteridge, J.M.C. (1984) Lipid peroxidation, oxygen radicals, cell damage and antioxidant therapy. *Lancet*, i: 1396 – 1397.

Halliwell, B. and Gutteridge, J.M.C. (1985a) *Free Radicals in Biology and Medicine*, Clarendon Press, Oxford.

Halliwell, B. and Gutteridge, J.M.C. (1985b) Oxygen radicals and the nervous system. *Trends Neurosci.*, 8: 22 – 26.

Halliwell, B. and Gutteridge, J.M.C. (1986) Oxygen free radicals and iron in relation to biology and medicine: some problems and concepts. *Arch. Biochem. Biophys.*, 246: 501 – 514.

Halliwell, B., Kaur, H. and Ingelman-Sundberg, M. (1991) Hydroxylation of salicylate as an assay for hydroxyl radicals: a cautionary note. *Free Radical Biol. Med.*, 10: 439 – 441.

Hasegawa, K. and Patterson, L.K. (1978) Pulse radiolysis studies in model lipid systems: formation and behavior of peroxy radicals in fatty acids. *Photochem. Photobiol.*, 28: 817 – 823.

Hayashi, N., Tsubokawa, T., Green, B.A., Watson, B.D. and Prado, R. (1990) A new mapping study of superoxide free radicals, vascular permeability and energy metabolism in central nervous system. *Acta Neurochirurg. Suppl.*, 51: 31 – 33.

Hicks, M. and Gebicki, J.M. (1978) A quantitative relationship between permeability and the degree of peroxidation in ufasome membranes. *Biochem. Biophys. Res. Commun.*, 80: 704 – 708.

Holman, R.T. and Burr, G.O. (1946) Spectrophotometric studies of the oxidation of fats. VI. Oxygen absorption and chromophore production in fatty esters. *J. Am. Chem. Soc.*, 68: 562 – 566.

Ikeda, Y. and Long, D.M. (1990) The molecular basis of brain injury and brain edema: the role of oxygen free radicals. *Neurosurgery*, 27: 1 – 11.

Imaizumi, S., Woolworth, V., Fishman, R.A. and Chan, P.H. (1990) Liposome-entrapped superoxide dismutase reduces cerebral infarction in cerebral ischemia in rats. *Stroke*, 21: 1312 – 1317.

Imlay, J.A. and Linn, S. (1988) DNA damage and oxygen radical toxicity. *Science*, 240: 1302 – 1309.

Itoh, T., Kawakami, M., Yamauchi, Y., Shimizu, S. and Nakamura, M. (1986) Effect of allopurinol on ischemia and reperfusion-induced cerebral injury in spontaneously hypertensive rats. *Stroke*, 17: 1284 – 1287.

Jackson, J.H., Gajewski, E., Schraufstatter, I.U., Hyslop, P.A., Fuciarelli, A.F., Cochrane, C.G. and Dizdarloglu, M. (1989) Damage to the bases in DNA induced by stimulated neutrophils. *J. Clin. Invest.*, 84: 1644 – 1649.

Kanamaru, K., Weir, B.K.A., Simpson, I., Witbeck, T. and Grace, M. (1991) Effect of 21-aminosteroid U74006F on lipid peroxidation in subarachnoid clot. *J. Neurosurg.*, 74:

454 – 459.

Kinouchi, H., Mizui, T., Carlson, E., Epstein, C.J. and Chan, P.H. (1991) Focal cerebral ischemia and the antioxidant system in transgenic mice overexpressing Cu-Zn superoxide dismutase. *J. Cereb. Blood Flow Metab.,* 11: S423.

Kinuta, Y., Kikuchi, H., Ishikawa, M., Kimura, M. and Itokawa, Y. (1989) Lipid peroxidation in focal cerebral ischemia. *J. Neurosurg.,* 71: 421 – 429.

Kirsch, J.R., Lange, D.G., Helfaer, M.A. and Traystman, R.J. (1991) Detection of free radicals in brain following ischemia/reperfusion using spin-trapping agents and electron paramagnetic resonance (EPR) techniques. *J. Cereb. Blood Flow Metab.,* 11: S207.

Klein, R.A. (1970) The detection of oxidation in liposome preparations. *Biochim. Biophys. Acta,* 210: 486 – 489.

Kogure, K., Watson, B.D., Busto, R. and Abe, K. (1982) Potentiation of lipid peroxides in rat brain by ischemia. *Neurochem. Res.,* 7: 437 – 454.

Kogure, K., Arai, H., Abe, K. and Nakano, M. (1985) Free radical damage to the brain following ischemia. *Prog. Brain Res.,* 63: 237 – 259.

Komara, J.S., Nayini, N.R., Bialick, H.A., Indrieri, R.J., Evans, A.T., Garritano, A.M., Hoehner, T.J., Jacobs, W.A., Huang, R.R., Krause, G.S., White, B.C. and Aust, S.D. (1986) Brain iron delocalization and lipid peroxidation following cardiac arrest. *Ann. Emerg. Med.,* 15: 384 – 389.

Kontos, H.A. (1987) Oxygen radicals from arachidonate metabolism in abnormal vascular responses. *Annu. Rev. Respir. Dis.,* 136: 474 – 477.

Kontos, H.A. (1989a) Oxygen radicals in CNS damage. *Chem.-Biol. Interact.,* 72: 229 – 255.

Kontos, H.A. (1989b) Oxygen radicals in cerebral ischemia. In: M.D. Ginsberg and W.D. Dietrich (Eds.), *Cerebrovascular Diseases – Sixteenth Research (Princeton) Conference,* Raven Press, New York, pp. 365 – 371.

Kukreja, R.C., Kontos, H.A., Hess, M.L. and Ellis, E.F. (1986) PGH synthase and lipoxygenase generate superoxide in the presence of NADH or NADPH. *Circ. Res.,* 59: 612 – 619.

Le, C.T., Hollaar, L., Van der Valk, E.J.M. and Van der Laarse, A. (1992) Effects of glucose, trolox-C, and glutathione disulphide on lipid peroxidation and cell death induced by oxidant stress in rat heart. *Cardiovasc. Res.,* 26: 133 – 142.

Liu, T.H., Beckman, J.S., Freeman, B.A., Hogan, E.L. and Hsu, C.Y. (1989) Polyethylene glycol-conjugated superoxide dismutase and catalase reduce ischemic brain injury. *Am. J. Physiol.,* 256: H589 – H593.

MacMillan, V. (1982) Cerebral Na^+,K^+-ATPase activity during exposure to and recovery from acute ischemia. *J. Cereb. Blood Flow Metab.,* 2: 457 – 465.

Markey, B.A., Phan, S.H., Varani, J., Ryan, U.S. and Ward, P.A. (1990) Inhibition of cytotoxicity by intracellular superoxide dismutase supplementation. *Free Radical Biol. Med.,* 9: 307 – 314.

McCord, J.M. (1985) Oxygen-derived free radicals in postischemic tissue injury. *N. Engl. J. Med.,* 312: 159 – 163.

McCord, J.M. (1987) Oxygen-derived radicals: a link between reperfusion injury and inflammation. *Fed. Proc.,* 46: 2402 – 2406.

Mickel, H.S., Vaishnav, Y.N., Kempski, O., von Lubitz, D., Weiss, J.F. and Feuerstein, G. (1987) Breathing 100% oxygen after global brain ischemia results in increased lipid peroxidation and increased mortality. *Stroke,* 18: 426 – 430.

Nakayama, H., Dietrich, W.D., Watson, B.D., Busto, R. and Ginsberg, M.D. (1988) Photothrombotic occlusion of rat middle cerebral artery: histopathological and hemodynamic sequlae of acute recanalization. *J. Cereb. Blood Flow Metab.,* 8: 357 – 366.

Nordstrom, C.-H., Rehncrona, S. and Siesjo, B.K. (1976) Restitution of cerebral energy state after complete and incomplete ischemia of 30 min duration. *Acta Physiol. Scand.,* 97: 270 – 272.

Noronha-Dutra, A.A. and Steen, E.M. (1982) Lipid peroxidation as a mechanism of injury in cardiac myocytes. *Lab. Invest.,* 47: 346 – 353.

Oh, S.M. and Betz, A.L. (1991) Interaction between free radicals and excitatory amino acids in the formation of ischemic brain edema in rats. *Stroke,* 22: 915 – 921.

Pasquali-Ronchetti, I., Bini, A., Botti, B., De Alojsio, G., Fornieri, C. and Vannini, V. (1980) Ultrastructural and biochemical changes induced by progressive lipid peroxidation on isolated microsomes and rat liver endoplasmic reticulum. *Lab. Invest.,* 42: 457 – 468.

Patt, A., Harken, A.H., Burton, L.K., Rodell, T.C., Piermattei, D., Schorr, W.J., Parker, N.B., Berger, E.M., Horeah, I.R., Terada, L.S., Linas, S.L., Cheronis, J.C. and Repine, J.E. (1988) Xanthine oxidase-derived hydrogen peroxide contributes to ischemia reperfusion-induced edema in gerbil brains. *J. Clin. Invest.,* 81: 1556 – 1652.

Pellegrini-Giampietro, D.E., Cherici, G., Alesiani, A., Carla, V. and Moroni, F. (1990) Excitatory amino acid release and free radical formation may cooperate in the genesis of ischemia-induced neuronal damage. *J. Neurosci.,* 10: 1035 – 1041.

Pompella, A., Maellaro, E., Casini, A.F. and Comporti, M. (1987) Histochemical detection of lipid peroxidation in the livers of bromobenzene-poisoned mice. *Am. J. Pathol.,* 129: 295 – 301.

Prado, R., Ginsberg, M.D., Dietrich, W.D., Watson, B.D. and Busto, R. (1988) Hyperglycemia increases infarct size in collaterally perfused but not end-arterial vascular territories. *J. Cereb. Blood Flow Metab.,* 8: 186 – 192.

Pulsinelli, W.A. and Brierley, J.B. (1979) A new model of bilateral hemispheric ischemia in the unanesthetized rat. *Stroke,* 10: 267 – 272.

Rehncrona, S., Folbergrova, J., Smith, D. and Siesjo, B.K. (1980) Influence of complete and pronounced incomplete cerebral ischemia and subsequent recirculation on cortical concentrations of oxidized and reduced glutathione in the rat. *J. Neurochem.,* 34: 477 – 486.

Rehncrona, S., Westerberg, E., Akesson, B. and Siesjo, B.K. (1982) Brain cortical fatty acids and phospholipids during and following complete and severe incomplete ischemia. *J. Neurochem.,* 38: 84–93.

Rothe, G. and Valet, G. (1990a) Flow cytometric analysis of respiratory burst activity in phagocytes with hydroethidine and 2′,7′-dichlorofluorescein. *J. Leukocyte Biol.,* 47: 440–448.

Rothe, G. and Valet, G. (1990b) Flow cytometric characterization of oxidative processes in neutrophils and monocytes with dihydrorhodamine 123, 2′,7′-dichlorofluorescein and hydroethidine. In: G. Burger, M. Oberholzer and G.P. Vooijs (Eds.), *Advances in Cellular Pathology,* Elsevier, Amsterdam, pp. 313–314.

Rusoff, I.I., Platt, J.R., Klevens, H.B. and Burr, G.O. (1945) Extreme ultraviolet absorption spectra of the fatty acids. *J. Am. Chem. Soc.,* 67: 675–678.

Saez, J.C., Kessler, J.A., Bennett, M.V.L. and Spray, D.C. (1987) Superoxide dismutase protects cultured neurons against death by starvation. *Proc. Natl. Acad. Sci. U.S.A.,* 84: 3056–3059.

Schmidley, J.W. (1990) Free radicals in central nervous system ischemia. *Stroke,* 21: 1086–1090.

Schraufstatter, I.U., Hinshaw, D.B., Hyslop, P.A., Spragg, R.G. and Cochrane, C.G. (1985) Glutathione cycle activity and pyridine nucleotide levels in oxidant-induced injury of cells. *J. Clin. Invest.,* 76: 1131–1139.

Schraufstatter, I.U., Hinshaw, D.B., Hyslop, P.A., Spragg, R.G. and Cochrane, C.G. (1986) Oxidant injury of cells. *J. Clin. Invest.,* 77: 1312–1320.

Sevanian, A. and Hochstein, P. (1985) Mechanisms and consequences of lipid peroxidation in biological systems. *Annu. Rev. Nutr.,* 5: 365–390.

Siesjo, B.K. (1981) Cell damage in the brain: a speculative synthesis. *J. Cereb. Blood Flow Metab.,* 1: 155–185.

Siesjo, B.K., Benedek, G., Koide, T., Westerberg, E. and Wieloch, T. (1985) Influence of acidosis on lipid peroxidation in brain tissues in vitro. *J. Cereb. Blood Flow Metab.,* 5: 253–258.

Smolen, J.E. and Shohet, S.B. (1974) Permeability changes induced by peroxidation in liposomes prepared from human erythrocyte lipids. *J. Lipid Res.,* 15: 273–280.

Stadtman, E.R. (1990) Metal-ion catalyzed oxidation of proteins: biochemical mechanism and biological consequences. *Free Radical Biol. Med.,* 9: 315–325.

Tappel, A.L. (1973) Lipid peroxidation damage to cell components. *Fed. Proc.,* 32: 1870–1874.

Thaw, H.H., Hamberg, H. and Brunk, U.T. (1983) Acute and irreversible injury following exposure of cultured cells to reactive oxygen metabolites. *Eur. J. Cell. Biol.,* 31: 46–54.

Thomas, C.E., Morehouse, L.A. and Aust, S.D. (1985) Ferritin and superoxide-dependent lipid peroxidation. *J. Biol. Chem.,* 260: 3275–3280.

Turrens, J.F., Alexandre, A. and Lehninger, A.L. (1985) Ubisemiquinone is the electron donor for superoxide formation by complex III of heart mitochondria. Arch. Biochem. Biophys., 237: 404–414.

Warso, M.A. and Lands, W.E.M. (1983) Lipid peroxidation in relation to prostacyclin and thromboxane physiology and pathopathology. *Br. Med. Bull.,* 39: 277–280.

Watson, B.D. (1989) What is the evidence for oxygen radical-mediated reperfusion injury in stroke? In: M.D. Ginsberg and W.D. Dietrich (Eds.), *Cerebrovascular Diseases – Sixteenth Research (Princeton) Conference,* Raven Press, New York, pp. 381–386.

Watson, B.D. (1990a) Oxygen free radicals in the central nervous system, Part 1: Origins, molecular interactions and microfocal consequences. In: P. Scheinberg (Eds), *Neurology and Neurosurgery Update Series,* Continuing Professional Education Center, Princeton, NJ, 8 (Lesson 20): 1–8.

Watson, B.D. (1990b) Oxygen free radicals in the central nervous system, Part 2: Microscopic and macroscopic effects and their mitigation. In: P. Scheinberg (Ed.), *Neurology and Neurosurgery Update Series,* Continuing Professional Education Center, Princeton, NJ, 8 (Lesson 21): 1–8.

Watson, B.D. and Busto, R. (1989) Ultrasensitive autofluorescence detection of conjugated diene and triene structures during brain ischemia and reperfusion. *J. Cereb. Blood Flow Metab.,* 9: S268.

Watson, B.D. and Ginsberg, M.D. (1988) Mechanisms of lipid peroxidation potentiated by ischemia in brain. In: B. Halliwell (Ed.), *Oxygen Radicals and Tissue Injury Symposium (Proceedings),* Federation of American Society for Experimental Biology, Bethesda, MD, pp. 81–91.

Watson, B.D. and Ginsberg, M.D. (1989) Ischemic injury in brain: role of oxygen radical-mediated processes. In: A.I. Barkai and N.G. Bazan (Eds.), *Arachidonic Acid in the Nervous System. Physiological and Pathological Significance – Ann. N.Y. Acad. Sci.,* 559: 269–281.

Watson, B.D., Busto, R., Goldberg, W.J., Santiso, M., Yoshida, S. and Ginsberg, M.D. (1984) Lipid peroxidation in vivo induced by reversible global ischemia in rat brain. *J. Neurochem.,* 42: 268–274.

Weiss, S.J. (1989) Tissue destruction by neutrophils. *N. Engl. J. Med.,* 320: 365–376.

White, B.C., Nayini, N.R., Krause, G.S., Aust, S.D., March, G.G., Bicknell, J.S. and Goosman, M. (1988) Effect on biochemical markers of brain injury of therapy with deferoxamine or superoxide dismutase following cardiac arrest. *Am. J. Emerg. Med.,* 6: 569–576.

White, B.C., DeGracia, D.J., Krause, G.S., Skjaerlund, J.M., O'Neil, B.J. and Grossman, L.I. (1991) Brain nuclear DNA survives cardiac arrest and reperfusion. *Free Radical Biol. Med.,* 10: 125–135.

Xue, D., Slivka, A. and Buchan, A. (1992) Tirilizad reduces cortical infarction after transient but not permanent focal cerebral ischemia in rats. *Stroke,* 23: 894–899.

Yagi, K. (1976) A simple fluorometric assay for lipoperoxide in blood plasma. *Biochem. Med.,* 15: 212 – 216.

Yagi, K., Ohkawa, H., Ohishi, N., Yamashita, M. and Nakashima, T. (1981) Lesions of aortic intima caused by intravenous administration of linoleic acid hydroperoxide. *J. Appl. Biochem.,* 3: 58 – 65.

Yoshida, S., Busto, R., Watson, B.D., Kogure, K. and Ginsberg, M.D. (1982) Influence of transient ischemia on lipid-soluble antioxidants, free fatty acids and energy metabolites in rat brain. *Brain Res.,* 245: 307 – 316.

Yoshida, S., Busto, R., Watson, B.D., Santiso, M. and Ginsberg, M.D. (1985) Postischemic cerebral lipid peroxidation in vitro: modification by dietary vitamin E. *J. Neurochem.,* 44: 1593 – 1601.

Young, J.D.-E. and Cohn, Z.A. (1988) How killer cells kill. *Sci. Am.,* 258: 38 – 44.

Young, W., Wojak, J.C. and DeCrescito, V. (1988) 21-aminosteroid reduces ion shifts and edema in the rat middle cerebral artery occlusion model of cerebral ischemia. *Stroke,* 19: 1013 – 1019.

Zucarello, M. and Anderson, D.K. (1989) Protective effect of a 21-aminosteroid on the blood-brain barrier following subarachnoid hemorrhage in rats. *Stroke,* 20: 367 – 371.

K. Kogure, K.-A. Hossmann and B.K. Siesjö (Eds.)
Progress in Brain Research, Vol. 96

CHAPTER 6

Role of superoxide dismutase in ischemic brain injury: reduction of edema and infarction in transgenic mice following focal cerebral ischemia

P.H. Chan[1,2], H. Kinouchi[1], C.J. Epstein [3,4], E. Carlson[3], S.F. Chen[1], S. Imaizumi[1] and G.Y. Yang[1]

Departments of [1]Neurology, [2]Neurosurgery, [3]Pediatrics and [4]Biochemistry and Biophysics, and the CNS Injury and Edema Research Center, University of California, School of Medicine, San Francisco, CA 94143-0114, U.S.A.

Introduction

During the past few decades, a large accumulated body of experimental data has indicated that the biological reduction of molecular oxygen can yield dangerously reactive free radicals (Fredovich, 1986). About 2 – 5% of the electron flow in isolated brain mitochondria produces superoxide ($O_2^{\cdot -}$) and hydrogen peroxide (H_2O_2) (Boveris and Chance, 1973). These constantly produced oxygen radicals are scavenged by endogenous antioxidants including antioxidative enzymes such as superoxide dismutases (SODs), catalase, glutathione peroxidase and non-enzymatic antioxidants such as reduced glutathione, ascorbic acid and α-tocopherol.

Superoxide dismutase scavenges superoxide radicals ($O_2^{\cdot -}$) at a rate close to diffusion, whereas glutathione peroxidase and catalase are specific scavengers for H_2O_2 and other lipid peroxides. Both enzymatic and non-enzymatic antioxidants are located in cellular membranes, cytoplasmic compartments and subcellular organelles such as mitochondria and peroxisomes (Freeman and Crapo, 1982). Based on the metal ion requirements and the anatomical distribution, two types of SOD exist in brain cells. CuZn-SOD is a cytosolic enzyme that requires both copper and zinc ions as cofactors, whereas manganese (Mn)-SOD is a mitochondrial enzyme with requirement for Mn^{2+} (Oberley, 1982). Recent studies have demonstrated that CuZn-SOD is primarily localized in peroxisomes, a subcellular organelle that also contains high levels of catalase in plants. Both CuZn-SOD and Mn-SOD from various sources have been fully characterized biochemically and the cDNAs of both human enzymes have been successfully cloned (Lieman-Hurwitz et al., 1982; Levanon et al., 1985). Furthermore, both cDNA and genomic DNA of human CuZn-SOD have been used to successfully generate transgenic mice (Epstein et al., 1987, 1992).

Although CNS tissue equips itself with high levels of antioxidants in scavenging the constantly formed free radicals such as $O_2^{\cdot -}$ and H_2O_2, pathological insults, including ischemia and trauma, perturb this defense mechanism and result in the overproduction of oxygen radicals (Kontos, 1985; Choi, 1988; Hall and Braughler, 1989; Siesjö et al., 1989; Chan, 1989). Due to technical difficulties, the level of oxygen free radicals in brain tissue following ischemic insults could only be indirectly assessed despite some recent success in measuring the hydroxyl free radicals as detected by salicylate hydroxylation in gerbil brains (Oliver et al., 1990). In most methods, the reduced levels of endogenous antioxidants are measured based on the assumption that the reduced levels of antioxidative compounds are due to their consumption by oxygen free radicals (Flamm et al., 1978; Demopoulos et al., 1982; Yoshida et al., 1982). Another commonly used method is to measure the level of lipid peroxidation, including thiobarbituric acid reactive substance, presumably malondialdehyde (MDA), fluorescence MDA, conjugated dienes and polyunsaturation of phospholipid lipids (Siesjö et al., 1981; Watson et al., 1984; Chan, 1989). In addition to the non-specific nature of some of these methods (i.e., MDA) in measuring a rather transient and minute amount of lipid peroxides in ischemic brain, the levels of lipid peroxidation may not be solely represented in the oxidative brain injury. Recent studies have demonstrated that oxidative damage of protein (enzyme in particular) could be an equally important, if not greater, account for the oxygen radical damage in ischemic brain injury (Carney et al., 1991). Furthermore, oxidative injury to DNA occurs in cells and can be quantitatively measured (Cathcart et al., 1984; Huang et al., 1992).

As specified, the free radical scavenger, superoxide dismutase, has been used extensively to reduce superoxide radical associated with ischemic brain injury. Unfortunately, the half life of CuZn-SOD in

TABLE I

Role of SOD on brain ischemia and trauma

Study	Animal species	SOD	Effects	Reference
Fluid percussion (arteriolar damage)	Cats	Free	+	Wei et al. (1981)
Hyperbaric O_2	Rats	Liposome + L-catalase	+	Yusa et al. (1984)
Intraventricular hemorrhage	Beagle puppy	Free	−	Ment et al. (1985)
Fluid percussion	Cats	Free	+	Kontos and Wei (1986)
Cold injury	Rats	Liposome	+	Chan et al. (1987)
Cardiac arrest	Dogs	Free + deferoxamine	+	Cerchiari et al. (1987)
Starvation	Neuronal culture	Free	+	Saez et al. (1987)
Kainic acid	Neuronal culture	Free	+	Dykens et al. (1987)
Complete cerebral ischemia	Dogs	Free + free catalase	−	Forsman et al. (1988)
Global cerebral ischemia	Rats	Free	+	Pigott et al. (1988)
Brain trauma	Rats	Liposome	+	Michelson et al. (1988)
Focal cerebral ischemia	Rats	PEG	+	Liu et al. (1989)
Cold injury	Rats	Derivative	+	Ando et al. (1989)
Cold injury, peritumoral edema	Cats	Free or PEG	−	Ikeda et al. (1989)
Fluid percussion	Rats	Free	+	Levasseur et al. (1989)
Hypoperfusion (survival)	Dogs	Free	+	Schettini et al. (1989)
Post-asphyxia hypoperfusion	Lambs (newborn)	PEG	+	Rosenberg et al. (1989)
Ischemia/reperfusion	Gerbils	Free	+	Uyama et al. (1990)
Focal cerebral ischemia	Rats	Liposome	+	Imaizumi et al. (1990)
2-V + hypotension	Rats	Free	−	Schurer et al. (1990)
Bilateral MCAO	Gerbils	Pyran	+	Kitagawa et al. (1990)
Glutamic acid	Cortical neurons (transgenic mice)	Transgene	+	Chan et al. (1990)
Acute hypertension	Rats	Free	+	Zhang and Ellis (1991)
Global ischemia/reperfusion	Piglets	PEG	−	Haun et al. (1991)
Cold injury	Transgenic mice	Transgene	+	Chan et al. (1991)
Ischemic/reperfusion	Dogs	Liposome	+	Phelan and Lange (1991)
Focal cerebral ischemia	Transgenic mice	Transgene	+	Kinouchi et al. (1991)

circulating blood is extremely short (6 min) and it is unable to pass the blood-brain barrier. Therefore, use has been made of chemically modified enzymes for work on cerebral injury and it has been found that polyethylene glycol-conjugated SOD (PEG-SOD) and PEG-catalase reduce the degree of cortical infarction resulting from focal cerebral ischemia (Liu et al., 1989). We have reported that liposome-entrapped CuZn-SOD which has a half life of 4.2 h (Yusa et al., 1984) and can pass through the blood-brain barrier, reduces the severity of traumatic and ischemic injuries (Chan et al., 1987; Imaizumi et al., 1990). Despite these successes, other investigators have obtained various degrees of success and failure when free, non-modified SOD was used in ameliorating ischemic brain injury (Table I). And in some instances, the modified SOD (i.e., PEG-SOD) has been used with a mixed result. Table I summarizes some representative studies using free, liposome SOD and PEG-SOD in ischemia and trauma.

To assess the direct role of SOD in the pathogenesis of brain edema and infarction in focal cerebral ischemia, we used human CuZn-SOD (SOD-1) transgenic mice overexpressing CuZn-SOD activity (Epstein et al., 1987). We have demonstrated recently that following a 30 sec cold traumatized injury, bot vasogenic edema and infarction were significantly reduced in these transgenic mice (Chan et al., 1990). The aim of this study was to test the hypothesis that the severity of focal cerebral ischemic injury would be reduced in SOD-1 transgenic mice, should superoxide radicals play a major role in their pathogenesis.

Materials and methods

Transgenic mice of strain TgHS/SF-218 carrying the human CuZn-SOD (h-SOD-1) gene, produced as described by Epstein and colleagues (Epstein et al., 1987), were used. The genome of this strain carries several copies of the h-SOD-1 gene, presumably in a tandem array. The founder mice has been bred to produce transgenic offspring expressing the h-SOD-1 genes. Transgenic mice were identified by Northern blot analysis for the presence of the messenger RNA (mRNA) of h-SOD-1, as well as by the detection of h-SOD-1 enzymatic activity in brain tissue using non-denaturing gel electrophoresis followed by nitroblue tetrazolium staining (Epstein et al., 1987; Chan et al., 1991). Direct enzyme activity was determined using the superoxide radical-dependent cytochrome C reduction assay (Chan et al., 1988). Male Tg and nTg mice were subject to focal cerebral ischemia according to the method used for rat models (Chen et al., 1986). The left middle cerebral artery (MCA) was occluded by electrical coagulation just proximal to the pyriform branch. Immediately following occlusion of the MCA, the left common carotid artery (CCA) was ligated and the right CCA was occluded for 1 h using a microaneurysmal clip. The cerebral blood flow, measured by [^{14}C] iodoantipyrine, is reduced to 6 – 12% in ipsilateral ischemic core (C.Y. Hsu, personal communication). This focal ischemia model provides a reproducible infarction volume (as measured by 2,3,5-triphenyl tetrazolium chloride (TTC) staining and by H and E histology) in ipsilateral cortex without affecting the subcortical area and striatum (Chen et al., 1986). The degree of neocortical infarct depends on the duration of the occlusion of the right CCA (Chen et al., 1986). The release of right CCA does not constitute a reperfusion manipulation, but rather it appears that the interruption of collateral flow to ipsilateral hemisphere is a critical manipulation for producing reproducible neocortical infarction in this particular rat and mouse model. Although cerebral infarction produced by this MCAo + CCAo model has been widely used and characterized, the selective vulnerability of certain neurons (i.e., NADPH diaphorase) which are known to be resistant to ischemic insults have not been determined in this model. Nevertheless, a significant and reproducible model of ischemic infarct can be obtained in ischemic core and in surrounding MCA territory at 24 h after the transient occlusion of the right CCA for 1 h (Chen et al., 1986; Liu et al., 1989; Imaizumi et al., 1990).

For our experiments, we have chosen the method using permanent occlusion of both MCA and left

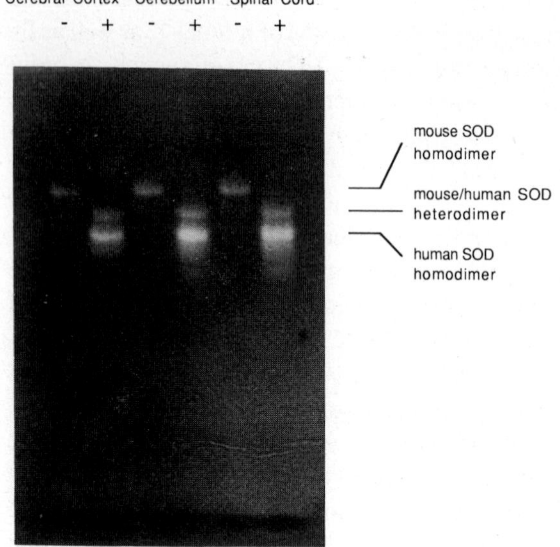

Fig. 1. Expression of human CuZn-SOD enzymatic activity in cerebral cortex, cerebellum and spinal cord of transgenic mice. Both mouse and human CuZn-SOD enzymatic activity were detected using non-denaturing gel electrophoresis followed by nitroblue tetrazolium staining. +, Transgenic mice; −, non-transgenic mice. Data obtained from Chan et al. (1991)

CCA plus 1 h transient occlusion of right CCA. At 24 h after ischemia, the brain was removed and the forebrain was cut coronally at 1 (plane A), 3 (plane B), 5 (plane C) and 7 (plane D) mm distal from the frontal pole using the Mouse Brain Matrix (Harvard Apparatus). The brain slices were stained for mitochondrial dehydrogenase activity using 2% 2,3,5-triphenyl tetrazolium chloride (TTC). In other experiments, brain tissues were dissected for water content measurements (Chan et al., 1987; Imaizumi et al., 1990). There were no observable phenotypic differences between transgenic mice (Tg) and non-transgenic (nTg) littermates.

Results

Fig. 1 shows the presence of human CuZn-SOD enzymatic activity in cerebral cortex, cerebellum and spinal cord resulting from the expression of h-SOD-1 transgenes in mice. In non-transgenic mice, only mouse CuZn-SOD activity was expressed, whereas in transgenic mice, human SOD homodimer activity as well as the human/mouse SOD heterodimer were found. The actual amount of total CuZn-SOD activity in cerebral cortices, cerebella and spinal cords of transgenic and non-transgenic mice are shown in Table II. The cortices and cerebella of transgenics had a near three-fold increase in CuZn-SOD activity as compared to that of non-transgenics.

There were no significant differences between Tg and nTg mice in mean arterial blood pressure, PaO_2, $PaCO_2$ and pH (data not shown). As shown in Figs. 2 and 3, the infarct sizes were significantly smaller in Tg than in nTg in planes B and C. The total infarct volumes, hemispheric volumes, infarct percentages and left/right hemisphere ratios of Tg and nTg are shown in Table III. The water content in the left hemisphere was increased 24 h after ischemia in both groups (Fig. 4). However, the increase in water content of MCA cortex and anterior cerebral artery (ACA) cortex was significantly less in Tg than in nTg.

Discussion

Oxygen-derived radicals, superoxide in particular, have been implicated in the pathogenesis of brain edema, microvascular abnormality and neuronal cell death following cerebral ischemia, trauma and other neurological disorders (Kontos, 1985; Choi,

TABLE II

CuZn-SOD levels in neural tissues of transgenic and non-transgenic mice

	SOD (units/mg protein)		
	nTg	Tg	T/N
Cerebral cortex	7.9 ± 0.5	22.7 ± 1.4[a]	2.9
Cerebellum	9.0 ± 2.0	25.8 ± 1.3[a]	2.9
Spinal cord	15.4 ± 2.0	34.9 ± 1.5[a]	2.3

Values are the mean ± S.E.M. of three mice $P < 0.001$, compared to the non-transgenic (nTg) group. T, Transgenic; N, non-transgenic. Data obtained from Chan et al. (1991)

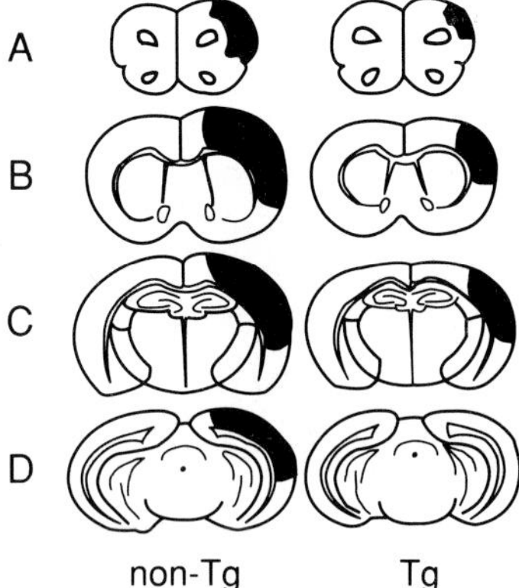

Fig. 2. The illustration of cortical infarction in brain of Tg and non-Tg mice stained by TTC following 24 h of ischemia. The sizes of cortical infarction (black area) in transgenic mice were significantly smaller than in non-transgenic mice. Data obtained from Kinouchi et al. (1991).

TABLE III

Total infarcted volume and hemispheric volume in Tg and nTg mice at 24 h of MCA occlusion

	nTg	Tg
Volume of left hemisphere	212.3 ± 5.2	189.4 ± 4.3*
Volume of right hemisphere	179.5 ± 2.5	176.6 ± 3.9*
Volume of infarction	39.9 ± 4.0	25.6 ± 2.1*
Percentage of infarction	18.4 ± 1.3	13.7 ± 0.8*
L/R hemisphere ratio	1.18 ± 0.02	1.07 ± 0.01*

Total volumes of infarction and of the left and the right hemispheres were calculated according Liu et al. (1989). Volumes are expressed in mm^3. Each value is mean ± S.E.M. of 15 animals. $*P < 0.001$, versus nTg, using Student's *t*-test. Data obtained from Kinouchi et al. (1991).

1988; Hall and Braughler, 1989; Siesjö et al., 1989; Chan, 1989). Both free and chemically modified superoxide dismutase have been used by many investigators to ameliorate tissue infarction in rats following focal cerebral ischemia (Table I). Though these studies may provide therapeutic potential in ischemic brain injury, the complicating issue that often confounds these approaches are permeability of the blood-brain barrier to the enzyme, its half life in blood and the potential systemic side effects of exogenously supplied enzyme.

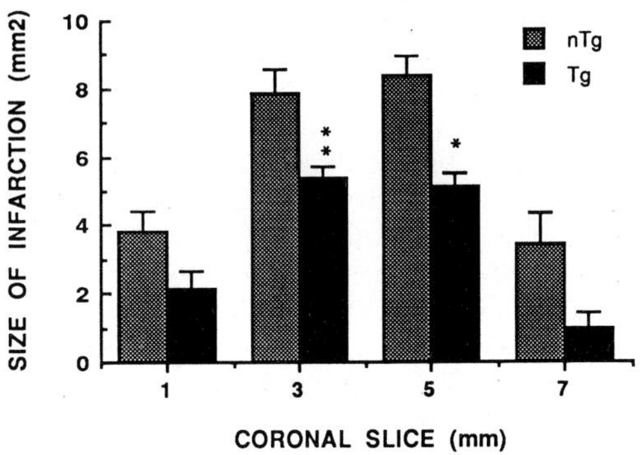

Fig. 3. Infarct size in Tg and nTg mice. Infarct areas determined by TTC staining were reduced in transgenic mice following 24 h of ischemia. There were significant differences in the coronal slices at 3 and 5 mm distal from the frontal pole. Number of determinations is 15 in each group. $^{*}P< 0.01$, $^{**}P< 0.05$, versus nTg, using Student's *t*-test. Data obtained from Kinouchi et al. (1991).

These potential problems could be eliminated by increasing the enzyme levels endogenously using genetic manipulation. Tg mice of strain Tg HS/SF-218 overexpressing CuZn-SOD have a 3.1-fold increased level of endogenous CuZn-SOD activity in brain. These transgenic mice have been successfully developed and maintained in our laboratory (Epstein et al., 1990a,b; Kinouchi et al., 1991).

Our studies showed that both brain edema (as indicated by water content) and infarct volume (as measured by TTC staining) were significantly reduced in Tg mice following focal cerebral ischemia. Our studies further indicated that the penumbra area (planes A and D) was spared from cortical infarction in Tg mice. Although we did not directly measure the level of brain superoxide radicals in the penumbra and MCA infarct areas, the data suggest that increased CuZn-SOD activities may provide an environment in the penumbra area resistant to ischemic injury. In order to test this hypothesis, we studied the levels of GSH/GSSG and ascorbic acid in the infarct area and penumbra in both nTg and Tg mice subjected to MCAo and CCAo. We have found that both GSH/GSSG and ascorbic acid levels maintained close to normal values in the penumbra area despite a significant drop in the in-

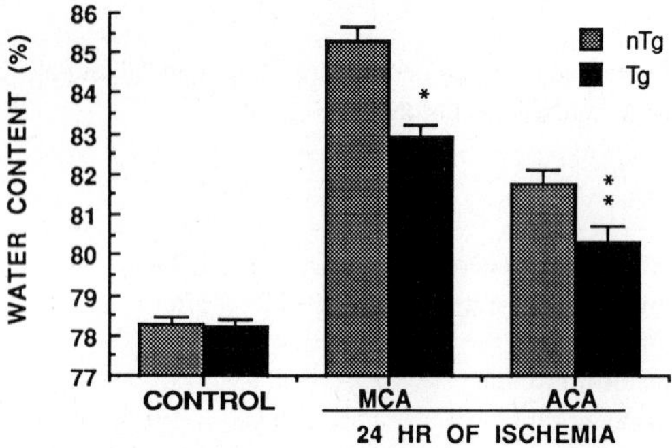

Fig. 4. Water content in the cortex in Tg and nTg mice before and 24 h after MCA occlusion. Water content of both MCA cortex and anterior cerebral artery (ACA) cortex increased significantly from control values ($n = 8$, $^{*}P < 0.01$, $^{**}P < 0.05$ versus nTg, using Student's t-test). Data obtained from Kinouchi et al. (1991).

farct area associated with the MCA core (Kinouchi et al., 1991). Overall, these observations suggest that increased endogenous SOD activity in Tg mice alters the antioxidant system so as to favor the cytoprotection of the brain against ischemic injury.

Besides the cytoprotective mechanism, other possibilities may exist to account for the observed differences in neuroprotection between Tg and nTg mice. One such factor is the difference in cerebral blood flow (CBF) between Tg and nTg mice. However, our preliminary studies suggest that there were no differences in CBF measured by laser-Doppler flowmetry, a semi-quantitative method for CBF between Tg and nTg mice, nor were there any morphological and anatomical differences in vascular supply in Tg mice. Therefore, we conclude that the reduced oxidative stress appears to be the major mechanism underlying the cytoprotection in Tg. In other studies using rats with the same focal cerebral ischemia model, we demonstrated that the levels of endogenous GSH and the degree of infarct sizes in ischemic brain are inversely related (Mizui et al., 1992). Furthermore, the reduction on the levels of GSH in ischemic core is dependent on the duration of CCA occlusion. These rat studies support the notion that oxidative stress is a key determinant contributing to the degree of infarction following a focal cerebral ischemia. Thus, the transgenic mice overexpressing human CuZn-SOD activity are valuable models for studying the potential role of free radicals and CuZn-SOD in neurological disorders, including trauma, aging, Alzheimer's disease and other forms of neurodegenerative diseases.

Acknowledgements

This work was supported in part by grants NS-25372, NS-14543 and AG-08938.

References

Ando, Y., Inoue, M., Hirota, M., Morino, Y. and Araki, S. (1989) Effect of a superoxide dismutase derivative on cold-induced brain edema. *Brain Res.*, 477: 286–291.

Boveris, A. and Chance, B. (1973) The mitochondrial generation of hydrogen peroxide. *Biochem. J.*, 134: 707–716.

Carney, J.M., Starke-Reed, P.E., Oliver, C.N., Landum, R.W., Cheng, M.S., Wu, J.F. and Floyd, R.A. (1991) Reversal of age-related increase in brain protein oxidation decrease in enzyme activity, and loss in temporal and spatial memory by chronic administration of the spin-trapping compound *N*-tert-butyl-L-phenylnitrone. *Proc. Natl. Acad. Sci. U.S.A.*, 88: 3633–3636.

Cathcart, R., Schwiers, E., Saul, R.L. and Ames, B.N. (1984) Thymine glycol and thymidine glycol in human and rat urine: a possible assay for oxidative DNA damage. *Proc. Natl. Acad. Sci. U.S.A.*, 81: 5633–5637.

Cerchiari, E.L., Hoel, T.M., Safar, P. and Sclabassi, R.J. (1987) Protective effects of combined superoxide dismutase and deferoxamine on recovery of cerebral blood flow and function after cardiac arrest in dogs. *Stroke*, 18: 869–878.

Chan, P.H. (1989) The role of oxygen radicals in brain injury and edema. In: C.K. Chow (Ed.), *Cellular Antioxidant Defense Mechanisms*, CRC Press, Boca Raton, FL, pp. 89–109.

Chan, P.H., Longar, S. and Fishman, R.A. (1987) Protective effects of liposome-entrapped superoxide dismutase on post-traumatic brain edema. *Ann. Neurol.*, 21: 540–547.

Chan, P.H., Chu, L. and Fishman, R.A. (1988) Reduction of activities of superoxide dismutase but not of glutathione peroxidase in rat brain regions following decapitation ischemia. *Brain Res.*, 439: 388–390.

Chan, P.H., Chu, L., Chen, S.F., Carlson, E.J. and Epstein, C.J. (1990) Reduced neurotoxicity in transgenic mice overexpressing human copper-zinc-superoxide dismutase. *Stroke*, 21: III80–III82.

Chan, P.H., Yang, G.Y., Chen, S.F., Carlson, E. and Epstein, C.J. (1991) Cold-induced brain edema and infarction are reduced in transgenic mice overexpressing CuZn-superoxide dismutase. *Ann. Neurol.*, 29: 482–486.

Chen, S.T., Hsu, C.Y., Hogan, E.L., Maricq, H. and Balentine, J.D. (1986) A model of focal ischemic stroke in the rat: reproducible extensive cortical infarction. *Stroke,* 17: 738 – 743.

Choi, D.W. (1988) Glutamate neurotoxicity and diseases of the nervous system. *Neuron,* 1: 623 – 634.

Demopoulos, H.B., Flamm, E., Seligman, M. and Pietronigro, D.D. (1982) Oxygen free radicals in central nervous system ischemia and trauma. In: A.P. Autor (Ed.), *Pathology of Oxygen,* Academic Press, New York, pp. 127 – 155.

Dykens, J.A., Stern, A. and Trenkner, E. (1987) Mechanism of kainate toxicity to cerebellar neurons in vitro is analogous to reperfusion tissue injury. *J. Neurochem.,* 49: 1222 – 1228.

Epstein, C.J., Avraham, K.B., Lovett, M., Smith, S., Elroy-Sein, O., Rotman, G., Bry, C. and Groner, Y. (1987) Transgenic mice with increased Cu/Zn-superoxide dismutase activity: animal model of dosage effects in Down syndrome. *Proc. Natl. Acad. Sci. U.S.A.,* 84: 8044 – 8048.

Epstein, C.J., Berger, C.N., Chan, P.H., Carlson, E.J. and Huang, T.T. (1990a) Models for Down syndrome: chromosome 21-specific genes in mice. In: D. Patterson and C.J. Epstein (Eds.), *Molecular Genetics of Chromosome 21 and Down Syndrome,* Wiley-Liss, New York, pp. 215 – 232.

Epstein, C.J., Huang, T.T., Chan, P.H. and Carlson, E. (1990b) The molecular biology of Down syndrome. In: K. Beyreuther and G. Schettle (Eds.), *Proceedings of the International Workshop on the Molecular Mechanisms of Aging,* Springer, Heidelberg, pp. 98 – 109.

Epstein, C.J., Chan, P.H., Cadet, J.L., Carlson, E., Chen, S., Chu, S., Farn, S., Jackson-Lewis, V., Kinouchi, H., Kostic, V., Kujirai, K., Mizui, T., Naini, A., Przedborski, S. and Yang, C.Y. (1992) Resistance of SOD-transgenic mice to oxidative stress. In: F. Gage and Y. Christen (Eds.), *Gene Transfer and Therapy in the Nervous System,* Springer, Berlin, pp. 106 – 117.

Flamm, E.S., Demopoulos, H.B., Seligman, M.L., Poser, R.G. and Ransohoff, J. (1978) Free radicals in cerebral ischemia. *Stroke,* 9: 445 – 447.

Forsman, M., Fleischer, J.E., Milde, J.H., Steen, P.A. and Michenfelder, J.D. (1988) Superoxide dismutase and catalase failed to improve neurologic outcome after complete cerebral ischemia in the dog. *Acta Anaesthesiol. Scand.,* 32: 152 – 155.

Fredovich, I. (1986) Biological effects of the superoxide radical. *Arch. Biochem. Biophys.,* 274: 1 – 11.

Freeman, B.A. and Crapo, J.D. (1982) Biology of disease: free radicals and tissue injury. *Lab. Invest.,* 47: 412 – 426.

Hall, E.D. and Braughler, J.M. (1989) Central nervous system trauma and stroke. II. Physiological and pharmacological evidence for involvement of oxygen radicals and lipid peroxidation. *Free Radicals Biol. Med.,* 6: 303 – 313.

Haun, S.E., Kirsch, J.R., Helfaer, M.A., Kubos, K.L. and Traystman, R.J. (1991) Polyethylene glycol-conjugated superoxide dismutase fails to augment brain superoxide dismutase activity in piglets. *Stroke,* 22: 655 – 659.

Huang, T.T., Carlson, E.J., Leadon, S.A. and Epstein, C.J. (1992) Relationship of resistance to oxygen free radicals to CuZn-superoxide dismutase activity in transgenic, transfected and trisomic cells. *FASEB J.,* 6: 903 – 910.

Ikeda, Y., Anderson, J.H. and Long, D.M. (1989) Oxygen free radicals in the genesis of traumatic and peritumoral brain edema. *Neurosurgery,* 24: 679 – 685.

Imaizumi, S., Woolworth, V., Fishman, R.A. and Chan, P.H. (1990) Liposome-entrapped superoxide dismutase reduces cerebral infarction in cerebral ischemia in rats. *Stroke,* 21: 1312 – 1317.

Kinouchi, H., Epstein, C.J., Mizui, T., Carlson, E., Chen, S.F. and Chan, P.H. (1991) Attenuation of focal cerebral ischemic injury in transgenic mice overexpressing CuZn-superoxide dismutase. *Proc. Natl. Acad. Sci. U.S.A.,* 88: 11158 – 11162.

Kitagawa, K., Matsumoto, M., Oda, T., Niinobe, M., Hata, R., Handa, N., Fukunaga, R., Isaka, Y., Kimura, K., Maeda, H., et al. (1990) Free radical generation during brief periods of cerebral ischemia may trigger delayed neuronal death. *Neuroscience,* 35: 551 – 558.

Kontos, H.A. (1985) Oxygen radicals in cerebral vascular injury. *Circ. Res.,* 57: 508 – 516.

Kontos, H.A. and Wei, E.P. (1986) Superoxide production in experimental brain injury. *J. Neurosurg.,* 64: 803 – 807.

Levanon, D., Lieman-Hurwitz, J., Dafni, N., Wigderson, M., Sherman, L., Bernstein, Y., Laver-Rudich, Z., Danciger, E., Stein, O. and Groner, Y. (1985) Architecture and anatomy of the chromosomal locus in human chromosome 21 encoding the Cu/Zn superoxide dismutase. *EMBO J.,* 4: 77 – 84.

Levasseur, J.E., Patterson Jr., J.L., Ghatak, N.R., Kontos, H.A. and Choi, S.C. (1989) Combined effect of respirator-induced ventilation and superoxide dismutase in experimental brain injury. *J. Neurosurg.,* 71: 573 – 577.

Lieman-Hurwitz, J., Dafni, N., Lavie, V. and Groner, Y. (1982) Human cytoplasmic superoxide dismutase cDNA clone: a probe for studying the molecular biology of Down syndrome. *Proc. Natl. Acad. Sci. U.S.A.,* 79: 2808 – 2811.

Liu, T.H., Beckman, J.S., Freeman, B.A., Hogan, E.L. and Hsu, C.Y. (1989) Polyethylene glycol-conjugated superoxide dismutase and catalase reduce ischemic brain injury. *Am. J. Physiol.,* 256: H589 – H593.

Ment, L.R., Stewart, W.B. and Duncan, C.C. (1985) Beagle puppy model of intraventricular hemorrhage. Effect of superoxide dismutase on cerebral blood flow and prostaglandins. *J. Neurosurg.,* 62: 563 – 569.

Michelson, A.M., Jadot, G. and Puget, K. (1988) Treatment of brain trauma with liposomal superoxide dismutase. *Free Radicals Res. Commun.,* 4: 209 – 224.

Mizui, T., Kinouchi, H. and Chan, P.H. (1992) Depletion of brain glutathione by buthionine sulfoximine enhances cerebral ischemic injury in rats. *Am. J. Physiol.,* 262: H313 – H317.

Oberley, L.W. (Ed.) (1982) *Superoxide Dismutase, Vol. 1,* CRC Press, Boca Raton, FL, pp. 1 – 141.

Oliver, C.N., Starke-Reed, P.E., Stadtman, E.R., Liu, G.J.,

Carney, J.M. and Floyd, R.A. (1990) Oxidative damage to brain proteins, loss of glutamine synthetase activity and production of free radicals during ischemia/reperfusion-induced injury to gerbil brain. *Proc. Natl. Acad. Sci. U.S.A.*, 87: 5144 – 5147.

Phelan, A.M. and Lange, D.G. (1991) Ischemia/reperfusion-induced changes in membrane fluidity characteristics of brain capillary endothelial cells and its prevention by liposomal-incorporated superoxide dismutase. *Biochim. Biophys. Acta*, 1067: 97 – 102.

Pigott, J.P., Donovan, D.L., Fink, J.A. and Sharp, W.V. (1988) Experimental pharmacologic cerebroprotection. *J. Vasc. Surg.*, 7: 625 – 630.

Rosenberg, A.A., Murdaugh, E. and White, C.W. (1989) The role of oxygen free radicals in postasphyxia cerebral hypoperfusion in newborn lambs. *Pediatr. Res.*, 26: 215 – 219.

Saez, J.C., Kessler, J.A., Bennett, M.V.L. and Spray, D. (1987) Superoxide dismutase protects cultured neurons against death by starvation. *Proc. Natl. Acad. Sci. U.S.A.*, 84: 3056 – 3059.

Schettini, A., Lippman, R.H. and Walsh, E.K. (1989) Attenuation of decompressive hypoperfusion and cerebral edema by superoxide dismutase. *J. Neurosurg.*, 71: 578 – 587.

Schürer, L., Grögaard, B., Gerdin, B. and Arfors, K.E. (1990) Superoxide dismutase does not prevent delayed hypoperfusion after incomplete cerebral ischemia in the rat. *Acta Neurochir.*, 103: 163 – 170.

Siesjö, B.K., Bendek, G., Koide, T., Westerberg, E. and Wieloch, T. (1981) Influence of acidosis on lipid peroxidation in brain tissues in vitro. *J. Cereb. Blood Flow Metab.*, 1: 155 – 185.

Siesjö, B.K., Ahardh, C-D. and Bengtsson, F. (1989) Free radicals and brain damage. *Cereb. Brain Metab. Rev.*, 1: 165 – 211.

Uyama, O., Shiratsuki, N., Matsuyama, T., Nakanishi, T., Matsumoto, Y., Yamada, T., Narita, M. and Sugita, M. (1990) Protective effects of superoxide dismutase on acute reperfusion injury of gerbil brain. *Free Radicals Biol. Med.*, 8: 265 – 268.

Watson, B.D., Busto, R., Goldberg, W.J., Santiso, M., Yoshida, S. and Ginsberg, M.D. (1984) Lipid peroxidation in vivo induced by reversible global ischemia in rat brain. *J. Neurochem.*, 42: 268 – 274.

Wei, E.P., Kontos, H.A., Dietrich, W.D., Povlishock, J.T. and Ellis, E.F. (1981) Inhibition by free radical scavengers and by cyclooxygenase inhibitors of pial arteriolar abnormalities from concussive brain injury in cats. *Circ. Res.*, 48: 95 – 103.

Yoshida, S., Abe, K., Busto, R., Watson, B.D., Kogure, K. and Ginsberg, M.D. (1982) Influence of transient ischemia on lipid-soluble antioxidants, free fatty acids and energy metabolites in rat brain. *Brain Res.*, 245: 307 – 315.

Yusa, T., Crapo, J.D. and Freeman, B.A. (1984) Liposome-mediated augmentation of brain SOD and catalase inhibits CNS O_2 toxicity. *J. Appl. Physiol.*, 57: 1674 – 1681.

Zhang, X.M. and Ellis, E.F. (1991) Superoxide dismutase decreases mortality, blood pressure, and cerebral blood flow responses induced by acute hypertension in rats. *Stroke*, 22: 489 – 494.

K. Kogure, K.-A. Hossmann and B.K. Siesjö (Eds.)
Progress in Brain Research, Vol. 96

CHAPTER 7

Glutamate receptor transmission and ischemic nerve cell damage: evidence for involvement of excitotoxic mechanisms

N.H. Diemer, E. Valente, T. Bruhn, M. Berg, M.B. Jørgensen and F.F. Johansen

Molecular Neuropathology Unit and PharmaBiotec Research Center, Institute of Neuropathology, University of Copenhagen, DK-2100 Copenhagen, Denmark

Introduction

Nerve cell loss in cerebral ischemia is characterized by selectivity; thus, within small regions one type of nerve cell can be resistant while another one is vulnerable. The varying vulnerability between even neighboring cells, such as hippocampal pyramidal neurons and interneurons (Johansen et al., 1983) eliminates local intra-ischemic and post-ischemic flow differences as being responsible for the selective neuron loss, since flow regulation influences groups of cells. Cerebral ischemia has been studied in a number of animal models, mainly with rats; although the most popular ones differ somewhat with respect to the neuropathological changes, often a hierarchy within the vulnerable cells can be identified. The development of morphological changes (acidophilia, eosinophilia) takes from a few hours (dentate hilus) to four days or longer (hippocampal CA1 region, delayed neuronal death) (Pulsinelli et al., 1982a; Smith et al., 1984). More severe ischemia (longer or complete occlusion) results in an earlier occurring eosinophilia and vice versa, the so-called maturation phenomenon (Ito et al., 1975). Even in the different rat models of complete forebrain ischemia, the neuropathological damage is variable, i.e., in the Siemkowicz-Hansen model (carotid artery occlusion plus hypovolemic hypotension) 14 min of ischemia result in the same damage to hippocampus (Diemer and Siemkowicz, 1981) as 20 min in the Pulsinelli-Brierley model (Pulsinelli and Brierley, 1979) (4-VO model). Since the neuronal damage induced by ischemia has a multifactorial pathogenesis, where each of the involved factors is capable of destroying vulnerable neurons, it is advisable to study as short periods of ischemia as possible when the effect of a single factor is to be evaluated. In studying the influence of the excitatory (glutamatergic) input on the ischemic neuronal damage, which is the main subject of the present review, the use of short ischemia is necessary (Diemer et al., 1987, 1990).

Selectivity of ischemic damage

Neuropathological examination some days after an episode of cerebral ischemia reveals that a number of cell types are involved. The hematoxylin-eosin stain or acid-fuchsin stain (Auer et al., 1984) are standard for the detection of eosinophilic neurons, but the Fink-Heimer impregnation (Fink and Heimer, 1967) is more suitable to show both dead nerve cell bodies as well as their axons and dendrites, and is the superior method if the distribution of ischemic damage must be mapped. Recently it was shown that ^{45}Ca-autoradiograms also can be used for mapping of the damage at a regional level (Dienel, 1984; Benveniste and Diemer, 1988; Araki et al., 1989).

Some of the most ischemia-sensitive nerve cell types are listed below (Ito et al., 1975; Diemer and Siemkowicz, 1981; Pulsinelli et al., 1982a): (a) somatostatin neurons and mossy cells of dentate hilus; (b) pyramidal neurons of subiculum; (c) pyramidal neurons of hippocampal CA1; (d) neurons of lateral reticular nucleus of thalamus; (e) septal neurons; (f) Purkinje cells; (g) medium-sized neurons of striatum; (h) neurons in neocortical layers 3 and 5; and (i) neurons in pars reticulata of substantia nigra.

One of the most studied brain regions is the hippocampal CA1 sector. In the rat, more than 3 – 4 min of ischemia destroys the pyramidal cells whereas the interneurons (which make up about 10 – 15% of the total neuronal population in this region) are resistant (Johansen et al., 1984). A moderate or pronounced loss of Purkinje cells is found in many cases of transient global ischemia in the human brain. In the cerebellum, the Purkinje cells and the basket cells are the most ischemia-vulnerable, but also loss of neurons from the cerebellar nuclei (especially the dentate nucleus) can be seen (Brierley and Graham, 1984). Most rodent models of cerebral ischemia comprise total forebrain ischemia, but partial ischemia of the brain-stem and the cerebellum, and Purkinje cell loss is only infrequently seen. Thus, in the original rat 4-vessel occlusion (4-VO) model devised by Pulsinelli and Brierley (1979) inconsistent Purkinje cell loss is found, and only after longer ischemia periods. In the 4-vessel occlusion model with hypotension to 60 – 70 mm Hg, there is no or only a slight Purkinje cell loss, but if the ischemic period is prolonged to 20 min, Purkinje cell loss is seen in all animals although the loss is much more variable than that of CA1 pyramidal cells. In the neck cuff plus hypotension model the Purkinje cell loss is prominent and less variable (Diemer and Siemkowicz, 1981). In the rat ischemia model with increased intracranial pressure, a Purkinje cell loss of up to 50% has been described (Kirino et al., 1988).

Concomitant with the nerve cell loss there is an increase in glial cell number, mainly attributable to invasion by microglial cells having a rod-shaped nucleus (Gehrmann et al., 1992). For neuropathological study of ischemia-induced damage, perfusion fixation is a prerequisite in order to avoid confusion between the dark neuron artifact of Cammermeyer (1961) and ischemically damaged (eosinophilic) neurons. A study of the different stages of ischemic cell injury in the gerbil (Ito et al., 1975) revealed the maturation phenomenon, i.e., the denser the ischemia, the faster the development of the ischemia changes. The size of the neurons does not determine the maturation speed; thus small-sized striatal neurons and large hilar neurons are among the first to disintegrate after ischemia. The maturation phenomenon is also seen in connection with the Purkinje cell loss induced by global cerebral ischemia, at least in moderately hypoglycemic rats (Diemer and Siemkowicz, 1981). Four days after 10 min of ischemia 82% of Purkinje cells were left but this decreased to 58% three weeks after ischemia.

Neuropathology of ischemic damage to the hippocampal CA1 region

As shown by Kirino (1982) in the gerbil, three different types of cell changes could be observed: in the hilus the cell changes were similar to the ischemic cell change and scattered nerve cell injury of dark type is seen within a few hours, at a time when the other hippocampal subregions are still intact (Kirino et al., 1988); in the CA2 sector there were changes of the reactive type (Ito et al., 1975) which resembles reactions seem after axotomy; this change, as seen in the gerbil, was termed "selective chromatolysis" by Brown et al. (1979). In the CA1 changes typical for delayed neuronal death after shorter periods of ischemia were found, whereas longer periods tended to produce ischemic cell change. After 24 h changes of ribosomes (disaggregation) and distended cisterns of endoplasmic reticulum begin to appear. Even in cases with total loss of CA1 pyramidal neurons, GABAergic interneurons (Johansen et al., 1989) and neurons with numerous stacks of endoplasmic reticulum are resistant to ischemia (Kirino and Sano, 1984). Four days after ischemia the stratum radiatum of CA1 shows electron microscopical damage to dendrites whereas the axons (and astrocytes) are spared (Johansen et al., 1984; Kirino et al., 1990). An ultrastructural study up to 72 h after 10 min of 2-vessel occlusion (2-VO) showed no dilatation of dendrites in the stratum radiatum and the mitochondria ultrastructure was preserved until neuronal disintegration began (Deshpande et al., 1992). The authors concluded that the ultrastructural changes found during the maturation period differed from those typical of programmed cell death (apoptosis). When the period of ischemia is prolonged the delay (maturation period) is shortened; theoretically it should be possible to change the pattern of ischemic damage in CA1 to that of "acute cell change", but the duration of the ischemic period necessary for this is incompatible with survival of the animals.

A somewhat similar pyramidal neuron loss, but developing rapidly, can be seen after i.v. injection of a glutamate analogue, kainic acid, which also results in sparing of axons and selective neuron death. This resemblance between the ischemic lesion and the kainic acid lesion fostered the idea that excitotoxic mechanisms might be operating in ischemia (Jørgensen and Diemer, 1982).

Hippocampal connections

The internal architecture of hippocampus is relatively similar in the frequently used rodents (mice, gerbils and rats) and in the human, and the vulnerability to ischemia is likewise strikingly similar. The macroscopic structure of hippocampus can be compared to a bent tube with the hippocampus and the dentate fascia being oriented in an interlocking fashion. Therefore a ventral and a dorsal component is seen on most coronal sections. In the majority of ischemia models only the dorsal part is damaged, probably due to differences in residual blood flow during ischemia between the two parts. Compared to neocortex, the light microscopical structure of hippocampus is much simpler; it has only three layers with a distinct organization of somata in stratum pyramidale and dendrites in stratum oriens and stratum radiatum/lacunosum moleculare.

The main wiring pattern of the hippocampal formation and the entorhinal cortex can be described as a "trisynaptic pathway" (Gottlieb and Cowan, 1973; Swanson et al., 1978). Neurons in the entorhinal cortex innervate the dentate granule cells via the perforant path. These in turn innervate the CA3 pyramidal cells via the mossy fibers. The CA3 neurons innervate the ipsilateral CA1 pyramidal cells via the Schaffer collaterals and the contralateral CA1 pyramidal cells via the commissural fibers. The most apical dendrites of the pyramidal cells, situated in the stratum lacunosum moleculare, are also directly innervated from the entorhinal cortex.

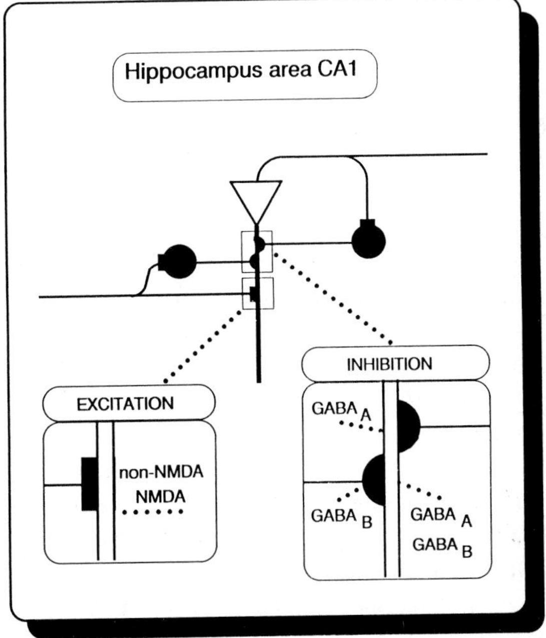

Fig. 1. Drawing of the main connection and transmitters in hippocampal CA1 zone. Triangular cell body is a pyramidal neuron; round cell bodies are belonging to interneurons. The Schaffer collateral coming from the CA3 cells innervates both CA1 pyramidal cells and the (NPY containing?) interneurons (feed-forward inhibition). The figure is kindly provided by Morten Skovgaard-Jensen, Institute of Physiology, Aarhus University, Denmark.

The output from CA1 is mainly directed towards the subiculum and septum. The morphological axis of the trisynaptic circuit is oriented perpendicular to the longitudinal axis of the hippocampal formation (lamellar structure). The border between the CA1 and CA3 regions is not always easy to distinguish in the Nissl (cresyl violet) stain, whereas the Timm stain for free zinc content shows that only CA3 has a mossy fiber input.

In the hippocampal CA1 region, two main types of neurons are found: pyramidal neurons with typical spiny dendrites, and interneurons, often with beaded processes. The interneurons, which are all supposed to use GABA as an inhibitory neurotransmitter, are also peptidergic, containing somatostatin, neuropeptide Y, cholecystokinin etc. Two subtypes of CA1 interneurons have been described (Fig. 1): one type (somatostatinergic) situated in the stratum oriens receives a glutamatergic collateral input from the CA1 pyramidal cells and another type (NPYergic), mainly localized in the stratum radiatum, receives a glutamatergic input from the CA3 pyramidal cells via the Schaffer collaterals. Most (all?) of the CA1 interneurons contain the calcium-binding protein parvalbumin; immunostaining for this protein visualizes also distinctly their dendrites which can be seen spanning the whole stratum radiatum like the pyramidal cell dendrites (Nitsch et al., 1989; Johansen et al., 1990).

Glutamate receptors

The ionotropic glutamate receptors are usually subdivided into three classes (Watkins and Evans, 1981), named after their agonists, *N*-methyl-D-aspartate (NMDA), kainate and quisqualate. The NMDA receptor can be blocked competitively by the selective ω-phosphonic acid homologues AP5 and AP7 (APH) and non-competitively by phencyclidine, ketamine, MK-801 (Dizocilpine) and a number of other compounds. Antagonists against the non-NMDA receptors (kainate and quisqualate type) were developed later and among such compounds especially the quinoxaline diones (Honoré et al., 1988) CNQX, DNQX and NBQX have attracted attention. Quisqualate, however, was discovered to bind to the kainate site as well as to a metabotropic glutamate receptor. The (ionotropic) quisqualate receptor was recently renamed the AMPA receptor since AMPA (α-amino-3-hydroxy-5-methyl-4-isoxazoleproprionic acid) is a more specific agonist with little affinity for the kainate site (Krogsgaard-Larsen et al., 1980). Besides these ionotropic receptors, a metabotropic type of glutamate receptor, coupled to phsophoinositol metabolism, has been found (Sugiyama et al., 1987); metabotropic receptors for other neurotransmitters have been known for some time, e.g., β-adrenergic, muscarinic cholinergic, histaminergic etc.

The distribution of the different ionotropic glutamate receptors is best known for the rat brain (Monaghan et al., 1983; Young and Fagg, 1990) but the human autoradiographical studies published up to now have not shown any major qualitative deviations from the pattern of distribution described in the rat brain.

NMDA receptors are numerous in hippocampus, neocortex, amygdala and septal nuclei and in striatum. In hippocampus, the density of NMDA receptors, as labeled with the non-competitive ligand [^{3}H]TCP, is especially high in the dendritic fields of CA1: stratum radiatum and stratum oriens. Kainate receptors, as labeled with [^{3}H]kainic acid (representing both high and low affinity binding), are concentrated in the stratum lucidum of CA3 in the rat hippocampus (where the mossy fibers innervate the CA3 pyramidal cells) and in the supragranular layer of the dentate fascia. In the dentate hilus, which contains 2 – 3 cell types vulnerable to ischemia, the most prominent glutamate receptor is of the kainate type.

The hippocampal distribution of the AMPA receptor almost overlaps with that of the NMDA receptor with the highest density corresponding to the dendritic fields of CA1. Autoradiographic studies after ischemia with total loss of CA1 pyramidal cells have shown a pronounced loss of both NMDA and AMPA binding sites (Diemer et al., 1987; Westerberg et al., 1987). Removal of the Schaffer collateral input to CA1 has shown no loss of NMDA or AMPA binding sites (Valente et al., unpublished results), indicating that these two glutamate receptor subtypes are not located on the presynaptic Schaffer collaterals or commissurals. It is reasonable to assume that a small fraction of the AMPA receptors is located on interneurons which constitute up to 10% of the CA1 neuron population (Johansen et al., 1983). On the other hand, binding of [^{3}H]-D-aspartate in CA1 is significantly increased four days after ischemia (Diemer et al., unpublished results). At this time, all pyramidal cells are lost and replaced by hypertrophied astrocytes. Thus, the [^{3}H]-D-aspartate binding most likely visualizes the astrocytic glutamate transporter.

The metabotropic glutamate receptor is the most recently described subtype of glutamate receptors. It does not gate an ion channel; glutamate or quisqualate stimulates the hydrolysis of polyphosphoinositide to inositoltrisphosphate (stimulating the release of calcium from endoplasmic reticulum via the IP_3 receptor) and diacylglycerol (activating protein kinase C) (Sladeczek et al., 1988) in a calcium-dependent way. The metabotropic glutamate receptor subtype is known also to activate phospholipase C (PLC) (Sladeczek et al., 1988) and this coupling has been shown to be increased after transient ischemia (Seren et al., 1989). During ischemia there is an early decrease in phosphatidylinositol 4,5,biphosphate (PIP_2) (Berridge, 1987) and an increase in its two PLC-catalyzed hydrolysis products, diacylglycerol (DAG) and inositoltrisphosphate (Ikeda et al., 1986; Yoshida et al., 1986; Sun et al., 1988). Also, there is a 50% decrease in IP_3 and DAG receptor binding (Jørgensen et al., 1989a, 1991a; Onodera and Kogure, 1989). A number of agonists to the metabotropic receptor exists; ibotenic and especially quisqualic acid are potent stimulators, but not very selective. The endogenous agonist is supposed to be L-glutamate. Recently a selective agonist was discovered: trans-ACPD (or more correctly 1_s,3_r-APCD, trans-1-aminocyclopentane-1,3-dicarboxylic acid), having about the same potency as ibotenic acid (Palmer et al., 1989). Only a few antagonists to the metabotropic receptor are known, e.g., AP3 which is a more useful antagonist than AP4. The latter is also acting on a presynaptic, inhibitory L-AP4 glutamate receptor. Stimulation of the metabotropic glutamate receptor with trans-APCD produces an increased firing in a number of neuron types, including hippocampal neurons. By means of autoradiography, the highest density of metabotropic receptors is found in neocortex, hippocampus, striatum and cerebellum. The metabotropic glutamate receptor was cloned by Masu et al. (1991) and shown to have a unique structure with no sequence similarity to conventional G protein-coupled receptors. Expression of the messenger RNA was pronounced in cerebellar Purkinje cells, hippocampus, granule cells, hilar cells, CA2 – 3 pyramidal cells and CA1 interneurons.

Infusion of trans-ACPD into rat striatum produces no excitotoxic lesion (Schoepp et al., 1990). However, after ischemia in neonatal and mature rats, an increase of quisqualate and ibotenate-induced phosphatidylinositol hydrolyse was found (Chen et al., 1988; Seren et al., 1989), but it is not known whether the metabotropic receptor participates in neurotoxic situations involving glutamate.

Ischemia-induced changes of regional glucose metabolism

The pattern of regional cell loss is not correlated to the value of pre-ischemic (normal) blood flow or glucose metabolism as shown by autoradiography (Reivich et al., 1969; Sokoloff et al., 1977), indicating that the pre-ischemic level of regional energy metabolism does not determine the ischemia vulnerability of a region. In the normal dorsal hippocampus in unesthetized animals, the CMRglu is about 60 mmol/100 g per minute in CA1 stratum radiatum, and 80 mmol/100 g per minute in CA1 stratum lacunosum moleculare (Sokoloff et al., 1977; Jørgensen et al., 1990). The largest drug-induced depression of glucose metabolism has been observed after barbiturate administration, where up to a 50% reduction of glucose metabolism was found (Sokoloff et al., 1977). In hippocampus, however, the reduction was about 30%. Blockade of the NMDA receptor-mediated excitatory transmission in hippocampus with ketamine showed only a modest reduction in stratum radiatum (Davies et al., 1988; Rischke et al., 1990). This can be an indication of the fact that in this layer, where the main innervation comes from the Schaffer collaterals, NMDA receptor-mediated transmission is only modest during normophysiological activity. On the other hand, ketamine increased the glucose metabolism in CA1 stratum lacunosum moleculare (Rischke et al., 1990). This could be a result of a presynaptic action of ketamine on the perforant path boutons terminating in this layer. It should be noted that the density of NMDA receptors, labeled for example with the non-competitive ligand [^{3}H]TCP, is lower in stratum lacunosum moleculare than in stratum radiatum (and stratum oriens) and the possibility exists that the NMDA receptors in this layer are located on GABAergic interneurons which gives rise to excitation in the layer via an interpositioned Ach-ergic terminal.

Concerning the other main glutamate receptor in the CA1 zone, the AMPA receptor (formerly termed quisqualate receptor), administration of the antagonist NBQX leads to a reduction of CMRglu in CA1 stratum radiatum (Berg et al., in preparation) of about 40%. This is in line with the observation that the fast excitation in stratum radiatum is mediated via AMPA receptors (Herreras et al., 1988).

It appears that all brain regions including white matter ones have the capability of developing increased deoxyglucose uptake immediately after focal ischemia or start of recirculation after global ischemia. However, after a shorter period of global ischemia certain regions are especially prone to develop this change.

Thus, immediately after post-ischemic recirculation is re-established ^{14}C-2-deoxyglucose (2-DG) autoradiograms show a striking pattern (Fieschi et al., 1978; Diemer and Siemkowicz, 1980a,b; Pulsinelli et al., 1982b). Using the carotid occlusion/hypotension 10 min ischemia model (normoglycemic rats) and an isotope circulation period from 5 to 15 min, increased accumulation of 2-DG was found in hippocampal CA1, cerebellar molecular layer, substantia nigra and globus pallidus (Diemer and Siemkowicz, 1980a,b). All other brain regions showed about the same accumulation. However, in hyperglycemic rats, the 2-DG accumulation pattern was totally uniform 15 min after ischemia.

Pulsinelli et al. (1982b) studied regional cerebral blood flow and glucose utilization serially after 30 min of 4-VO. They found an initial 5 – 15 min period of hyperemia in hippocampus, probably related to the increased deoxyglucose uptake described above. Regional glucose utilization 1 h after ischemia was depressed in all brain regions exposed to moderate or severe ischemia, except for the hippocampal CA1 zone (and some cerebellar and brainstem structures) which had an unchanged utilization. At 6 h post-ischemia CA1 followed the generally decreased pattern of most forebrain regions, which was still present at 48 h.

Jørgensen et al. (1990) calculated values of the glucose metabolism after 20 min 4-VO ischemia, using a circulation time period from 15 to 60 min after ischemia. Glucose utilization was still decreased four days after ischemia by 50% in neocortex except in hippocampal stratum radiatum where the decrease was about 30% (Jørgensen et al., 1990).

Pappius (1988) found that the general decrease in glucose metabolism after brain injury (freezing lesion) was due to an increase of serotonin metabolism and that p-chlorophenylalanine, a 5-HT synthesis blocker, normalized the cortical LCGU in the traumatized hemisphere. It was also found that the noradrenergic system was involved by using the noradrenergic blocker, prazosine. These findings indicate an inhibitory role of serotonin and noradrenaline in cerebral cortex after certain injuries, maybe also including ischemia.

In several situations where activation of brain regions lead to increased glucose utilization, there is also an expression of *c-fos* mRNA (Dragunow et al., 1987) and production of the *c-fos* protein at the cellular level.

The *c-fos* proto-oncogene can be regarded as a third messenger. It is an immediate early gene in which the protein product is involved in gene regulation. It thus regulates long-term responses of cells to various short-term stimuli (Curran, 1988). Since it is induced in neurons following both sensory stimulation (Hunt et al., 1987) and seizure activity (Morgan et al., 1987; Dragunow et al., 1987), its expression can be used as a marker of metabolic activity.

If the ischemic necrosis of the cells were preceded by increased excitation, it would be reflected by an increased *c-fos* expression. Instead, a delayed increase in *c-fos* mRNA (Jørgsen et al., 1989b) and protein (Jørgensen et al., 1991b) has been found in the CA1 pyramidal layer after 2 – 3 days of recirculation. It was particularly clear in the latter study that the increase precedes the necrosis (karyorhexis and gliosis). Also, at early recirculation times, *c-fos* mRNA expression has been found (after 1 – 3 h) in several hippocampal regions (Nowak et al., 1990) and in neocortex (Onodera et al., 1989). Probably due to post-ischemic impairment of protein synthesis (Cooper et al., 1977; Thilmann et al., 1986) there is no early *c-fos* protein increase (Jørgensen et al., 1991b). The *c-fos* induction is of course not necessarily due to a general increase in metabolism. *c-Fos* induction has been shown to depend on calcium influx (Morgan and Curran, 1986) and could be secondary to the calcium increase at the time of necrosis (Dienel, 1984; Despande et al., 1987).

Ischemia-induced damage in the dentate hilus

Ischemic damage of neurons located in the dentate hilus has been demonstrated both in humans surviving an episode of cardiac arrest (Petito et al., 1987) and in animals subjected to experimental cerebral ischemia (Ito et al., 1975; Smith et al., 1984). In a rat model of transient incomplete global ischemia (Johansen et al., 1992), hilar neuron damage is present following episodes of ischemia as short as 8 min. This damage can be demonstrated during the first 6 h of post-ischemic reflow using acid-fuchsin staining of ischemic cell changes or Fink-Heimer silver impregnation of necrotic neurons (Johansen et al., 1992). When the length of the ischemic episode is increased from 8 to 12, 16, 20, 30 and 40 min, damage to two different populations of hilar neurons can be demonstrated in Fink-Heimer impregnated sections (Johansen et al., 1987, 1992). Thus, damage to one population with projections to the outer molecular layers of the dentate gyrus is seen even after short episodes of ischemia, whereas damage to another neuron population with projections to the inner molecular layer is infrequently seen among animals subjected to ischemic episodes shorter than 30 min. The neuron population with ipsilateral projections to the outer molecular layers contains the neuropeptide somatostatin (SS) (Bakst et al., 1986), while the mossy cell population with bilateral projections to the inner molecular layer (Sloviter, 1991) does not contain any identified neuropeptide (Fig. 2). Investigations of Fink-Heimer sections also demonstrated that ischemic necrosis of mossy cells was delayed in relation to the fast maturation of ischemic cell death of the SS neurons (Johansen et al., 1987, 1992).

Amaral (1978) has identified as many as 21 cell types with different morphological characteristics in the dentate hilus. Various subpopulations of hilar neurons can be identified using antibodies against glutamic acid decarboxylase (GAD), parvalbumin, SS, neuropeptide Y (NPY) and cholecystokinin (CCK). Changes in immunoreactivity of these immunocytochemical markers have been examined in the ischemic dentate hilus. Within the first two days after ischemia one observes a significant 50 – 80% loss of SS and NPY immunoreactivity in hilar cell bodies (Johansen et al., 1987, 1989, 1992). GAD immunoreactivity is transiently increased around the fourth post-ischemic day (Johansen et al., 1989), whereas parvalbumin immunoreactivity is transiently decreased at this time of survival (Johansen et al., 1990). Finally, CCK immunoreactivity is unchanged following ischemia (Johansen et al., 1987).

The hilar SS neurons have been investigated electron-microscopically after ischemia (Johansen et al., 1992). Irreversible ischemic cell changes were demonstrated. It is concluded that the majority of hilar SS neurons necrotizes shortly after ischemia. A high degree of colocalization of SS and NPY has

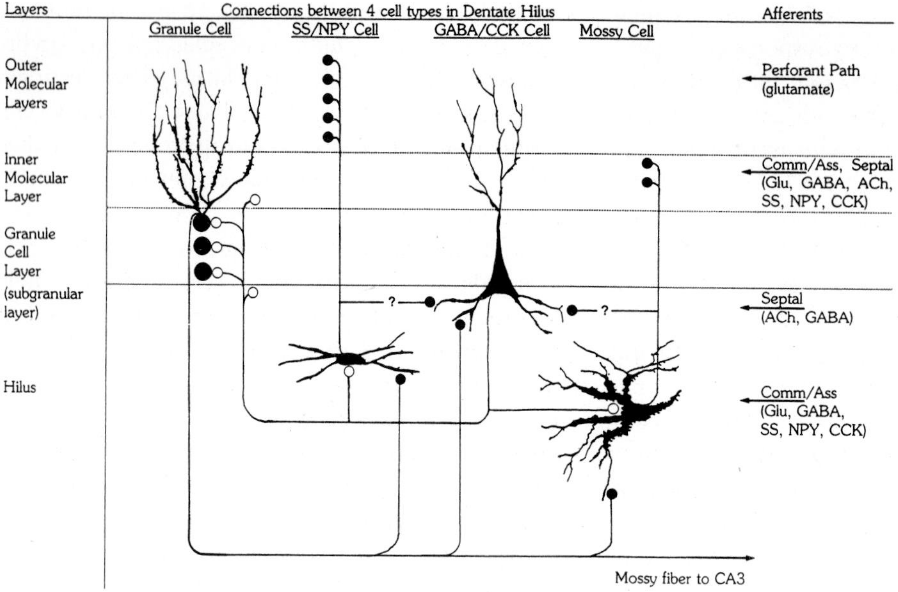

Fig. 2. Interpretation of neuronal circuits and transmitters/modulators in dentate gyrus. Granule cells activate (○) GABA/CCK basket cell interneurons mediating feedback inhibition (●) to their cell bodies and inhibition to axon-initial-segments located on both sides of the granule cell layer. Granule cells may also activate SS/NPY neurons and mossy cells in hilus. These two cell types may both be excitatory cells activating (?) the GABA/CCK interneurons and, thus, be interposed in the loop mediating inhibition to granule cells. Mossy cells most likely mediate excitation of dentate inhibitory interneurons. SS/NPY neurons may mediate feedback excitation in the outer molecular layers to granule cells, whereas mossy cells activate granule cells and/or GABA/CCK interneurons on dendrites in inner molecular layer. It is speculated that loss of SS/NPY neurons in this circuit leads to decreased feedback excitation of granule cells and, thus, to increased granule cell inhibition.

been demonstrated in hilar neurons (Köhler et al., 1987), and it has been suggested that those NPY neurons that costore SS also necrotize after ischemia. Finally, it is suggested that the reversible changes of GAD and parvalbumin immunoreactivity occur in the hilar neurons surviving ischemia (Johansen et al., 1989, 1990). Some of these neurons may also contain CCK (Johansen et al., 1987).

The impact of ischemic loss of hilar SS/NPY neurons and partial loss of mossy cells on granule cell excitability is difficult to predict. Chang et al. (1989) have demonstrated that ischemia is followed by a decreased in granule cell excitability, i.e., increase inhibition, but it is unknown whether mossy cells were damaged in their ischemia model. On the other hand, Sloviter (1987, 1991) has demonstrated a decreased granule cell inhibition following 24 h intermittent perforant path stimulation. This "epilepsia model" demonstrated substantial loss of SS/NPY cells and mossy cells, whereas the GABA-ergic neurons survived as in ischemia. Sloviter (1987, 1991) suggested that the decreased granule cell inhibition may be in part caused by a loss of bilateral mossy cell stimulation of the surviving GABAergic dentate basket cells. The "in vitro" electrophysiology has been studied in hippocampus slices taken from animals surviving 20 min of ischemia (Jensen et al., 1991). No signs of hippocampal hyperexcitability were found supporting the "in vivo" recordings by Chang et al. (1989). We conclude that following 20 min of cerebral ischemia and loss of 60 – 80% of the hilar neurons, granule cell inhibition is unchanged or even decreased. Thus, no evidence supports the assumption that a rapid ischemic loss of hilar SS/NPY neurons leads to hyperexcitability in the dentate gyrus, which through an "epileptic" process might be responsible for the delayed death of mossy cells and CA3c and

CA1 pyramidal cells. Whether episodes of 30 and 40 min of ischemia lead to major mossy cell loss and loss of granule cell inhibition remains to be clarified.

Post-ischemic changes in kainic acid receptors and AMPA receptors have been investigated autoradiographically in the dentate gyrus. In animals surviving 20 min of ischemia for three weeks a significant increase in AMPA binding is demonstrated in the outer molecular layers (Valente and Diemer, 1989, personal communication), whereas the kainic acid binding in the inner molecular layer is unchanged (Westerberg et al., 1987). This is in agreement with the major loss of terminals from the SS/NPY cells in the outer molecular layers and suggests that these cells may be excitatory cells activating AMPA receptors. Furthermore, the lack of changes in kainic acid receptors in the inner molecular layer accords with evidence suggesting that mossy cells are excitatory cells activating kainic acid receptors, and thus with the suggestion that the majority of mossy cells survive 20 min of ischemia.

We have previously demonstrated that ischemic damage to hilar SS neurons is accompanied by a decrease in chelatable zinc in the presynaptic mossy fibers, and that concomitantly there is an accumulation of zinc in or on the rapidly dying SS neurons (Tønder et al., 1990). In contrast to this, no zinc is accumulated in or on the CA3c and CA1 pyramidal cells showing delayed ischemic death. Following kainic acid seizures, reduced contents of mossy fiber zinc is also demonstrated, but in contrast to ischemia, zinc is accumulated in or on hilar neurons as well as in CA3 pyramidal cells (Frederickson et al., 1989). In this connection, it would be interesting to examine whether episodes of 30 and 40 min of ischemia could lead to zinc accumulation in CA3c pyramidal cells.

Release of excitatory amino acids during and after ischemia

During cerebral ischemia in rats there is a pronounced release of glutamate and aspartate in hippocampus (Benveniste et al., 1984; Hagberg et al., 1985; Korf et al., 1988; Benveniste et al., 1989; Christensen et al., 1991; Mitani et al., 1991) as well as in striatum (Globus et al., 1988; Korf et al., 1988) and cerebral cortex (Shimada et al., 1990). The increase measured by microdialysis ranges from 3.5- to 15-fold in the hippocampus. Calculations of the extracellular glutamate concentration gave values of $[\text{glutamate}]_e$ up to 1 mM (Benveniste et al., 1989), taking into account the extracellular space shrinkage of 50% of the normal value during ischemia, the tortuosity factor (non-linearity of the extracellular diffusion path) and the in vitro recovery of the fiber. Cell culture studies have shown that exposure to 100 μM glutamate for more than 5 min is lethal (Choi et al., 1987). The concentration of glutamate and aspartate normalizes within 10 – 20 min of recirculation. In most studies, EAA concentrations have only been followed for less than an hour, but a recent study by Andiné et al. (1991), using chronically implanted microdialysis fibers, showed a 5.5-fold increase of aspartate and a two-fold increase of glutamate at 8 h post-ischemia. This was paralleled by an increase of multiple unit activity to 140% of baseline level. On the other hand, Buszàki et al. (1989) found no neurophysiological signs of spontaneous or evoked neuronal hyperexcitability at any time during a period of eight days after 15 or 20 min of 4-VO in rats.

Since there are several glutamate pools, as indicated above, the question arises from which compartment(s) glutamate is released during ischemia (see Fig. 3): (presynaptic) cytoplasm, vesicles, neuronal soma, astrocytes, etc.

Release of glutamate from the transmitter pool is calcium-dependent, most probably dependent on N-channel activation (Meyer et al., 1989) but ATP is also required and the release is therefore arrested within a few minutes after start of ischemia (Siesjö, 1981; see also Siesjö, 1988, 1990). Furthermore, the high-affinity uptake processes will attempt to cope with the increased release. Approximately 2 min after induction of ischemia/anoxia extracellular $[K^+]$ increases steeply to 60 – 80 mM (for a review, see Hansen, 1985) with an accompanying decrease in both extracellular sodium and chloride. This

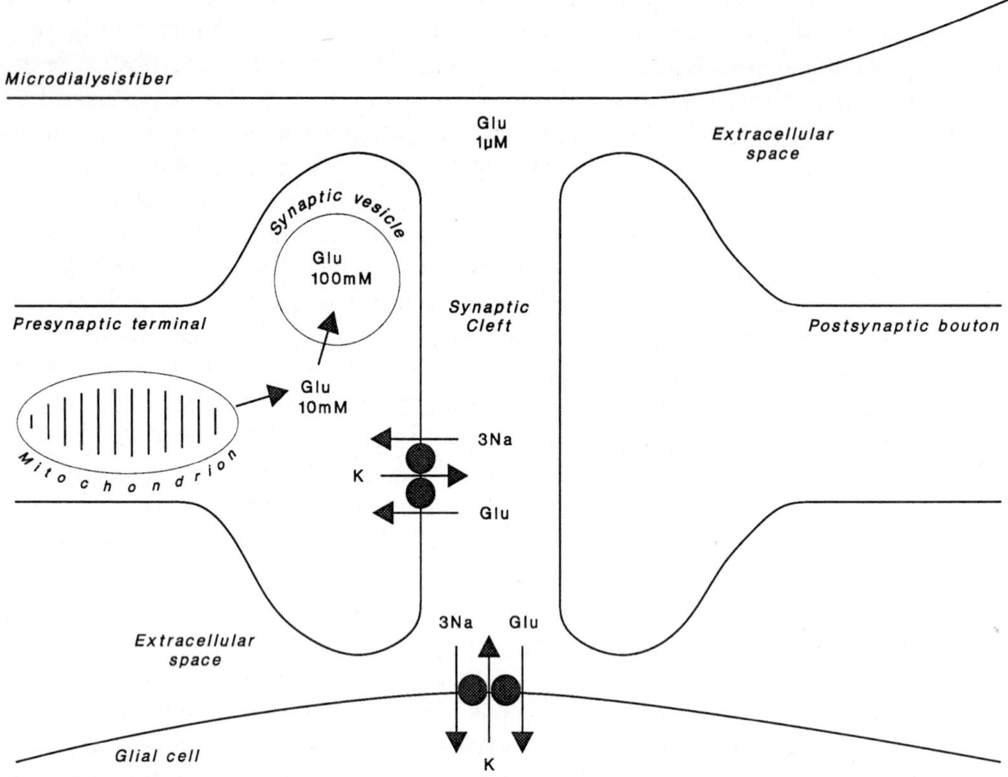

Fig. 3. Schematic drawing of five of the compartments involved in glutamate metabolism and transmission (synaptic vesicles, presynaptic cytoplasm, postsynaptic terminal (dendritic spine), astrocyte, extracellular space). Concentrations in the extracellular space, presynaptic terminal and vesicles are as indicated by Nicholls and Atwell (1990). High affinity uptake mechanisms for glutamate (glutamate transporters) are located to the presynaptic membrane and astrocyte membrane.

drastic change of the $[K^+]/[Na^+]$ ratio reverses the glutamate uptake carriers in astrocytes and presynaptic terminals (for a review, see Nicholls and Atwell, 1990). It is not known which of these two compartments contributes most to the extracellular increase. In hippocampus, the volume of presynaptic terminals is about 20% and the volume fraction of astrocytes is 6% (von Lubitz and Diemer, 1982); with a presynaptic glutamate concentration of 10 mM (Nicholls and Atwell, 1990) and an astrocytic concentration of 5 mM (Schousboe et al., 1975), it seems reasonable to assume that the presynaptic terminals and astrocytes are contributing most to the extracellular glutamate increase. Studies by Drejer et al. (1985) showed that substitution of the 1 mM $CaCl_2$ with 10 mM $CoCl_2$ in the microdialysis fiber perfusate starting 40 min before 10 min ischemia impaired the ischemia-induced increase of glutamate. This was interpreted as indicating that glutamate released during ischemia is coming from the transmitter (vesicle) pool. However, in a number of later studies, both on in vivo (Ikeda et al., 1989) and in vitro (Kauppinen et al., 1988; Sánchez-Prieto and Gonzales, 1988; Ikeda et al., 1989) ischemia/anoxia, it has been repeatedly shown that the glutamate and aspartate released during ischemia are calcium-independent.

There is some indirect evidence showing that the glutamate initially released during ischemia, before ATP is depleted, might originate from a transmitter pool. Thus, stereological analysis of the number of synaptic vesicles in stratum radiatum of the rat hippocampal CA1 region 10 min after reperfusion was significantly decreased (von Lubitz and Diemer, 1982). However, stimulated Ca^{2+}-dependent release of glutamate and aspartate is always accompanied by a reduction of extracellular glutamine (Lehmann et al., 1983; Bruhn et al., 1992) and this is not the case during cerebral ischemia (Benveniste et al., 1984, 1989; Hagberg et al., 1985). The reason for the impairment of ischemia-induced release by cobalt (Drejer et al., 1985) is presently unexplained, but it is known that Co^{2+} can enter neurons and thereby influence glutamate metabolism.

Effect of selective pathway cuttings

Because of its relatively simple trilaminar structure, hippocampus (archicortex) is one of the most frequently used regions for denervation studies. The ischemia-vulnerable CA1 cells can be (subtotally) denervated by a parasagittal cut of Schaffer collaterals and commissurals or after destruction of CA3 (with kainic acid, ibotenic acid, etc). Bilateral lesion of CA3, as it is seen after intraventricular injection of kainic acid, removes about 80% of the presynaptic terminals on the CA1 dendrites. As mentioned earlier, the apical tips of the CA1 pyramidal cells are innervated by the perforant path, and this innervation can be eliminated by a cut through the angular bundle or removal of the proper parts of entorhinal cortex. Franck et al. (1988) reported that the CA1 pyramidal neurons became hyperexcitable after a CA3 lesion; however, up to several months after a CA3 lesion, no damage to CA1 cells was observed (Jørgensen and Diemer, unpublished results).

Using receptor autoradiography we studied changes in [^{3}H]kainic acid binding in rat hippocampal subregions after removal of pre- or postsynaptic components. This was achieved using ischemia-induced loss of CA1 neurons, colchicine-induced loss of dentate granule cells and kainic acid-induced loss of CA3 pyramidal cells (Valente et al., unpublished results). After ischemia there was no change in the total kainate binding in CA1 (Fig. 4), although there was a 90% loss of pyramidal cells in this region. Elimination of dentate granule cells showed a total loss of supragranular kainate binding but no changes in CA1 and CA3. Animals subjected to both lesion of the granule cells and 20 min 4-VO ischemia showed a decrease in the kainate binding in CA1 and a striking redistribution of binding in CA3 (Fig. 4). These results as well as post-ischemic changes in [^{3}H]AMPA binding demonstrate plasticity or aberrant innervation processes taking place in hippocampus, especially after severe ischemia, which might be involved in post-ischemic epileptogenesis.

Effect of denervation of loss of CA1 pyramidal cells after ischemia

The first study on the effect of denervation on excitatory transmitter-mediated nerve cell damage was done by Köhler et al. (1978). In rats, an injection of kainic acid into the dentate fascia produced loss of granule cells. If the animals had a perforant path transsection, the injection caused no loss. Since the lesion produced by ischemia has similarities to that produced by i.v. kainic acid, a further proof of the excitatory hypothesis would be a protective effect of a denervation of CA1. The first lesion we studied in the 4-VO animals with 20 min ischemia was unilateral injection of kainic acid in the CA3 region, at three different places. It turned out that some of the animals had a protective effect of this lesion (Diemer, unpublished results). However, further studies were needed because the lesion had a protective effect in only some of the animals.

In 1984, Wieloch and coworkers described a protective effect of removal of some of the input from the entorhinal cortex, the angular bundle. We also studied other lesions of the trisynaptic pathway, such as removal of the granule cells (Johansen et al., 1984) and of the entorhinal cortex (Jørgensen et al., 1987) finding 80 and 85% protection, respectively, after 20 min of 4-VO ischemia. Both the pre-ischemic Schafferotomy and the degranulation reduced the CA1 pyramidal cell loss from about 90% (the remaining 5 – 10% neurons in the pyrami-

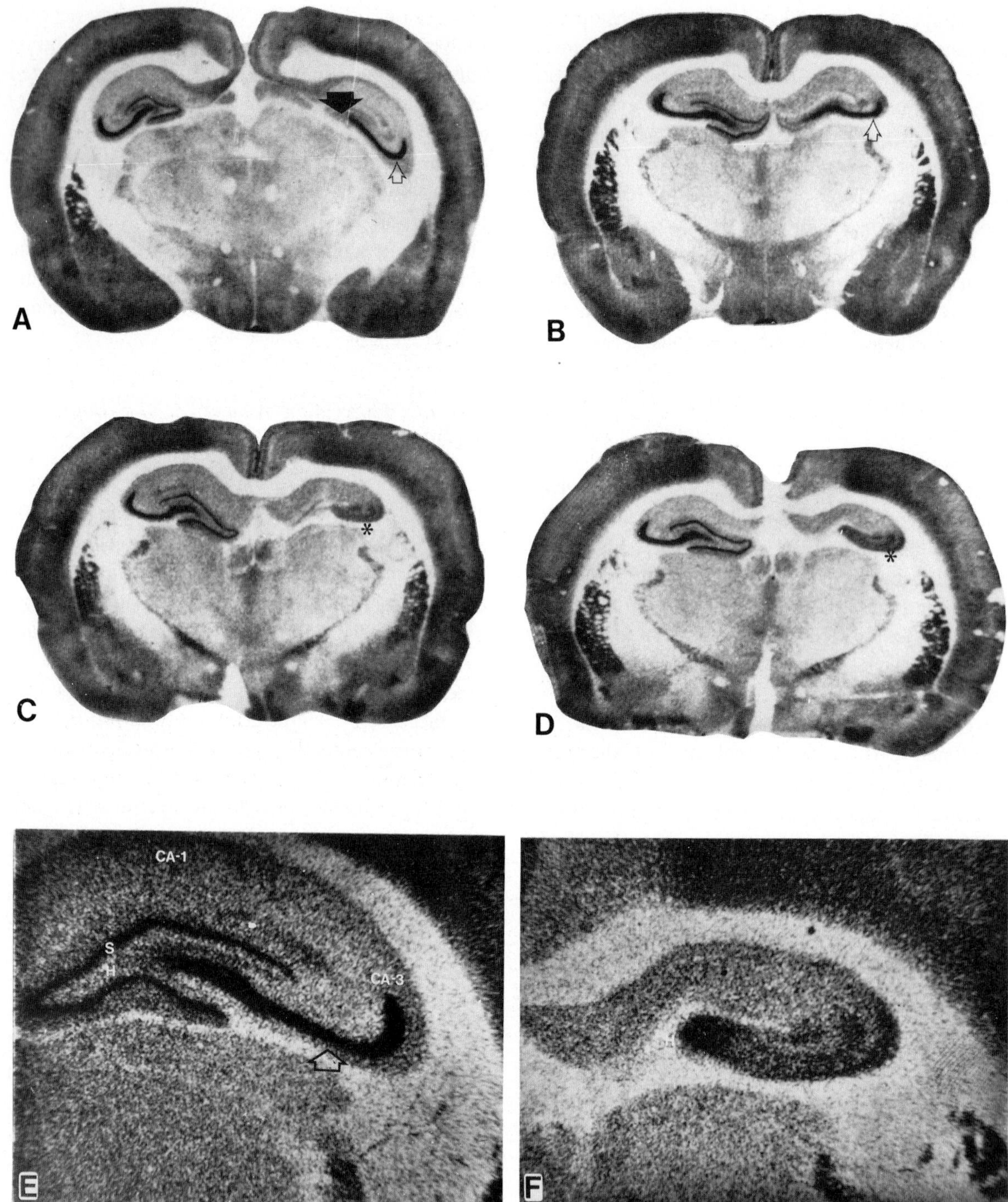

Fig. 4. Representative autoradiograms of [^{3}H]kainic acid binding to sections of rat brains injected with colchicine in the right dentate gyrus (arrow). *A*. Loss of [^{3}H]kainate binding in an animal with total loss of granule cells (degranulated). *B*. Degranulated animal one day after ischemia; no differences from *A*. *C*. Degranulated animal three days following ischemia. *D*. Twenty-one days after ischemia showing redistribution of kainate binding sites in CA3. *E*. Larger magnification from control rat. *F*. Larger magnification from *D* (*).

dal cell layer are interneurons) to about 20% (Diemer et al., 1987).

Effect of denervation on transmitter release in hippocampus

One of the parameters contributing to hippocampal ischemic damage is the release of the excitatory amino acids glutamate and aspartate. They are released (together with GABA and taurine) in both hippocampus and striatum, whereas it is not known whether they are released in non-vulnerable regions. There is both a calcium-dependent and a calcium-independent component, but during the first 10 min of ischemia only the calcium-dependent pool is released (transmitter glutamate); later also glutamate from the metabolic pool is released (see Kauppinen et al., 1988). It takes 5 – 10 min before extracellular glutamate is cleared (Benveniste et al., 1989).

In the denervated rat (kainic acid-induced destruction of CA3 and its axons to CA1), 10 min of ischemia did not produce the dramatic increase of extracellular glutamate or aspartate seen in non-lesioned animals (Benveniste et al., 1984) and extracellular calcium did not decrease significantly (Benveniste and Diemer, 1988). However, GABA showed a similar pronounced increase as in non-lesioned ischemic rats, illustrating that GABA (stored in interneurons) can be released by potassium, which is released slowly during ischemia in the denervated rats (Benveniste et al., unpublished results).

Protection against ischemia-induced damage with glutamate antagonists

Pharmacological blockade of the transmission at glutamatergic synapses has been the subject of a number of studies. With regard to the three main groups of ionotropic glutamate receptors (NMDA, AMPA and kainate), most antagonists available until recently were of the NMDA type, competitive and non-competitive. Studies of their efficacy in cerebral ischemia experiments have been reviewed by Meldrum (1990) and Buchan (1990). A number of studies have shown that the volume of a cortical infarct can be reduced significantly by NMDA an-

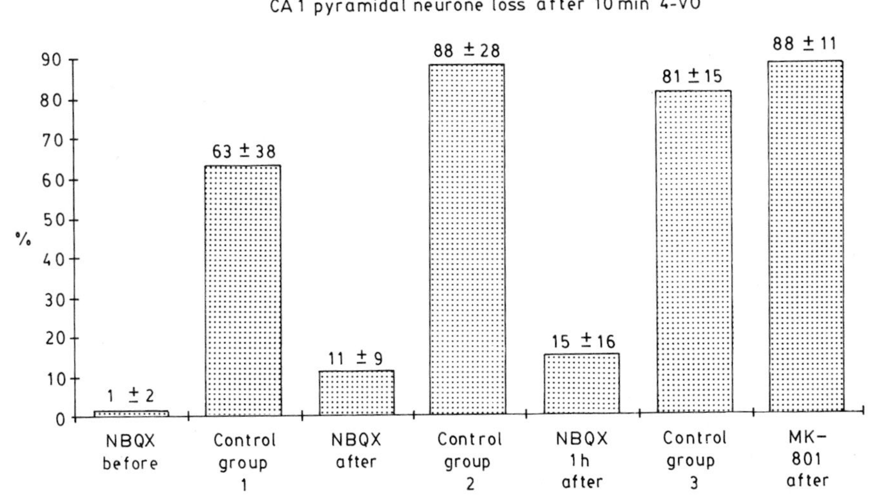

Fig. 5. Per cent loss of CA1 pyramidal cells six days after 10 min of 4-VO ischemia plus hypotension. Three groups of animals were given the AMPA antagonist NBQX (30 mg/kg i.p.) before, immediately after and 1 h after ischemia with three untreated groups serving as controls. All the NBQX treated groups showed a significant protection. One group of rats was given the NMDA antagonist MK-801 (5 mg/kg i.v.) immediately after ischemia. The CA1 neuron loss in this group was not different from that of the control group.

tagonists, also if given after the vascular occlusion. Their effect in reducing global ischemia is controversial (Fig. 5; Meldrum, 1990; Buchan, 1990; Diemer et al., 1992), and in studies in which a protective effect has been reported, the effect of a deranged temperature control due to the combination of ischemia plus an NMDA antagonist cannot be excluded (Buchan, 1990). Recently, an AMPA antagonist, NBQX, which penetrates the blood-brain barrier in sufficient amounts became available. In gerbils subjected to 5 min of ischemia it had a pronounced protective effect on the CA1 pyramidal cells, when given immediately or 2 h after ischemia (Sheardown et al., 1990). Also in rats with 4-VO plus hypotension (Fig. 5; Diemer et al., 1992) and rats with 2-VO plus hypotension, the protective effect was striking, not only in hippocampus but also in cortex and striatum (Nellgård and Wieloch, 1992). Even when NBQX was administered 6 h after 5 min ischemia in the gerbil, there was a clear protective effect (Sheardown et al., 1990). Further, NBQX has been tested in rat models of focal ischemia and also in such cases a protective effect was found (Gill and Lodge, 1991). Another AMPA antagonist, AMOA (Krogsgaard-Larsen et al., 1991), which was given intracerebroventricularly, also offered a pronounced protection of CA1 pyramidal cells after 10 min of 4-VO plus hypotension (Diemer et al., 1992). When tested in rats with 20 min of 4-VO, NBQX and GYKI-52466 produced a marked protection in striatum, cortex and in the CA3 area, whereas no protection was observed in CA1, CA2 and CA4 (Le Peillet et al., 1991).

Another prominent, ischemia-vulnerable neuron is the Purkinje cell which is GABAergic and innervates the inferior olivary nucleus. It receives its main excitatory (glutamatergic) input from the cerebellar granule cells. Its dendritic field is located in the molecular layer. Also, in the rat, the density of NMDA receptors is low in this layer, whereas the AMPA binding density is high. Whether this neuron type can be protected by AMPA antagonists is not known at present. The Purkinje cell content of the calcium-binding protein parvalbumin (Heizmann, 1984) exemplifies that this protein is not an indicator of non-vulnerability to cerebral ischemia.

A tentative explanation for the protective mechanism of AMPA antagonists is that vulnerable nerve cells (all of which have AMPA receptors?) are sensitized by the high extracellular glutamate concentration during ischemia. Although the glutamate (and aspartate) levels are close to pre-ischemic values after ischemia, the normal physiological glutamatergic excitation of sensitized neurons leads to irreversible damage. This is supported by both the protective effect of post-ischemic Schafferotomy (Johansen et al., 1987) and delayed administration of the AMPA antagonist, NBQX (Sheardown et al., 1990). Whether the AMPA receptor-mediated pathology is due to post-ischemic increase of the AMPA receptor transduction, or the cell is not able to sequester normal calcium influx (Siesjö, 1990) are nearby possibilities, which could explain the glutamate-mediated cell death.

References

Amaral, D.G. (1978) A Golgi study of the cell types in the hilar region of the hippocampus in the rat. *J. Comp. Neurol.,* 182: 851 – 914.

Andiné, P., Orwar, O., Jacobson, I., Sandberg, M. and Hagberg, H. (1991) Changes in extracellular amino acids and spontaneous neuronal activity during ischemia and extended reflow in the CA1 of the rat hippocampus. *J. Neurochem.,* 57: 222 – 229.

Araki, T., Kato, H. and Kogure, K. (1989) Selective neuronal vulnerability following transient cerebral ischemia in the gerbil: distribution and time course. *Acta Neurol. Scand.,* 80: 548 – 553.

Auer, R.N., Wieloch, T., Olsson, B. and Siesjö, B.K. (1984) The distribution of hypoglycemic brain damage. *Acta Neuropathol. (Berl.),* 64: 177 – 191.

Bakst, I., Avendano, C., Morrison, J.H. and Amaral, D.G. (1986) An experimental analysis of the origins of somatostatin-like immunoreactivity in the dentate gyrus of the rat. *J. Neurosci.,* 6(5): 1452 – 1462.

Benveniste, H. and Diemer, N.H. (1988) Early postischemic ^{45}Ca accumulation in rat dentate hilus. *J. Cereb. Blood Flow Metab.,* 8: 713 – 719.

Benveniste, H., Drejer, J., Schousboe, A. and Diemer, N.H. (1984) Elevation of extracellular concentrations of glutamate and aspartate in rat hippocampus during transient cerebral ischemia monitored by intracerebral microdialysis. *J. Neurochem.,* 43: 1369 – 1374.

Benveniste, H., Jørgensen, M.B., Sandberg, M., Hagberg, H. and Diemer, N.H. (1989) Ischemic damage in hippocampal CA1 is dependent on glutamate-release and intact innervation from CA3. *J. Cereb. Blood Flow Metab.,* 9: 629 – 639.

Berridge, M.J. (1987) Inositol trisphosphate and diacylglycerol: two interacting second messengers. *Annu. Rev. Biochem.,* 56: 615 – 649.

Brierley, J.B. and Graham, D.I. (1984) Hypoxia and vascular disorders of the central nervous system. In: *Greenfields Neuropathology,* Edward Arnold, London, pp. 125 – 207.

Brown, A.W., Levy, D.E., Kublik, M., Harrow, J., Plum, F. and Brierley, J.B. (1979) Selective chromatolysis of neurons in the gerbil brain: a possible consequence of "epileptic" activity produced by common carotid artery occlusion. *Ann. Neurol.,* 5: 127 – 138.

Bruhn, T., Cobo, M., Berg, M. and Diemer, N.H. (1992) Limbic seizure-induced changes in extracellular amino acid levels in the hippocampal formation: a microdialysis study on freely moving rats. (Submitted.)

Buchan, A. (1990) Do NMDA antagonists protect against cerebral ischemia: are clinical trials warranted? *Cerebrovasc. Brain Metab. Rev.,* 2: 1 – 26.

Buzsáki, G., Freund, T.F., Bayardo, F. and Somogyi, P. (1989) Ischemia-induced changes in the electrical activity of the hippocampus. *Exp. Brain Res.,* 78: 268 – 278.

Cammermeyer, J. (1961) The importance of avoiding "dark" neurons in experimental neuropathology. *Acta Neuropathol. (Berl.),* 1: 245 – 270.

Chang, H.S., Steward, O. and Kassel, N.F. (1989) Decreases in excitatory transmission and increases in recurrent inhibition in the rat dentate gyrus after transient cerebral ischemia. *Brain Res.,* 505: 220 – 224.

Chen, C.-K., Silverstein, F.S., Fisher, S.K., Statman, D. and Johnston, M. (1988) Perinatal hypoxic-ischemic brain injury enhances quisqualic acid-stimulated phosphoinositide turnover. *J. Neurochem.,* 51: 353 – 359.

Choi, D.W., Maulucci-Gedde, M. and Kriegstein, A.R. (1987) Glutamate neurotoxicity in cortical cell culture. *J. Neurosci.,* 7: 357 – 368.

Christensen, T., Bruhn, T., Diemer, N.H. and Schousboe, A. (1991) Effect of phenylsuccinate on potassium- and ischemia-induced release of glutamate in rat hippocampus monitored by microdialysis. *Neurosci. Lett.,* 134: 71 – 74.

Cooper, H.K., Zalewska, T., Kawakami, S., Hossmann, K.-A. and Kleihues, P. (1977) The effect of ischemia and recirculation on protein synthesis in the rat brain. *J. Neurochem.,* 28: 929 – 934.

Curran, T. (1988) The fos oncogene. In: E.P. Reddy, A.M. Skalka and T. Curran (Eds.), *The Oncogene Handbook,* Elsevier, Amsterdam, pp. 307 – 325.

Davies, S.N., Alford, S.T., Coan, E.J., Lester, R.A.J. and Collingridge, G.L. (1988) Ketamine blocks an NMDA receptor-mediated component of synaptic transmission in rat hippocampus in a voltage-dependent manner. *Neurosci. Lett.,* 92: 213 – 217.

Deshpande, J.K., Siesjö, B.K. and Wieloch, T. (1987) Calcium accumulation and neuronal damage in the rat hippocampus following cerebral ischemia. *J. Cereb. Blood Flow Metab.,* 7: 89 – 95.

Deshpande, J.K., Bergstedt, K., Lindén, T., Kalimo, H. and Wieloch, T. (1992) Ultrastructural changes in the hippocampal CA1 region following transient cerebral ischemia: evidence against programmed cell death. *Exp. Brain Res.,* 88: 91 – 105.

Diemer, N.H. and Siemkowicz, E. (1980a) Increased 2-deoxyglucose uptake in hippocampus, globus pallidus and substantia nigra after cerebral ischemia. *Acta Neurol. Scand.,* 61: 56 – 63.

Diemer, N.H. and Siemkowicz, E. (1980b) Regional glucose metabolism and nerve cell damage after cerebral ischemia in normo- and hypoglycemic rats. In: M. Spatz, B.B. Mrsjulja, L.J. Rakic and W.D. Lust (Eds.), *Circulatory and Developmental Aspects of Brain Metabolism,* Plenum, New York, pp. 23 – 32.

Diemer, N.H. and Siemkowicz, E. (1981) Regional neurone damage after cerebral ischemia in the normo- and hypoglycemic rat. *Neuropathol. Appl. Neurobiol.,* 7: 217 – 227.

Diemer, N.H., Jørgensen, M.B. and Johansen, F.F. (1987) Significance on intra- and postischemic pathophysiological processes for development of ischemic nerve cell loss. In: M.E. Raichle and W.J. Powers (Eds.), *Cerebrovascular Diseases,* Raven Press, New York.

Diemer, N.H., Johansen, F.F. and Jørgensen, M.B. (1990) *N*-Methyl-D-aspartate and non-*N*-methyl-D-aspartate antagonists in global cerebral ischemia. *Stroke,* 21 (Suppl. III): III-39 – III-42.

Diemer, N.H., Jørgensen, M.B., Johansen, F.F., Sheardown, M. and Honoré, T. (1992) Protection against hippocampal CA1 damage in the rat with a new non-NMDA antagonist, NBQX. *Acta Neurol. Scand.,* in press.

Dienel, G.A. (1984) Regional accumulation of calcium in postischemic rat brain. *J. Neurochem.,* 43: 913 – 925.

Dragunow, M. and Robertson, H.A. (1987) Kindling stimulation induces *c-fos* protein(s) in granule cells of the rat dentate gyrus. *Nature,* 329: 441 – 442.

Drejer, J., Benveniste, H., Diemer, H. and Schousboe, A. (1985) Cellular origin of ischemia-induced glutamate release from brain tissue in vivo and in vitro. *J. Neurochem.,* 45: 145 – 151.

Fieschi, C., Sakurada, O. and Sokoloff, L. (1978) Local cerebral glucose utilization during resolution of embolic experimental ischemia. In: J. Cervos-Navarro et al. (Eds.), *Advances of Neurology, Vol. 20,* Raven Press, New York, pp. 223 – 229.

Fink, R.P. and Heimer, L. (1967) Two methods for selective silver impregnation of degenerating axons and their synaptic endings in the central nervous system. *Brain Res.,* 4: 369 – 374.

Franck, J.E., Kunkel, D.D., Baskin, D.G. and Schwartzkroin,

P.A. (1988) Inhibition in kainate-lesioned hyperexcitable hippocampi: physiologic, autoradiographic and immunocytochemical observations. *J. Neurosci.,* 8: 1991 – 2002.

Frederickson, C.J., Hernandez, M.D. and McGinty, J.F. (1989) Translocation of zinc may contribute to seizure-induced death of neurons. *Brain Res.,* 480: 317 – 321.

Gehrmann, J., Bonnekoh, P., Miyazawa, T., Hossmann, K.-A. and Kreutzberg, G.W. (1992) Immunocytochemical study of an early microglial activation in ischemia. *J. Cereb. Blood Flow Metab.,* 12: 257 – 269.

Gill and Lodge (1991) The neuroprotective action of 2,3-dihydro-6-nitro-7-sulfamoyl-benzo(F)quinoxaline (NBQX) in a rat focal ischemia model. *Br. J. Physiol.,* 102: 61P.

Globus, M.Y.T., Busto, R., Dietrich, D., Martinez, E., Valdes, I. and Ginsberg, M.D. (1988) Effect of ischemia on the in vivo release of striatal dopamine, glutamate and γ-aminobutyric acid studied by intracerebral microdialysis. *J. Neurochem.,* 51: 1455 – 1464.

Gottlieb, D.I. and Cowan, W.M. (1973) Autoradiographic studies of the commisural and ipsilateral association connections of the hippocampus and dentate of the rat. *J. Comp. Neurol.,* 149: 393 – 422.

Hagberg, H., Lehmann, A., Sandberg, M., Nyström, B., Jacobson, I. and Hamberger, A. (1985) Ischemia-induced shift of inhibitory and excitatory amino acids from intra- to extracellular compartments. *J. Cereb. Blood Flow Metab.,* 5: 413 – 419.

Hansen, A.J. (1985) Effect of anoxia on ion distribution in the brain. *Physiol. Rev.,* 65: 101 – 148.

Heizmann, C.W. (1984) Parvalbumin, an intracellular calcium binding protein; distribution, properties and possible roles in mammalian cells. *Experientia,* 40: 910 – 921.

Herreras, O., Menendez, N., Herranz, A., et al. (1989) Synaptic transmission at the Schaffer-CA1 synapse is blocked by 6,7-dinitro-quinoxaline-2,3-dione. An in vivo brain dialysis study in the rat. *Neurosci. Lett.,* 99: 119 – 124.

Honoré, T., Davis, S.N., Drejer, J., Fletcher, J.E., Jacobsen, P., Lodge, D. and Nielsen, F.E. (1988) Quinoxaline diones: potent competitive non-NMDA glutamate receptor antagonists. *Science,* 241: 701 – 703.

Hunt, P.H., Pini, A. and Evan, G. (1987) Induction of *c-fos*-like protein in spinal cord neurons following sensory stimulation. *Nature,* 328: 632 – 634.

Ikeda, M., Yoshida, S., Busto, R., Santiso, M. and Ginsberg, M.D. (1986) Polyphosphoinositides as a probable source of brain free fatty acids accumulated at the onset of ischemia. *J. Neurochem.,* 47: 123 – 132.

Ikeda, M., Nakazawa, T., Abe, K., Kaneko, T. and Yamatsy, K. (1989) Extracellular accumulation of glutamate in the hippocampus induced by ischemia is not calcium dependent – in vitro and in vivo evidence. *Neurosci. Lett.,* 96: 202 – 206.

Ito, U., Spatz, M., Walker Jr., J.T. and Klatzo, I. (1975) Experimental cerebral ischemia in Mongolian gerbil. I. Light microscopic observations. *Acta Neuropathol. (Berl.),* 32: 209 – 233.

Jensen, M.S., Lambert, J.D.C. and Johansen, F.F. (1991) Electrophysiological recordings from rat hippocampus slices following in vivo brain ischemia. *Brain Res.,* 554: 166 – 175.

Johansen, F.F. and O'Hare, M.M.T. (1989) Loss of neuropeptide Y immunoreactivity in the rat hippocampus following transient cerebral ischaemia. *J. Neurosurg. Anesthesiol.,* 1(4): 339 – 345.

Johansen, F.F., Jørgensen, M.B. and Diemer, N.H. (1983) Resistance of hippocampal CA1 interneurons to 20 min of transient cerebral ischemia in the rat. *Acta Neuropathol. (Berl.),* 61: 135 – 140.

Johansen, F.F., Jørgensen, M.B., von Lubitz, D.K.J.E. and Diemer, N.H. (1984) Selective dendrite damage in hippocampal CA1 stratum radiatum with unchanged axon ultrastructure and glutamate uptake after transient cerebral ischemia in the rat. *Brain Res.,* 291: 373 – 377.

Johansen, F.F., Jørgensen, M.B. and Diemer, N.H. (1986) Ischemia-induced delayed neuronal death in the CA1 hippocampus is dependent on intact glutamatergic innervation. In: T.P. Hicks, D. Lodge and H. McLennan (Eds.), *Excitatory Amino Acid Transmission. Neurology and Neurobiology,* Alan R. Liss, New York, pp. 245 – 248.

Johansen, F.F., Zimmer, J. and Diemer, N.H. (1987) Early damage of somatostatin neurons in dentate hilus after cerebral ischaemia in the rat precedes CA-1 pyramidal cell loss. *Acta Neuropathol. (Berl.),* 73: 110 – 114.

Johansen, F.F., Lin, C.-T., Schousboe, A. and Wu, J.-Y. (1989) Immunocytochemical investigation of L-glutamic acid decarboxylase in the rat hippocampal formation: the influence of transient cerebral ischaemia. *J. Comp. Neurol.,* 281: 40 – 53.

Johansen, F.F., Tønder, N., Zimmer, J., Baimbridge, K.G. and Diemer, N.H. (1990) Short-term changes of parvalbumin and calbindin immunoreactivity in the rat hippocampus following cerebral ischaemia. *Neurosci. Lett.,* 120: 171 – 174.

Johansen, F.F., Sørensen, T., Tønder, N., Zimmer, J. and Diemer, N.H. (1992) Ultrastructure of neurons containing somatostatin in the dentate hilus of the rat hippocampus after cerebral ischemia, and a note on their commissural connections. *Neuropathol. Appl. Neurobiol.,* 18: 145 – 147.

Jørgensen, M.B. and Diemer, N.H. (1982) Selective neuron loss after cerebral ischemia in the rat: possible role of transmitter glutamate. *Acta Neurol. Scand.,* 66: 536 – 546.

Jørgensen, M.B., Johansen, F.F. and Diemer, N.H. (1987) Removal of the entorhinal cortex protects hippocampal CA1 neurons from ischemic damage. *Acta Neuropathol. (Berl.),* 73: 189 – 194.

Jørgensen, M.B., Deckert, J. and Wright, D.C. (1989a) The binding of second messenger ligands IP3 and PDBU to rat hippocampus following transient global ischemia: a quantitative autoradiographic study. *Neurosci. Lett.,* 103: 219 – 224.

Jørgensen, M.B., Deckert, J., Wright, D.C. and Gehlert, D.R. (1989b) Delayed *c-fos* proto-oncogene expression in the rat hippocampus induced by transient global cerebral ischemia:

an in situ hybridization study. *Brain Res.*, 484: 393 – 398.

Jørgensen, M.B., Wright, D.C. and Diemer, N.H. (1990) Postischemic glucose metabolism is modified in the hippocampal CA1 depleted of excitatory input or pyramidal cells. *J. Cereb. Blood Flow Metab.*, 10: 243 – 251.

Jørgensen, M.B., Jensen, C.V. and Diemer, N.H. (1991a) The binding of [^{3}H]inositoltrisphosphate to kainic acid lesioned and postischemic rat hippocampus. *Brain Res.*, 538: 246 – 250.

Jørgensen, M.B., Johansen, F.F. and Diemer, N.H. (1991b) Postischemic and kainic acid induced *c-fos* protein expression in the rat brain. *Acta Neurol. Scand.*, in press.

Kauppinen, R.A., McMahon, H.T. and Nicholls, D.G. (1988) Ca^{2+}-dependent and Ca^{2+}-independent glutamate release, energy status and cytosolic free Ca^{2+} concentration in isolated nerve terminals following metabolic inhibition: possible relevance to hypoglycemia and anoxia. *Neuroscience*, 27: 175 – 182.

Kirino, T. (1982) Delayed neuronal death in the gerbil hippocampus following ischemia. *Brain Res.*, 239: 235 – 244.

Kirino, T. and Sano, K. (1984) Selective vulnerability in the gerbil hippocampus following transient ischemia. *Acta Neuropathol. (Berl.)*, 62: 201 – 208.

Kirino, T., Tamura, A. and Sano, K. (1988) Early and late neuronal damage following cerebral ischemia. In: G. Somjen (Ed.), *Mechanisms of Cerebral Hypoxia and Stroke*, Plenum Press, New York, pp. 23 – 34.

Kirino, T., Tamura, A. and Sano, K. (1990) Chronic maintenance of presynaptic terminals in gliotic hippocampus following ischemia. *Brain Res.*, 239: 57 – 69.

Kobayashi, M., Lust, W.D. and Passoneau, J.V. (1977) Concentrations of energy metabolites and cyclic nucleotides during and after bilateral ischemia in the gerbil cerebral cortex. *J. Neurochem.*, 29: 53 – 59.

Köhler, C., Schwarz, R. and Fuxe, K. (1978) Perforant path transections protect hippocampal granule cells from kainate lesion. *Neurosci. Lett.*, 10: 241 – 246.

Köhler, C., Eriksson, L.G., Davis, S. and Chan-Palay, V. (1987) Co-localization of neuropeptide tyrosine and somatostatin immunoreactivity in neurons of individual subfields of the rat hippocampal region. *Neurosci. Lett.*, 78: 1 – 6.

Korf, J., Klein, H.C., Venema, K. and Postema, F. (1988) Increases in striatal and hippocampal impedance and extracellular levels of amino acids by cardiac arrest in freely moving rats. *J. Neurochem.*, 50: 1087 – 1096.

Krogsgaard-Larsen, P., Honoré, T., Hansen, J.J., Curtis, D.R. and Lodge, D. (1980) New class of glutamate agonists structurally related to ibotenic acid. *Nature*, 284: 64 – 66.

Krogsgaard-Larsen, P., Ferkany, J.W., Nielsen, E.Ø., Madsen, U., Ebert, B., Johansen, J.S., Diemer, N.H., Bruhn, T., Beattie, D.T. and Curtis, D.R. (1991) Novel class of amino acid antagonists at non-*N*-methyl-D-aspartic acid excitatory amino acid receptors. Synthesis, in vitro and in vivo pharmacology, and neuroprotection. *J. Med. Chem.*, 34: 123 – 130.

Lehmann, A., Isacsson, H. and Hamberger, A. (1983) Effects of in vivo administration of kainic acid on the extracellular amino acid pool in the rabbit hippocampus. *J. Neurochem.*, 40: 1314 – 1320.

Le Peillet, E., Arvin, B., Moncada, C. and Meldrum, B.S. (1991) Protection by 2 non-NMDA antagonists, NBQX and GYKI-52466, against selective cell loss following transient global ischaemia (4VO) in the rat. In: *The Role of Neurotransmitters in Brain Injury, Key West, June 7 – 9,* Abstracts, p. 21.

Masu, M., Tanabe, Y., Tsuchida, K., Shigemoto, R. and Nakanishi, S. (1991) Sequence and expression of a metabotropic glutamate receptor. *Nature*, 349: 760 – 765.

Meldrum, B. (1990) Protection against neuronal damage by drugs acting on excitatory neurotransmission. *Cerebrovasc. Brain Metab. Rev.*, 2: 27 – 57.

Meyer, F.B., Anderson, R.E. and Sundt Jr., T.M. (1989) Calcium, neuronal hyperexcitability and ischemic neuronal injury. In: A. Hartmann and W. Kuschinsky (Eds.), *Cerebral Ischemia and Calcium,* Springer, Berlin, Heidelberg, pp. 429 – 439.

Mitani, A. and Kataoka, K. (1991) Critical levels of extracellular glutamate mediating gerbil hippocampal delayed neuronal death during hypothermia: brain microdialysis study. *Neuroscience*, 42: 661 – 670.

Monaghan, D.T., Holets, R.V., Toy, D.W. and Cotman, C.W. (1983) Anatomical distributions of four pharmacologically distinct ^{3}H-glutamate binding sites. *Nature*, 306: 176 – 179.

Morgan, J.I. and Curran, T. (1986) Role of ion flux in the control of *c-fos* expression. *Nature*, 322: 552 – 554.

Morgan, J.I., Cohen, D.R., Hemstead, J.L. and Curran, T. (1987) Mapping patterns of *c-fos* in the central nervous system after seizure. *Science*, 237: 192 – 197.

Nellgård, B. and Wieloch, T. (1992) Differential protection by 2,3-dihydro-6-nitro-7-silfamoyl-benzo(F)quinoxaline (NBQX) and dizocilpine (MK-801) following complete ischemia and insulin-induced hypoglycemia in the rat. *J. Cereb. Blood Flow Metab.*, 12: 2 – 11.

Nicholls, D. and Atwell, D. (1990) The release and uptake of excitatory amino acids. In: D. Lodge and D. Collingridge (Eds.), *The Pharmacology of Excitatory Amino Acids – Trends in Pharmacological Sciences,* Elsevier, Cambridge, pp. 68 – 73.

Nitsch, C., Scotti, A., Sommacal, A. and Kalt, G. (1979) GABAergic hippocampal neurons resistant to ischemia-induced neuronal death contain the Ca^{2+} binding protein parvalbumin. *Neurosci. Lett.*, 105: 263 – 268.

Nowak Jr., T.S., Ikeda, J. and Nakajima, T. (1990) 70 Kilodalton heat shock protein and *c-fos* gene expression following transient ischemia. *J. Neurochem.*, 54: 451 – 458.

Onodera, H. and Kogure, K. (1989) Mapping second messengers in the rat hippocampus after transient forebrain ischemia: in vitro [^{3}H]forskolin and [^{3}H]inositol 1,4,5-trisphosphate binding. *Brain Res.*, 487: 343 – 349.

Onodera, H., Kogure, K., Ono, Y., Igarashi, K., Kiyota, Y. and Nagaoka, A. (1989) Proto-oncogene *c-fos* is transiently induced in the rat cerebral cortex after forebrain ischemia. *Neurosci. Lett.*, 98: 101 – 104.

Palmer, E., Monaghan, D.T. and Cotman, C.W. (1989) Trans-ACPD, a selective agonist of the phosphoinositide-coupled excitatory amino acid receptors. *Eur. J. Pharmacol.*, 166: 585 – 587.

Pappius, H.M. (1988) Significance of biogeneic amines in functional disturbances resulting from brain injury. *Metab. Brain Dis.*, 3: 303 – 310.

Petito, C.K., Feldmann, E., Pulsinelli, W.A. and Plum, F. (1987) Delayed hippocampal damage in humans following cardiorespiratory arrest. *Neurology*, 37: 1281 – 1286.

Pulsinelli, W. and Brierley, J.B. (1979) A new model of bilateral hemispheric ischemia in the unanesthetized rat. *Stroke*, 10: 267 – 272.

Pulsinelli, W., Brierley, J. and Plum, F. (1982a) Temporal profile of neuronal damage in a model of transient forebrain ischemia. *Ann. Neurol.*, 11: 491 – 498.

Pulsinelli, W.A., Levy, D.E. and Duffy, T.E. (1982b) Regional cerebral blood flow and glucose metabolism following transient forebrain ischemia. *Ann. Neurol.*, 11: 499 – 509.

Reivich, M., Jehle, J., Sokoloff, L. and Kety, S.S. (1969) Measurement of regional cerebral blood flow with antipyrine-^{14}C in awake cats. *J. Appl. Physiol.*, 27: 296 – 300.

Rischke, R., Rami, A., Bachmann, U., Rabié, A. and Krieglstein, J. (1990) Different vulnerability to ischemia of pre- and postsynaptic terminals in rat hippocampus. In: J. Krieglstein and H. Oberpichler (Eds.), *Pharmacology of Cerebral Ischemia*, Wissenschaftliche Verlagsgesellschaft mbH, Stuttgart, pp. 129 – 134.

Sagar, S.M., Sharp, F.R. and Curran, T. (1988) Expression of *c-fos* protein in brain: metabolic mapping at the cellular level. *Science*, 240: 1328 – 1331.

Sánchez-Prieto, J. and González, P. (1988) Occurrence of a large Ca^{2+}-independent release of glutamate during anoxia in isolated nerve terminals (synaptosomes). *J. Neurochem.*, 50: 1322 – 1324.

Schoepp, D., Bockaert, J. and Sladecek, F. (1990) Pharmacological and functional characteristics of metabotropic excitatory amino acid receptors. *Trends Pharmacol. Sci.*, 11: 508 – 515.

Schousboe, A., Fosmark, H. and Hertz, L. (1975) High content of glutamate and of ATP in astrocytes cultured from rat brain hemispheres: effect of serum withdrawal and of cyclic AMP. *J. Neurochem.*, 25: 909 – 911.

Seren, M.S., Aldino, C., Zanoni, R., Leon, A. and Nicoletti, F. (1989) Stimulation of inositol phospholipid hydrolysis by excitatory amino acids is enhanced in brain slices from vulnerable regions after transient global ischemia. *J. Neurochem.*, 53: 1700 – 1705.

Sheardown, M.J., Nielsen, E.Ø., Hansen, A.J., Jacobsen, P. and Honoré, T. (1990) 2,3-Dihydro-6-nitro-7-sulfamoyl-benzo(f)quinoxaline: a neuroprotectant for cerebral ischemia. *Science*, 247: 571 – 574.

Shimada, N., Graf, R., Rosner, G. and Heiss, W.-D. (1990) Differences in ischemia-induced accumulation of amino acids in the cat cortex. *Stroke*, 21: 1445 – 1451.

Siesjö, B.K. (1981) Cell damage in the brain: a speculative synthesis. *J. Cereb. Blood Flow Metab.*, 1: 155 – 185.

Siesjö, B.K. (1988) Mechanisms of ischemic brain damage. *Crit. Care Med.*, 16: 954 – 963.

Siesjö, B.K. (1990) Calcium, excitotoxins and brain damage. *News Physiol. Sci.*, 5: 120 – 125.

Sladeczek, F., Recasens, M. and Bockaert, J. (1988) A new mechanism for glutamate receptor action: phosphoinositide hydrolysis. *Trends Neurosci.*, 11: 545 – 549.

Sloviter, R.S. (1987) Decreased hippocampal inhibition and a selective loss of interneurons in experimental epilepsy. *Science*, 235: 73 – 76.

Sloviter, R.S. (1991) Permanently altered hippocampal structure, excitability, and inhibition after experimental status epilepticus in the rat: the "dormant basket cell" hypothesis and its possible relevance to temporal lobe epilepsia. *Hippocampus*, 1(1): 41 – 66.

Smith, M.L., Bendek, G., Dahlgren, N., Rosén, I., Wieloch, T. and Siesjö, B.K. (1984) Models for studying long-term recovery following forebrain ischemia in the rat. 2. A 2-vessel occlusion model. *Acta Neurol. Scand.*, 69: 385 – 401.

Sokoloff, L., Reivich, M., Kennedy, C., Des Rosiers, M.H., Patlak, C.S., Pettigrew, K.D., Sakurada, O. and Shinohara, M. (1977) The [^{14}C] deoxyglucose method for the measurement of local cerebral glucose utilization: theory, procedure, and normal values in the conscious and anesthetized albono rat. *J. Neurochem.*, 28: 897 – 916.

Sugiyama, H., Ito, I. and Hirono, C. (1987) A new type of glutamate receptor linked to inositol phospholipid metabolism. *Nature*, 325: 531 – 533.

Sun, G.Y., Huang, H.M. and Chandrasekhar, R. (1988) Turnover of inositol phosphates in brain during ischemia-induced breakdown of polyphosphoinositides. *Neurochem. Int.*, 13: 63 – 68.

Swanson, L.W., Wyss, J.M. and Cowan, W.M. (1978) An autoradiographic study of the organisation of intrahippocampal association pathways in the rat. *J. Comp. Neurol.*, 172: 49 – 84.

Thilmann, R., Xie, Y., Kleihues, P. and Kiessling, M. (1986) Persistent inhibition of protein synthesis precedes delayed neuronal death in the gerbil. *Acta Neuropathol. (Berl.)*, 71: 88 – 93.

Tønder, N., Johansen, F.F., Frederickson, C.J., Zimmer, J. and Diemer, N.H. (1990) Possible role of zinc in the selective degeneration of dentate hilar neurons after cerebral ischaemia in the adult rat. *Neurosci. Lett.*, 109: 247 – 252.

Von Lubitz, D.K.J.E. and Diemer, N.H. (1982) Complete cerebral ischemia in the rat: an ultrastructural and stereological analysis of the distal stratum radiatum in the hippocampal CA-1 region. *Neuropathol. Appl. Neurobiol.*, 8: 197 – 215.

Watkins, J.C. and Evans, R.H. (1981) Excitatory amino acid transmitters. *Annu. Rev. Pharmacol. Toxicol.,* 21: 165 – 204.

Westerberg, E., Monaghan, D.T., Cotman, C.W. and Wieloch, T. (1987) Excitatory amino acid receptors and ischemic brain damage in the rat. *Neurosci. Lett.,* 73: 119 – 124.

Wieloch, T., Lindvall, O., Blomquist, P. and Gage, F.H. (1984) Evidence for amelioration of ischemic neuronal damage in the hippocampal formation by lesions of the perforant path. *Neurol. Res.,* 7: 24 – 26.

Yoshida, S., Ikeda, M., Busto, R., Santiso, M., Martinez, E. and Ginsberg, M.D. (1986) Cerebral phosphoinositide, triacylglycerol, and energy metabolism in reversible ischea: origin and fate of free fatty acids. *J. Neurochem.,* 47: 744.

Young, A.B. and Fagg, G.E. (1990) Excitatory amino acid receptors in the brain: membrane binding and receptor autoradiographic approaches. In: D. Lodge and G. Collingridge (Eds.), *The Pharmacology of Excitatory Amino Acids – Trends in Pharmacological Sciences,* Elsevier, Cambridge, pp. 18 – 21.

K. Kogure, K.-A. Hossmann and B.K. Siesjö (Eds.)
Progress in Brain Research, Vol. 96

CHAPTER 8

Antagonism of the NMDA and non-NMDA receptors in global versus focal brain ischemia

William Pulsinelli, Abigail Sarokin and Alastair Buchan[1]

Cerebrovascular Disease Research Center, Department of Neurology and Neuroscience, Cornell University Medical College, New York, N.Y. 10021, U.S.A., and [1]Neuroscience Research, Ottawa Civic Hospital, Ottawa, Ont., K1Y4E9 Canada

Introduction

Research into the pathogenesis of a variety of neurologic diseases changed focus in the late 1970s due largely to John Olney's excitotoxic theory (Olney, 1978). Olney's theory, that neuronal death was caused by pathologic stimulation of excitatory amino acids spearheaded the move towards examining the common role of excitatory amino acids in brain damage caused by epilepsy, stroke and neurodegenerative disease. Several laboratories substantiated the excitotoxic theory with in vitro studies (Rothman, 1985; Garthwaite and Garthwaite, 1986; Choi, 1987) while others focused on the imbalance between neuronal excitation and inhibition in in vivo models of global brain ischemia (Meldrum, 1981; Francis and Pulsinelli, 1982; Jørgensen and Diemer, 1982). Since then, many articles have been published on excitatory/inhibitory neurotransmitters and their role in brain damage from cardiac arrest and stroke (see for reviews, Buchan, 1990; Meldrum, 1990).

Much of this research has focused on the *N*-methyl-D-aspartate (NMDA) receptor/channel's function in injury from global and focal brain ischemia since this channel is known to be permeable to calcium ions. However, while there is largely a consensus among investigators that antagonists of the NMDA receptor/channel reduce infarction volume in animal models of focal (moderate) brain ischemia, there is a lack of agreement as to their effectiveness in models of transient but severe forebrain ischemia. This disagreement may soon become overshadowed by a new class of antagonists, selective for the non-NMDA receptors, which appear to offer superior protection from transient severe ischemia. Accordingly, the purpose of this chapter is: (1) to review the existing data from both the literature and our own laboratories concerning the role of the NMDA receptor/channel in ischemic stroke studies, and to propose an explanation for the disparate results associated with its use in animal models of global brain ischemia; and (2) to present recent data on AMPA receptor blockade and highlight why these new antagonists may become the most important therapeutic agents to date in attenuating neuronal damage caused by stroke.

Methods

Transient forebrain ischemia

The modified 4-vessel occlusion model (4-VO) was used to produce transient but severe forebrain ischemia in adult Wistar rats (Pulsinelli and Duffy, 1983; Pulsinelli and Buchan, 1988). After anesthetizing the rats with halothane, reversible clasps were placed loosely around both common carotid arteries. Using electrocauterization, the vertebral arteries were permanently occluded at the first cervical vertebra and a suture was inserted encircling the cervical muscles. During the next 18 – 24 h the animals recovered from the anesthesia; food was withheld during this period. Following the recovery phase both the carotid artery clasps and the suture encircling the paracervical muscles were tightened to produce 5, 10 or 15 min of severe forebrain ischemia. The carotid clasps and cervical suture were released at the end of the ischemic interval. Until the animals regained thermal homeostasis, and throughout the forebrain ischemia/recirculation period, rectal temperature was monitored and maintained at 37 ± 0.5 C. Tail artery blood samples taken from a separate group of rats were used to measure physiological variables such as mean arterial pressure, PO_2, PCO_2 and pH.

Focal cerebral ischemia

Adult spontaneously hypertensive (SH) rats were either subjected to permanent (Brint et al., 1988) or reversible (Buchan et al., 1992a) focal ischemia. The rats were anesthetized with halothane and the right CCA was occluded with a suture. A burr hole made beneath the temporalis muscle allowed access to the distal right MCA. Irreversible ischemia was produced by permanently occluding both the middle cerebral artery (MCA) and the ipsilateral common carotid arteries (CCA). Reversible ischemia was achieved by permanently occluding the CCA and reversibly occluding the MCA. Halothane anesthesia was discontinued just prior to, or immediately after, MCA/CCA occlusion. During surgery and until the animals regained thermal homeostasis during the post-surgery period, rectal temperature was monitored and maintained at 37 ± 0.5 C. Tail artery blood samples from selected animals were used to measure mean arterial blood pressure, PO_2, PCO_2 and pH.

Histopathology

After a survival period of 3 – 7 days, the animals subjected to transient 4-VO ischemia were reanesthetized and killed by perfusion fixation. Paraffin brain sections (7 μm in thickness) were prepared and stained with hematoxylin and eosin. A blinded observer counted normal-appearing neurons from two separate dorsal CA1 hippocampal sections and

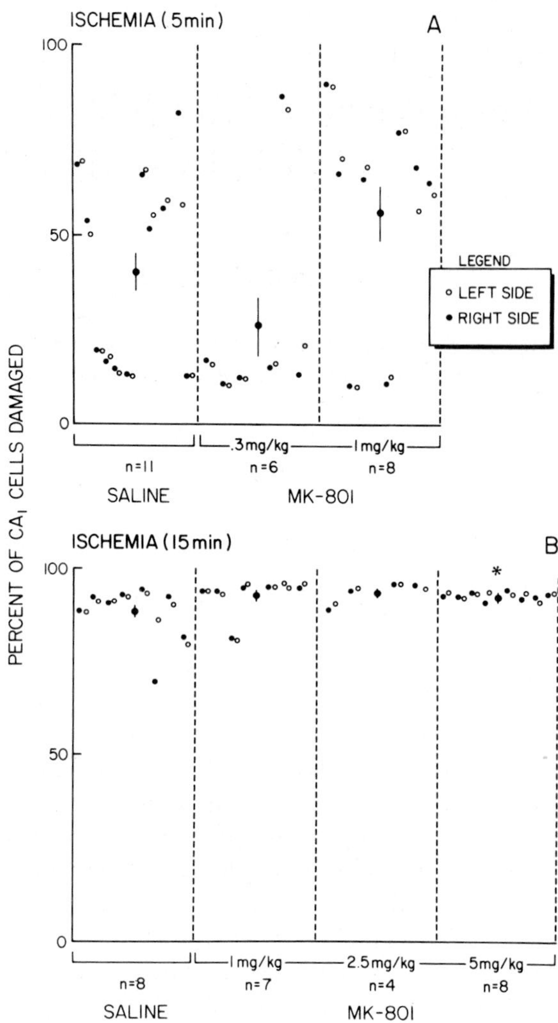

Fig. 1. Percent dead CA1 hippocampal neurons after a single i.p. dose of saline or MK-801 in rats subjected to 5 min (*A*) or 15 min (*B*) of 4-VO ischemia. The open and filled small circles represent the percent dead neurons in the left and right hippocampus of each animal, respectively. The larger filled circles with error bars represent the group mean ± S.E. Asterisk denotes $P < 0.05$ compared to saline-treated controls. (Data from Buchan et al., 1991b; reprinted with permission from Pulsinelli et al., 1992.)

this number was subtracted from a previously determined value for the number of normal neurons at this hippocampal level. Results are reported as percent dead neurons in the CA1 zone.

After a 24 h survival period, those animals subjected to focal cerebral ischemia were anesthetized and decapitated. Their brains were frozen in freon or isopentane over dry ice and 20 μm thick sections were cut every 500 μm at −25°C. The frozen sections were dried and stained with hematoxylin and eosin. Lightly stained tissue clearly identified the infarct margins. An image analyzer totalled infarct volumes for all serial brain sections; infarct volumes are reported as mm^3.

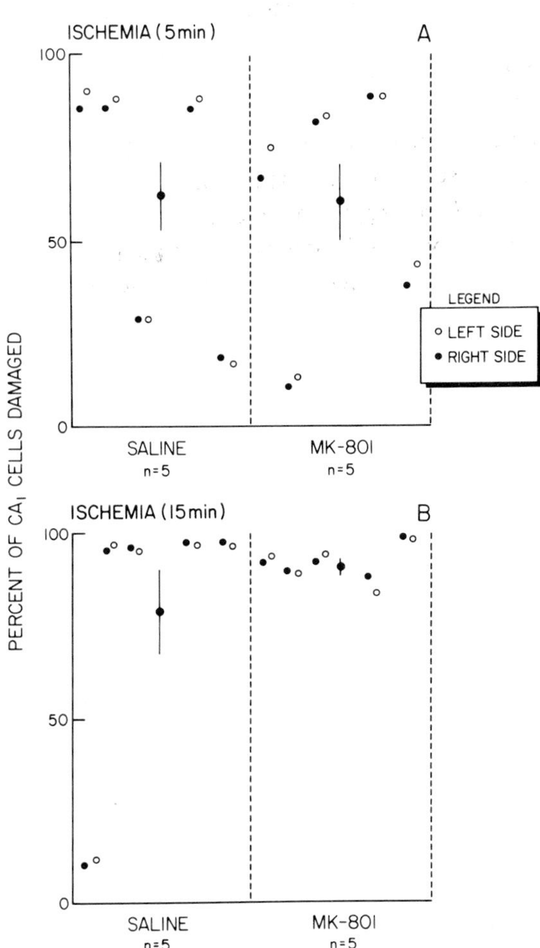

Fig. 2. Percent dead CA1 hippocampal neurons after multiple doses of saline or MK-801 (see text) in rats subjected to 5 min (*A*) or 15 min (*B*) of 4-VO ischemia. The open and filled small circles represent the percent dead neurons in the left and right hippocampus of each animal, respectively. The larger filled circles with error bars represent the group mean ± S.E. (Data from Buchan et al., 1991b; reprinted with permission from Pulsinelli et al., 1992.)

Results

NMDA antagonists in transient forebrain ischemia

Experimental rats received a single-dose intraperitoneal (i.p.) injection of either 0.3, 1, 2.5 or 5 mg/kg of MK-801 1 h prior to 5 or 15 min of 4-VO ischemia; control animals received an i.p. injection of saline (0.1 ml/100 g) 1 h prior to ischemia. Fig. 1 presents the results of this experimental paradigm. No attenuation of injury was found in any of the MK-801-treated groups although the group of animals subjected to 15 min 4-VO and 5 mg/kg of MK-801 showed slightly, but significantly ($P < 0.05$), greater hippocampal damage than their saline-treated counterpart (Buchan et al., 1991b). In the 5 min ischemia groups, the percent dead neurons was less, and the variance greater, than in the 15 min ischemia groups.

In a multiple-dose treatment paradigm rats were treated with MK-801 (5 mg/kg i.p.) or saline immediately after 15 min of 4-VO and again with 2.5 mg/kg MK-801 after approximately 8 and 20 h. Rats subjected to 5 min of ischemia were treated with MK-801 (5 mg/kg i.p.) or saline 1 h before 4-VO and again with 2.5 mg/kg at 8 and 16 h after cerebral recirculation (Buchan et al., 1991b). Fig. 2 presents the results of these studies. Again, no attenuation of CA1 hippocampal injury was found in either multiple-dose MK-801-treated groups. The 15 min ischemia group had significantly more neuronal damage than the 5 min group; variance in the 5 min group was greater than that in the 15 min group.

We used an a priori power analysis with $\alpha = 0.05$ and $\beta = 0.20$ (80% power) on the 5 min data due to the high variance of CA1 damage in rats subjected to 5 min of 4-VO ischemia. This analysis determined that 60 animals in each group were needed to detect a 15% difference between the saline- and MK-801-treated rats. Accordingly, we conducted a study in which 60 rats were treated with 1 mg/kg of MK-801 (or 1 ml of saline) 1 h prior to 4-VO ischemia and again at 8 and 16 h after cerebral recirculation. Fig. 3 presents the results of this study. The severity of CA1 hippocampal damage was the same in both the

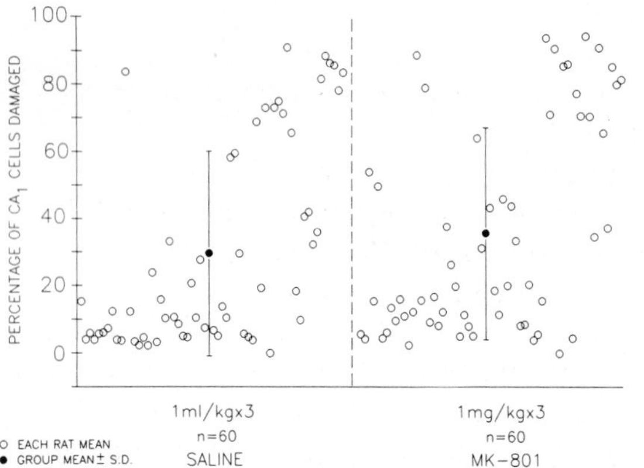

Fig. 3. Percent dead CA1 hippocampal neurons after multiple doses of saline or MK-801 (1 mg/kg × 3) in rats subjected to 5 min of 4-VO ischemia. Open circles are the average left and right percent dead neurons in each rat. The filled circles with error bars are the group mean ± S.D. (Reprinted with permission from Buchan et al., 1991b.)

MK-801- and saline-treated groups. An analysis of the two group's physiological values showed several statistically significant, but biologically unimportant, differences (Buchan et al., 1991b).

NMDA antagonists in permanent focal cerebral ischemia

MK-801 (5 mg/kg i.p.) was administered to adult SH rats 30 min before the initiation of MCA/CCA occlusion and 2.5 mg/kg MK-801 was administered again at 8 and 16 h after the ischemic insult. These data are presented in Table I. MK-801 reduced infarction volume between 18 and 29% in three separate studies (Dirnagl et al., 1990; Buchan et al., 1992b). Mean arterial blood pressure was significantly higher in saline-treated controls at 8 and 16 h after cerebral recirculation. The lower arterial blood pressure associated with the MK-801-treated group could have reduced the full neuroprotective effect of MK-801.

AMPA receptor antagonists in transient forebrain ischemia

We tested the AMPA antagonist, 2,3-dihydroxy-6-nitro-7-sulfamoyl-benzoquinoxaline (NBQX) in the 4-VO model of transient forebrain ischemia (Buchan et al., 1991a) Adult Wistar rats were subjected to 10 min of 4-VO. Immediately upon cerebral reperfusion, and again after 15 and 30 min of recirculation, the rats were treated i.p. with the lithium salt of NBQX (30 mg/kg) or LiCl vehicle. Data showed that the number of damaged neurons was significantly less ($P < 0.01$) in the CA1 hippocampal zone of rats receiving NBQX after 10 min of transient forebrain ischemia (see Fig. 4).

AMPA receptor antagonists in transient focal cerebral ischemia

Adult SH rats subjected to 2 h of reversible focal cerebral ischemia were treated i.p. with saline or NBQX (30 mg/kg) 90 min into the ischemic insult, at the time of reperfusion, and again after 30 min of recirculation (Buchan et al., 1991d). Infarct volume analysis performed at 24 h after reperfusion revealed that the NBQX-treated group showed a significant ($P < 0.001$) reduction in infarct volume (Fig. 5).

TABLE I

NMDA antagonists in permanent focal cerebral ischemia

	Means ± S.D. volume of cortical infarction (mm_3)		
	Study 1*	Study 2*	Study 3**
Saline control	231 ± 22 (n = 5)	169 ± 34 (n = 8)	226 ± 43 (n = 9)
MK-801	165 ± 63 (n = 7)	134 ± 58 (n = 8)	185 ± 34 (n = 10)
Volume reduction	29%	20%	18%
P Value	0.016	0.016	< 0.05

* Data are from Dirnagl et al. (1990).
** Data are from Buchan et al. (1992b).

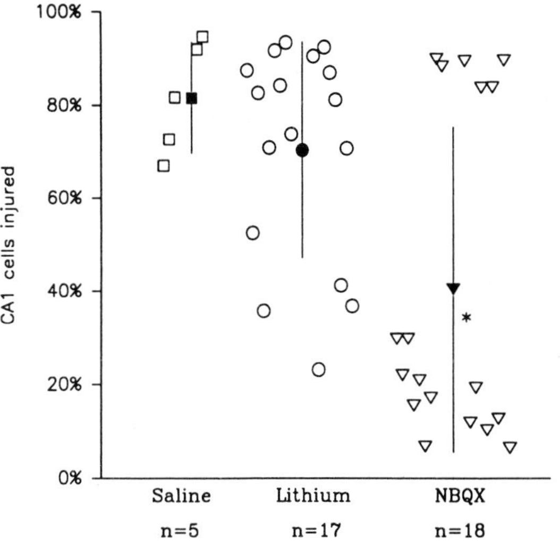

Fig. 4. Percent level CA1 pyramidal neurons following post-ischemic treatment with saline (squares), lithium (1 mg i.p. × 3) (circles) and NBQX (30 mg/kg i.p. × 3) (triangles). Open squares, circles and triangles represent the average percent of dead cells in the left and right hippocampi for each animal. The filled square, circle and triangle each with error bars represent the mean ± S.D. for each group ($*P < 0.01$) (Reprinted with permission from Buchan et al., 1991a.)

Discussion

NMDA receptor antagonists in focal and global ischemia

Through our own research efforts and a review of the relevant literature, we conclude that the NMDA receptor/channel plays little or no role in the pathogenesis of necrosis to selectively vulnerable neurons caused by transient severe ischemia. To support this conclusion we will demonstrate from the available data that there exists a poor correlation between the distribution of NMDA receptors and ischemia-sensitive neurons in rodent brain. Further, we will show that neither pharmacologic blockade of the NMDA receptor/channel with non-competitive antagonists nor antagonizing the channel through modulation of the extracellular H^+ ion concentration alters damage to ischemia-vulnerable neurons. This thesis and supporting data pertain to the relationship of the NMDA receptor/channel in severe ischemia; we do not dispute the role that excitatory neurotransmitters and the NMDA receptor/channel may play in brain damage from focal (moderate) ischemia (see below).

Histopathology of selective ischemic necrosis and NMDA receptor distribution

The term "selective ischemic necrosis of neurons" refers to the lack of uniform sensitivity to ischemic injury among neurons. This lack of uniformity is well exemplified in the hippocampus where the CA1 pyramidal neurons and the CA4 neurons are equally vulnerable to ischemic injury, but neurons within the dentate gyrus of the hippocampus are highly resistant to ischemia. Other neurons vulnerable to ischemia include: the neurons within layers 3, 5 and 6 of the neocortex, the medium-sized neurons which lie within the striatum and the cerebellar Purkinje cell.

Interestingly, in rat brain, the distribution of these vulnerable neuron populations does not correlate well with the distribution density of the NMDA receptor. Again this point is well illustrated

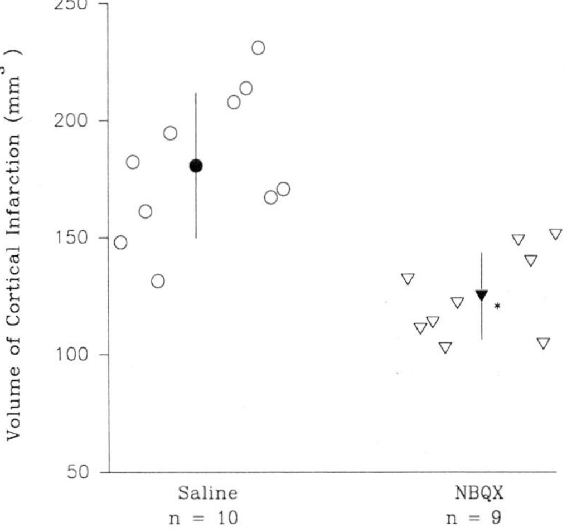

Fig. 5. Volumes of neocortical infarction for each rat following 2 h of transient MCA occlusion and 11 h of reperfusion. Open circles represent the infarct volume for each animal given three doses of saline, and open triangles those given three doses of NBQX (30 mg/kg). The filled circle and triangle show the mean ± S.D. for the two groups. ($*P < 0.001$). (Reprinted with permission from Buchan et al., 1991d.)

in the hippocampus where although the CA1 pyramidal cells and the CA4 neurons share an equal vulnerability to ischemia (Pulsinelli, 1985), the former group of cells has a large number of NMDA receptors while the latter appears to have relatively few. Moreover, the dentate granule neurons in the hippocampus are ischemia-resistant, yet possess a concentration of NMDA receptors equal to that found in the ischemia-sensitive CA1 pyramidal cells. There is also a weak correlation between NMDA receptor density and sensitivity to ischemia in layers 5 and 6 of neocortex and in the striatum. The Purkinje cell, however, offers the most dramatic evidence of this weak correlation: while this cell is highly vulnerable to ischemia it is virtually devoid of NMDA receptors (Crepel et al., 1982). The lack of consistency between an area's sensitivity to ischemia and its concentration of NMDA receptors makes it unlikely that the NMDA receptor is the single determinant in classically defined selective ischemic necrosis.

We used Monaghan et al.'s (1988) color-coded autoradiographs of [^{3}H]glutamate and [^{3}H]CPP binding in rat brain to make the above observations. These autoradiographs represent selective binding of glutamate to NMDA receptors since the [^{3}H]glutamate binding was examined in the presence of non-NMDA receptor antagonists which will also bind glutamate. The distribution density of [^{3}H]glutamate binding differed from that found with the binding of the selective and competitive NMDA antagonist, [^{3}H]CPP. These data led Monaghan et al. (1988) to conclude that the NMDA receptor is heterogeneous, existing in both agonist and antagonist preferring forms. The combination of the [^{3}H]glutamate and [^{3}H]CPP autoradiographs provides a reliable representation of NMDA receptor distribution density (see Fig. 1; Monaghan et al., 1988).

H^+ Ion antagonism of the NMDA receptor

It seems reasonable to conclude that if NMDA receptor/channel-mediated mechanisms singularly influence the severity of brain damage caused by transient severe ischemia, then their blockade would influence neurological outcome from the ischemic insult. However, results from studies using two mechanistically distinct, NMDA receptor/channel antagonists (H^+ ions and the non-competitive NMDA channel blocker, MK-801) indicate that the NMDA receptor/channel is not causally related to the pathophysiology of selective ischemic necrosis of neurons.

Using whole cell patch techniques, Morad et al. (1988) and Tang et al. (1989) demonstrated that NMDA-mediated currents virtually stopped when the extracellular, but not the intracellular, pH of tissue culture neurons was lowered from 7.3 to 6.6. Finding that membrane voltage and H^+ ion antagonism were independent of each other, and that protons had little effect on glutamate binding, they further concluded that the change in glycine binding caused by H^+ ions was too small to account for the marked NMDA receptor antagonism produced by moderate extracellular acidosis. Both Giffard et al. (1990) and Traynelis and Cull-Candy (1990) confirmed these electrophysiological properties of the NMDA receptor/channel in vivo. Additionally, Giffard et al. (1990) demonstrated that by reducing the extracellular pH to approximately 6.4, the neurotoxicity of glutamate in cortical cultures was noticeably reduced. In fact, the neurotoxicity produced by 6 h of anoxia-aglycemia was eliminated in hippocampal cultures when the extracellular pH was reduced to 6.5 (Tombaugh and Sapolsky, 1990).

Based on the aforementioned in vitro studies clearly showing that the NMDA receptor is effectively antagonized in a pH environment below 7.0, speculation arose as to its effect during in vivo ischemia. Would extracellular H^+ ions similarly modify NMDA receptor currents in vivo? If so, it should follow that Ca^{2+} influx and current transduction would be limited during ischemia-induced cerebral acidosis. It has been suggested (Tombaugh and Sapolsky, 1990) that it may be activation of the NMDA receptor upon cerebral recirculation that is more important to cell injury than is glutamate elevation during this interval. However, it requires approximately the same amount of time to normalize extracellular pH following transient cerebral ischemia (Siemkowicz and Hansen, 1981; Smith et al., 1986; Kraig and Petito, 1989) as it does to normalize extracellular glutamate concentrations (Benveniste et al., 1984; Hagberg et al., 1985; Globus et al., 1988). Therefore, during the ischemic insult and throughout early post-ischemic recirculation, the NMDA receptor will experience considerable inhibition through extracellular acidosis.

Whether H^+ ions effectively antagonize the NMDA receptor during in vivo ischemia is speculative; however, there are experimental data regarding this question. In the early 1980s, Diemer and Siemkowicz (1981) and Pulsinelli et al. (1982) lowered brain glucose concentrations prior to the onset of transient severe forebrain ischemia to examine the effects of reduced ischemic cerebral lactic acidosis. The expected result based on the in vitro studies of H^+ ion blockade of the NMDA channel would be an exacerbation of damage due to the facilitated NMDA-mediated Ca^{2+} flux caused by the reduced acidosis. However, Pulsinelli et al. (1982) reported no change in the severity of ischemic necrosis to CA1 neurons and Diemer and Siemkowicz (1981) noted a slight reduction of damage in studies where cerebral lactate was reduced by 50%. These data also support the thesis that the NMDA receptor has little influence on the degree of brain injury produced by transient severe ischemia, since they clearly show that manipulation of NMDA receptor/channel function had little impact on the severity of selective ischemic necrosis.

Antagonists of the NMDA receptor/channel in global and focal brain ischemia

Using the modified 4-vessel occlusion model of forebrain ischemia, we examined the effects of the potent and selective non-competitive NMDA channel antagonist, MK-801 in rats (Buchan et al., 1991b). Despite brief (5 min) ischemic periods, several pre- and post-treatment paradigms, and a wide dose range MK-801 failed to alter CA1 hippocampal damage in this model.

Our observations differ markedly from others (Simon et al., 1984; Gill et al., 1987; Swan et al., 1988) showing that NMDA antagonists offer protection to the hippocampus from forebrain ischemia. We believe, however, that two factors largely explain these varied results. The first factor is body temperature. Body temperature was not considered a variable in many, but not all, of the studies reporting NMDA receptor antagonist protection, and was therefore neither monitored nor maintained at a constant degree. This factor appears especially important in bilateral carotid artery occlusion studies in which gerbils were used. Our data (Buchan and Pulsinelli, 1990) indicated that in the gerbil a decline in body temperature of $2-3°C$ lasting 7 h or more is produced by the combination of 5 min of forebrain ischemia and the administration of MK-801. Moreover, the neuroprotective effect presumably achieved by the administration of MK-801 was not evident when MK-801- and vehicle-treated controls were maintained at normal body temperature during and after bilateral carotid artery occlusion. We infer from these data that the neuroprotective effect of MK-801 seen in other studies of global brain ischemia does not result principally from the drug's effect on receptor-mediated hippocampal mechanisms, but rather from hypothermia.

The second factor which we believe explains the discrepancy between our data and those demonstrating neuroprotection from MK-801 administration in global ischemia is the lack of a consistent degree of forebrain ischemia among the studies. In studies such as Swan et al. (1988) where bilateral carotid artery occlusion plus hypotension induced only moderate ischemia, NMDA antagonism offered neuroprotection. However, negative results were consistently reported from laboratories using models where blood flow to brain was severely reduced (Block and Pulsinelli, 1987; Wieloch et al., 1988; Fleischer et al., 1989; Michenfelder et al., 1989).

It is probably the NMDA receptor/channel antagonist's inability to block neurotoxic levels of calcium which accumulate via mechanisms independent of the NMDA-regulated Ca^{2+} channel that accounts for its inability to protect the brain against severe ischemia. Calcium uptake by the mitochondria and endoplasmic reticulum, as well as the Na^+/Ca^{2+} exchange (a membrane pump that extrudes Ca^{2+}) are either directly or indirectly energy-dependent. Since ATP is depleted in severe ischemia, these mechanisms fail, leading to lethal calcium ion levels in the cytoplasm. However, some or all of these mechanisms may still function in moderate ischemia since ATP is partially preserved (Selman et al., 1987; Kaplan and Pulsinelli, 1989). This renders calcium movement through the NMDA-regulated channel more critical to cell injury and accordingly, NMDA channel blockade would be neuroprotective under circumstances of moderate ischemia (Siesjö and Bengtsson, 1989; Wieloch et al., 1989).

AMPA receptor antagonists in focal and global brain ischemia

Remarkable results have been obtained from laboratories using the AMPA receptor antagonist (NBQX) to attenuate ischemic injury to neurons (Sheardown et al., 1990; Buchan et al., 1991a,d). Not only does this compound appear to decrease selective ischemic necrosis of neurons, but it appears to be effective even when first administered *after* cerebral circulation has resumed. If this attribute of the compound proves unalterable it would represent a major advance in cerebrovascular disease research and could lead to successful therapeutic intervention in those patients suffering brain damage following cardiac arrest. Additionally, the compound's success in mitigating brain damage from ischemia when initially administered during recirculation substantiates the hypothesis that irreversible mechanisms of brain injury do not begin until after this period has begun.

Research and much speculative thought is currently focused on how the AMPA receptor attenuates brain damage at the cellular level. If a necessary element of ischemic cell injury is the disturbance of intracellular calcium homeostasis, then blockade of the AMPA receptor could conceivably reduce Na^+/K^+ membrane currents and block secondarily voltage-regulated calcium channels and/or voltage-dependent NMDA receptor-regulated calcium channels, thereby moderating the effects from an intracellular rise in Ca^{2+}. This conjecture, however, is weakened by the inability of potent NMDA antagonists (Block and Pulsinelli, 1987; Wieloch et al., 1988; Buchan et al., 1991b) and voltage-regulated calcium channel antagonists (Vibulsresth et al., 1987) to shield hippocampal neurons from the effects of transient severe ischemia.

Recent molecular studies involving the expression of kainate/AMPA receptor/ionophore subunits in oocytes and electrophysiological studies in other in vitro preparations suggest another mechanism. Data from these studies (Iino et al., 1990; Gilbertson et al., 1991; Hollmann et al., 1991) have shown that specific combinations of subunit molecules are permeable to calcium ions and data from others have shown that hippocampal neurons as well as other neurons have similar subunit types. This raises the possibility that during cerebral recirculation, specific second messenger systems directly involved in irreversible ischemic injury to neurons are activated by calcium flux through this particular AMPA-regulated ionophore.

In summary, we have shown that the correlation between NMDA receptor distribution density and a brain region's vulnerability to selective ischemic necrosis is poor. Several instances of this poor correlation were cited, but the most revealing example perhaps was that of the cerebellar Purkinje cell. This cell is one of the neurons most vulnerable to ischemic injury, yet it completely lacks the NMDA receptor. The role of the NMDA receptor in influencing the outcome from transient forebrain ischemia was further questioned by our review of data from various studies where the NMDA receptor/channel was inhibited. Neither the administration of the non-competitive NMDA channel antagonist, MK-801, nor the manipulation of extracellular H^+ ions which suppress the NMDA receptor/channel demonstrably altered the severity or distribution pattern of selective ischemic necrosis in rodent models of transient forebrain ischemia. We conclude, therefore, that not only does the NMDA receptor/channel have at best a minimal role in the pathophysiology of classic selective ischemic necrosis but that efforts to pharmacologically block the NMDA receptor/channel will have at best minimal success in protecting the human brain from the effects of cardiac arrest.

Alternatively, the protection from moderate ischemia provided by the NMDA receptor antagonist as well as the protection afforded by the AMPA antagonist in paradigms of both moderate and severe transient ischemia indicate that the pathogenesis of some forms of ischemic brain injury is caused by abnormalities between excitatory amino acid neurotransmitters and their receptors. Due to the AMPA antagonist's ability to attenuate damage from severe ischemia when administered during the recirculation period, we conclude that pathophysiological events mediated by AMPA during recirculation are directly involved in causing selective ischemic necrosis. In moderate ischemia, however, both the AMPA and the NMDA receptor antagonists appear to influence neurological outcome.

Regarding clinical applicability, we conclude that although both the NMDA and AMPA receptor antagonists may prove effective in combatting the effects of focal brain ischemia (stroke), the AMPA receptor antagonist alone appears to offer hope for treating the effects of global brain ischemia (cardiac arrest).

References

Benveniste, H., Drejer, J., Schousboe, A. and Diemer, N. (1984) Elevation of extracellular concentrations of glutamate and aspartate in rat hippocampus during transient cerebral ischemia monitored by intracerebral microdialysis. *J. Neurochem.,* 43: 1369 – 1374.

Block, G. and Pulsinelli, W. (1987) *N*-Methyl-D-aspartate receptor antagonists: failure to prevent ischemia-induced selective neuronal damage. In: M. Raichle and W. Powers (Eds.), *Cerebrovascular Diseases – Fifteenth Conference, Princeton, NJ,* Raven Press, New York, pp. 37 – 42.

Brint, S., Jacewicz, M., Kiessling, M., Tanabe, J. and Pulsinelli, W. (1988) Focal brain ischemia in the rat: methods for reproducible infarction using tandem occlusion of the distal middle cerebral and ipsilateral common carotid arteries. *J. Cereb. Blood Flow Metab.,* 8: 474 – 485.

Buchan, A. (1990) Do NMDA antagonists protect against cerebral ischemia: are clinical trials warranted? *Cerebrovasc. Brain Metab. Rev.,* 2: 1 – 26.

Buchan, A. and Pulsinelli, W. (1990) Hypothermia but not the *N*-methyl-D-aspartate antagonist, MK-801, attenuates neuronal damage in gerbils subjected to transient global ischemia. *J. Neurosci.,* 10: 311 – 316.

Buchan, A., Li, H., Cho, S.-H. and Pulsinelli, W. (1991a) Blockade of the AMPA receptor prevents CA1 hippocampal injury following severe but transient forebrain ischemia in adult rats. *Neurosci. Lett.,* 132: 255 – 258.

Buchan, A., Li, H. and Pulsinelli, W. (1991b) The *N*-methyl-D-aspartate antagonist, MK-801, fails to protect against neuronal damage caused by transient, severe forebrain ischemia in adult rats. *J. Neurosci.,* 11: 1049 – 1056.

Buchan, A., Xue, D., Huang, Z., Smith, K. and Lesiuk, H. (1991d) Delayed AMPA receptor blockade reduces cerebral infarction induced by focal ischemia. *Neuro-Report,* 2: 473 – 476.

Buchan, A., Slivka, A. and Xue, D. (1992a) A new model of focal stroke in the rat. Stroke, 23: 273 – 279.

Buchan, A., Silvka, A. and Xue, D. (1992b) The effect of the NMDA receptor antagonist, MK-801, on CBF and infarct volume in experimental focal stroke. *Brain Res.,* 574: 171 – 177.

Choi, D.W. (1987) Ionic dependence of glutamate neurotoxicity. *J. Neurosci.,* 7: 369 – 379.

Crepel, F., Dhanjal, S. and Sears, T. (1982) Effect of glutamate aspartate, and related derivatives on cerebellar Purkinje cell dendrites in the rat: an in vitro study. *J. Physiol. (Lond.),* 329: 297 – 317.

Diemer, N. and Siemkowicz, E. (1981) Regional neuron damage after cerebral ischemia in the normo- and hypoglycemic rat. *Neuropathol. Appl. Neurobiol.,* 7: 217 – 227.

Dirnagl, U., Tanabe, J. and Pulsinelli, W. (1990) Pre- and post-treatment with MK-801 but not pretreatment alone reduces neocortical damage after focal cerebral ischemia in the rat. *Brain Res.,* 527: 62 – 68.

Fleischer, J., Tateishi, A., Drummond, C., Scheller, M., Grafe, M., Zornow, M., Shearman, G. and Shapiro, H. (1989) MK-801, an excitatory amino acid antagonist does not improve neurologic outcome following cardiac arrest in cats. *J. Cereb. Blood Flow Metab.,* 9: 805 – 811.

Francis, A. and Pulsinelli, W. (1982) Response of *GABA*ergic and cholinergic neurons to transient forebrain ischemia. *Brain Res.,* 243: 271 – 278.

Garthwaite, G. and Garthwaite, J. (1986) Neurotoxicity of excitatory amino acid receptor agonists in rat cerebellar slices: dependence on calcium concentration. *Neurosci. Lett.,* 66: 193 – 198.

Giffard, R., Monyer, H., Christine, C. and Choi, D. (1990) Acidosis reduces NMDA receptor activation, glutamate neurotoxicity and oxygen-glucose deprivation neuronal injury in cortical cultures. *Brain Res.,* 506: 339 – 342.

Gilbertson, T., Scobey, R. and Wilson, M. (1991) Permeation of calcium ions through non-NMDA glutamate channels in retinal bipolar cells. *Science,* 251: 1613 – 1615.

Gill, R., Foster, A. and Woodruff, G. (1987) Systemic administration of MK-801 protects against ischemia-induced hippocampal neurodegeneration in the gerbil. *J. Neurosci.,* 7: 3345 – 3349.

Globus, M., Busto, R., Dietrich, W.D., Martinez, E., Valdes, I. and Ginsberg, M.D. (1988) Effect of ischemia on the in vivo release of striatal dopamine, glutamate, and gamma-aminobutyric acid studied by intracerebral microdialysis. *J. Neurochem.,* 51: 1455 – 1464.

Hagberg, H., Lehmann, A., Sandberg, M., Nystrom, B., Jacobson, I. and Hamberger, A. (1985) Ischemia-induced shift of inhibition and excitatory amino acids from intra- to extracellular compartments. *J. Cereb. Blood Flow Metab.,* 5: 413 – 419.

Hollmann, M., Hartley, M. and Heinemann, S. (1991) Ca^{2+} permeability of KA-AMPA-gated glutamate receptor channels depend on sub-unit composition. *Science,* 252: 851 – 853.

Iino, M., Ozawa, S. and Tsuzuki, K. (1990) Permeation of calcium through excitatory amino acid receptor channels in cultured rat hippocampal neurons. *J. Physiol. (Lond.),* 424: 151 – 165.

Jørgensen, M. and Diemer, N. (1982) Selective neuron loss after cerebral ischemia in the rat: possible role of transmitter glutamate. *Acta Neurol. Scand.,* 66: 536 – 546.

Kaplan, B. and Pulsinelli, W. (1989) Energy metabolites in the ischemic penumbra. *Soc. Neurosci. Abstr.,* 15: 855.

Kraig, R. and Petito, C. (1989) Interrelation of proton and volume regulation in astrocytes. In: M. Ginsberg and W.D. Dietrich (Eds.), *Cerebrovascular Diseases – Sixteenth Research Conference, Princeton, NJ,* Raven Press, New York, pp. 239 – 246.

Meldrum, B. (1981) Metabolic effects of prolonged epileptic seizures and the causation of epileptic brain damage. In: F. Rose (Ed.), *Metabolic Disorders of the Nervous System,* Pitman, London, pp. 175 – 187.

Meldrum, B. (1990) Protection against ischemic neuronal damage by drugs acting on excitatory neurotransmission. *Cerebrovasc. Brain Metab. Rev.,* 2: 27 – 57.

Michenfelder, J., Lanier, W., Scheithauer, B., Perkins, W., Shearman, G. and Milde, J. (1989) Evaluation of the glutamate antagonist dizocilipine maleate (MK-801) on the neurologic outcome in a canine model of complete cerebral ischemia: correlation with hippocampal histopathology. *Brain Res.,* 481: 228 – 234.

Monaghan, D., Olverman, H., Nguyen, L., Watkins, J. and Cotman, C. (1988) Two classes of *N*-methyl-D-aspartate recognition sites: differential distribution and differential regulation by glycine. *Proc. Natl. Acad. Sci. U.S.A.,* 85: 9836 – 9840.

Morad, M., Dichter, M. and Tang, C. (1988) The NMDA activated current in hippocampal neurons is highly sensitive to $[H^+]$. *Soc. Neurosci. Abstr.,* 14: 791.

Olney, J.W. (1978) Neurotoxicity of excitatory amino acids. In: E.G. McGeer, J.W. Olney and P.L. McGeer (Eds.), *Kainic Acid as a Tool in Neurobiology,* Raven Press, New York, pp. 37 – 70.

Pulsinelli, W. (1985) Selective neuronal vulnerability: morphological and molecular characteristics. *Prog. Brain Res.,* 63: 29 – 37.

Pulsinelli, W. and Buchan, A. (1988) The four-vessel occlusion rat model: methods for complete occlusion of vertebral arteries and control of collateral circulation. *Stroke,* 19: 913 – 914.

Pulsinelli, W. and Duffy, T. (1983) Regional energy balance in rat brain after transient forebrain ischemia. *J. Neurochem.,* 40: 1500 – 1503.

Pulsinelli, W., French, J., Rawlinson, D. and Plum, F. (1982) Cerebral ischemia damages neurons despite lowered brain lactate levels. *Ann. Neurol.,* 12: 86.

Pulsinelli, W., Dirnagl, W., Jacewicz, M. and Buchan, A. (1992) Antagonists of excitatory amino acid neurotransmitter: a comparison of their effects on global versus focal ischemia. In: A. Schousboe, N. Diemer and H. Kofod (Eds.), *Drug Research Related to Neuroactive Amino Acids,* Munksgaard, Copenhagen.

Rothman, S. (1985) The neurotoxicity of excitatory amino acids is produced by passive chloride influx. *Neuroscience,* 5: 1483 – 1489.

Selman, W., VanDerVeer, C., Whittingham, T., LaManna, J., Lust, W. and Ratcheson, R. (1987) Visually defined zones of focal ischemia in the rat brain. *Neurosurgery,* 21: 825 – 830.

Sheardown, M., Nielsen, E., Hansen, A., Jacobsen, P. and Honoré, T. (1990) 2,3-Dihydroxy-6-nitro-7-sulfamoyl-benzo(F)quinoxaline: a neuroprotectant for cerebral ischemia. *Science,* 247: 571 – 574.

Siemkowicz, E. and Hansen, E. (1981) Brain extracellular ion composition and EEG activity following ten minutes ischemia in normo- and hyperglycemic rats. *Stroke,* 12: 236 – 240.

Siesjö, B. and Bengtsson, F. (1989) Calcium fluxes, calcium antagonists and calcium-related pathology in brain ischemia, hypoglycemia and spreading depression: a unifying hypothesis. *J. Cereb. Blood Flow Metab.,* 9: 127 – 140.

Simon, R., Swan, J., Griffith, T. and Meldrum, B. (1984) Blockade of *N*-methyl-D-aspartate receptors may protect against ischemic damage in the brain. *Science,* 226: 850 – 852.

Smith, M.-L., von Hanwehr, R. and Siesjo, B.K. (1986) Changes in extra- and intracellular pH in the brain during and following ischemia in hyperglycemic and in moderately hypoglycemic rats. *J. Cereb. Blood Flow Metab.,* 6: 574 – 583.

Swan, J., Evans, M. and Meldrum, B. (1988) Long-term development of selective neuronal loss and the mechanism of protection by 2-amino-7-phosphonoheptanoic acid in a rat model of incomplete forebrain ischemia. *J. Cereb. Blood Flow Metab.,* 8: 64 – 78.

Tang, C., Dichter, M. and Morad, M. (1989) Mechanism of NMDA channel modulation by H^+ at near physiological pH. *Soc. Neurosci. Abstr.,* 15: 326.

Tombaugh, G. and Sapolsky, R. (1990) Mild acidosis protects

hippocampal neurons from injury induced by oxygen and glucose deprivation. *Brain Res.,* 506: 343 – 345.

Traynelis, S. and Cull-Candy, S. (1990) Proton inhibition of *N*-methyl-D-aspartate receptors in cerebellar neurons, *Nature,* 345: 347 – 350.

Vibulsresth, S., Dietrich, D., Busto, R. and Ginsberg, M. (1987) Failure of nimodipine to prevent ischemic neuronal damage in rats. *Stroke,* 18: 210 – 216.

Wieloch, T., Gustafson, I. and Westerberg, E. (1988) Effects of non-competitive NMDA receptor antagonist MK-801 on ischemic and hypoglycemic brain damage. In: L. Turski, E. Lehmann and E. Cavalheiro (Eds.), *Neurology and Neurobiology – Frontiers of Excitatory Amino Acid Research, Vol. 46,* Alan R. Liss, New York, pp. 715 – 722.

Wieloch, T., Gustafson, I. and Westerberg, E. (1989) The NMDA antagonist, MK-801, is cerebro-protective in situations where some energy production prevails but not under conditions of complete energy deprivation. *J. Cereb. Blood Flow Metab. (Suppl.),* 9: S6 – S7.

K. Kogure, K.-A. Hossmann and B.K. Siesjö (Eds.)
Progress in Brain Research, Vol. 96

CHAPTER 9

NMDA receptors and AMPA/kainate receptors mediate parallel injury in cerebral cortical cultures subjected to oxygen-glucose deprivation

Dennis W. Choi

Department of Neurology, Washington University School of Medicine, St. Louis, MO 63110, U.S.A.

Introduction

Growing evidence has suggested that glutamate neurotoxicity may contribute to brain injury after certain acute insults, including hypoxia-ischemia (Meldrum, 1985; Rothman and Olney, 1987; Choi, 1988). Consistent with a substantial experience in animal models of focal ischemia (reviewed in Buchan, 1990; Albers et al., 1992), antagonists of the *N*-methyl-D-aspartate (NMDA) subtype of glutamate receptors markedly improve neuronal survival in cortical cell cultures subjected to trauma, hypoxia, glucose deprivation, or oxygen-glucose deprivation (Choi, 1990, 1991). In contrast, NMDA antagonists appear to be of limited value when used alone in global ischemia (Buchan, 1990). Two distinct hypotheses can be considered to explain a greater value of NMDA antagonists as neuroprotective agents in focal ischemia compared with global ischemia:

(1) The toxic potential of NMDA receptor overactivation is small, and is only a critical factor in neuronal death under certain special conditions, such as in the partial energy depletion associated with the focal ischemic penumbra.

(2) The toxic potential of NMDA receptor overactivation is large, but limited by endogenous mechanisms especially active in global ischemia. Only when NMDA receptor-mediated toxicity is suppressed does a more slowly triggered toxicity of AMPA/kainate receptors become apparent.

The critical difference between these two hypotheses is the rank order of NMDA versus AMPA/kainate receptors, with respect to excitotoxic potential. In both hypotheses, the occurrence of calcium overload is suggested to trigger neurodegeneration (Siesjö et al., 1989; Choi, 1990a). Hypothesis nr. 1 has been proposed by Siesjö and Bengtsson (1989), who have concomitantly emphasized the high potential toxicity of AMPA/kainate receptor overactivation. Since these receptor families mediate most fast excitatory synaptic transmission throughout the CNS (Mayer and Westbrook, 1987), they may contribute heavily to sodium overload during and after an ischemic insult, leading subsequently to calcium overload. Hypothesis nr. 2, at least on neocortical neurons, is favored by cell culture studies of excitotoxic injury (Choi, 1990a, 1991). As discussed further below, hypothesis nr. 2 does not suggest that AMPA/kainate receptor overstimulation is benign, but simply that lethal damage can be more rapidly induced by NMDA receptor activation than by AMPA/kainate receptor activation.

Excitotoxicity in cortical cultures

Glutamate receptor-mediated neuronal injury in

murine cortical cell culture systems occurs in two main patterns: (1) rapidly triggered excitotoxicity induced by the brief intense stimulation of large numbers of NMDA receptors; and (2) slowly triggered excitotoxicity induced by the prolonged stimulation of AMPA/kainate receptors (or the low level stimulation of NMDA receptors).

Three to five minutes of exposure to high concentrations of glutamate is sufficient to induce widespread neuronal degeneration by the next day. This injury can be separated into two components. The first, minor, component, is marked by immediate neuronal swelling. It depends on the presence of extracellular Na^+, as well as extracellular Cl^-, and most likely reflects Na^+ influx through ligand-gated and voltage-gated channels, accompanied by passive Cl^- and water influx. The second, major, component, is marked by delayed cell degeneration. It depends on the presence of extracellular Ca^{2+} and is likely triggered by excessive Ca^{2+} influx.

Acute neuronal swelling, like neuronal excitation, can be produced by either NMDA or kainate. Glutamate-induced neuronal swelling is only weakly attenuated by saturating levels of NMDA antagonists; a larger partial attenuation is produced by high levels of 6-nitro-7-cyano-quinoxaline-2,3-dion (CNQX) in the presence of 1 mM glycine, a treatment exhibiting good selectivity for AMPA/kainate receptor-mediated toxicity in our system (Koh and Choi, 1991). The combination of MK-801 with CNQX plus glycine completely blocks glutamate-induced immediate neuronal swelling. Thus activation of metabotropic receptors or other presently undefined types of glutamate receptors appears neither necessary nor sufficient for this acute toxic response.

In contrast, the late neuronal degeneration induced by intense glutamate exposure is mediated mainly by NMDA receptors. This event can be triggered also by a 5 min exposure to selective NMDA agonists, such as homocysteate, but most cortical neurons do not degenerate following 5 min exposure to even high concentrations of kainate or AMPA. As noted above, neurons exposed to kainate develop prominent immediate swelling, but when exposure is terminated after a few minutes, most cortical neurons regain their normal morphology and survive.

These agonist experiments are supported by counterpart experiments with glutamate antagonists. Selective antagonism of NMDA receptors with either competitive or non-competitive antagonists virtually suffices to eliminate the late neuronal death induced by brief exposure to glutamate; in contrast, mostly late death is not blocked by CNQX plus glycine (Koh and Choi, 1991). NMDA antagonists can substantially reduce glutamate-induced late neuronal death even if added after glutamate wash-out, suggesting that the injury initially incurred during brief exposure to exogenous glutamate may be augmented subsequently by the activation of NMDA receptors by endogenously released glutamate.

The dependence of this late neuronal death on extracellular Ca^{2+} may reflect a requirement for Ca^{2+} influx through the NMDA receptor-gated ionophore. The pattern of delayed cortical neuronal degeneration can also be induced by the Ca^{2+} ionophore, A23187. Furthermore, cortical neurons exposed briefly to high concentrations of glutamate or selective NMDA agonists accumulate large amounts of $^{45}Ca^{2+}$ during the exposure period, and this NMDA receptor-induced $^{45}Ca^{2+}$ accumulation correlates quantitatively with subsequent degeneration. Both the neuronal degeneration and the $^{45}Ca^{2+}$ influx induced by brief glutamate exposure can be reduced to near baseline levels by selective blockade of NMDA receptors; only minor attenuation of degeneration or $^{45}Ca^{2+}$ influx is produced by even 100 μM nifedipine (Hartley and Choi, unpublished results).

Excessive Ca^{2+} influx and resultant cellular Ca^{2+} overload may be cytotoxic for several reasons (Choi, 1988), including the activation of catabolic enzymes and, in particular, the production of free radicals (Siesjö 1989; Monyer et al., 1990). Free radicals might be linked to loss of calcium homeostasis in several ways, including : (1) calcium activation of phospholipase A_2, leading to the liberation of arachidonic acid and subsequent free radical production (Chan et al., 1985); (2) calcium triggering the conversion of xanthine dehydrogenase to xanthine oxidase, a rich enzymatic source of free radicals (Dykens et al., 1987); and (3) stimulation of NMDA receptors leading to the release of nitric oxide (Garthwaite et al., 1988), which can react with superoxide to form peroxynitrite and ultimately promote the production of hydroxyl radicals (Beckman et al., 1990). In addition, Murphy and Coyle have suggested that glutamate exposure may produce cytotoxicity by inhibition of cystine uptake, resulting in reduced glutathione production and increased oxidative stress (Murphy et al., 1989). Once free radicals are formed, they may promote further excitotoxic injury by promoting glutamate release (Pellegrini-Giampietro et al., 1988).

A dominant contribution of NMDA receptors to injury following brief intense glutamate exposure does not imply that AMPA/kainate receptors cannot also participate in excitotoxic injury, as emphasized in other studies (Frandsen et al., 1989). While high concentrations of glutamate or other potent NMDA agonists can trigger degeneration of cultured mouse cortical neurons after an exposure time of only 3 – 5 min, AMPA or kainate require exposure times exceeding several hours to induce comparable widespread neuronal damage. If exposure time is extended to 24 h, 10 – 20 μM concentrations of either AMPA or kainate can produce widespread neuronal death.

This slowly triggered excitotoxicity may also involve excessive Ca^{2+} influx. As most channels gated by AMPA/kainate receptors have limited Ca^{2+} permeability, the main route of Ca^{2+} entry may be indirect; for example, involving voltage-gated Ca^{2+} channels, reverse operation of the Na^{+}-Ca^{2+} exchanger, membrane stretch-activated conductances or leak conductances by cell swelling (Choi, 1991). However, recent studies have indicated that some AMPA/kainate receptors may gate channels permeable to Ca^{2+}, perhaps reflecting a molecular composition lacking the Glu-R2/Glu-RB subunit (reviewed in Sommer and Seeburg, 1992). Direct evidence for extracellular Ca^{2+} dependence of AMPA/kainate receptor-mediated toxicity has been demonstrated on other neuronal types, including hippocampal (Rothman et al., 1987) and cerebellar neurons (Garthwaite and Garthwaite, 1986).

Several mechanisms may amplify resultant elevations in intracellular free Ca^{2+}, including the release of Ca^{2+} from intracellular stores, the activation of certain enzyme families – e.g., C kinases, calmodulin-regulated enzymes, calpains and phospholipases – and the effects of immediate early gene expression. These mechanisms may induce a lasting enhancement of excitatory synaptic efficacy and circuit excitability that exacerbates excitotoxicity, especially submaximal, slowly triggered excitotoxicity. In addition, glutamate efflux from injured neurons may contribute to the further propagation of excitotoxic injury. With intense activation of NMDA receptors, initial intracellular Ca^{2+} accumulation and free Ca^{2+} elevation may reach lethal levels with little need for subsequent augmentation. Supporting the idea that AMPA/kainate receptor-mediated toxicity may merge mechanistically with NMDA receptor-mediated toxicity, kainate toxicity (in the presence of MK-801) can be partially reduced by a 21-aminosteroid free radical scavenger (Hartley and Choi, unpublished results). A diagram summarizing the above putative injury mechanisms is shown in Fig. 1.

Parallel occurrence of NMDA receptor-mediated and AMPA/kainate receptor-mediated excitotoxicity in oxygen-glucose deprivation neuronal injury

Consistent with a dominant participation of NMDA receptor-mediated rapidly triggered excitotoxicity in the injury induced by combined oxygen-glucose deprivation, cultures exposed to this insult for 45 – 60 min develop widespread neuronal injury that can be mostly prevented by adding any of several NMDA antagonists to the exposure medium. In contrast, adding the AMPA/kainate

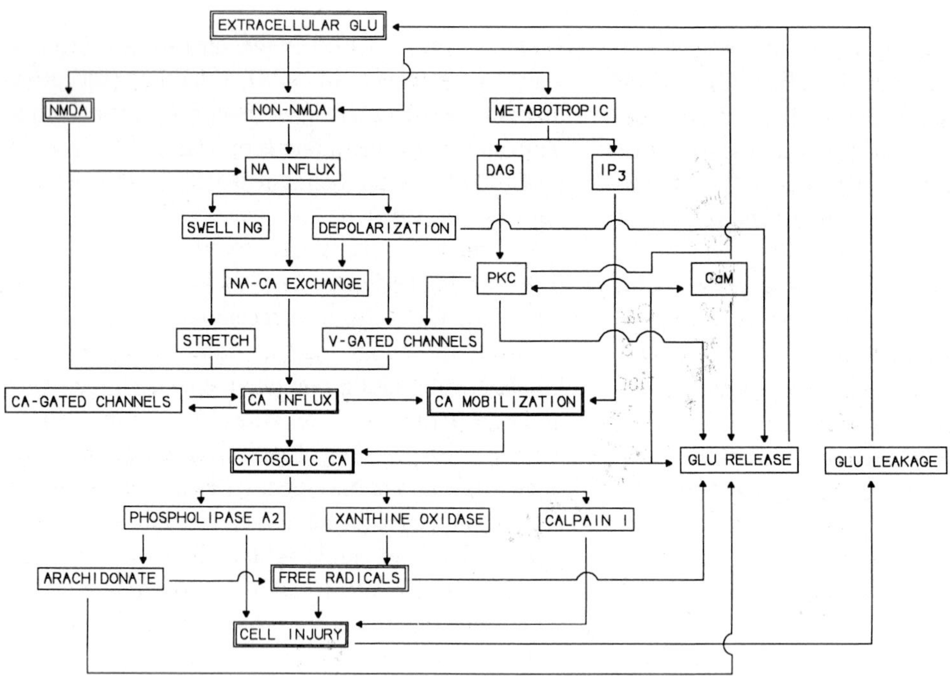

Fig. 1. Speculative diagram outlining some of the major processes that may contribute to excitotoxic neuronal death. In this scheme, a key role is assigned to Ca^{2+} influx leading to free radical overproduction. Metabotropic glutamate receptor activation triggers formation of diacylglycerol (DAG) and inositol 1,4,5-trisphosphate (IP_3). Protein kinase C (PKC) and calmodulin (CaM) may participate in up-regulating AMPA/kainate receptors, and glutamate efflux due to enhanced release/leakage may feed back to further evoke additional excitotoxic injury. (Taken from Choi, 1990a.)

antagonist CNQX or high concentrations of nifedipine produces little benefit (Kaku et al., 1991; also Goldberg and Choi, unpublished results). Given a difference in speed between NMDA receptor-mediated injury and AMPA/kainate receptor-mediated injury, it is possible that a sustained overavailability of extracellular glutamate may lead quickly to death mediated by NMDA receptors, rendering irrelevant any injury subsequently triggered by AMPA/kainate receptors overactivation (Fig. 2).

To unmask AMPA/kainate receptor participation in cultures subjected to oxygen-glucose deprivation, we added 10 μM MK-801 to the exposure medium, and then increased the insult duration to 100 min, an insult sufficient to override partially the protective effect of MK-801. Under these circumstances, with NMDA receptor-mediated injury eliminated with MK-801, the addition of $1-100$ μM CNQX produced a substantial improvement in neuronal survival (Fig. 3); further increases in NMDA receptor blockade did not reproduce this additional protective effect (Kaku et al., 1991).

Endogenous mechanisms limiting NMDA receptor-mediated injury

Several endogenous factors might limit rapidly triggered NMDA receptor-mediated excitotoxicity in vivo, especially under conditions of global ischemia:

(1) Extracellular acidity. In cell culture, reducing the pH to 6.4 decreases glutamate neurotoxicity, hypoxia-induced $^{45}Ca^{2+}$ accumulation and hypoxic neuronal degeneration (Morad et al., 1988; Giffard et al., 1990; Tombaugh and Sapolsky, 1990).

(2) Extracellular zinc. Zn^{2+} is co-released with glutamate and may reduce NMDA receptor-mediated current by both a voltage-independent

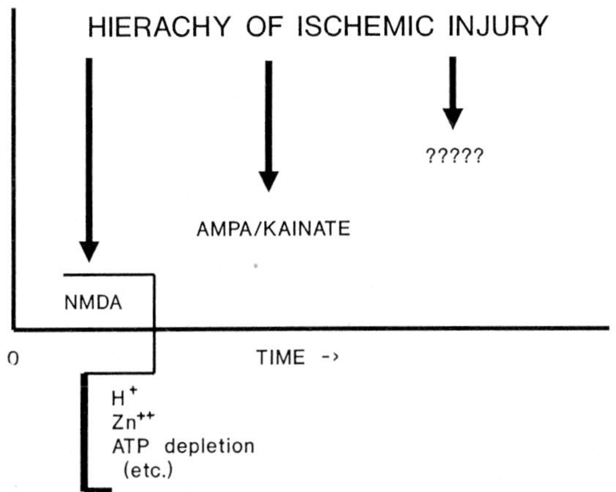

Fig. 2. Injury hierachy. There may be an intrinsic hierarchy of neuronal injury mechanisms operative in the neocortex under conditions of hypoxia-ischemia. NMDA receptor-mediated injury may reach lethal threshold first, unless it is attenuated by endogenous or exogenous antagonists. If NMDA receptor-mediated injury is not stopped, it will mask – render irrelevant – other injury mechanisms such as AMPA/kainate receptor-mediated injury. AMPA/kainate receptor-mediated injury is just as lethal as NMDA receptor-mediated injury, but is more slowly triggered. If both glutamate receptor-mediated mechanisms are prevented, then other even more slowly triggered mechanisms eventually produce neuronal death.

reduction of channel opening frequency and a voltage-dependent fast flicker channel block (Westbrook and Mayer, 1987; Christine and Choi, 1990).

(3) Extracellular GABA. This would help keep the membrane hyperpolarized and maintain the Mg^{2+} block of the NMDA receptor-gated channel.

(4) Extracellular Ca^{2+} depletion. Rapid influx of Ca^{2+} from the extracellular space may transiently deplete available extracellular Ca^{2+} and thus limit NMDA receptor-mediated Ca^{2+} influx.

(5) Oxygen free radicals. Although these are highly destructive and may generally be downstream mediators of excitotoxicity (see above), these may also alter the redox state of the NMDA receptor-channel complex and reduce NMDA receptor-mediated currents (Aizenman et al., 1989).

(6) Intracellular energy depletion. Loss of intracellular high energy phosphates and dephosphorylation of the NMDA receptor-channel complex may reduce currents (Mody et al., 1988).

The down-modulation of NMDA receptors due to the above factors, perhaps especially extracellular acidity, may be more complete in global ischemia than in the penumbra of focal ischemia, or in hypoglycemia, providing a potential explanation why NMDA antagonists have been reported more consistently to be beneficial in the latter two conditions than in global ischemia.

It is noteworthy that the alpha-amino-3-hydroxy-5-methyl-isoxazole-4-propionate (AMPA)/kainate receptor antagonist, 2,3-dihydroxy-6-nitro-7-sulfamoyl-benzo(F)quinoxaline (NBQX), has shown protective efficacy in initial studies of either global or focal ischemia (Sheardown et al., 1990; Xue et al., 1991), suggesting that AMPA/kainate receptor

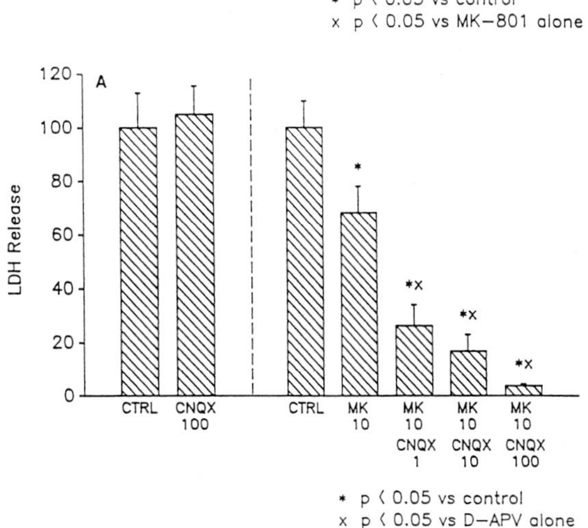

Fig. 3. CNQX combined with MK-801 enhances neuroprotection against oxygen-glucose deprivation. Murine cortical cell cultures were deprived of oxygen and glucose for 100 min, alone (control, CTRL) or in the presence of CNQX, MK-801 (MK) or both as indicated. Values represent mean LDH + S.E.M. ($n = 4$), measured 20 – 24 h after exposure, scaled to the mean LDH of controls (= 100). Results shown to the left and right of the dashed line are from two separate experiments, each scaled to their own control. Numbers below drugs indicate micromolar concentration. Significant difference ($P < 0.05$) from control (*) or from 10 μM MK-801 alone (×) was determined by ANOVA and Student-Neuman-Keuls test. (From Kaku et al., 1991.)

overactivation may be of broad importance in mediating injury following hypoxia-induced sustained elevations in extracellular glutamate. A critical role of AMPA/kainate receptors in global ischemia is highly consistent with the above arguments: if NMDA receptors are turned off but extracellular glutamate concentrations remain high, neuronal death could be due predominantly to injury triggered more slowly by overactivation of AMPA/kainate receptors (Fig. 1). In addition, Pellegrini-Giampietro et al. (1992) have recently reported that global ischemia can induce a selective reduction in the level of mRNA for the Glu-R2/Glu-RB subunit, raising the very intriguing possibility that AMPA/kainate receptors may be modified following global ischemia in a manner that enhances the Ca^{2+} permeability of the associated membrane channel, and thus enhances the contribution of AMPA/kainate receptors to neuronal injury.

As a result of this modification, or other factors yet to be defined, AMPA/kainate receptors may also play a critical role in focal ischemic neuronal injury. Such a critical role for AMPA/kainate receptors is compatible with a similarly critical role for NMDA receptors. It is possible that the overactivation of both NMDA and AMPA/kainate receptors are needed to achieve widespread excitotoxic death in focal ischemia, so that blockade of either leads to reduced brain injury. This situation could reflect a non-specific summation of injury to reach a critical threshold. NMDA receptor overactivation and AMPA/kainate receptor overactivation could independently injure the same neurons, or even different neurons; only when summed together would these events cause massive neuronal death and changes in the cellular microenvironment promoting pannecrosis. Alternatively, this situation could reflect a direct mechanistic interaction between the injury processes, for example, if AMPA/kainate receptor-induced sodium entry was needed to reduce NMDA receptor blockade by extracellular Mg^{2+}, or to disable extrusion of NMDA receptor-induced Ca^{2+} influx through the sodium-calcium exchanger.

References

Albers, G.A., Goldberg, M.P. and Choi, D.W. (1992) Do NMDA antagonists prevent neuronal injury? Yes. *Arch. Neurol.*, 49: 418 – 420.

Aizenman, E., Lipton, S.A. and Loring, R.H. (1989) Selective modulation of NMDA responses by reduction and oxidation. *Neuron*, 2: 1257 – 1263.

Beckman, J.S., Beckman, T.W., Chen, J., Marshall, P.A. and Freeman, B.A. (1990) Apparent hydroxyl radical production by peroxynitrite: implications for endothelial injury from nitric oxide and superoxide. *Proc. Natl. Acad. Sci. U.S.A.*, 87: 1620 – 1624.

Buchan, A.M. (1990) Do NMDA antagonists protect against cerebral ischemia: are clinical trials warranted? *Cereb. Brain Metab. Rev.*, 2: 1 – 26.

Chan, P.H., Fishman, R.A., Longar, S., Chen, S. and Yu, A. (1985) Cellular and molecular effects of polyunsaturated fatty acids in brain ischemia and injury. *Prog. Brain Res.*, 63: 227 – 235.

Choi, D.W. (1988) Glutamate neurotoxicity and diseases of the nervous system. *Neuron*, 1: 623 – 634.

Choi, D.W. (1990a) Methods for antagonizing glutamate neurotoxicity. *Cerebrovasc. Brain Metab. Rev.*, 2: 105 – 147.

Choi, D.W. (1990b) Cerebral hypoxia – some new approaches and unanswered questions. *J. Neurosci.*, 10: 2493 – 2501.

Choi, D.W. (1991) Excitotoxicity. In: B.S. Meldrum (Ed.), *Excitatory Amino Acid Antagonists*, Oxford University Press, Blackwell Scientific Publications, Oxford, pp. 216 – 236.

Christine, C.W. and Choi, D.W. (1990) Effect of zinc on NMDA receptor-mediated channel currents in cortical neurons. *J. Neurosci.*, 10: 108 – 116.

Dykens, J.A., Stern, A. and Trenkner, E. (1987) Mechanism of kainate toxicity to cerebellar neurons in vitro is analogous to reperfusion tissue injury. *J. Neurochem.*, 49: 1222 – 1228.

Frandsen, A., Drejer, J. and Schousboe, A. (1989) Direct evidence that excitotoxicity in cultured neurons is mediated via *N*-methyl-D-aspartate (NMDA) as well as non-NMDA receptors. *J. Neurochem.*, 53: 297 – 299.

Garthwaite, G. and Garthwaite, J. (1986) Neurotoxicity of excitatory amino acid receptor agonists in rat cerebellar slices: dependence on calcium concentration. *Neurosci. Lett.*, 66: 193 – 198.

Garthwaite, J., Charles, S.L. and Chess-Williams, R. (1988) Endothelium-derived relaxing factor release on activation of NMDA receptors suggests role as intercellular messenger in the brain. *Nature*, 336: 385 – 387.

Giffard, R.G., Monyer, H., Christine, C.W. and Choi, D.W. (1990) Acidosis reduces NMDA receptor activation, glutamate neurotoxicity, and oxygen-glucose deprivation neuronal injury in cortical cultures. *Brain Res.*, 506: 339 – 342.

Kaku, D.A., Goldberg, M.P. and Choi, D.W. (1991) Antagonism of non-NMDA receptors augments the neuroprotective effect of NMDA receptor blockade in cortical cultures subjected to prolonged deprivation of oxygen and glucose. *Brain Res.*, 554: 344 – 347.

Koh, J. and Choi, D.W. (1991) Selective blockade of non-NMDA receptors does not block rapidly triggered glutamate-induced neuronal death. *Brain Res.*, 548: 318 – 321.

Mayer, M.L. and Westbrook, G.L. (1987) The physiology of excitatory amino acids in the vertebrate central nervous system. *Prog. Neurobiol.*, 28: 197 – 276.

Meldrum, B. (1985) Possible therapeutic applications of antagonists of excitatory amino acid neurotransmitters. *Clin. Sci.*, 68: 113 – 122.

Mody, I., Salter, M.W. and MacDonald, J.F. (1988) Requirement of NMDA receptor/channels for intracellular high-energy phosphates and the extent of intraneuronal calcium buffering in cultured mouse hippocampal neurons. *Neurosci. Lett.*, 93: 73 – 78.

Monyer, H., Hartley, D.M. and Choi, D.W. (1990) 21-Aminosteroids attenuate excitotoxic neuronal injury in cortical cell cultures. *Neuron*, 5: 121 – 126.

Morad, M., Dichter, M. and Tang, C.M. (1988) The NMDA activated current in hippocampal neurons is highly sensitive to $[H^+]_o$. *Soc. Neurosci. Abstr.*, 14: 791.

Murphy, T.H., Miyamoto, M., Sastre, A., Schnaar, R.L. and Coyle, J.T. (1989) Glutamate toxicity in a neuronal cell line involves inhibition of cystine transport leading to oxidative stress. *Neuron*, 2: 1547 – 1558.

Pellegrini-Giampietro, D.E., Cherici, G., Alesiani, M., Carla, V. and Moroni, F. (1988) Excitatory amino acid release from rat hippocampal slices as a consequence of free-radical formation. *J. Neurochem.*, 51: 1960 – 1963.

Pellegrini-Giampietro, D.E., Friedman, L.K., Moshe, S.L., Pulsinelli, W.A., Bennett, M.V.L. and Zukin, R.S. (1992) Glutamate receptor gene expression in epilepsy and ischemia rat models: a subunit "switch" controls Ca^{2+} permeability through kainate/AMPA receptors. In: *Excitatory Amino Acids, 1992* (poster abstracts), p. 35.

Rothman, S.M. and Olney, J.W. (1987) Excitotoxicity and the NMDA receptor. *Trends Neurosci.*, 10: 299 – 302.

Rothman, S.M., Thurston, J.H. and Hauhart, R.E. (1987) Delayed neurotoxicity of excitatory amino acids in vitro. *Neuroscience*, 22: 471 – 480.

Sheardown, M.J., Nielsen, E.O., Hansen, A.J., Jacobsen, P. and Honoré, T. (1990) 2,3-Dihydroxy-6-nitro-7-sulfamoyl-benzo(F)quinoxaline: a neuroprotectant for cerebral ischemia. *Science*, 247: 571 – 574.

Siesjö, B.K. (1989) Free radicals and brain damage. *Cerebrovasc. Brain Metab. Rev.*, 1: 165 – 211.

Siesjö, B.K. and Bengtsson, F. (1989) Calcium fluxes, calcium antagonists, and calcium-related pathology in brain ischemia, hypoglycemia, and spreading depression: a unifying hypothesis. *J. Cereb. Blood Flow Metab.*, 9: 127 – 140.

Siesjö, B.K., Bengtsson, F., Grampp, W. and Theander, S. (1989) Calcium, excitotoxins, and neuronal death in the brain. *Ann. N.Y. Acad. Sci.*, 568: 234 – 251.

Sommer, B. and Seeburg, P.H. (1992) Glutamate receptor channels: novel properties and new clones. *Trends Pharmacol. Sci.*, 13: 291 – 296.

Tombaugh, G.C. and Sapolsky, R.M. (1990) Mild acidosis protects hippocampal neurons from injury induced by oxygen and glucose deprivation. *Brain Res.*, 506: 343 – 345.

Westbrook, G.L. and Mayer, M.L. (1987) Micromolar concentrations of Zn^{2+} antagonize NMDA and GABA responses of hippocampal neurons. *Nature*, 328: 640 – 643.

Xue, D., Huang, Z.G., Smith, K.E., Lesiuk, H. and Buchan, A.M. (1991) Delayed treatment with NBQX attenuates neocortical infarction. *Soc. Neurosci. Abstr.*, 17: 1266.

SECTION III

Polyamine and Protein Metabolism

K. Kogure, K.-A. Hossmann and B.K. Siesjö (Eds.)
Progress in Brain Research, Vol. 96

CHAPTER 10

Ischemia-induced disturbances of polyamine synthesis

Wulf Paschen[1], Mathias Cleef[1], Gabriele Röhn[1], Michael Müller[2] and Antti E.I. Pajunen[3]

[1]*Max-Planck Institute for Neurological Research, Department of Experimental Neurology, Cologne, Germany;* [2]*Institute for Neurobiology and Brain Research, Department of Neuromorphology, Magdeburg, Germany; and* [3]*Biocenter and Department of Biochemistry, University of Oulu, Oulu, Finland*

Introduction

Polyamine synthesis plays a key role in cellular growth processes including neonatal growth, cell proliferation and differentiation as well as neoplastic growth (for reviews see: Jänne et al., 1978; Canellakis et al., 1979; Williams-Ashman and Canellakis, 1979; Heby, 1981; Seiler and Shaw, 1981; Pegg and McCann, 1982; Pegg et al., 1982; Tabor and Tabor, 1984; Pegg, 1986). Involvement of polyamine synthesis during the phase of perinatal growth is indicated by the high activity of ornithine decarboxylase (ODC, the first key enzyme in polyamine synthesis) and high cerebral levels of putrescine (the product of ODC reaction) at birth, and by the observation that brain development can be retarded considerably by treating animals with the irreversible ODC inhibitor α-difluoromethyl-ornithine (DFMO) (Jasper et al., 1982; Slotkin et al., 1982; Bartolome et al., 1985; Bell et al., 1986; Slotkin and Bartolome, 1986).

In the adult brain polyamine synthesis can be activated by different physiological stimuli: a moderate but significant activation is already produced by saline injection (Dienel and Cruz, 1984; Porcella et al., 1991). ODC activity is sensitive to trophic factors and hormones such as nerve growth factor, bovine growth hormone, insulin, vasopressin, angiotensin II, or glucocorticoids such as corticosterone or dexamethasone (Lewis et al., 1978; Ikeno and Guroff, 1979; Cousin et al., 1982), all of which induce an increase in ODC activity.

Polyamines and particularly putrescine has been shown to activate an influx of calcium ions and release of excitotoxic amino acids from nerve endings (Iqbal and Koenig, 1985; Bondy and Walker, 1986; Komulainen and Bondy, 1987) and thus to be putatively neurotoxic when high levels of this compound are present in nerve endings, as has been observed recently after cerebral ischemia (see Röhn et al., 1990). Polyamines and particularly putrescine play a role in disturbances of the blood-brain barrier in different pathological states (Koenig et al., 1983a, 1989a-c; Sears et al., 1985; Trout et al., 1986): blood-brain barrier disturbances were almost completely prevented by treating animals with the ODC inhibitor DFMO (Koenig et al., 1983a, 1989b; Sears et al., 1985). DFMO could also prevent *N*-methyl-D-aspartate (NMDA) toxicity in tissue culture (Markwell et al., 1990), and the neurotoxic effects of chlordecone (Tilson et al., 1986), thus implying that the polyamine system is involved. In addition, evidence has been presented that T-lymphocyte-mediated cytolysis is evoked by polyamines (Chayen et al., 1990) and that the cytotoxicity of aziridinylbenzoquinone or cis-diamminedichloro-platinum (II) is considerably reduced by DFMO thus illustrating that the polyamine system plays a role in these pathological processes, too (Oredsson et al., 1982; Alhonen-Hongisto et al., 1984). Finally, polyamines released from cells into the extracellular compartment may bind to the NMDA receptor and may thus cause a pathological overactivation of this receptor complex: the NMDA receptor complex exhibits a polyamine recognition site which upon binding with polyamines induces an increase in the activity of the receptor (Gotti et al., 1988; Ransom and Stec, 1988; Reynolds and Miller, 1989; Sacaan and Johnson, 1989, 1990; Williams et al., 1989; Schoemaker et al., 1990; Singh et al., 1990; Sprosen and Woodruff, 1990; for review, see also Williams et al., 1991). Finally, polyamines when applied to neuronal cell cultures or injected intraventricularly into animals potentiate the NMDA-induced whole cell currents (Sprosen and Woodruff, 1990) and potentiate, dose-dependently, the seizure activity of *N*-methyl-DL-aspartate or pentylenetetrazol (Singh et al., 1990). All these observations indicate that under certain pathological conditions polyamines may be neurotoxic, a view which has been discussed recently by Coffino and Poznanski (1991).

Polyamine synthesis is markedly activated in different pathological states of the brain such as seizures (Pajunen et al., 1979; Baudry et al., 1986; Tilson et al., 1986; Martinez et al., 1991), electrical stimulation (Russell et al., 1974; Pajunen et al., 1978; Bondy et al., 1987; Arai et al., 1990; Zawia and Bondy, 1990), lesions (Agnati et al., 1985; Ali et al., 1987; Desiderio et al., 1988; Walsh et al., 1989), excitotoxic conditions (Reed and de Belleroche, 1989, 1990; Gardiner and de Belleroche, 1990; Porcella et al., 1991), ischemia (Kleihues et al., 1975; Dienel et al., 1985; Paschen et al., 1987a,b, 1988e; Dempsey et al., 1988a,b), hypoglycemia (Paschen et al., 1991c) and conditions under which the integrity of the blood-brain barrier is disturbed (Koenig et al., 1983a; Sears et al., 1985). From these observations it becomes evident that activation of polyamine synthesis is related to cellular stress, the activation of polyamine synthesis (increase in ODC activity and putrescine levels) being most pronounced following severe metabolic stress such as that produced by transient cerebral ischemia.

The present review will summarize what is known about ischemia-induced disturbances in polyamine synthesis. The following topics will be discussed in more detail: (a) the periods of time during which changes take place; (b) the relationship of changes in polyamine synthesis to the duration of ischemia; (c) the exact cellular location of these disturbances; (d) the relationship between post-ischemic changes in polyamine synthesis and density of neuronal cell death; and (e) pharmacological interventions reducing ischemia-induced disturbances in polyamine synthesis. In the discussion emphasis will be put on the possible role of ischemia-induced alterations in polyamine metabolism either in the process of recovery from the metabolic stress produced by cerebral ischemia or in the manifestation of neuronal necrosis. In fact, results of previous studies permit both conclusions to be drawn. However, as will be discussed below, we favor the assumption that post-ischemic disturbances in polyamine metabolism play a role in the development of neuronal cell damage.

Temporal profile of ischemia-induced changes in polyamine synthesis

Changes in polyamine synthesis induced by transient forebrain ischemia have been studied in different animal species, including monkeys, cats, rats and Mongolian gerbils, by measuring the activity of the key enzymes ornithine decarboxylase (ODC) and S-adenosylmethionine decarboxylase (SAMDC) and the levels of the polyamines putrescine, spermidine and spermine (Kleihues et al., 1975; Dempsey et al., 1985, 1988a,b; Dienel et al., 1985; Paschen et al., 1987a,b, 1988a; Koenig et al., 1990). Global cerebral ischemia affected neither ODC nor SAMDC activity immediately, independent of the animal species used and the duration of vascular occlusion (Kleihues et al., 1975; Dienel et al., 1985; Paschen et al., 1988a). The observation that ODC and SAMDC activity did not change during ischemia is indicative of a "metabolically frozen" state of the tissue during which protein synthesis and degradation are suppressed (Kleihues et al., 1975). During the first 60 – 120 min of reperfusion the activity of both enzymes decreased, most likely as a result of a suppressed protein synthesis and increased degradation (Kleihues et al., 1975; Dienel et al., 1985). Later ODC activity returned to control values and then sharply increased in animals in which the recirculation time was extended to more than 3 h (Kleihues et al., 1975; Dienel et al., 1985). SAMDC activity remained depressed for several hours after ischemia (Kleihues et al., 1975; Dienel et al., 1985).

ODC and SAMDC are key enzymes in polyamine synthesis. Ischemia-induced changes in enzyme activity should, therefore, influence polyamine levels considerably: the high post-ischemic ODC activity should accelerate decarboxylation of ornithine to putrescine and the low SAMDC activity should suppress the interconversion of putrescine into spermidine and spermine. Indeed, putrescine levels were sharply increased after cerebral ischemia (Paschen et al., 1987a,b, 1990b). Spermidine and spermine levels were less affected by ischemia. A decrease could only be observed in animals at a time when cell damage had already developed (Paschen et al., 1987a,b, 1988b).

A typical example of the changes in polyamine metabolism produced by global cerebral ischemia is given in Fig. 1. Ischemia of 5 min duration was produced in Mongolian gerbils. ODC activity was sharply increased after 8 h of recirculation but it returned to control levels when the recirculation was extended to 24 h. SAMDC activity, in contrast, was decreased throughout the whole recirculation time studied. Putrescine levels were sharply increased after 8 h and even more pronounced after 24 h of recirculation. Spermidine and spermine levels were not significantly changed.

Little information is available about changes in polyamine synthesis in focal cerebral ischemia (Dempsey et al., 1985; Paschen et al., 1991a). In the cat brain, middle cerebral artery occlusion produced a significant increase in ODC activity in the penumbra region in which blood flow was only moderately reduced (Dempsey et al., 1985). This increase could only be found 6 h after vascular occlusion. During

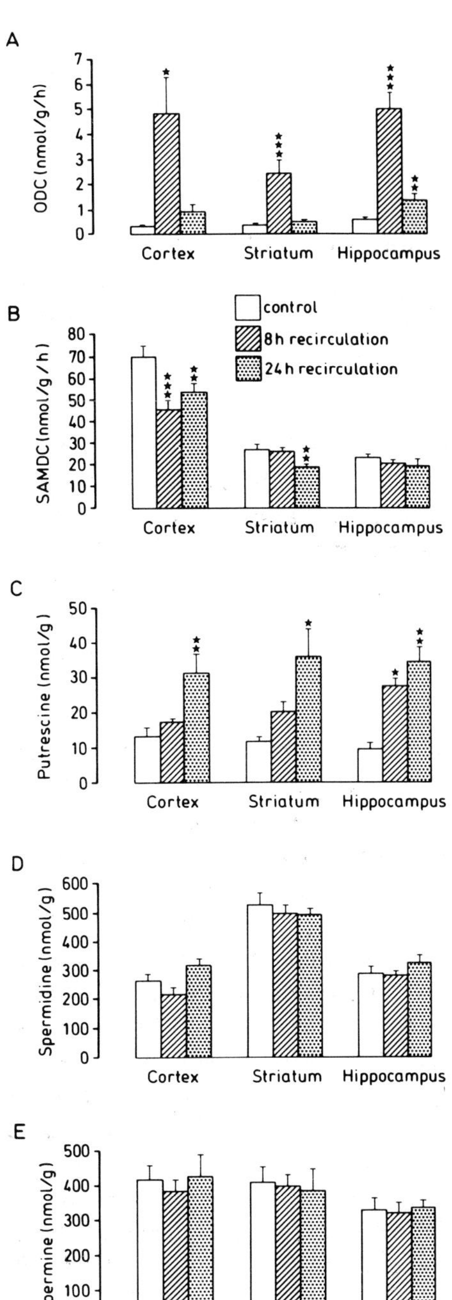

Fig. 1. Ischemia-induced changes in ODC (*A*) and SAMDC (*B*) activity and putrescine (*C*), spermidine (*D*) and spermine (*E*) levels in the cerebral cortex, striatum and hippocampus of Mongolian gerbils. Ischemia was produced by occluding both common carotid arteries for 5 min. (From Paschen et al., 1987b, 1990a; and Röhn et al., 1992, with modifications.)

embolization of the middle cerebral artery in the rat brain, spermidine levels were significantly reduced in the ipsilateral cerebral cortex and striatum and spermine levels in the ipsilateral cortex (Paschen et al., 1991a). The changes could be reversed during recirculation. ODC activity and putrescine levels did not change during focal cerebral ischemia but after reflow; a significant increase in ODC activity was observed after 4 h of recirculation and the highest putrescine levels (about five-fold over control values) were found after 24 h of recirculation (Paschen et al., 1991a).

In summary, ischemia-induced changes in polyamine synthesis exhibit the following features: in all but one study of transient forebrain ischemia (exception: Koenig et al., 1990) ODC and SAMDC activity and polyamine levels were stable during ischemia. During the first 2 h of recirculation the activity of both enzymes dropped. After prolonged recirculation SAMDC activity remained severely suppressed for several days (exception: monkey study, Kleihues et al., 1975) and ODC activity increased sharply peaking at 8 – 10 h of recirculation. Post-ischemic putrescine levels were markedly increased. Spermidine and spermine levels were found to be decreased but only after prolonged recirculation in severely damaged areas. In focal cerebral ischemia spermidine and, to a lesser extent, spermine levels were already reduced during vascular occlusion in the ischemic territory. Values normalized after recirculation. Post-ischemic changes in polyamine profiles are most probably the result of the marked increase in ODC activity and decrease in SAMDC activity and thus arising from a pathological disturbance of polyamine synthesis, because only the first step (ODC-step) is activated whereas the second step (SAMDC-step) is markedly suppressed.

Location of changes in polyamine synthesis

For a discussion of the physiological or pathological role of ischemia-induced changes in polyamine synthesis the exact location of these changes is of importance: (a) the brain areas which are affected; (b) within a given area the cells which respond; and finally (c) the cellular compartment involved and whether these changes take place in the intracellular compartment only or both in the intra- and extracellular compartment. These three topics will be discussed below.

As regards (a): all brain areas supposed to be ischemic during vascular occlusion responded to transient cerebral ischemia with an increase in ODC and decrease in SAMDC activity and a sharp rise in putrescine levels (Dienel et al., 1985; Paschen et al., 1987a,b, 1988a; Röhn et al., 1991). These changes did not differ much in the various forebrain structures studied. It is, therefore, not possible to identify brain structures vulnerable to cerebral ischemia by a specific pattern. However, in vulnerable brain structures such as the hippocampal CA1 subfield, putrescine levels remained high for several days after cerebral ischemia but levels returned to control values in areas which are not vulnerable to short-term ischemia such as the cortex or thalamus (Paschen et al., 1987b).

As regards (b): the biochemical techniques available for measuring ODC and SAMDC activity and polyamine levels do not permit these parameters to be studied at the cellular level. Instead, immunohistochemical approaches have been used to identify the cellular location of post-ischemic changes in ODC protein (Dempsey et al., 1988a,b). In a recent series of experiments performed in our laboratory (Müller et al., 1991) ODC activity and immunoreactivity were studied in the cerebral cortex, striatum and hippocampus of gerbils subjected to 5 min forebrain ischemia and 8 h of recirculation (Fig. 2). In control animals both ODC activity and immunoreactivity were low. Immunoreactivity was found in neurons but not in glial cells. After ischemia ODC immunoreactivity increased sharply in all brain structures studied. The highest density of the reaction product was observed in the stratum pyramidale of the hippocampal CA1-subfield (Fig. 2). This observation is surprising because transient cerebral ischemia produces a severe activation in ODC protein synthesis but, on the other hand, autoradiographic measurements in gerbils have established that transient cerebral ischemia leads to a severe depression of protein synthesis in the hippocampal CA1-subfield (Bodsch et al., 1985; Thilman et al., 1986). The assumption that ODC is newly synthezised after cerebral ischemia is corroborated by the observation that the post-ischemic increase in ODC activity can be suppressed by blocking protein synthesis (Dienel et al., 1985), and that ischemia evokes an activation of ODC gene expression (Dempsey et al., 1991). Remarkably, results from previous studies indicate that in the hippocampal CA1-subfield the development of ischemic cell damage can be prevented by blocking protein synthesis with cycloheximide (Goto et al., 1990), thus implying that proteins synthesized during recirculation contribute to the pathological process.

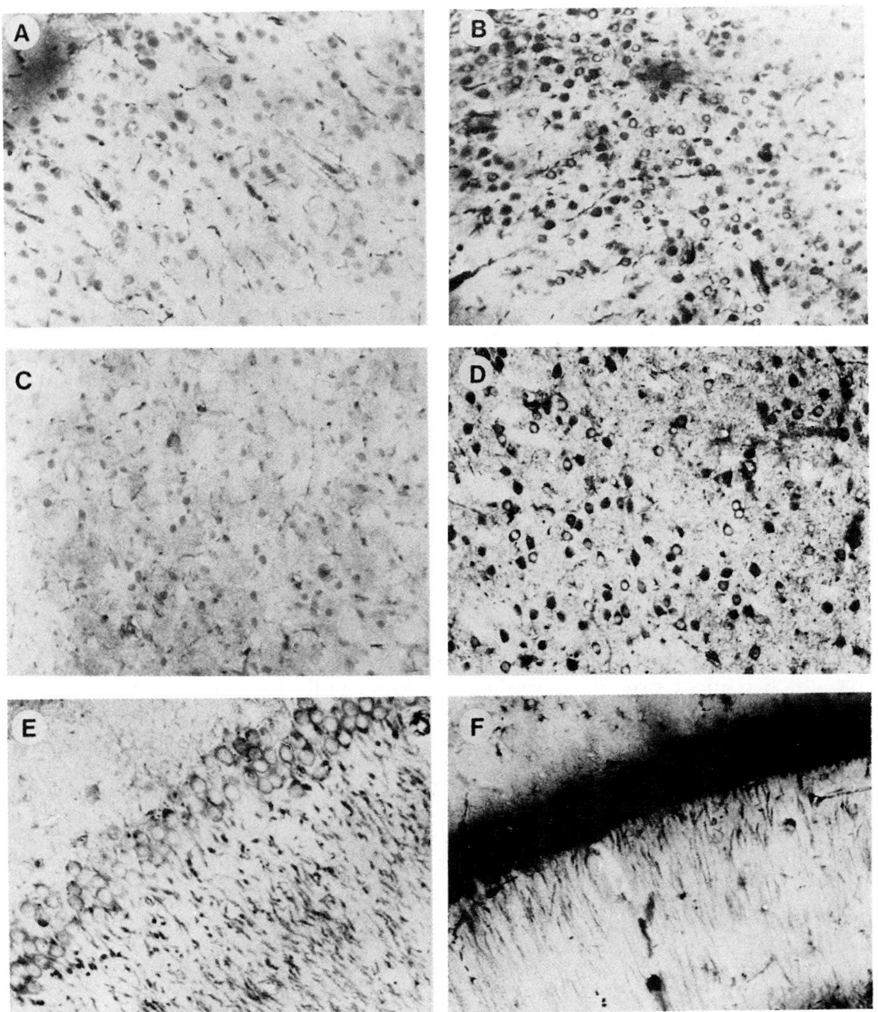

Fig. 2. ODC immunoreactivity studied in the cerebral cortex (*A,B*), striatum (*C,D*) and hippocampal CA1-subfield (*E,F*) of control gerbils (*A,C,E*) and animals subjected to 5 min transient cerebral ischemia (occlusion of both common carotid arteries) and 8 h of recirculation. Transient cerebral ischemia induced a marked increase in ODC immunoreactivity in all brain structures studied, changes being most prominent in the CA1-subfield of the hippocampus. The increase in ODC immunoreactivity was most pronounced in the perinuclear cytoplasm.

As regards (c): as illustrated by the neuronal distribution of ODC immunoreactivity (see above), polyamine synthesis is a cellular event. Post-ischemic changes in polyamine levels take, therefore, most likely place in the intracellular compartment. However, it has already been shown that polyamines are released under in vitro conditions from cells into the extracellular compartment: from cortical slices after potassium-induced depolarization (Harman and Shaw, 1981) and from hippocampal slices upon incubation under ischemia-like conditions (Djuricic et al., 1990). Any decrease of the tissue polyamine levels results most probably from a release of polyamines from neurons into the extracellular compartment and clearance into the blood. Such changes have in fact been observed in transient cerebral ischemia in two different phases (see above): during focal cerebral ischemia within the ischemic territory (Paschen et al., 1991a) and after transient forebrain ischemia in severely damaged areas (Paschen et al., 1987b, 1988b, 1990a).

In summary, ischemia-induced changes in polyamine synthesis are confined to transiently ischemic brain regions and are most pronounced and prolonged in structures known to be vulnerable to cerebral ischemia such as the striatum and hippocampus. The post-ischemic increase in ODC activity results from an activation of ODC gene expression and protein synthesis. It is a neuronal response to transient ischemia which is most pronounced in the hippocampal CA1-subfield. Changes in polyamine synthesis are mainly intracellular events but polyamines may also be released from neurons during ischemia and after prolonged recirculation in severely damaged regions.

Post-ischemic changes in polyamine synthesis in relation to the duration of ischemia

In a recent study performed in our laboratory the post-ischemic changes in ODC and SAMDC activity were investigated in Mongolian gerbils subjected to 2, 4, 6, 8 or 10 min ischemia and 8 h or 24 h of recirculation (Fig. 3; see also Röhn et al., 1991, 1992). Interestingly, after 8 h of recirculation ODC activity correlated closely with the duration of ischemia in animals in which the carotid arteries were occluded for a few minutes only. However, ODC activity leveled off when the duration of ischemia was prolonged. In the hippocampus this occurred after only 4 min of vascular occlusion and in the cerebral cortex and striatum after 8 min of ischemia. SAMDC activity was decreased after ischemia but only slightly. This change was most pronounced in the cortex in which the activity was highest in control animals. In absolute terms the lowest SAMDC activity was observed after 24 h of recirculation in the hippocampus.

The post-ischemic changes in polyamine profiles are produced by a sharp increase in ODC activity and decrease in SAMDC activity. Thus, the SAMDC/ODC ratio is a suitable index of the extent of these changes. From the results of Röhn et al. (1991, 1992) the SAMDC/ODC ratio can be calculated. In control animals this ratio ranged between 52 and 162 indicating that SAMDC activity exceeded ODC activity considerably. After only 4 min ischemia and 8 h of recirculation the SAMDC/ODC ratio was sharply reduced in the hippocampus to 2 but it was still above 12 in the cortex, striatum and thalamus. These results, thus, illustrate that after short-term cerebral ischemia disturbances in polyamine synthesis are most marked in the vulnerable hippocampus.

In the gerbil brain post-ischemic putrescine levels correlated closely with the duration of ischemia: after 5 min ischemia and 24 h of recirculation average putrescine levels amounted to 31.3, 35.8, 34.5 and 18.4 nmol/g in the cerebral cortex, striatum, hippocampal CA1-subfield and thalamus, respectively (Paschen et al., 1987b). After 10 min ischemia and 24 h of recirculation average putrescine contents were 58.0, 76.4, 46.7 and 27.5 nmol/g, respectively, indicating that prolonging the duration of ischemia from 5 to 10 min produced a two-fold increase in putrescine levels.

In summary, after short-term ischemia and 8 h of recirculation ODC activity correlates with the duration of ischemia. However, post-ischemic enzyme activity levels off after only 4 min of ischemia in the

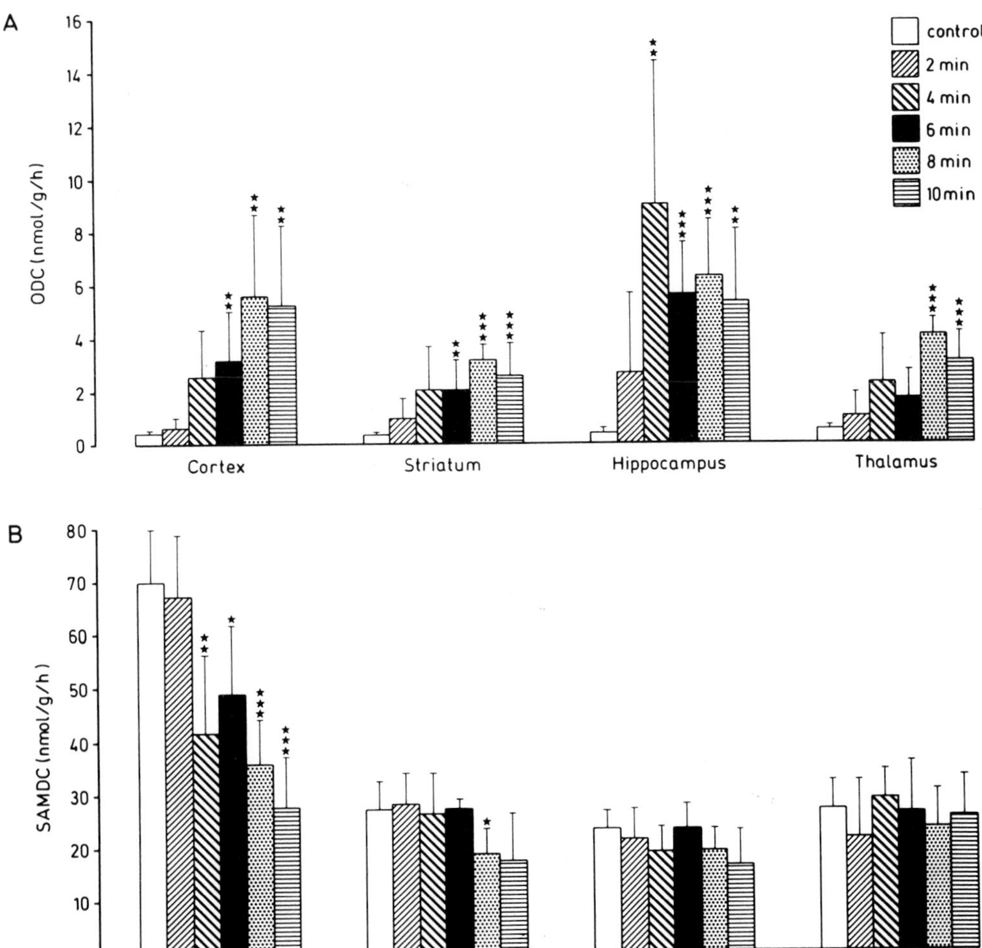

Fig. 3. Post-ischemic changes in ODC (*A*) and SAMDC (*B*) activity after 8 h recirculation in relation to the duration of ischemia. Cerebral ischemia was produced in Mongolian gerbils by occluding both common carotid arteries. (From Röhn et al., 1992, with permission.)

hippocampus and after 8 min in the cortex, striatum and thalamus. SAMDC activity is reduced after cerebral ischemia in relation to the duration of vascular occlusion, the lowest values being found in the hippocampus. Post-ischemic putrescine levels correlate closely with the duration of ischemia. It is suggested that the sharp increase in putrescine levels is the result of an increase in ODC and decrease in SAMDC activity. Thus, the SAMDC/ODC activity ratio and putrescine levels can be used as an indicator of the extent of ischemia-induced disturbances in polyamine synthesis.

Density of neuronal cell damage in relation to the extent of post-ischemic disturbances in polyamine synthesis

One prerequisite for a role of polyamines in the manifestation of ischemic cell damage is that the disturbances in polyamine metabolism are most pronounced in animals exhibiting a high density of injured neurons. This prerequisite is indeed fulfilled. In the gerbil brain after 5 min ischemia and 96 h of recirculation a close threshold relationship could be established between cell death and putrescine levels in the hippocampal CA1-subfield (Paschen et al., 1988c,d). In animals in which putrescine levels were below 20 nmol/g less than 10% of neurons of the stratum pyramidale were damaged, whereas in animals with putrescine levels above 30 nmol/g more than 90% of neurons were injured. A similar threshold has been established recently in the lateral striatum of gerbils after 5 min ischemia and 24 h of recirculation. Notably, in animals exhibiting a high density of injured neurons putrescine levels were above 60 nmol/g (60.7 – 81.5 nmol/g) in the lateral striatum while in animals in which only a few neurons were affected in this area putrescine levels were between 15.8 and 51.9 nmol/g. These results indicate that in the lateral striatum the threshold of putrescine is about twice as high as in the hippocampal CA1-subfield.

In summary, a threshold putrescine level for the manifestation of neuronal cell death has been established at a period of recirculation when cell damage is fully developed, i.e., after 24 h or 96 h of recirculation in the lateral striatum and hippocampal CA1-subfield, respectively. These thresholds amounted to putrescine levels of about 25 nmol/g for the CA1-subfield and of about 55 nmol/g for the lateral striatum.

The effects of pharmacological intervention on ischemia-induced disturbances in polyamine synthesis

Several studies have been performed to investigate the basic mechanisms underlying the ischemia-induced activation and disturbance of polyamine synthesis (Dempsey et al., 1988a,b, 1991; Paschen et al., 1988a – d, 1989, 1990a; Koenig et al., 1990). The following drugs have been used: barbiturate (Paschen et al., 1988b – d, 1990a; Dempsey et al., 1991), the calcium antagonist nimodipine (Paschen et al., 1988b,c), the glutamate antagonist MK-801 (Koenig et al., 1990; Dempsey et al., 1991), and α-difluoromethylornithine (DFMO, Dempsey et al., 1988; Paschen et al., 1988a, 1989; Koenig et al., 1990) which is an enzyme-activated (suicidal) irreversible inhibitor of ODC (Metcalf et al., 1978).

It has been shown previously that barbiturate treatment suppresses the development of ischemia-induced neuronal necrosis (Hallmeyer et al., 1985; Kirino et al., 1986; Paschen et al., 1988b,c). In gerbils barbiturate produced different effects on ODC gene expression, ODC activity and putrescine levels. Interestingly, barbiturate suppressed the ischemia-induced activation of ODC gene expression (Dempsey et al., 1991) but it had no effect on ODC activity (Paschen et al., 1990a): in barbiturate-treated gerbils the post-ischemic increase in ODC activity was even higher than in untreated ones. In contrast, putrescine levels were significantly reduced by barbiturate treatment (Paschen et al., 1990a). It has been suggested that the sharp post-ischemic rise in putrescine levels arises from an increase in ODC and decrease in SAMDC activity, the latter being caused by a post-ischemic suppression of overall protein synthesis (see above). The observation that barbiturate did not affect ODC activity but produced a significant reduction in putrescine levels suggests that SAMDC activity may be influenced by this drug. In fact, in barbiturate-treated animals protein synthesis recovers after ischemia even in the vulnerable hippocampal CA1-subfield (Xie et al., 1987; for a discussion of the relationship between ischemia-induced disturbances in protein and polyamine metabolism, see also Paschen et al., 1991b).

Treating gerbils with the calcium antagonist nimodipine suppressed the development of neuronal necrosis and the ischemia-induced increase in putrescine levels in the lateral striatum but this drug had no significant effect on cell damage and polyamine synthesis in the hippocampal CA1-subfield (Paschen et al., 1988b,c). The glutamate antagonist MK-801, on the other hand, had no effect in gerbils on the ischemia-induced activation of ODC gene expression (Dempsey et al., 1991) but suppressed the post-ischemic increase in ODC activity and putrescine levels almost completely (Koenig et al., 1990).

The ODC inhibitor DFMO had different effects on the post-ischemic increase in ODC activity and putrescine levels (Paschen et al., 1988a): in the rat brain after 30 min forebrain ischemia and 8 h of recirculation the rise in ODC activity was almost completely suppressed by DFMO but the effect on putrescine levels was considerably weaker. This discrepancy was most pronounced in the hippocampus where ODC activity remained at control values in treated animals but putrescine levels were unaffected. Obviously, under these experimental conditions, the reduction in SAMDC activity may be the main cause of the overshoot in putrescine levels. One study investigated the effect of DFMO on cell necrosis (Paschen et al., 1989). DFMO did not produce a significant effect on neuronal necrosis in the hippocampal CA1-subfield. However, in treated animals spermine levels were markedly below those of untreated gerbils. Since spermine plays an important function in the calcium buffering capacity of mitochondria (Nicchitta and Williamson, 1984; Jensen et al., 1987; Kröner, 1988; Rottenberg and Marbach, 1990) the DFMO-induced decrease in spermine levels might be viewed as a complicating factor.

In summary, the results discussed above suggest that activation of the NMDA receptor complex and an overflow of calcium ions into neurons during ischemia are responsible for the post-ischemic activation of polyamine synthesis. The differences in the effect of barbiturate and MK-801 on ODC gene expression and ODC activity indicate that transient cerebral ischemia may influence both transcription and translation. This remains to be elucidated in further investigations.

Polyamines: neuroprotective or neurotoxic?

The features of the post-ischemic disturbances in polyamine synthesis summarized above (e.g., the close relationship between density of cell necrosis and putrescine levels) suggest that the overshoot in putrescine formation contributes to the manifestation of cell damage. However, it has been shown that in the recovery of peripheral nerves from injury polyamines may be neuroprotective (Gilad and Gilad, 1983a,b; Dornay et al., 1986; Kanje et al., 1986; Wells, 1986), a concept which has been questioned by others (Kohsaka et al., 1982; Wong and Mattox, 1991). Recently evidence has been presented indicating that polyamines are also neuroprotective in a model of transient forebrain ischemia (Gilad and Gilad, 1991): the density of neuronal necrosis in the hippocampal CA1-subfield of gerbils subjected to 5 min transient forebrain ischemia was significantly reduced after intraperitoneal injection of either putrescine, spermidine or spermine. However, there was no conclusive evidence presented that the observed neuroprotective activity was a direct effect of polyamines acting in the tissue after passage through the blood-brain barrier.

Polyamine-induced neurotoxicity could arise in four different ways: (a) a damaging effect produced by the overshoot in putrescine formation resulting in a putrescine-sensitive influx of calcium ions and efflux of excitatory neurotransmitters from nerve endings (Koenig et al., 1983a – c; Iqbal and Koenig, 1985; Bondy and Walker, 1986; Komulainen and Bondy, 1987); (b) disturbance of intracellular calcium homeostasis owing to a reduced calcium buffering capacity of mitochondria in regions in which spermine levels are low; (c) cytotoxic effects caused by H_2O_2 formation: the post-ischemic overshoot in putrescine may in part result from an activation of the interconversion of spermidine into putrescine as in other pathological conditions such as carbon tetrachloride-induced liver cell damage (Persson and Pegg, 1984). This interconversion is produced by the enzymes spermidine N-acetyltransferase and polyamine oxidase, where H_2O_2 is formed during the oxidase-catalyzed reaction; and (d) cell damage induced by an overactivation of the NMDA-receptor complex in regions in which polyamines are released from neurons and bound to the polyamine recognition site of the NMDA receptor complex at cells in close vicinity.

A promising approach for determining whether ischemia-induced activation of polyamine synthesis is a physiological or a pathological response to cellular stress is to study changes in ODC activity under conditions known to influence the development of neuronal necrosis. In the gerbil brain after

5 min transient cerebral ischemia most neurons of the hippocampal CA1-subfield develop neuronal necrosis after about four days of recirculation. ODC activity as well as ODC immunoreactivity is sharply increased in this brain region after 8 h of recirculation, i.e., at a time when the cells are still viable. In a recent publication Kirino and co-workers (1991) presented evidence that in the hippocampal CA1-subfield after 5 min transient ischemia neuronal necrosis can be considerably reduced by pretreating animals 3 – 4 days earlier with a sublethal ischemia of 2 min duration. This illustrates that a sublethal form of stress protects against subsequent, otherwise lethal, stress. We have used this experimental paradigm to further investigate the possible role of polyamine synthesis in either cell damage or regeneration of cells from stress (unpublished observations). Assuming a role of polyamine synthesis in cell regeneration, a sublethal ischemia of 2 min duration should cause a further increase in ODC activity after the second 5 min period of ischemia because regeneration is activated. On the other hand, assuming a role of polyamine synthesis in the development of cell necrosis, the 2 min period of ischemia should suppress the increase in ODC activity after the second ischemia of 5 min duration because the manifestation of cell necrosis is inhibited. Indeed, in gerbils the sublethal 2 min period of ischemia preceding the second period of ischemia by three days almost completely suppressed the increase in ODC activity evoked by 5 min ischemia: in the hippocampus ODC activity in pretreated (2 min ischemia) and non-pretreated animals amounted to 1.5 ± 0.76 and 7.0 ± 5.45 nmol/g per hour, respectively (means ± S.D., $P < 0.05$). These results, thus, corroborate the assumption that the post-ischemic activation of polyamine synthesis plays a role in the manifestation of ischemia-induced neuronal cell death.

In summary, transient cerebral ischemia causes a disturbance of polyamine synthesis which is characterized by a sharp increase in ODC and decrease in SAMDC activity. The result is an overshoot in putrescine formation and a reduction in spermine levels. In addition, evidence is presented that polyamines are released from the intracellular compartment during ischemia and following prolonged recirculation in severely damaged areas. Because of the main features of ischemia-induced disturbances in polyamine synthesis and the reactions known to be influenced by these altered polyamine profiles it is suggested that these changes play a role in the manifestation of ischemia-induced neuronal necrosis. Since similar disturbances in polyamine synthesis are a common response to severe cellular stress, studying polyamine synthesis in transient cerebral ischemia may help to elucidate the molecular mechanisms which are involved in the development of neuronal necrosis under different pathological conditions.

Acknowledgements

The excellent technical assistance of Änne Pribliczki is gratefully acknowledged. This work was supported by the Deutsche Forschungsgemeinschaft, Grant Pa 266/3-2.

References

Agnati, L.F., Fuxe, K., Davalli, P., Zini, I., Corti, A. and Zoli, M. (1985) Striatal ornithine decarboxylase activity following neurotoxic and mechanical lesions of the mesostriatal dopamine system of the male rat. *Acta Physiol. Scand.*, 125: 173 – 175.

Alhonen-Hongisto, L., Deen, D.F. and Marton, L.J. (1984) Decreased cytotoxicity of aziridinylbenzoquinone caused by polyamine depletion in 9L rat brain tumor cells in vitro. *Cancer Res.*, 44: 39 – 42.

Ali, S.F., Newport, G.D., Slikker Jr., W. and Bondy, S.C. (1987) Effect of trimethyltin on ornithine decarboxylase in various regions of the mouse brain. *Toxicol. Lett.*, 36: 67 – 72.

Arai, A., Baudry, M., Staubli, U., Lynch, G. and Gall, C. (1990) Induction of ornithine decarboxylase by subseizure stimulation in the hippocampus in vivo. *Mol. Brain Res.*, 7: 167 – 169.

Bartolome, J.V., Schweitzer, L., Slotkin, T.A. and Nadler, J.V. (1985) Impaired development of cerebellar cortex in rats treated postnatally with α-difluoromethylornithine. *Neuroscience,* 15: 203 – 213.

Baudry, M., Lynch, G. and Gall, C. (1986) Induction of ornithine decarboxylase as a possible mediator of seizure-elicited changes in genomic expression in rat hippocampus. *J. Neurosci.*, 6: 3430 – 3435.

Bell, J.M., Whitmore, W.L. and Slotkin, T.A. (1986) Effects of α-difluoromethylornithine, a specific irreversible inhibitor of ornithine decarboxylase, on nucleic acids and proteins in developing rat brain: critical perinatal periods for regional selectivity. *Neuroscience,* 17: 399 – 407.

Bodsch, W., Takahashi, K., Barbier, A., Grosse Ophoff, B. and Hossmann, K.-A. (1985) Cerebral protein synthesis and ischemia. *Prog. Brain Res.,* 63: 197 – 210.

Bondy, S.C. and Walker, C.H. (1986) Polyamines contribute to calcium-stimulated release of aspartate from brain particulate fraction. *Brain Res.,* 371: 96 – 100.

Bondy, S.C., Mitchell, C.L., Rahmaan, S. and Mason, G. (1987) Regional variation in the response of cerebral ornithine decarboxylase to electroconvulsive shock. *Neurochem. Pathol.,* 7: 129 – 141.

Canellakis, E.S., Viceps-Madore, D., Kyriakidis, D.A. and Heller, J.S. (1979) The regulation and function of ornithine decarboxylase and of polyamines. *Curr. Top. Cell. Regul.,* 15: 155 – 202.

Chayen, J., Pitsillides, A.A., Bitenski, L., Muir, I.H., Taylor, P.M. and Askonas, B.A. (1990) T-cell mediated cytolysis: evidence for target-cell suicide. *J. Exp. Pathol.,* 71: 197 – 208.

Coffino, P. and Poznanski, A. (1991) Killer polyamines? *J. Cell. Biochem.,* 45: 54 – 58.

Cousin, M.A., Lando, D. and Moguilewsky, M. (1982) Ornithine decarboxylase induction by glucocorticoids in brain and liver of adrenalectomized rats. *J. Neurochem.,* 38: 1296 – 1304.

Dempsey, R.J., Roy, M.W., Meyer, K., Tai, H. and Olson, J.W. (1985) Polyamine and prostaglandine markers in focal cerebral ischemia. *Neurosurgery,* 17: 635 – 640.

Dempsey, R.J., Roy, M.W., Cowen, D.E. and Combs, D. (1988a) Polyamine inhibition preserves somatosensory evoked potential activity after transient cerebral ischaemia. *Neurol. Res.,* 10: 141 – 145.

Dempsey, R.J., Maley, B.E., Cowen, D. and Olson, J.W. (1988b) Ornithine decarboxylase and immunohistochemical location in postischemic brain. *J. Cereb. Blood Flow Metab.,* 8: 843 – 847.

Dempsey, R.J., Carney, J.M. and Kindy, M.S. (1991) Modulation of ornithine decarboxylase mRNA following transient ischemia in the gerbil brain. *J. Cereb. Blood Flow Metab.,* 11: 979 – 985.

Desiderio, M.A., Zini, I., Davalli, P., Zoli, M., Corti, A., Fuxe, K. and Agnati, L.F. (1988) Polyamines, ornithine decarboxylase, and diamine oxidase in the substantia nigra and striatum of the male rat after hemitransection. *J. Neurochem.,* 51: 25 – 31.

Dienel, G.A. and Cruz, N.F. (1984) Induction of brain ornithine decarboxylase during recovery from metabolic, mechanical, thermal, or chemical injury. *J. Neurochem.,* 42: 1053 – 1061.

Dienel, G.A., Cruz, N.F. and Rosenfeld, S.J. (1985) Temporal profiles of proteins responsive to transient ischemia. *J. Neurochem.,* 44: 600 – 610.

Djuricic, B., Assaf, H.M., Lust, W.D. and Drewes, L.R. (1990) Release of polyamines from hippocampal slices occurs during in vitro ischemia. *Yugoslav. Physiol. Pharmacol. Acta,* 26: 361 – 367.

Dornay, M., Gilad, V.H., Shiller, I. and Gilad, G.M. (1986) Early polyamine treatment accelerates regeneration of rat sympathetic neurons. *Exp. Neurol.,* 92: 665 – 674.

Gardiner, I.M. and de Belleroche, J. (1990) Reversal of neurotoxin-induced ornithine decarboxylase activity in rat cerebral cortex by nimodipine. A potential neuroprotective mechanism. *Stroke,* 21 (Suppl. IV): IV-93 – IV-94.

Gilad, G.M. and Gilad, V.H. (1983a) Early rapid and transient increase in ornithine decarboxylase activity within sympathetic neurons after axonal injury. *Exp. Neurol.,* 81: 158 – 166.

Gilad, G.M. and Gilad, V.H. (1983b) Polyamine biosynthesis is required for survival of sympathetic neurons after axonal injury. *Brain Res.,* 273: 191 – 194.

Gilad, G.M. and Gilad, V.H. (1991) Polyamines can protect against ischemia-induced nerve cell death in gerbil forebrain. *Exp. Neurol.,* 111: 349 – 355.

Goto, K., Ishige, A., Sekiguchi, K., Iizuka, S., Sugimoto, A., Yuzurihara, M., Aburada, N., Hosoya, E. and Kogure, K. (1990) Effects of cycloheximide on delayed neuronal death in rat hippocampus. *Brain Res.,* 534: 299 – 302.

Gotti, B., Duverger, D., Bertin, J., Carter, C., DuPont, R., Frost, J., Gaudilliere, B., MacKenzie, E.T., Rousseau, J., Scatton, B. and Wick, A. (1988) Ifenprodil and SL 82.0715 as cerebral anti-ischemic agents. I. Evidence for efficacy in models of focal cerebral ischemia. *J. Pharmacol. Exp. Ther.,* 247: 1211 – 1221.

Hallmayer, J., Hossmann, K.-A. and Mies, G. (1985) Low dose of barbiturates for prevention of hippocampal lesions after brief ischemic episodes. *Acta Neuropathol. (Berl.),* 68: 27 – 31.

Harman, R.J. and Shaw, G.G. (1981) The spontaneous and evoked release of spermine from rat brain in vitro. *Br. J. Pharmacol.,* 73: 165 – 174.

Heby, O. (1981) Role of polyamines in the control of cell proliferation and differentiation. *Differentiation,* 19: 1 – 20.

Ikeno, T. and Guroff, G. (1979) The effect of vasopressin on the activity of ornithine decarboxylase in rat brain and liver. *J. Neurochem.,* 33: 973 – 975.

Iqbal, Z. and Koenig, N.H. (1985) Polyamines appear to be second messengers in mediating Ca^{2+} fluxes and neurotransmitter release in potassium-stimulated synaptosomes. *Biochem. Biophys. Res. Commun.,* 133: 563 – 573.

Jänne, J., Pösö, H. and Raina, A. (1978) Polyamines in rapid growth and cancer. *Biochim. Biophys. Acta,* 473: 241 – 293.

Jasper, T.W., Luttge, W.G., Benton, T.B. and Garnica, A.D. (1982) Polyamines in the developing mouse brain. *Dev. Neurosci.,* 5: 233 – 242.

Jensen, J.R., Lynch, G. and Baudry, M. (1987) Polyamines stimulate mitochondrial calcium transport in rat brain. *J. Neurochem.,* 48: 765 – 772.

Kanje, M., Fransson, I., Edström, A. and Löwkvist, B. (1986) Ornithine decarboxylase activity in dorsal root ganglia of regenerating frog sciatic nerve. *Brain Res.,* 381: 24 – 28.

Kirino, T., Tamura, A. and Sano, K. (1986) A reversible type of neuronal injury following ischemia in the gerbil. *Stroke,* 17: 455 – 459.

Kirino, T., Tsujita, Y. and Tamura, A. (1991) Induced tolerance to ischemia in gerbil hippocampal neurons. *J. Cereb. Blood Flow Metab.,* 11: 299 – 307.

Kleihues, P., Hossmann, K.-A., Pegg, A.E., Kobayashi, K. and Zimmermann, V. (1975) Resuscitation of the monkey brain after one hour complete ischemia. III. Indications of metabolic recovery. *Brain Res.,* 95: 61 – 73.

Koenig, H., Goldstone, A.D. and Lu, C.Y. (1983a) Blood-brain barrier breakdown in brain edema following cold injury is mediated by microvascular polyamines. *Biochem. Biophys. Res. Commun.,* 116: 1039 – 1048.

Koenig, H., Goldstone, A. and Lu, C.Y. (1983b) β-Adrenergic stimulation of Ca^{2+}-fluxes, endocytosis, hexose transport, and amino acid transport in mouse kidney is mediated by polyamine synthesis. *Proc. Natl. Acad. Sci. U.S.A.,* 80: 7210 – 7214.

Koenig, H., Goldstone, A. and Lu, C.Y. (1983c) Polyamines regulate calcium fluxes in a rapid membrane response. *Nature,* 305: 530 – 534.

Koenig, H., Goldstone, A.D. and Lu, C.Y. (1989a) Blood-brain barrier breakdown in cold-injured brain is linked to a biphasic stimulation of ornithine decarboxylase activity and polyamine synthesis: both are coordinately inhibited by verapamil, dexamethasone, and aspirin. *J. Neurochem.,* 52: 101 – 109.

Koenig, H., Goldstone, A.D. and Lu, C.Y. (1989b) Polyamines mediate the reversible opening of the blood-brain barrier by the intracarotid infusion of hyperosmolal manitol. *Brain Res.,* 483: 110 – 116.

Koenig, H., Goldstone, A.D., Lu, C.Y. and Trout, J.J. (1989c) Polyamines and Ca^{2+}-mediated hyperosmolal opening of the blood-brain barrier: in vitro studies in isolated rat cerebral capillaries. *J. Neurochem.,* 52: 1135 – 1142.

Koenig, H., Goldstone, A.D., Lu, C.Y. and Trout, J.J. (1990) Brain polyamines are controlled by *N*-methyl-D-aspartate receptors during ischemia and recirculation. *Stroke,* 21 (Suppl. III): III-98 – III-102.

Kohsaka, S., Heacock, A.M., Klinger, P.D., Porta, R. and Agranoff, B.W. (1982) Dissociation of enhanced ornithine decarboxylase activity and optic nerve regeneration in goldfish. *Dev. Brain Res.,* 4: 149 – 156.

Komulainen, H. and Bondy, S.C. (1987) Transient elevation of intrasynaptosomal free calcium by putrescine. *Brain Res.,* 401: 50 – 54.

Kröner, H. (1988) Spermine, another specific allosteric activator of calcium uptake in rat liver mitochondria. *Arch. Biochem. Biophys.,* 267: 205 – 210.

Lewis, M.E., Lakshmanan, J., Nagaiah, K., MacDonnell, P.C. and Guroff, G. (1978) Nerve growth factor increases activity of ornithine decarboxylase in rat brain. *Proc. Natl. Acad. Sci. U.S.A.,* 75: 1021 – 1023.

Markwell, M.A., Berger, S.P. and Paul, S.M. (1990) The polyamine synthesis inhibitor α-difluoromethylornithine blocks NMDA-induced neurotoxicity. *Eur. J. Pharmacol.,* 182: 607 – 609.

Martinez, E., de Vera, N. and Artigas, F. (1991) Differential response of rat brain polyamines to convulsant agents. *Life Sci.,* 48: 77 – 84.

Metcalf, B.W., Bey, P., Danzin, C., Jung, M.J., Casara, P. and Vevert, J.P. (1978) Catalytic irreversible inhibition of mammalian ornithine decarboxylase (E.C. 4.1.1.17) by substrate and product analogues. *J. Am. Chem. Soc.,* 100: 2551 – 2553.

Müller, M., Cleef, M., Röhn, G., Bonnekoh, P., Pajunen, A.E.I., Bernstein, H.-G. and Paschen, W. (1991) Ornithine decarboxylase in reversible cerebral ischemia: an immunohistochemical study. *Acta Neuropathol. (Berl.),* 83: 39 – 45.

Nicchitta, C. and Williamson, J.R. (1984) Spermine: a regulator of mitochondrial calcium cycling. *J. Biol. Chem.,* 259: 12978 – 12983.

Oredsson, S.M., Deen, D.F. and Marton, L.J. (1982) Decreased cytotoxicity of cis-diamminedichloroplatinum(II) by α-difluoromethylornithine depletion of polyamines in 9L rat brain tumor cells in vitro. *Cancer Res.,* 42: 1296 – 1299.

Pajunen, A.E.I., Hietala, O.A., Vibransalo, E.-L. and Piha, R.S. (1978) Ornithine decarboxylase and adenosylmethionine decarboxylase in mouse brain – effect of electrical stimulation. *J. Neurochem.,* 30: 281 – 283.

Pajunen, A.E.I., Hietala, O.A., Baruch-Virransalo, E.-L. and Piha, R.S. (1979) The effect of DL-allalglycine on polyamine and GABA metabolism in mouse brain. *J. Neurochem.,* 32: 1401 – 1408.

Paschen, W., Schmidt-Kastner, R., Djuricic, B., Meese, C., Linn, F. and Hossmann K.-A. (1987a) Polyamine changes in reversible cerebral ischemia. *J. Neurochem.,* 49: 35 – 37.

Paschen, W., Hallmayer, J. and Mies, G. (1987b) Regional profiles of polyamines in reversible cerebral ischemia of Mongolian gerbils. *Neurochem. Pathol.,* 7: 143 – 156.

Paschen, W., Röhn, G., Meese, C.O., Djuricic, B. and Schmidt-Kastner, R. (1988a) Polyamine metabolism in reversible cerebral ischemia: effect of α-difluoromethylornithine. *Brain Res.,* 453: 9 – 16.

Paschen, W., Hallmayer, J. and Röhn, G. (1988b) Regional changes of polyamine profiles after reversible cerebral ischemia in Mongolian gerbils: effects of nimodipine and barbiturate. *Neurochem. Pathol.,* 8: 27 – 41.

Paschen, W., Hallmayer, J. and Röhn, G. (1988c) Relationship between putrescine content and density of ischemic cell damage in the brain of Mongolian gerbils: effect of nimodipine and barbiturate. *Acta Neuropathol. (Berl.),* 76: 388 – 394.

Paschen, W., Röhn, G., Hallmayer, J. and Mies, G. (1988d) Polyamine metabolism in reversible cerebral ischemia of

Mongolian gerbils. *Metab. Brain. Dis.,* 3: 297 – 302.

Paschen, W., Schmidt-Kastner, R., Hallmayer, J. and Djuricic, B. (1988e) Polyamines in cerebral ischemia. *Neurochem. Pathol.,* 9: 1 – 20.

Paschen, W., Hallmayer, J., Meese, C.O. (1989) Effects of α-difluoromethylornithine on post-ischaemic changes in regional polyamine profiles. *Yugoslav. Physiol. Pharmacol. Acta,* 25: 475 – 483.

Paschen, W., Hallmayer, J., Mies, G. and Röhn, G. (1990a) Ornithine decarboxylase activity and putrescine levels in reversible cerebral ischemia of Mongolian gerbils: effect of barbiturate. *J. Cereb. Blood Flow Metab.,* 10: 236 – 242.

Paschen, W., Kocher, M. and Hossmann, K.-A. (1990b) Relationship between changes in putrescine and energy metabolites during early recirculation following ischemia of rat brain. *Circ. Metab. Cerveau,* 7: 29 – 40.

Paschen, W., Csiba, L., Röhn, G. and Bereczxi, D. (1991a) Polyamine metabolism in transient focal ischemia of rat brain. *Brain Res.,* 566: 354 – 357.

Paschen, W., Xie, Y., Röhn, G., Hallmayer, J. and Hossmann, K.-A. (1991b) Protein and polyamine metabolism in reversible cerebral ischemia of gerbil. In: H. Takeshita, B.K. Siesjö and J.D. Miller (Eds.), *Brain Resuscitation,* Springer, Tokyo, pp. 99 – 114.

Paschen, W., Bengtsson, F., Röhn, G., Bonnekoh, P., Siesjö, B.K. and Hossmann, K.-A. (1991c) Cerebral polyamine metabolism in reversible hypoglycemia of rat: relationship to energy metabolites and calcium. *J. Neurochem.,* 57: 204 – 215.

Pegg, A.E. (1986) Recent advances in the biochemistry of polyamines in eukaryotes. *Biochem. J.,* 234: 249 – 262.

Pegg, A.E. and McCann, P.P. (1982) Polyamine metabolism and function. *Am. J. Physiol.,* 243: C212 – C221.

Pegg, A.E., Seely, J.E., Pösö, H., Della Ragiona, F. and Zagon, I.S. (1982) Polyamine biosynthesis and interconversion in rodent tissue. *Fed. Proc.,* 41: 3065 – 3072.

Persson, L. and Pegg, A.E. (1984) Studies of the induction of spermidine/spermine N^1-acetyltransferase using specific antiserum. *J. Biol. Chem.,* 259: 12364 – 12367.

Porcella, A., Carter, C., Fage, D., Voltz, C., Lloyd, K.G., Serrano, A. and Scatton, B. (1991) The effects of *N*-methyl-D-aspartate and kainate lesions of the rat striatum on striatal ornithine decarboxylase activity and polyamine levels. *Brain Res.,* 549: 205 – 212.

Ransom, R.W. and Stec, N.L. (1988) Cooperative modulation of [^{3}H] MK-801 binding to the *N*-methyl-D-aspartate receptor-ion complex by L-glutamate, glycine and polyamines. *J. Neurochem.,* 51: 830 – 836.

Reed, L.J. and de Belleroche, J. (1989) Excitotoxines induce ornithine decarboxylase activity in the rat central nervous system. *Biochem. Soc. Trans.,* 17: 715 – 716.

Reed. L.J. and de Belleroche, J. (1990) Induction of ornithine decarboxylase in cerebral cortex by excitotoxin lesion of nucleus basalis: association with postsynaptic responsiveness and *N*-methyl-D-aspartate receptor activation. *J. Neurochem.,* 55: 780 – 787.

Reynolds, I.J. and Miller, R.J. (1989) Ifenprodil is a novel type of *N*-methyl-D-aspartate receptor antagonist: interaction with polyamines. *Mol. Pharmacol.,* 36: 758 – 765.

Röhn, G., Kocher, M., Oschlies, U., Hossmann, K.-A. and Paschen, W. (1990) Putrescine content and structural defects in isolated fractions of rat brain after reversible cerebral ischemia. *Exp. Neurol.,* 107: 249 – 255.

Röhn, G., Schlenker, M. and Paschen, W. (1991) Activity of ornithine decarboxylase (ODC) and S-adenosylmethionine decarboxylase (SAMDC) in reversible cerebral ischemia of Mongolian gerbils. *J. Cereb. Blood Flow Metab.,* 11 (Suppl. 2): S504.

Röhn, G., Schlenker, M. and Paschen, W. (1992) Activity of ornithine decarboxylase and S-adenosylmethionine decarboxylase in reversible cerebral ischemia of Mongolian gerbils. *Exp. Neurol.,* 117: 210 – 215.

Rottenberg, H. and Marbach, M. (1990) Regulation of Ca^{2+} transport in brain mitochondria. I. The mechanism of spermine enhancement of Ca^{2+} uptake and retention. *Biochim. Biophys. Acta,* 1016: 77 – 86.

Russell, D.H., Gfeller, E., Marton, L.J. and LeGendre, S.M. (1974) Distribution of putrescine, spermidine, and spermine in rhesus monkey brain: decrease in spermidine and spermine concentrations in motor cortex after electrical stimulation. *J. Neurobiol.,* 5: 349 – 354.

Sacaan, A.I. and Johnson, K.M. (1989) Spermine enhances binding to the glycine site associated with the *N*-methyl-D-aspartate receptor complex. *Mol. Pharmacol.,* 36: 836 – 839.

Sacaan, A.I. and Johnson, K.M. (1990) Characterization of the stimulatory and inhibitory effects of polyamines on [^{3}H] *N*-(1-[thienyl]cyclohexyl) piperidine binding to the *N*-methyl-D-aspartate receptor ionophore complex. *Mol. Pharmacol.,* 37: 572 – 577.

Schoemaker, H., Allen, J. and Langer, S.Z. (1990) Binding of [^{3}H]ifenprodil, a novel NMDA antagonist, to a polyamine-sensitive site in the rat cerebral cortex. *Eur. J. Pharmacol.,* 176: 249 – 250.

Sears, E.S., McCandless, D.W. and Chandler, M.D. (1985) Disruption of the blood-brain barrier in hyperammonemic coma and the pharmacologic effects of dexamethasone and difluoromethyl ornithine. *J. Neurosci. Res.,* 14: 255 – 261.

Seiler, N. and Shaw, G.C. (1981) Polyamine metabolism and function in brain. *Neurochem. Int.,* 3: 95 – 110.

Singh, L., Oles, R. and Woodruff, G. (1990) In vivo interaction of a polyamine with the NMDA receptor. *Eur. J. Pharmacol.,* 180: 391 – 392.

Slotkin, T.A. and Bartolomé, J. (1986) Role of ornithine decarboxylase and the polyamines in nervous system development: a review. *Brain Res. Bull.,* 17: 307 – 320.

Slotkin, T.A., Barnes, G., Lauf, C., Seidler, F.J., Trepanier, P., Weigel, S.J. and Whitmore, W.L. (1982) Development of polyamine and biogenic amine systems in brains and hearts of neonatal rats given dexamethasone: role of biochemical alterations in cellular maturation for producing deficits in ontogeny of neurotransmitter levels, uptake, storage and turnover. *J. Pharmacol. Exp. Ther.*, 221: 686 – 693.

Sprosen, T.M. and Woodruff, G.N. (1990) Polyamines potentiate NMDA induced whole-cell currents in cultured striatal neurons. *Eur. J. Pharmacol.*, 179: 477 – 478.

Tabor, C.W. and Tabor, H. (1984) Polyamines. *Annu. Rev. Biochem.*, 53: 749 – 790.

Thilmann, R., Xie, Y., Kleihues, P. and Kiessling, M. (1986) Persistent inhibition of protein synthesis precedes delayed neuronal death in postischemic gerbil hippocampus. *Acta Neuropathol. (Berl.)*, 71: 88 – 93.

Tilson, H.A., Emerich, D. and Bondy, S.C. (1986) Inhibition of ornithine decarboxylase alters neurological responsiveness to a tremorigen. *Brain Res.*, 379: 147 – 150.

Trout, J.J., Koenig, H., Goldstone, A.D. and Lu, C.Y. (1986) Blood-brain barrier breakdown by cold injury: polyamine signals mediate acute stimulation of endocytosis, vesicular transport, and microvillus formation in rat cerebral capillaries. *Lab. Invest.*, 55: 622 – 631.

Walsh, T.J., Emerich, D.F. and Bondy, S.C. (1989) Destruction of specific hippocampal cell fields increase ornithine decarboxylase activity: modulation of the biochemical but not the histological changes by ganglioside GM1. *Exp. Neurol.*, 105: 54 – 61.

Wells, M.R. (1986) Autoradiographic measurement of relative changes in ornithine decarboxylase in axotomized superior cervical ganglion neurons. *Exp. Neurol.*, 92: 445 – 450.

Williams, K., Romano, C. and Molinoff, P.B. (1989) Effects of polyamines on the binding of [^{3}H]MK-801 to the *N*-methyl-D-aspartate receptor: pharmacological evidence for the existence of a polyamine recognition site. *Mol. Pharmacol.*, 36: 575 – 581.

Williams, K., Romano, C., Dichter, M.A. and Molinoff, P.B. (1991) Modulation of the NMDA receptor by polyamines. *Life Sci.*, 48: 469 – 498.

Williams-Ashman, H.G. and Canellakis, Z.N. (1979) Polyamines in mammalian biology and medicine. *Perspect. Biol. Med.*, 22: 421 – 438.

Wong, B.J.F. and Mattox, D.E. (1991) The effects of polyamines and polyamine inhibitors on rat sciatic and facial nerve regeneration. *Exp. Neurol.*, 111: 263 – 266.

Xie, Y., Hossmann, K.A., Munekata, K. and Seo, K. (1987) Prolonged suppression of protein synthesis after brief cerebral ischemia in gerbils. In: J. Cervos-Navarro and R. Ferszt (Eds.), *Stroke and Microcirculation,* Raven Press, New York, pp. 135 – 141.

Zawia, N.H. and Bondy, S.C. (1990) Electrically stimulated rapid gene expression in the brain: ornithine decarboxylase and *c-fos*. *Mol. Brain Res.*, 7: 243 – 247.

K. Kogure, K.-A. Hossmann and B.K. Siesjö (Eds.)
Progress in Brain Research, Vol. 96

CHAPTER 11

Disturbances of cerebral protein synthesis and ischemic cell death

K.-A. Hossmann

Max-Planck-Institute for Neurological Research, Department of Experimental Neurology, D-5000 Cologne, Germany

Introduction

The development of rational therapeutical strategies for the treatment of cerebrovascular disease depends crucially on the understanding of the pathophysiology and pathobiochemistry of ischemic brain damage. The discovery of post-ischemic hemodynamic disturbances (Ames et al., 1968) and the development of therapeutic interventions for the reversal of such disturbances (Hossmann et al., 1973) led to the observation that neurons are able to survive complete circulatory arrest for 60 min if blood flow and energy metabolism are promptly restored after the circulatory arrest (Hossmann et al., 1973, 1977). Only in the selectively vulnerable areas of the brain – in particular the hippocampus – a delayed type of ischemic cell death occurred despite normalization of blood flow and energy metabolism (Schmidt-Kastner et al., 1990). These lesions are not life-threatening but they are likely to interfere with higher mental function. More disturbing, such lesions are not restricted to prolonged ischemia but may already appear after ischemic episodes of 5 min or shorter (Kirino, 1982). They may, therefore, affect a great number of patients suffering from transient cardiac or cerebrovascular disorders.

During the past years a substantial amount of experimental evidence has accumulated which suggests that ischemic lesions may result from functional disturbances, in particular the massive release of neurotransmitters and the associated changes of calcium homeostasis (Siesjö et al., 1990). Aspects of this pathophysiology will be discussed in detail by several authors of this volume. However, it has not been established how these functional disturbances interfere with neuronal integrity, and why neuronal death may be delayed for up to several days after the ischemic impact.

In the following, the possible role of disturbances of protein biosynthesis will be discussed. One of the main arguments for such a role is the persisting inhibition of protein synthesis despite recovery of energy metabolism in the areas destined to die. There is also evidence of a relationship between disturbances of calcium homeostasis and global protein synthesis on one hand, and between abnormalities of signal transduction and selective genomic expression on the other. The understanding of the mechanisms responsible for post-ischemic disturbances of protein synthesis may, therefore, contribute to the elucidation of the mechanisms of ischemic cell death.

Global ischemia

Reversible alterations of protein synthesis

The first investigations on the effect of brain ischemia on protein synthesis were carried out to study the potentials of post-ischemic recovery after prolonged cerebrocirculatory arrest (Kleihues and Hossmann, 1971, 1973). Since these studies are of importance for the present discussion of this topic, they will be briefly reviewed. The reason for these investigations was the observation that energy metabolism and certain electrophysiological functions such as evoked potentials and EEG recovered after 1 h complete ischemia in normothermia if care was taken to prevent post-ischemic disturbances of recirculation (Hossmann et al., 1973, 1977). Since these observations were in sharp contrast to the previous assumption that normothermic neurons die after a few minutes of circulatory arrest, measurements of protein synthesis were performed to find out if more complex biochemical functions were also restored. It turned out that this was the case but the recovery of protein synthesis – expressed as the incorporation of labeled amino acids into brain proteins – progressed much slower than that of energy metabolism or the restoration of ion homeostasis. In fact, in normothermic cats and monkeys submitted to 1 h complete ischemia, recovery of protein synthesis up to 50% required more than 6 h and recovery to normal about 24 h (Kleihues and Hossmann, 1971; Bodsch et al., 1986). Energy state and ion homeostasis, in contrast, began to recover within a few minutes of recirculation and returned to near normal in less than 1 h (Hossmann et al., 1973, 1977). Electron-micrographs and polysomal density gradients further showed that polyribosomes remained intact during ischemia but transiently disaggregated after the beginning of recirculation in parallel with the post-ischemic inhibition of protein synthesis (Kleihues and Hossmann, 1971).

The biochemical assays of protein synthesis were supplemented by autoradiographic studies in order to establish the anatomical pattern of post-ischemic recovery (Kleihues and Hossmann, 1973; Bodsch et al., 1986; Hossmann et al., 1987). These studies revealed that after up to 1 h complete ischemia protein synthesis recovered within 24 h in the vast majority of neurons except the selectively vulnerable regions (see below). After one year survival the anatomical pattern of amino acid incorporation was essentially the same as after 24 h, indicating that recovery of protein synthesis was permanent. Post-ischemic restoration of protein synthesis, in consequence, is a reliable predictor of post-ischemic cell survival (Fig. 1).

These observations have been confirmed in various animal species and models of global ischemia. Wasterlain (1974) reduced cerebral blood flow in rats by increasing intracranial pressure to 1500 mm water for 30 min and observed a reversible disaggregation of polyribosomes and an inhibition of in vitro protein synthesis. Carai et al. (1979) occluded a carotid artery in gerbils for up to 3 h and

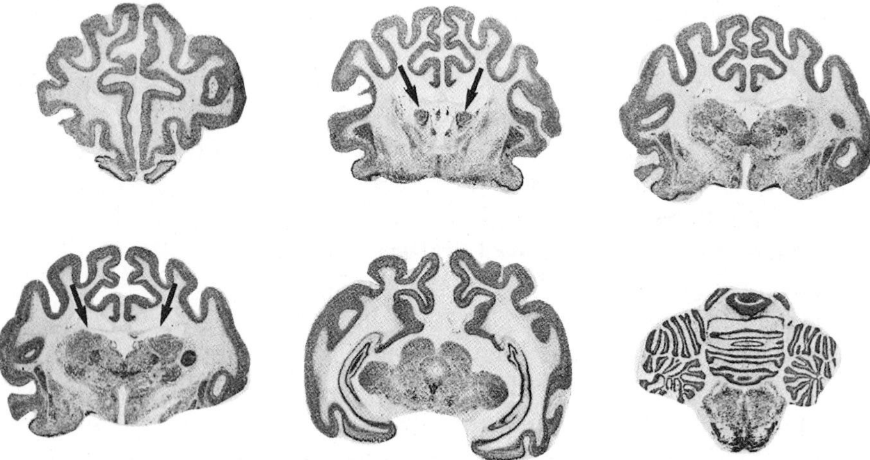

Fig. 1. Autoradiograms of ^{14}C-leucine incorporation into brain proteins of a cat submitted to 1 h complete cerebrocirculatory arrest. Measurement was carried out one year after the ischemia. Note the excellent preservation of most anatomical structures except the selectively vulnerable parts of the hippocampus and striatum (arrows). (Reproduced with permission from Hossmann et al., 1987).

observed a reversible disaggregation of polyribosomes and a reduction of amino acid incorporation into brain proteins. Yanagihara (1976) incubated brain slices in vitro under anoxic conditions for 3 – 30 min and found a gradual decline of protein synthesis in parallel with the disaggregation of ribosomes. Dienel et al. (1980) submitted rats to 10 or 30 min four-vessel occlusion followed by recirculation for up to two days. Protein synthesis measured in vitro was severely suppressed after ischemia but returned to control after 4 h following 10 min and after 2 – 4 days following 30 min ischemia. Chavko et al. (1987) produced partial spinal cord ischemia by occluding the abdominal aorta for 40 min. They described disaggregation of polyribosomes and inhibition of in vitro protein synthesis after 10 min recirculation, followed by gradual recovery within one day. Many investigators also confirmed the dissociation between the rapid post-ischemic recovery of energy metabolism and the much slower restoration of protein synthesis (Dienel et al., 1980; Nowak et al., 1985; Raley and Lipton, 1990). Moreover, it was pointed out that the maximal effect on protein synthesis was produced already by 5 min ischemia, and that there was little further change when ischemia was prolonged to 20 min (Nowak et al., 1985).

The analysis of these observations suggests the following sequel of events. During ischemia protein synthesis is completely suppressed because energy-rich phosphates required for acylation of transfer RNA and the formation of peptide bounds are rapidly depleted (Lowry et al., 1964). Despite this suppression polyribosomes remain intact during ischemia because all steps of mRNA translation, i.e., initiation, elongation and termination come to a halt ("ischemic freeze", Kleihues et al., 1975). When the brain is recirculated with oxygenated blood, energy metabolism recovers. As a consequence acylation of transfer RNA is resumed, and the elongation and termination of polypeptide chains that have been initiated before the ischemic event continues. However, initiation of new polypeptide chains does not immediately recover and polyribosomes transiently disaggregate. A degradation of mRNA by increased RNAse activity is less likely because polysomal density gradients showed a separation of monosomes into the small and large subunits (Kleihues et al., 1975).

The post-ischemic disaggregation of polyribosomes and the associated inhibition of protein synthesis is not irreversible, even after 1 h complete cerebrocirculatory arrest in normothermia. However, reaggregation after this long ischemia depends on the prevention of a no-reflow phenomenon and requires about one day for completion (Kleihues et al., 1975; Bodsch et al., 1986).

The post-ischemic inhibition of polypeptide chain initiation is presumably due to the post-ischemic inactivation of polypeptide chain initiation factors. In vitro incorporation studies of ribosomes sampled during and at various times after global ischemia revealed that ribosomes isolated from rat cerebral cortex after 30 min complete ischemia were aggregated, and when suspended in a medium containing an energy-generating system, exhibited the same protein synthesizing capacity as control ribosomes (Cooper et al., 1977). After a few minutes of recirculation following 30 min ischemia, ribosomes disaggregated and in vitro protein synthesis sharply declined. Addition of the specific inhibitor of polypeptide chain initiation, Poly (I), did not result in a further reduction of protein synthesis, indicating that the initiation factors were inactivated. With increasing recirculation time in vitro protein synthesis slowly recovered in parallel with the gradual reaggregation of polyribosomes, and the inhibitory effect of Poly (I) returned. An inactivation of polypeptide chain initiation factors has also been suggested by Chavko et al. (1987) who demonstrated that post-ischemic inhibition of protein synthesis could be partially reversed by adding the eukaryotic initiation factor eIF-2 to the incubation mix.

In conclusion, the post-ischemic inhibition of overall protein synthesis seems to be a functional disturbance at the translational level which develops after a few minutes of ischemia and which is probably due to the inactivation of polypeptide chain initiation factors. The disturbance recovers much more slowly than energy metabolism but it is reversed in most parts of the brain even after ischemia of as long as 1 h if care is taken to prevent a no-reflow phenomenon.

Irreversible alterations of protein synthesis

Although most of the earlier studies on protein synthesis were carried out to explore the resistance of the brain to prolonged circulatory arrest, more recent investigations have focused on the potential role of protein synthesis for the manifestation of selective brain injury. This development was initiated by the observation of Ito et al. (1975) that a few minutes of ischemia may cause selective neuronal death in some circumscribed regions such as the CA1 sector of hippocampus although the rest of the brain remained intact. Hemodynamic disturbances or disturbances of energy metabolism could be excluded as mechanisms of this injury (Munekata and Hossmann, 1987; Mies et al., 1990); therefore, the question arose whether post-ischemic disturbances of protein synthesis may be involved.

The first to report such a relationship were Dienel et al. (1980). These authors submitted rats to four-vessel occlusion of 10 – 30 min duration, followed by post-ischemic recirculation for up to 48 h. Autoradiographic assays of protein synthesis revealed a gradual recovery to normal in all parts of the brain except the vulnerable CA1 sector. In gerbils the same pattern of persisting inhibition of protein synthesis in the selectively vulnerable areas of the brain was observed already after an ischemia time of 5 min (Bodsch et al., 1985; Thilmann et al., 1986a; Widmann et al., 1991) or even 2 min (Araki et al., 1990). Interestingly, these short ischemia times also induced a transient inhibition of protein synthesis (Thilmann et al., 1986a; Widman et al., 1991) and a transient disaggregation of ribosomes (Munekata et al., 1987) in the resistant parts of the brain (see above). However, in contrast to the selectively vulnerable areas, disturbances in these regions recovered within 3 – 6 h. Selective vulnerability, in consequence, is not the result of the selective inhibition of protein synthesis but of the selective failure of recovery (Fig. 2).

The close relationship between recovery of protein synthesis and cellular survival is also supported by histoautoradiographic studies. Neurons exhibiting the typical morphological pattern of ischemic cell injury fail to incorporate amino acids into proteins (Kleihues and Hossmann, 1973). Removal of the endogenous adenosine action by

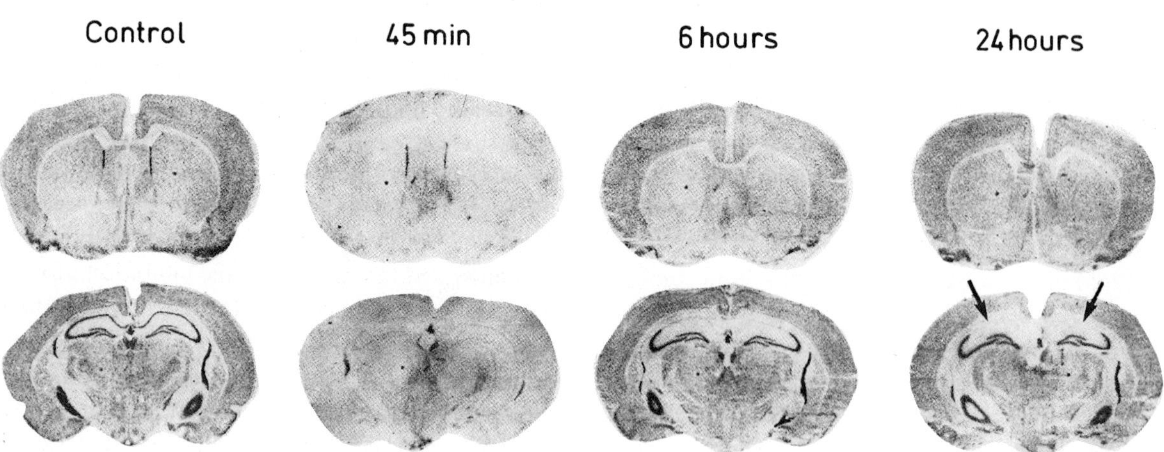

Fig. 2. Autoradiograms of ^{14}C-leucine incorporation into brain proteins in gerbil submitted to 5 min forebrain ischemia followed by recirculation times of 45 min, 6 h and 24 h (above: coronal section at the level of striatum; below: level of dorsal hippocampus). During early recirculation protein synthesis is severely inhibited throughout the forebrain but it recovers to normal in all parts except CA1 sector of hippocampus (arrows). (By courtesy of R. Widmann.)

treatment with the receptor antagonist theophylline aggravates the disaggregation of ribosomes and shortens the ischemic period which can be tolerated without subsequent damage in gerbil (Dux et al., 1990). Conversely, neurons destined to survive including the resistant interneurons in the selectively vulnerable CA1 sector of hippocampus recover their protein synthesizing capacity (Johansen and Diemer, 1990).

Recently, the importance of protein synthesis for cell survival has also been documented after repetitive ischemia. Tomida et al. (1987) reported that repetition of brief episodes of ischemia at 1 h intervals results in a substantial aggravation of ischemic injury even in brain regions outside the vulnerable areas. Autoradiographic studies confirmed that in these regions protein synthesis failed to recover (Widmann et al., 1992). Conversely, prevention of neuronal death in the selectively vulnerable areas by barbiturates or hypothermia was associated with a reaggregation of ribosomes and a normalization of protein synthesis (Xie et al., 1989c; Miyazawa et al., 1991; Bonnekoh et al., 1992). Interestingly, neither these nor the equally efficient treatment with the glutamate antagonist 2-3dihydroxy-6-nitro-7-sulfamoyl-benzo(F)triox-aline (NBQX) were able to prevent the initial post-ischemic inhibition of protein synthesis (Bergstedt and Wieloch, 1991). This is in line with the conclusion that the failure of recovery and not the initial inhibition of protein synthesis determines neuronal death after ischemia.

Selective gene expression

Although the close association between suppression of protein synthesis and ischemic cell death has now been firmly established, its causal relationship remains to be clarified. On the first sight it is attractive to relate the delay of ischemic cell death in the selectively vulnerable brain regions to the long half-life of proteins. In fact, the mean half-life of brain proteins is about three days which could reasonably explain the maturation interval of 2 – 4 days in the CA1 sector of hippocampus (Kirino, 1982). However, the vulnerable neurons in the dorsolateral part of striatum exhibit morphological injury already after 24 h (Petito and Pulsinelli, 1984). Moreover, the half-life of brain proteins after ischemia may be longer than under normal conditions, because amino acid recycling slows down (Widmann et al., 1991).

There are, however, distinct qualitative changes in the pattern of newly synthesized proteins during the post-ischemic recovery phase. Kleihues et al. (1975) noted that following 1 h ischemia the synthesis of the short-lived proteins ornithin decarboxylase (ODC, half-life 11 – 21 min) and S-adenosylmethionine decarboxylase (SAMDC, half-life 35 – 120 min) began to recover after 1.5 and 6 h recirculation, respectively, i.e., after an interval at which global protein synthesis was still distinctly reduced. With longer recirculation times ODC markedly increased above normal and reached a peak of more than 300% of control after 12 h. A marked post-ischemic increase of ODC was also described by Dienel et al. (1985) at 10 h after 30 min four-vessel occlusion in rat, and by Paschen et al. (1990) and Müller et al. (1991) at 8 h after 5 min bilateral carotid artery occlusion in gerbil. Interestingly, ODC was synthesized not only in the resistant but also in vulnerable parts of the brain although inhibition of global protein synthesis was more pronounced in this region (see above).

A selective pattern of post-ischemic protein synthesis was also observed by Chavko et al. (1981) who reported that the post-ischemic inhibition of protein synthesis affected mainly proteins with molecular weight above 100 kDa whereas proteins with a molecular weight of 50 kDa increased and a new peak of proteins with a molecular weight of 40 kDa appeared. A more detailed analysis of the pattern of newly synthesized proteins by two-dimensional electrophoresis was carried out by Dienel et al. (1986) and Kiessling et al. (1986). Dienel et al. (1986) harvested polyribosomes from the rat cortex after 30 min four-vessel occlusion and 3 h recirculation, and translated them in vitro in a reticulocyte system with initiation capacity. They observed a new family of 70 kDa proteins that co-migrated with the 68 – 70 kDa heat stress protein, and an increase of the 93 and 110 kDa stress protein. A parallel in vivo study of regional protein synthesis after 3 h and 18 h recirculation following 30 min ischemia revealed a uniform elevation of the 27, 65 and 70 and 110 kDa stress proteins after 3 h, and of the 50 kDa protein after 18 h recirculation in all brain regions investigated. In the hippocampus the 70 kDa heat stress protein (hsp 70) remained selectively increased throughout the observation period of 18 h. The authors, therefore, suggested that this change might be related to the neuronal injury observed in this region a few days later.

Synthesis of the 70 kDa heat stress protein was also observed by Nowak (1985) in the gerbil brain after 5 min ischemia and 8 h recirculation but he pointed out that quantitatively this was not the major synthesized protein. However, in view of the important biological role of this protein, he and others undertook a detailed analysis of both hsp70 transcription and translation (Vass et al., 1988a; Dwyer et al., 1989, Nowak et al., 1990; Nowak, 1991; Takemoto et al., 1991; Abe et al., 1991c; Gonzales et al., 1991; Sharp et al., 1991; Simon et al., 1991). The results can be summarized as follows: 1 h after ischemia, hsp70 mRNA is expressed in the dentate gyrus and after about 3 h in the other layers of hippocampus. Hsp mRNA returns to normal within 12 h in the dentate gyrus and within 24 h in the other sectors of hippocampus except the CA1 sector where it remains elevated until the cells die. The translation of heat-shock proteins is markedly delayed in relation to hsp transcription. In the CA3 sector and dentate gyrus hsp protein appears after about 24 h and peaks after 48 h, and it does not appear at all in the CA1 sector of hippocampus except after brief periods of oligemia which probably are too short to induce irreversible ischemic injury (Simon et al. 1991; Gonzales et al., 1991).

The dissociation between induction and expression of heat shock proteins after ischemia is obviously the result of the global post-ischemic inhibition of protein synthesis at the translational level. In fact, expression of the hsp protein parallels the recovery of global protein synthesis and, therefore, remains low in the CA1 sector and other regions where global protein synthesis is not restored (Vass et al., 1988a). Synthesis of the hsp protein, in turn, feeds back on the induction of hsp mRNA expression after ischemia. As demonstrated by DiDomenico et al. (1982) induction of hsp mRNA is prolonged by preventing the accumulation of the hsp protein. Conversely, hsp mRNA begins to decline as soon as protein synthesis is restored, i.e., first in the dentate gyrus and then in the CA3 sector. In the CA1 sector in which protein synthesis is not restored, mRNA remains elevated until the neurons die, that is throughout the post-ischemic maturation period of cell injury (Nowak, 1991).

The synthesis of heat-shock proteins in the resistant parts of the hippocampus has led to the hypothesis that this protein has a protective effect against ischemic injury (Vass et al., 1988a). Although heat-shock proteins are known to alleviate injury induced by a variety of stress situations, their effect on cell survival after ischemia is less clear. Sharp et al. (1991) observed expression of hsp protein in neurons of regions known to be injured. Induction of the hsp protein in the CA1 sector by hyperthermia or a brief, non-lethal ischemia protected against injury of this sector after a second interruption of blood flow in gerbils (Kirino et al., 1991; Kitagawa et al., 1991a,b) but not in rats (Mima et al., 1991). Conversely, hypothermia suppresses the induction of heat-shock protein but it improves neuronal survival (Li et al., 1991). MK-801 attenuates the induction of hsp mRNA in the resistant parts of the hippocampus (Nowak, 1988) but it does not promote injury in these regions. Finally, the hsp protein is little expressed outside the hippocampus although these parts of the brain are much less vulnerable. These observations clearly demonstrate that the presence or abscence of heat-shock proteins per se does not predict ischemic neuronal injury.

The analysis of recent data on the induction of immediate-early or primary response genes leads to a similar conclusion. These genes are characterized by the rapid induction of their mRNAs by external stimuli such as neurotransmitters, growth factors, differentiation-inducing agents or cell membrane depolarizations (for review, see Doucet et al., 1990). The best studied genes of this group include the *fos* and *jun* proto-oncogenes and, more recently, the zinc finger gene *zif/268*. Their respective proteins fos, jun and zif/268 are components of transcription factors and, as such, regulatory elements at the genomic level. They act as third messengers in the stimulus-transcription coupling that transduces extracellular stimuli to long-term genomic responses and cellular adaptations.

An early response of the neuron to ischemia is cell membrane depolarization and a massive release of neurotransmitters. It is, therefore, not surprising that ischemia leads to the induction of immediate early response genes. However, the localization and the time at which the transcription products appear after ischemia, vary considerably under different experimental conditions. Onodera et al. (1989) observed a transient increase of *c-fos* mRNA in cerebral cortex between 30 and 90 min after 20 min four-vessel occlusion in rat. Jørgensen et al. (1989) described, after the same duration of ischemia, a more delayed response, i.e., the appearance of some scattered neurons expressing *c-fos* mRNA after 24 h recirculation, and a more intense reaction in the CA1 sector after 72 h. Nowak (1991) reported induction of c-*fos* mRNA in dentate gyrus and to a lesser degree in the CA1 – CA3 sectors already after 15 min following 5 min ischemia in gerbil, and Dempsey et al. (1990) found an increase in whole brain homogenates after 20 min ischemia and 2 h recirculation. A transient increase of *c-jun* and *c-fos* mRNA with peaks after 15 and 30 min recirculation, respectively, was observed in gerbils submitted to 10 min ischemia (Kindy et al., 1991). Abe et al. (1991b) studied the induction of *zif/268* (i.e., the nerve growth factor inducible protein-A, NGFI-A mRNA), and described a transient increase after 1 h recirculation following 30 min middle cerebral artery occlusion in rat.

The synthesis of the corresponding immediate early response gene products is clearly restricted to neurons that are resistant to the ischemic injury. Takemoto et al. (1991) and Suga and Nowak (1991) reported the transient appearance in CA3 and dentate gyrus of the fos protein after 3 – 6 h, and of jun after 3 – 24 h recirculation. Uemura et al. (1991a) observed induction in dentate gyrus and the CA3 and CA4 regions from 2 to 8 h after transient ischemia. The abscence of an expression in the vulnerable CA1 sector as well as the delay between induction and expression in the resistant parts of the hippocampus are presumably due to the overall inhibition of protein synthesis, as described above. Popovici et al. (1990) stressed the difference between the marked induction of the fos protein after seizures as compared to the much slighter expression after ischemia and concluded that the latter is seizure- and not hypoxia-related. It, therefore, remains unclear whether stimulus-transcription mechanisms are of pathophysiological importance for the production of ischemic cell death during the critical phase of early post-ischemic recirculation.

There is also little positive evidence at the present that other genomic responses are involved in the manifestation of neuronal injury. Using in situ hybridization techniques we investigated the expression of four mRNAs which represent different classes of functional and structural cell proteins, i.e., cytochrome c oxidase sequences, ribosomal sequences, β-actin sequences and the amyloid A4 precursor protein (Xie et al., 1989a). After 5 min global ischemia of the gerbil brain none of these mRNAs exhibited major changes until CA1 injury became manifest. Abe et al. (1991a) confirmed that the total amount of tubulin mRNA and amyloid-precursor protein mRNA did not change after 10 min ischemia in gerbil but they reported a selective induction of an amyloid-precursor subspecies containing a protease inhibitor domain at 1 – 21 days following permanent middle cerebral artery occlusion in rats. However, this protein may be involved in reparative processes rather than in the production of cerebral infarction. Finally, induction of copper zinc superoxide dismutase (CuZn SOD) mRNA has been described in gerbil hippocampus after 5 min ischemia and 30 min recirculation (Matsuyama et al., 1991). This response could be of functional importance because superoxide dismutase is involved in the scavenging of free radicals, and the enhancement of SOD levels in transgenic mice has been shown to increase the resistance of these animals to ischemia (Kinouchi et al., 1991). However, induction of CuZn SOD mRNA was most prominent in the vulnerable CA1 sector, indicating that either the message was not translated or the protein product was not able to prevent cell injury.

An indirect argument that has been raised in favor of a genomic component for the manifestation of ischemic cell death is the protective effect of inhibitors of protein synthesis on neuronal survival. Thilmann et al. (1986b) reported that delayed CA1 injury following 5 min bilateral carotid artery occlusion in gerbil was prevented by pre- or post-ischemic application of cycloheximide but they cautioned that this effect might be due to the associated hypothermia. More recently, Goto et al. (1990) observed a similar effect in rats submitted to 10 min four-vessel occlusion although normothermia was maintained during ischemia and the initial 4 h of recirculation. They, therefore, concluded that the drug inhibited the synthesis of a putative killer protein involved in an endogenous active death program. However, this view has been challenged by Kiessling et al. (1991) who reported that the effect of cycloheximide was reversed when normothermia was maintained throughout the post-ischemic survival of the animal. These data, therefore, do not support the hypothesis of the post-ischemic synthesis of a protein that induces selective neuronal death in analogy to the process of apoptosis during the ontogenesis of the central nervous system.

In conclusion, global cerebral ischemia – even of very short duration – results in irreversible inhibition of protein synthesis in the vulnerable neurons destined to suffer ischemic cell death. Global ischemia also causes the selective expression of immediate early response genes, stress proteins and various other proteins, but the localization correlates only marginally with the vulnerable or resistant parts of the brain. Selective responses at the genomic level, therefore, seem to be of lesser importance for the manifestation of ischemic cell death than the overall disturbance of protein synthesis at the translational level.

Focal ischemia

Disturbances of protein synthesis have also been described after focal reduction of cerebral blood flow (Yanagihara, 1976, 1978; Morimoto et al., 1978; Orunesu et al., 1980; Morimoto and Yanagihara, 1981a,b; Hossmann et al., 1985; Dwyer et al., 1987; Yoshimine et al., 1987; Abe et al., 1988; Xie et al., 1988, 1989b). Extent and severity of these disturbances are less predictable than after global ischemia because they depend not only on the duration of ischemia and recirculation but also on the severity of flow reduction.

Permanent vascular occlusion

After permanent occlusion of a major cerebral artery the local density of ischemia depends on the collateral blood supply to the territory of the occluded vessel. In accordance with the threshold concept of ischemic injury (Astrup et al., 1981), protein synthesis is a function of blood flow. Two hours after combined middle cerebral and carotid artery occlusion in rat, reduction of blood flow to 50 – 80 ml/100 g per minute led to a modest and further reduction to 40 – 50 ml/100 g per minute to the complete cessation of the synthesis of most proteins (Jacewicz et al., 1986). Xie et al. (1989b) investigated this relationship in more detail in gerbils, using double tracer autoradiography for the regional measurement of blood flow and protein synthesis. They noted a decline of amino acid incorporation beginning at flow values below 100 ml/100 g per minute, and a complete cessation at values below 40 ml/100 g per minute. These flow values are substantially higher than the threshold required to maintain a normal brain energy state which in the gerbil amounts to about 20 ml/100 g per minute (Paschen et al., 1991). During permanent focal ischemia inhibition of protein synthesis may, therefore, occur in the absence of energy failure (Fig. 3).

On the other hand, persisting inhibition of protein synthesis may cause a gradual deterioration of the energy state, as revealed by sequential measurements of the flow/metabolism threshold relationship (Mies et al., 1991). In rats submitted to permanent middle cerebral artery occlusion, the threshold for suppression of protein synthesis (defined as the flow value at which 50% of the investigated volume elements exhibit complete metabolic suppression) remained at a remarkably constant level of about 55 ml/100 g per minute over a period of 12 h. The threshold of energy state, in contrast, rose from 18 ml/100 g per minute after 1 h to 23 ml/100 g per minute after 6 h and further to 34 ml/100 g per minute after 12 h vascular occlusion. In the stroke-prone spontaneously hypertensive rat in which measurements of blood flow and metabolism were carried out under conditions of chronic infarction, the region of ATP depletion and inhibition of protein synthesis was identical (Paschen et al., 1985). These observations demonstrate that under chronic conditions of focal ischemia the thresholds of protein synthesis and energy metabolism converge.

The site of the inhibition of protein synthesis during focal ischemia has not been investigated but there are indirect observations that it may occur at the translational level. Yanagihara (1976) and Abe et al. (1988) reported that the inhibition of protein synthesis in focal ischemia is not the result of an inhibition of RNA synthesis, and Hartmann and Becker (1973) and Morimoto et al. (1981a,b) provided evidence of ribosomal disaggregation in the ischemic territory. It is, therefore, reasonable to assume that during focal ischemia – similarly as following global ischemia – protein synthesis is inhibited at the translational level.

Despite the global depression of protein synthesis selective gene expressions may occur in the periphery of an infarct, i.e., in regions in which blood flow does not decrease below the threshold of energy failure. Jacewicz et al. (1986) reported selective expression of 27 kDa proteins at flow values between 50 and 80 ml/100 g per minute, and of a variety of other proteins which most likely comprise heat-shock or stress proteins, when flow further decreased to below 40 ml/100 g per minute. More recently Welsh et al. (1992) used in situ hybridization for imaging of induction of hsp70 mRNA and c-*fos* mRNA after permanent middle cerebral artery occlusion in rats. They observed a transient (15 min – 3 h) increase of c-*fos* mRNA throughout the affected hemisphere, followed by a lasting (1 – 24 h) increase of hsp70 mRNA within the ischemic territory. Uemura et al. (1991b) and Diemer et al. (1991), in the same experimental model, studied the localization of the translational product of c-*fos* mRNA, the fos protein, by immunohistochemistry and found an increase between 2 h and 24 h in the periphery of the infarct but not in the infarct itself. The time lag between transcription and translation of c-*fos* and heat shock genes in the reversibly injured peripheral zone, as well as the failure of mRNA translation in the irreversibly damaged core of the infarct is similar to the findings in the resistant and vulnerable parts of the hippocampus after tran-

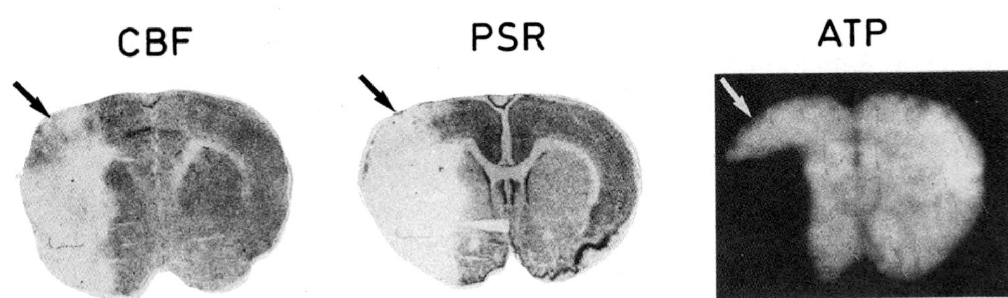

Fig. 3. Multiparametric imaging of blood flow, protein synthesis and the tissue content of ATP at 1 h after middle cerebral artery occlusion in rat. Blood flow was measured with ^{131}I-iodoantipyrine and protein synthesis with ^{14}C-leucine using double tracer autoradiography. ATP was assessed on the adjacent tissue section by substrate-induced bioluminescence. Note the dissociation between preserved ATP and depressed protein-incorporated ^{14}C radioactivity in the low perfusion region of the left parietal cortex (arrow). (By courtesy of G. Mies).

sient ischemia and suggests that the same molecular mechanisms may be involved.

Reversible vascular occlusion

Disturbances of protein synthesis after reversible focal ischemia have only occasionally been described but the pattern observed reflects features of both focal and global ischemia. Morimoto et al. (1981b) occluded the right common carotid artery in gerbils for 30 min or 3 h, followed by 3 h recirculation. During ischemia polyribosomes remained intact and the protein synthesizing capacity tested in vitro was not impaired. Recirculation resulted in the disaggregation of polyribosomes and a severe suppression of protein synthesis which slowly recovered after 30 min but not after 3 h ischemia. Post-ischemic aggravation of the disturbance of the protein synthesizing capacity of isolated polyribosomes was also observed by Orunesu et al. (1980) who used the same experimental model for induction of reversible ischemia. Xie et al. (1988) embolized monkeys with fragments of autologous blood clots which produce transient episodes of multifocal brain ischemia. They demonstrated sharply demarcated areas of complete inhibition of protein synthesis which clearly outlasted the ischemic episodes because they were still present after 2 h following the embolization although the electrophysiological alterations had already recovered.

An interesting observation was reported by Abe et al. (1988) who occluded the middle cerebral artery of rat for 1 h followed by 2 h to seven days reperfusion. These authors demonstrated that protein synthesis recovered in the territory of the middle cerebral artery but they also found that it remained irreversibly suppressed in the neurons of the CA1 sector of hippocampus although this area was outside the territory of the occluded artery. Obviously, the posterior cerebral artery was also occluded in these animals. The difference of recovery in the vulnerable and non-vulnerable parts of the hippocampus, therefore, indicates that the pattern of selective vulnerability is preserved after reversible focal ischemia.

The only investigation of protein synthesis during spontaneous collateral recirculation after permanent vascular occlusion has been carried out in our laboratory (Hossmann et al., 1985). In this study the cat transorbital middle cerebral artery occlusion model was used which is characterized by a heterogeneous flow pattern due to spontaneous focal recirculation. Two hours after the vascular occlusion the regional pattern of protein synthesis was correlated with various hemodynamic and metabolic variables, using multiparametric imaging techniques. The area of reduced protein synthesis was much larger than that in which ATP or glucose utilization were suppressed, and it included regions of reduced, normal or increased blood flow. This finding supports the contention that protein synthesis is dissociated from energy metabolism and that it remains suppressed for extended periods irrespective of the individual post-ischemic flow pattern.

Mechanisms of ischemic disturbances of protein synthesis

Up to now few experiments have been carried out to elucidate the mechanisms of disturbances of protein synthesis after global or focal ischemia. The following discussion is highly speculative and the concept proposed requires experimental validation. However, the comparison of the pattern and the time course of the metabolic disturbance with the known pathophysiological events associated with either focal or global ischemia converge in a rather simple concept that is able to explain most of the observed phenomena. This concept differentiates between selective gene expression at the transcriptional level and the unselective suppression of protein synthesis at the translational level.

Unselective suppresion of RNA translation

Complete cessation of blood flow in the normothermic brain results in the rapid cessation of the energy-producing metabolism and, in consequence, the breakdown of all endergonic processes including mRNA translation. It does not cause a breakdown of the protein synthesizing machinery, as evidenced by the undisturbed synthesis rate of ribosomes incubated in vitro after a period of ischemia (Cooper et al., 1977). The breakdown of this machinery occurs either during the recirculation after reversible global ischemia, or in the periphery of a focal ischemia, i.e., in the presence of energy metabolites: during post-ischemic recirculation as soon as energy metabolism has recovered or in the periphery of an infarct where blood flow remains above the threshold of energy depletion. The failure of protein synthesis is associated with a disaggregation of ribosomes, indicating that the disturbance is due to an inhibition of peptide chain initiation.

A critical step in peptide chain initiation is the formation of a stable ternary complex consisting of met-tRNA, GTP and the eukaryotic initiation factor eIF-2. This complex is inactivated by phosphorylation of eIF-2 which, in turn, is mediated by at least four different protein kinases (for review, see Jagus et al., 1981). One of these is the calcium/phospholipid-dependent protein kinase C which phosphorylates the β-subunit of eIF-2 (Schatzman et al., 1983; Alcazar et al., 1988). In fact, addition of calcium ions to heme-stabilized reticulocyte lysates leads to a dose-dependent translational inhibition by as much as 92% (De Haro et al., 1983).

If a similar inactivation by calcium ions of peptide chain initiation occurs in the brain, most if not all of the here described phenomena can be explained. During complete ischemia intracellular calcium activity increases due to the opening of agonist- and voltage-gated calcium channels and the release from intracellular calcium stores (for review, see Siesjö et al., 1990). Peptide chain initiation factors are not immediately phosphorylated because ATP declines before calcium increases. This explains that ribosomes sampled after the onset of ischemia maintain their protein-synthesizing capacity. Inactivation of polypeptide chain initiation occurs during post-ischemic recirculation because ATP is quickly restored. Intracellular calcium activity, in contrast, remains elevated for some time because the restoration of the intra/extracellular calcium homeostasis requires extensive ion pumping and – probably more important – because the elevated levels of extracellular excitatory amino acids prevent the closure of receptor-operated ion channels (Benveniste et al., 1984; Hagberg et al., 1985). As a result, elongation and termination (but not initiation) of peptide chains recover and ribosomes disaggregate.

This concept is confirmed by a recent study of Raley-Susman and Lipton (1990) who investigated protein synthesis in the rat hippocampal slice following "in vitro" ischemia. They observed that exposure of the slices to buffer lacking calcium and containing the NMDA receptor blocker ketamine prevented both the inhibition of protein synthesis and the morphological changes in the neurons. Conversely, the rapid flooding of the cytosol with calcium after the onset of ischemia (Harris et al., 1981) could explain that maximal inhibition of protein synthesis is produced already after 5 min circulatory arrest (Nowak et al., 1985).

The post-ischemic recovery process depends on the normalization of transmitter and calcium homeostasis. In the resistant parts of the brain intracellular calcium normalizes and protein synthesis recovers within a few hours after 5 min of ischemia, and within one day if ischemia is prolonged to 1 h. In the selectively vulnerable parts of the brain, in contrast, the disturbance of calcium homeostasis persists, and peptide chain initiation is not reversed. Persisting disturbances of ion homeostasis may also be responsible for the irreversible inhibition of protein synthesis after repetitive ischemia (Widmann et al., 1992). This would be in line with the observation that repetitive ischemia enhances disturbances of electrolyte homeostasis and, in consequence, post-ischemic brain edema (Vass et al., 1988b). Finally, this concept could explain that protein synthesis of selectively vulnerable neurons may transiently begin to recover before it is irreversibly suppressed (Bodsch et al., 1986; Thilmann et al., 1986a; Johansen and Diemer, 1990; Widmann et al., 1991). In fact, electron-microscopic evaluation of mitochondrial calcium sequestration – which parallels the alterations of cytosolic calcium activity (Nicholls, 1985) – revealed a triphasic pattern in

CA1 neurons: the massive calcium deposits visible 15 min after 5 min ischemia transiently disappeared between 30 min and 2 h but started to accumulate again after 6 h in parallel with the secondary suppression of protein synthesis (Dux et al., 1987). The temporal and topical pattern of the post-ischemic impairment of protein synthesis can, therefore, be readily associated with the known post-ischemic alterations of ion and transmitter homeostasis.

A similar scenario can be drawn for the alterations during and after focal ischemia. In the center of the ischemic focus protein synthesis is inhibited due to energy failure. In the peripheral parts of the infarct or in regions in which spontaneous recirculation occurs, energy metabolism is preserved but intracellular calcium homeostasis is disturbed because ischemia generates spreading depression like waves (Nedergaard and Astrup, 1986; Iijima et al., 1992) and because excitatory amino acids which are released in the center of the infarct (Shimada et al., 1989) diffuse into the surrounding tissue. This explains that protein synthesis begins to decline at much higher flow values than energy metabolism. Recovery of protein synthesis, and hence cell survival, depends on the normalization of ion homeostasis which, in turn, is closely associated with the normalization of transmitter homeostasis and/or the cessation of peri-infarct spreading depression. This may be the reason that the reversal of these disturbances by glutamate and calcium antagonists reduces the size of an infarct although blood flow does not improve (Park et al., 1988, 1989; Nakayama et al., 1988; Dirnagl et al., 1990).

Selective gene expression

The interpretation of the pattern of selective gene expression is less straightforward. At the onset of focal or global ischemia the depolarization of cell membranes and the release of neurotransmitters are signals for the induction of immediate early response genes (for review, see Doucet et al., 1990). As a result *fos, jun* and *zif* mRNAs are expressed but the synthesis of the corresponding proteins is inhibited at the translational level. With the reversal of the translational block in the non-vulnerable cells of the brain, fos, jun and zif proteins are synthesized and may induce the transcription of other genes, such as superoxide dismutase, ornithine decarboxylase or stress proteins. The persisting translational block in the vulnerable parts of the brain explains that both the immediate early response and stress proteins are only synthesized in regions destined to survive (Vass et al., 1988a; Gonzales et al., 1991; Takemoto et al., 1991; Uemura et al., 1991a,b). Conversely, superinduction of mRNA in the absence of the translation of the corresponding protein explains that these mRNAs are preferentially expressed in the vulnerable parts of the brain (Jørgensen et al., 1989; Nowak, 1990, 1991; Nowak et al., 1990).

However, there are other proteins which do not fit into this general concept. The most conspicuous one is ornithine decarboxylase (ODC) which is synthesized in the CA1 sector after 8 h recirculation despite the persisting inhibition of protein synthesis. ODC is a protein with a remarkably short half-life; it is possible that such proteins are less sensitive to the translational block and, therefore, escape the overall inhibition of protein synthesis (see also Paschen et al., 1988, and this volume).

Relationship to ischemic cell death

Inhibition of overall protein synthesis, as reflected by the reduced incorporation of labeled amino acids into brain proteins, is closely associated with neuronal death. In all experimental situations that have been reviewed in this article, the morphological manifestation of neuronal injury in or outside the selectively vulnerable areas was preceded by a severe reduction of amino acid incorporation. Conversely, recovery of protein synthesis consistently predicted neuronal survival throughout the brain, i.e., not only within the hippocampus, and therapeutic interventions which were able to restore protein synthesis also prevented neuronal injury.

This clear correlation between protein synthesis and neuronal vulnerability differs from most other putative mediators of ischemic injury. Following a brief period of global ischemia glutamate is released and cytosolic calcium increases throughout the brain but neurons are damaged only in the selectively vulnerable parts of the brain. Putrescine, another putative mediator of ischemic injury, increases to a higher level in the vulnerable areas but the difference to the resistant parts is not as sharp as the difference in protein synthesis. Similarly, the various regional patterns of receptor densities or selective gene inductions may allow a differentiation between vulnerable and non-vulnerable neurons within a given anatomical structure such as hippocampus or striatum, but not throughout the brain. It is, therefore, rather unlikely that any of these mediators injures the neurons by a simple dose-response relationship.

The much closer correlation of neuronal survival with overall protein synthesis suggests that the protein-synthesizing machinery is a more critical part in the cascade of pathogenetic events leading to ischemic cell death. However, it will not be easy to find out whether the failure of this machinery is the cause or the consequence of ischemic injury. This question is of more than academic interest because a causal role of protein synthesis for cell survival would imply that the effects of the various mediators of ischemic cell death could be reversed if ways are found to reactivate this machinery. A strong argument in favor of a causal role is the long delay which may elapse between the end of ischemia and the manifestation of cell death. Another one is the prevention of cell death when protein synthesis is restored by pharmacological interventions. The transient synthesis of some proteins like ornithine decarboxylase in neurons destined to die demonstrates that the overall depression of protein synthesis cannot be explained by an unselective destruction of the protein-synthesizing machinery. It rather suggests that protein synthesis is dysregulated which is in line with the concept of a functional disturbance. A dysregulation would imply that the neurons do not necessarily die because of an overall decline of their protein contents; they may suffer from the failure of the synthesis from specific proteins or peptides, or from disturbances of the equilibrium of specific enzymatic systems such as the one leading to the post-ischemic increase of putrescine (for details, see Paschen, this volume).

These arguments certainly do not rule out the possibility that post-ischemic inhibition of protein synthesis is an epiphenomenon of other more important pathological events, such as calcium-induced activations of proteases or the genomic induction of programmed cell death (see other chapters of this volume). However, at the present there is no compelling evidence in favor or against any of these or other molecular mechanisms of ischemic injury. Further detailed studies, therefore, are required to clarify this important matter.

References

Abe, K., Araki, T. and Kogure, K. (1988) Recovery from edema and of protein synthesis differs between the cortex and caudate following transient focal cerebral ischemia in rats. *J. Neurochem.*, 51: 1470 – 1476.

Abe, K., Tanzi, R.E. and Kogure, K. (1991a) Selective induction of Kunitz-type protease inhibitor domain-containing amyloid precursor protein mRNA after persistent focal ischemia in rat cerebral cortex. *Neurosci. Lett.*, 125: 172 – 174.

Abe, K., Kawagoe, J., Sato, S., Sahara, M. and Kogure, K. (1991b) Induction of the "zinc finger" gene after transient focal ischemia in rat cerebral cortex. *Neurosci. Lett.*, 123: 248 – 250.

Abe, K., Tanzi, R.E. and Kogure, K. (1991c) Induction of hsp70 mRNA after transient ischemia in gerbil brain. *Neurosci. Lett.*, 125: 166 – 168.

Alcazar, A., Mendez, E., L-Fando, J. and Salinas, M. (1988) Specific phosphorylation of the beta subunit of eIF-2 factor from brain by three different protein kinases. *Biochem. Biophys. Res. Commun.*, 153: 313 – 320.

Ames III, A., Wright, R.L., Kowada, M., Thurston, J.M. and Majno, G. (1968) Cerebral ischemia. II. The no-reflow phenomenon. *Am. J. Pathol.*, 52: 437 – 453.

Araki, T., Kato, H., Inoue, T. and Kogure, K. (1990) Regional impairment of protein synthesis following brief cerebral ischemia in the gerbil. *Acta Neuropathol. (Berl.)*, 79: 501 – 505.

Astrup, J., Siesjö, B.K. and Symon, L. (1981) Thresholds in cerebral ischemia. The ischemic penumbra. *Stroke*, 12: 723 – 725.

Benveniste, H., Drejer, J., Schousboe, A. and Diemer, N.H. (1984) Elevation of the extracellular concentrations of glutamate and aspartate in rat hippocampus during transient cerebral ischemia monitored by intracerebral microdialysis. *J. Neurochem.*, 43: 1369 – 1374.

Bergstedt, K. and Wieloch, T. (1991) Effect of hypothermia and postischemic NBQX administration of ^{14}C-leucine incorporation into proteins in the rat brain following 15-minute transient 2-VO ischemia. *J. Cereb. Blood Flow Metab.*, 11, (Suppl. 2): 118.

Bodsch, W., Takahashi, K., Barbier, A., Grosse Ophoff, B. and Hossmann, K.-A. (1985) Cerebral protein synthesis and ischemia. *Progr. Brain Res.*, 63: 197 – 210.

Bodsch, W., Barbier, A., Oehmichen, M., Grosse Ophof, B. and Hossmann, K.-A. (1986) Recovery of monkey brain after prolonged ischemia. II. Protein synthesis and morphological alterations. *J. Cereb. Blood Flow Metab.*, 6: 22 – 33.

Bonnekoh, P., Kuroiwa, T., Oschlies, U. and Hossmann, K.-A. (1992) Barbiturate promotes post-ischemic reaggregation of polyribosomes in gerbil hippocampus. *Neurosci. Lett.*, 146: 75 – 78.

Carai, A.M., Orunesu, G., Pau, A.M., Sehrbundt Viale, E., Turtas, S. and Viale, G.L. (1979) Untersuchungen über die Ribosomen in dem ischämischen und postischämischen Gehirn des Gerbils. Zentralbl. Neurochir., 40: 151 – 158.

Chavko, M., Kluchova, D. and Marsala, J. (1981) Incorporation of ^{14}C-leucine into the proteins of spinal ganglia in vivo under conditions of partial ischaemia. *Physiol. Bohemoslov.*, 30: 267 – 274.

Chavko, M., Danielisova, V. and Marsala, J. (1987) Molecular mechanisms of ischemic damage of spinal cord. *Gerontology*, 33: 220 – 226.

Cooper, H.K., Zalewska, T., Kawakami, S., Hossmann, K.-A. and Kleihues, P. (1977) The effect of ischaemia and recirculation on protein synthesis in the rat brain. *J. Neurochem.*, 28: 929 – 934.

DeHaro, C., de Herreros, A.G. and Ochoa, S. (1983) Activation of the heme-stabilized translational inhibitor of reticulocyte lysates by calcium ions and phospholipid. *Proc. Natl. Acad. Sci. U.S.A.*, 80: 6843 – 6847.

Dempsey, R.J., Kindy, M., Combs, D.J. and Carney, J. (1990) Induction of the proto-oncogene *c-fos* in reperfused brain after transient ischemia: relationship to development of brain edema. *J. Neurosurg.*, 72: 346A.

DiDomenico, B.J., Bugaisky, G.E. and Lindquist, S. (1982) The heat shock response is self-regulated at both the transcriptional and posttranscriptional levels. *Cell*, 31: 593 – 603.

Diemer, N.H., Valente, E. and Jorgensen, M.B. (1991) Induction of *c-fos* protein around the infarct following MCA-occlusion in the rat. *J. Cereb. Blood Flow Metab.*, 11 (Suppl. 2): 214.

Dienel, G.A., Pulsinelli, W.A. and Duffy, T.E. (1980) Regional protein synthesis in rat brain following acute hemispheric ischemia. *J. Neurochem.*, 35: 1216 – 1226.

Dienel, G.A., Cruz, N.F. and Rosenfeld, S.J. (1985) Temporal profiles of proteins responsive to transient ischemia. *J. Neurochem.*, 44: 600 – 610.

Dienel, G.A., Kiessling, M., Jacewicz, M. and Pulsinelli, W.A. (1986) Synthesis of heat shock proteins in rat brain cortex after transient ischemia. *J. Cereb. Blood Flow Metab.*, 6: 505 – 510.

Dirnagl, U., Jacewicz, M. and Pulsinelli, W. (1990) Nimodipine posttreatment does not increase blood flow in rats with focal cortical ischemia. *Stroke*, 21: 1357 – 1361.

Doucet, J.P., Squinto, S.P. and Bazan, N.G. (1990) Fos-Jun and the primary genomic response in the nervous system. Possible physiological role and pathophysiological significance. *Mol. Neurobiol.*, 4: 27 – 55.

Dux, E., Mies, G., Hossmann, K.-A. and Siklos, L. (1987) Calcium in the mitochondria following brief ischemia of gerbil brain. *Neurosci. Lett.*, 78: 295 – 300.

Dux, E., Fastbom, J., Ungerstedt, U., Rudolphi, K. and Fredholm, B.B. (1990) Protective effect of adenosine and a novel xanthine derivative propentofylline on the cell damage after bilateral carotid occlusion in the gerbil hippocampus. *Brain Res.*, 516: 248 – 256.

Dwyer, B.E., Nishimura, R.N., Powell, C.L. and Mailheau, S.L. (1987) Focal protein synthesis inhibition in a model of neonatal hypoxic-ischemic brain injury. *Exp. Neurol.*, 95: 277 – 289.

Dwyer, B.E., Nishimura, R.N. and Brown, I.R. (1989) Synthesis of the major inducible heat shock protein in rat hippocampus after neonatal hypoxia-ischemia. *Exp. Neurol.*, 104: 28 – 31.

Gonzales, M.F., Lowenstein, D., Fernyak, S., Hisanaga, K., Simon, R. and Sharp, F.R. (1991) Induction of heat shock protein 72-like immunoreactivity in the hippocampal formation following transient global ischemia. *Brain Res. Bull.*, 26: 241 – 250.

Goto, K., Ishige, A., Sekiguchi, K., Iizuka, S., Sugimoto, A., Yuzurihara, M., Aburada, M., Hosoya, E. and Kogure, K. (1990) Effects of cycloheximide on delayed neuronal death in rat hippocampus. *Brain Res.*, 534: 299 – 302.

Hagberg, H., Lehmann, A., Sandberg, M., Nyström, B., Jacobson, I. and Hamberger, A. (1985) Ischemia-induced shift of inhibitory and excitatory amino acids from intra- to extracellular compartments. *J. Cereb. Blood Flow Metab.*, 5: 413 – 429.

Harris, R.J., Symon, L., Branston, N.M. and Bayhan, M. (1981) Changes in extracellular calcium activity in cerebral ischaemia. *J. Cereb. Blood Flow Metab.*, 1: 203 – 209.

Hartmann, J.F. and Becker, R.A. (1973) Disaggregation of polyribosomes in intact gerbils following ischemia. An ultrastructural study. *Stroke*, 4: 964 – 968.

Hossmann, K.-A., Lechtape-Grüter, H. and Hossmann, V. (1973) The role of cerebral blood flow for the recovery of the brain after prolonged ischemia. *Z. Neurol.*, 204: 281 – 299.

Hossmann, K.-A., Sakaki, S. and Zimmerman, V. (1977) Cation activities in reversible ischemia of the cat brain. *Stroke*, 8: 77 – 81.

Hossmann, K.-A., Mies, G., Paschen, W., Csiba, L., Bodsch, W., Rapin, J.R., Le Poncin-Lafitte, M. and Takahashi, K. (1985) Multiparametric imaging of blood flow and metabolism after middle cerebral artery occlusion in cats. *J. Cereb. Blood Flow Metab.*, 5: 97 – 107.

Hossmann, K.-A., Schmidt-Kastner, R. and Grosse Ophoff, B. (1987) Recovery of integrative central nervous function after one hour global cerebrocirculatory arrest in normothermic cat. *J. Neurol. Sci.,* 77: 305 – 320.

Iijima, T., Mies, G. and Hossmann, K.-A. (1992) Repeated negative DC deflections in rat cortex following middle cerebral artery occlusion are abolished by MK-801: effect on volume of ischemic injury. *J. Cereb. Blood Flow Metab.,* 12: 727 – 733.

Ito, U., Spatz, M., Walker Jr., J.T. and Klatzo, I. (1975) Experimental cerebral ischemia in mongolian gerbils. I. Light microscopic observations. *Acta Neuropathol. (Berl.),* 32: 209 – 223.

Jacewicz, M., Kiessling, M. and Pulsinelli, W.A. (1986) Selective gene expression in focal cerebral ischemia. *J. Cereb. Blood Flow Metab.,* 6: 263 – 272.

Jagus, J., Anderson, W.F. and Safer, B. (1981) The regulation of initiation of mammalian protein synthesis. *Prog. Nucleic Acid Res.,* 25: 127 – 185.

Johansen, F.F. and Diemer, N.H. (1990) Temporal profile of interneuron and pyramidal cell protein synthesis in rat hippocampus following cerebral ischemia. *Acta Neuropathol. (Berl.),* 81: 14 – 19.

Jørgensen, M.B., Deckert, J., Wright, D.C. and Gehlert, D.R. (1989) Delayed *c-fos* proto-oncogene expression in the rat hippocampus induced by transient global cerebral ischemia: an in situ hybridization study. *Brain Res.,* 484: 393 – 398.

Kiessling, M., Dienel, G.A., Jacewicz, M. and Pulsinelli, W.A. (1986) Protein synthesis in postischemic rat brain: a two-dimensional electrophoretic analysis. *J. Cereb. Blood Flow Metab.,* 6: 642 – 649.

Kiessling, M., Xie, Y., Ulrich, B. and Thilmann, R. (1991) Are the neuroprotective effects of the protein synthesis inhibitor cycloheximide due to prevention of apoptosis? *J. Cereb. Blood Flow Metab.,* 11 (Suppl. 2): 357.

Kindy, M.S., Carney, J.P., Dempsey, R.J. and Carney, J.M. (1991) Ischemic induction of proto-oncogene expression in gerbil brain. *J. Mol. Neurosci.,* 2: 217 – 228.

Kinouchi, H., Mizui, T., Carlson, E., Epstein, C.J. and Chan, P.H. (1991) Focal cerebral ischemia and the antioxidant system in transgenic mice overexpressing CuZn-superoxide dismutase. *J. Cereb. Blood Flow Metab.,* 11 (Suppl. 2): 423.

Kirino, T. (1982) Delayed neuronal death in the gerbil hippocampus following ischemia. *Brain Res.,* 239: 57 – 69.

Kirino, T., Tsujita, Y. and Tamura, A. (1991) Induced tolerance to ischemia in gerbil hippocampal neurons. *J. Cereb. Blood Flow Metab.,* 11: 299 – 307.

Kitagawa, K., Matsumoto, M., Kuwabara, K., Tagaya, M., Ohtsuki, T., Hata, R., Ueda, H., Handa, N., Kimura, K. and Kamada, T. (1991a) "Ischemic tolerance" phenomenon detected in various brain regions. *Brain Res.,* 561: 203 – 211.

Kitagawa, K., Matsumoto, M., Tagaya, M., Kuwabara, K., Hata, R., Handa, N., Fukunaga, R., Kimura, K. and Kamada, T. (1991b) Hyperthermia-induced neuronal protection against ischemic injury in gerbils. *J. Cereb. Blood Flow Metab.,* 11: 449 – 452.

Kleihues, P. and Hossmann, K.-A. (1971) Protein synthesis in the cat brain after prolonged cerebral ischemia. *Brain Res.,* 35: 409 – 418.

Kleihues, P. and Hossmann, K.-A. (1973) Regional incorporation of L-[^{3}H]tyrosine into cat brain proteins after one hour of complete ischemia. *Acta Neuropathol. (Berl.),* 25: 313 – 324.

Kleihues, P., Hossmann, K-A., Pegg, A.E., Kobayashi, K. and Zimmermann, V. (1975) Resuscitation of the monkey brain after one hour complete ischemia. III. Indications of metabolic recovery. *Brain Res.,* 95: 61 – 73.

Li, Y., Chopp, M., Levine, S.R., Dereski, M.O., Garcia, J.H. and Welch, K.M.A. (1991) Hypothermia prevents 70-kDa heat shock protein induction in rat brain after ischemia. *Stroke,* 22: 130.

Lowry, O.H., Passonneau, J.V., Hasselberger, F.X. and Schulz, D.W. (1964) Effect of ischemia on known substrates and cofactors of the glycolytic pathway in brain. *J. Biol. Chem.,* 239: 18 – 30.

Matsuyama, T., Uyama, O., Michishita, H., Nakamura, H., Matsumoto, Y., Yamamoto, Y., Furuyama, J. and Sugita, M. (1991) Alteration in expression of copper-zinc superoxide dismutase mRNA in gerbil hippocampus after transient cerebral ischemia. *J. Cereb. Blood Flow Metab.,* 11 (Suppl. 2): 217.

Mies, G., Paschen, W. and Hossmann, K.-A. (1990) Cerebral blood flow, glucose utilization, regional glucose, and ATP content during the maturation period of delayed ischemic injury in gerbil brain. *J. Cereb. Blood Flow Metab.,* 10: 638 – 645.

Mies, G., Ishimaru, S., Xie, Y., Seo, K., and Hossmann, K.-A. (1991) Ischemic thresholds of cerebral protein synthesis and energy state following middle cerebral artery occlusion in rat. *J. Cereb. Blood Flow Metab.,* 11: 753 – 761.

Mima, T., Halaby, I., Petito, C. and Pulsinelli, W. (1991) Induction of heat shock proteins fails to attenuate ischemic damage to CA1 hippocampus in rats. *J. Cereb. Blood Flow Metab.,* 11 (Suppl. 2): 216.

Miyazawa, T., Widmann, R. and Hossmann, K.-A. (1991) Effect of brain temperature on selective vulnerability and protein synthesis after 30 min forebrain ischemia in rats. *J. Cereb. Blood Flow Metab.,* 11 (Suppl. 2): 844.

Morimoto, K. and Yanagihara, T. (1981a) Cerebral ischemia in gerbils: polyribosomal function during progression and recovery. *Stroke,* 12: 105 – 110.

Morimoto, K. and Yanagihara, T. (1981b) Cerebral ischemia in gerbils: polyribosomal function during progression and recovery. *Stroke,* 12: 105 – 110.

Morimoto, K., Brengman, J. and Yanagihara, T. (1978) Further evaluation of polypeptide synthesis in cerebral anoxia, hypoxia and ischemia. *J. Neurochem.,* 31: 1277 – 1282.

Müller, M., Cleef, M., Röhn, G., Bonnekoh, P., Pajunen, A.E.I., Bernstein, H.-G. and Paschen, W. (1991) Ornithine decarboxylase in reversible cerebral ischemia: an immunohistochemical study. *Acta Neuropathol. (Berl.),* 83: 39 – 45.

Munekata, K. and Hossmann, K.-A. (1987) Effect of 5-minute ischemia on regional pH and energy state of the gerbil brain: relation to selective vulnerability of the hippocampus. *Stroke,* 18: 412 – 417.

Munekata, K., Hossmann, K.-A., Xie, Y., Seo, K. and Oschlies, U. (1987) Selective vulnerability of hippocampus: ribosomal aggregation, protein synthesis, and tissue pH. In: W.J. Powers and M.E. Raichle (Eds.), *Cerebrovascular Diseases,* Raven Press, New York, pp. 107 – 117.

Nakayama, H., Ginsberg, M.D. and Dietrich, W.D. (1988) (S)-Emopamil, a novel calcium channel blocker and serotonin S_2 antagonist, markedly reduces infarct size following middle cerebral artery occlusion in the rat. *Neurology,* 38: 1667 – 1673.

Nedergaard, M. and Astrup, J. (1986) Infarct rim: effect of hyperglycemia on direct current potential and [^{14}C]2-deoxyglucose phosphorylation. *J. Cereb. Blood Flow Metab.,* 6: 607 – 615.

Nicholls, D.G. (1985) A role for the mitochondrion in the protection of cells against calcium overload? In: K. Kogure, K.-A. Hossmann, B.K. Siesjö and F.A. Welsh (Eds.), *Progress in Brain Research, Vol. 63,* Elsevier Science Publishers B.V. (Biomedical Division), Amsterdam, pp. 97 – 106.

Nowak Jr., T.S. (1985) Synthesis of a stress protein following transient ischemia in the gerbil. *J. Neurochem.,* 45: 1635 – 1641.

Nowak Jr., T.S. (1988) NMDA-receptor antagonist MK-801 blocks postischemic HSP70 induction: evidence that the heat shock (stress) response is a component of excitotoxic pathology in gerbil hippocampus. *J. Neuropathol. Exp. Neurol.,* 47: 363.

Nowak Jr., T.S. (1990) Protein synthesis and the heat shock/stress response after ischemia. *Cerebrovasc. Brain Metab. Rev.,* 2: 345 – 366.

Nowak Jr., T.S. (1991) Localization of 70 kDa stress protein mRNA induction in gerbil brain after ischemia. *J. Cereb. Blood Flow Metab.,* 11: 432 – 439.

Nowak Jr., T.S., Fried, R.L., Lust, W.D. and Passonneau, J.V. (1985) Changes in brain energy metabolism and protein synthesis following transient bilateral ischemia in the gerbil. *J. Neurochem.,* 44: 487 – 494.

Nowak Jr., T.S., Bond, U. and Schlesinger, M.J. (1990) Heat shock RNA levels in brain and other tissues after hyperthermia and transient ischemia. *J. Neurochem.,* 54: 451 – 458.

Onodera, H., Kogure, K., Ono, Y., Igarashi, K., Kiyota, Y. and Nagaoka, A. (1989) Proto-oncogene *c-fos* is transiently induced in the rat cerebral cortex after forebrain ischemia. *Neurosci. Lett.,* 98: 101 – 104.

Orunesu, G., Pau, A., Sehrbundt Viale, E., Turtas, S. and Viale, G.L. (1980) Amino acid incorporation into polyribosomes of ischemic and reperfused gerbil brain. *Acta Neurochir. (Wien),* 51: 247 – 252.

Park, C.K., Nehls, D.G., Graham, D.I., Teasdale, G.M. and McCulloch, J. (1988) Focal cerebral ischaemia in the rat: treatment with the glutamate antagonist MK-801 after induction of ischaemia. *J. Cereb. Blood Flow Metab.,* 8: 757 – 762.

Park, C.K., Nehls, D.G., Teasdale, G.M. and McCulloch, J. (1989) Effect of the NMDA antagonist MK-801 on local cerebral blood flow in focal cerebral ischaemia in the rat. *J. Cereb. Blood Flow Metab.,* 9: 617 – 622.

Paschen, W., Mies, G., Bodsch, W., Yamori, Y. and Hossmann, K.-A. (1985) Regional cerebral blood flow, glucose metabolism, protein synthesis, serum protein extravasation, and content of biochemical substrates in stroke-prone spontaneously hypertensive rats. *Stroke,* 16: 841 – 845.

Paschen, W., Schmidt-Kastner, R., Hallmayer, J. and Djuricic, B. (1988) Polyamines in cerebral ischemia. *Neurochem. Pathol.,* 9: 1 – 20.

Paschen, W., Hallmayer, J., Mies, G. and Röhn, G. (1990) Ornithine decarboxylase activity and putrescine levels in reversible cerebral ischemia of mongolian gerbils: effect of barbiturate. *J. Cereb. Blood Flow Metab.,* 10: 236 – 242.

Paschen, W., Mies, G. and Hossmann, K.-A. (1991) Threshold relationship between cerebral blood flow, glucose utilization and energy metabolites during development of stroke in gerbils. *Exp. Neurol.,* 117: 325 – 333.

Petito, C.K. and Pulsinelli, W.A. (1984) Sequential development of reversible neuronal damage following cerebral ischemia. *J. Neuropathol. Exp. Neurol.,* 43: 141 – 153.

Popovici, T., Represa, A., Crépel, V., Barbin, G., Beaudoin, M. and Ben-Ari, Y. (1990) Effects of kainic acid-induced seizures and ischemia on *c-fos*-like proteins in rat brain. *Brain Res.,* 536: 183 – 194.

Raley, K.M. and Lipton, P. (1990) NMDA receptor activation accelerates ischemic energy depletion in the hippocampal slice and the demonstration of a threshold for ischemic damage to protein synthesis. *Neurosci. Lett.,* 110: 118 – 123.

Raley-Susman, K.M. and Lipton, P. (1990) In vitro ischemia and protein synthesis in the rat hippocampal slice: the role of calcium and NMDA receptor activation. *Brain Res.,* 515: 27 – 38.

Schatzman, R.C., Grifo, J.A., Merrick, W.C. and Kuo, J.F. (1983) Phospholipid-sensitive Ca^{2+}-dependent protein kinase phosphorylates the beta subunit of eukaryotic initiation factor 2 (eIF-2). *FEBS Lett.,* 159: 167 – 170.

Schmidt-Kastner, R., Grosse Ophof, B. and Hossmann, K.-A. (1990) Pattern of neuronal vulnerability in the cat hippocampus after one hour of global cerebral ischemia. *Acta Neuropathol. (Berl.),* 79: 444 – 455.

Sharp, F.R., Lowenstein, D., Simon, R. and Hisanaga, K. (1991) Heat shock protein hsp72 induction in cortical and striatal astrocytes and neurons following infarction. *J. Cereb. Blood Flow Metab.,* 11: 621 – 627.

Shimada, N., Graf, R., Rosner, G., Wakayama, A., George, C.P. and Heiss, W.-D. (1989) Ischemic flow threshold for extracellular glutamate increase in cat cortex. *J. Cereb. Blood Flow Metab.*, 9: 603 – 606.

Siesjö, B.K., Bengtsson, F., Grampp, W. and Theander, S. (1990) Calcium, excitotoxins, and neuronal death in the brain. *Ann. N.Y. Acad. Sci.*, 568: 234 – 251.

Simon, R.P., Cho, H., Gwinn, R. and Lowenstein, D.H. (1991) The temporal profile of 72-kDA heat-shock protein expression following global ischemia. *J. Neurosci.*, 11: 881 – 889.

Suga, S. and Nowak Jr., T.S. (1991) Localization of immunoreactive fos and jun proteins in gerbil brain: effect of transient ischemia. *J. Cereb. Blood Flow Metab.*, 11 (Suppl. 2): 352.

Takemoto, O., Tomimoto, H. and Yanagihara, T. (1991) Induction of *c-fos* and *c-jun* gene products and heat shock protein after transient cerebral ischemia in gerbils. *Stroke*, 22: 131.

Thilmann, R., Xie, Y., Kleihues, P. and Kiessling, M. (1986a) Persistent inhibition of protein synthesis precedes delayed neuronal death in postischemic gerbil hippocampus. *Acta Neuropathol. (Berl.)*, 71: 88 – 93.

Thilmann, R., Xie, Y., Kleihues, P. and Kiessling, M. (1986b) Delayed ischemic cell death in gerbil hippocampus: suppression and recovery of protein synthesis and the protective effect of cycloheximide. *Clin. Neurol.*, 5: 107.

Tomida, S., Nowak Jr., T.S., Vass, K., Lohr, J.M. and Klatzo, I. (1987) Experimental model for repetitive ischemic attacks in gerbil: the cumulative effect of repeated ischemic insults. *J. Cereb. Blood Flow Metab.*, 7: 773 – 782.

Uemura, Y., Kowall, N.W. and Beal, M.F. (1991a) Global ischemia induces NMDA receptor-mediated *c-fos* expression in neurons resistant to injury in gerbil hippocampus. *Brain Res.*, 542: 343 – 347.

Uemura, Y., Kowall, N.W. and Moskowitz, M.A. (1991b) Focal ischemia in rats causes time-dependent expression of *c-fos* protein immunoreactivity in widespread regions of ipsilateral cortex. *Brain Res.*, 552: 99 – 105.

Vass, K., Welch, W.J. and Nowak Jr., T.S. (1988a) Localization of 70-kDa stress protein induction in gerbil brain after ischemia. *Acta Neuropathol. (Berl.)*, 77: 128 – 135.

Vass, K., Tomida, S., Hossmann, K.-A., Nowak Jr., T.S. and Klatzo, I. (1988b) Microvascular disturbances and edema formation after repetitive ischemia of gerbil brain. *Acta Neuropathol. (Berl.)*, 75: 288 – 294.

Wasterlain, C.G. (1974) Brain ribosomes in intracranial hypertension. *J. Neurochem.*, 23: 253 – 259.

Welsh, F.A., Moyer, D.J. and Harris, V.A. (1992) Regional expression of heat shock protein-70 mRNA and *c-fos* mRNA follwing focal ischemia in rat brain. *J. Cereb. Blood Flow Metab.*, 12: 204 – 212.

Widmann, R., Kuroiwa, T., Bonnekoh, P. and Hossmann, K.-A. (1991) [^{14}C]leucine incorporation into brain proteins in gerbils after transient ischemia: relationship to selective vulnerability of hippocampus. *J. Neurochem.*, 56: 789 – 796.

Widmann, R., Weber, C., Bonnekoh, P., Schlenker, M. and Hossmann, K.-A. (1992) Neuronal damage after repeated 5 min ischemia in the gerbil is preceded by prolonged impairment of protein metabolism. *J. Cereb. Blood Flow Metab.*, 12: 425 – 433.

Xie, Y., Munekata, K., Seo, K. and Hossmann, K.-A. (1988) Effect of autologous clot embolism on regional protein biosynthesis of monkey brain. *Stroke*, 19: 750 – 757.

Xie, Y., Herget, T., Hallmayer, J., Starzinski-Powitz, A. and Hossmann, K.-A. (1989a) Determination of RNA content in postischemic gerbil brain by in situ hybridization. *Metab. Brain Dis.*, 4: 239 – 251.

Xie, Y., Mies, G. and Hossmann, K.-A. (1989b) Ischemic threshold of brain protein synthesis after unilateral carotid artery occlusion in gerbils. *Stroke*, 20: 620 – 626.

Xie, Y., Seo, K. and Hossmann, K.-A. (1989c) Effect of barbiturate treatment on post-ischemic protein biosynthesis in gerbil brain. *J. Neurol. Sci.*, 92: 317 – 328.

Yanagihara, T. (1976) Cerebral anoxia: effect on neuron-glia fractions and polysomal protein synthesis. *J. Neurochem.*, 27: 539 – 543.

Yanagihara, T. (1978) Experimental stroke in gerbils: effect on translation and transcription. *Brain Res.*, 158: 435 – 444.

Yoshimine, T., Hayakawa, T., Kato, A., Yamada, K., Matsumoto, K., Ushio, Y. and Mogami, H. (1987) Autoradiographic study of regional protein synthesis in focal cerebral ischemia with TCA wash and image subtraction techniques. *J. Cereb. Blood Flow Metab.*, 7: 387 – 393.

K. Kogure, K.-A. Hossmann and B.K. Siesjö (Eds.)
Progress in Brain Research, Vol. 96

CHAPTER 12

Protein phosphorylation and the regulation of mRNA translation following cerebral ischemia

Tadeusz Wieloch, Kerstin Bergstedt and Bing Ren Hu

Laboratory for Experimental Brain Research, Department of Neurobiology, Clinical Research Center, Lund Hospital, S-221 85 Lund, Sweden

Introduction

During the last seven years we have witnessed a dramatic development in the pharmacology of cerebral ischemia. Significant and successful efforts devoted to the exploration of new drug candidates have yielded cerebro-protective compounds modulating neurotransmitter receptor and ion channel activities, or possessing free radical scavenging properties. Presently, the glutamate receptor antagonists directed towards the AMPA receptor subtype seem to be most promising, diminishing neuronal damage following both a transient severe global cerebral ischemia (Sheardown et al., 1990; Buchan et al., 1991a; Le Peillet et al., 1992; Nellgård and Wieloch, 1992) and focal cerebral ischemia (Gill and Lodge, 1991; Buchan et al., 1991b). The concept of an imbalance between excitatory, detrimental and inhibitory, protective transmitter systems in the post-ischemic phase (Wieloch, 1985; Wieloch et al., 1986; Mattson et al., 1989), further extended the development of neuro-protective compounds to receptor modulators such as adenosine analogues (DeLeo et al., 1987), noradrenaline (Gustafson et al., 1989) or trophic factors (Shigeno et al., 1991). Modulation of neuronal damage by many of these receptor ligands is observed when the compounds are administered in the reperfusion following ischemia, demonstrating that receptor activation in the post-ischemic phase is of pathogenetic importance. This suggests that ischemia modifies the processes involved in the post-ischemic receptor activation, which becomes detrimental to vulnerable neurons (Nellgård and Wieloch, 1992). Such processes could include an enhanced ligand release, changes in receptor characteristics, or changes in the intracellular signal transduction chain downstream from the activated receptor. The latter processes encompass changes in the concentration of second messengers, activation of protein kinases, protein phosphatases, proteases and lipases, resulting in a final covalent modification of target proteins. The covalent modifications could be irreversible such as proteolysis and lipolysis or reversible such as phosphorylation, acetylation or myristylation. In the present context, protein phosphorylation is of particular interest since, due to the reversibility, it provides a possibility to prevent potentially harmful events with therapeutical interventions.

One strategy of future ischemia research should be to define the intracellular mechanisms whereby activation of the plasma membrane receptors modulate ischemic cell death. This knowledge could spur further development of new and more efficient anti-ischemic drug candidates. One such process, minutely regulated by phosphorylation (Morley and Thomas, 1991) and thus a target for receptor-mediated influence, is cerebral protein synthesis which is rapidly inhibited following transient cerebral ischemia and thus constitutes a biochemical correlate to ischemic neuronal death (Hossman, this volume). In this article we will review the changes in protein phosphorylation following ischemia, with particular reference to the regulation of the initiation of protein synthesis.

Protein phosphorylation

Protein phosphorylation is a general mechanism whereby most cellular processes are regulated (Edelman et al., 1987). Phosphorylation leads to either activation or inhibition of the function of the phosphorylated protein, and the extent of the phosphorylation state is determined by the net effect of two enzymatic activities: protein kinases and protein phosphatases. The majority of protein kinases such as protein kinase C (PKC), the calcium-calmodulin kinase II (CaMKII) and the cAMP-dependent kinase (PKA) phosphorylate serines (Ser) and/or threonines (Thr) on target proteins (Edelman et al., 1987), while a minor, but very important class of protein kinases, the tyrosine kinases (PTK), phosphorylate tyrosine (Tyr) residues (Hunter and Cooper, 1985). In the central nervous system, protein kinases such as PKA, CaMKII and PKC often regulate processes associated with metabolism and neuronal functions such as excitability and transmitter release, while the PTKs are coupled to, or are part of, plasma membrane receptors activated by mitogens such as growth factors (Hunter, 1989). There is an extensive "cross talk" among protein kinases (Houslay, 1991). Protein kinases may autophosphorylate or phosphorylate another protein kinase, thereby modulating its own activity or the activities of other protein kinases, respectively. Also, different protein kinases may phosphorylate a protein at one or several, similar or different sites, affecting the properties of the phosphorylated protein differently. Protein kinases are activated by second messengers such as cAMP, calcium or diglycerides (PKA, CaMKII, PKA), or, in the case of tyrosine kinases, by conformational changes induced by the ligand receptor interaction. The protein phosphatases – enzymes that remove the phosphate groups on proteins – most probably are as numerous as the protein kinases but their regulation is not as well understood as the regulation of the kinases (Shenolikar and Nairn, 1991).

Since receptor activation is important for the outcome following an ischemic insult, and since receptor blockade provides a significant protection against ischemic damage it seems reasonable to assume that protein kinases and phosphatases play a central role in the intracellular response to an ischemic insult (Saitoh et al., 1991).

Protein kinases in cerebral ischemia

The effects of ischemia on PKC, CaMKII and PKA have been studied in some detail. Protein kinase C is a cytosolic enzyme that is translocated to the cell membranes upon increased levels of calcium ions, and that is activated in the presence of diglycerides and arachidonate (Huang, 1989). Ischemia is associated with an increase in intracellular calcium ion levels, and elevated levels of diglycerides and arachidonate (Siesjö, 1988), conditions that favor activation of protein kinase C. Several reports have demonstrated that PKC is translocated to cell membranes during ischemia (Louis et al., 1988; Wieloch et al., 1991). However, during reperfusion PKC is inhibited and its levels decrease probably due to proteolytic degradation (Kochhar et al., 1989; Wieloch et al., 1991). The translocation and down-regulation of PKC may be important for delayed neuronal death after ischemia. The enzyme regulates several important cell functions such as ion channel activity, transmitter release, receptor function and gene expression (Nishizuka, 1986). For example, PKC is known to activate a calcium ion channel and inhibit a potassium conductance, which could lead to increased neuronal excitability and enhanced accumulation of intracellular calcium ions (Alkon and Rasmussen, 1988). Also, PKC may regulate the activity of the G-protein-coupled receptor (Dumuis et al., 1990), and PKC is involved in the intracellular response to growth factor receptor activation (Hama et al., 1986). The late post-ischemic down-regulation of PKC may thus impair neuronal excitability and the influence of growth factors on vulnerable neurons (Araki et al., 1990a).

The CaMKII is activated by elevated intracellular levels of calcium and its activity may be stimulated in the post-ischemic period provided that the calcium levels are elevated. However, following transient cerebral ischemia in the rat and gerbil, the CaMKII activity decreases (Churn et al., 1990; Onodera et al., 1990; Yamamoto et al., 1992), although the level of the enzyme is not affected. The activity of CaMKII following spinal cord ischemia is also markedly decreased (Kochhar et al., 1989). The decrease in CaMKII activity could lead to a decrease in the phosphorylation of synapsin I and mobilization of synaptic vesicles leading to a depressed neurotransmitter release (Llinas et al., 1985). This is in agreement with the findings that synaptic vesicles accumulate and aggregate in nerve endings in the CA1 region following ischemia (Kirino and Sano, 1984). Also, since CaMKII is part of the postsynaptic densities (Rostas et al., 1986), neuronal activation may be depressed following ischemia.

The post-ischemic decrease in CaMKII (Yamamoto et al., 1992) and PKC activity (Cardell et al., 1990; Wieloch et al., 1991) in both vulnerable as well as resistant brain regions, suggests that a general inhibition of these protein kinases occurs in the post-ischemic phase, not specifically affecting selectively vulnerable brain regions. Since PKC and CaMKII influence neuronal excitability and transmitter release, the decrease in their activities could explain the observed depression of post-ischemic cerebral metabolism (Pulsinelli et al., 1982; Kozuka et al., 1989), and the absence of post-ischemic neuronal hyperactivity (Buszaki et al., 1989; Chopp et al., 1989). The depression of PKC activity may also lead to a decreased feed-back inhibition of phospholipase C, increasing the mobilization of intracellular calcium (Kirino et al., 1992). The down-regulation of PKC and CaMKII, affecting all parts of the brain, may not by themselves be decisive factors in causing neuronal damage, but in concert with other detrimental influences could lead to cell death. Intra-ischemic hypothermia is sofar the most efficient measure to prevent neuronal damage following cerebral ischemia (Busto et al., 1987; Boris-Möller et al., 1989). The intracellular mechanism underlying the protective effect of hypothermia is not fully understood, but it was recently demonstrated that the down-regulation of both PKC (Cardell et al., 1990) and CaMKII (Churn et al., 1990) following cerebral ischemia was prevented by intra-ischemic hypothermia. Preservation of protein kinases in the post-ischemic phase could be one explanation for the protection exerted by hypothermia.

Growth factors are required for normal cell development and maturation, and in the CNS these peptides have been implicated for neuronal survival following neuronal injury (Kromer, 1987; Gage et al., 1989; Shigeno et al., 1991). The intracellular signaling pathway downstream from the growth factor receptors is still not fully understood, but tyrosine kinases are activated by growth factor receptor stimulation (Hunter, 1989). The integrity of the intracellular growth factor receptor-stimulated reaction cascade could be important for the post-ischemic survival of neurons, in particular since growth factors influence gene expression and anabolic processes such as protein synthesis (Heidenreich and Toledo, 1989).

Post-ischemic protein synthesis

Which cellular processes, influenced by receptor activation and phosphorylation-dephosphorylation reactions, are persistently affected in selectively vulnerable brain areas in the post-ischemic phase, and may be related to cell death? The intracellular chaos caused by the decrease in ATP during an ischemic episode affects most physiological processes. However, the disturbances inflicted on the brain by transient ischemia are mostly reversible. For example, energy metabolism is rapidly restored (Pulsinelli and Duffy, 1983) in the post-ischemic phase, and even the vulnerable CA1 neurons show only minor or no ultrastructural changes of mitochondria until frank neuronal degeneration is evident (Petito and Pulsinelli, 1984; Deshpande et al., 1992). The ionic gradients across the plasma membrane are quickly normalized during reperfusion (Hansen, 1985), and glutamate overflow appearing during the ischemic insult is back to baseline values within minutes of recirculation (Boris-Möller, in preparation). Also the dramatic elevation of arachidonate occurring during an ischemic insult, returns to pre-ischemic levels soon after reperfusion (Yoshida et al., 1980).

Accumulation of dark material and a rapid dissolution of ribosomal rosettes into pinpoint like monosomes are two ultrastructural features that are characteristic of the degenerating CA1 neurons (Petito and Pulsinelli, 1984; Munekata et al., 1987; Deshpande et al., 1992). These changes are indicative of disturbances in protein turnover, and the polysomal disaggregation is a sign of inhibition of protein synthesis. As mentioned above, inhibition of protein synthesis is a biochemical correlate to ischemic cell death. Ultracentrifugation studies demonstrated disaggregation of polyribosomes within the first hour of reperfusion following ischemia suggesting that the initiation step of protein synthesis is inhibited (Cooper et al., 1977). The polysomal profile is unaffected at the end of ischemia indicating that reperfusion and functional recovery of the neurons is needed for inhibition to be instituted. Global protein synthesis measured as the incorporation of radioactive amino acids in the rat and gerbil brain exposed to transient cerebral ischemia is also significantly depressed (Bodsch et al., 1985; Thilmann et al., 1987; Araki et al., 1990b; Widmann et al., 1991). Using the 2-vessel occlusion model of cerebral ischemia, we found that [^{14}C]leucine incorporation is persistently inhibited in the selectively vulnerable areas such as the CA1 region of the hippocampus, while reversibly inhibited in the relatively ischemia resistant hippocampal CA3 region and dentate gyrus (Fig. 1). Most studies on protein synthesis following ischemia have been focused on investigations of radioactive amino acid incorporation (Dienel et al., 1980, 1985; Bodsch et al., 1985; Thilmann et al., 1987; Araki et al., 1990b; Widmann et al., 1991), while the mechanisms underlying the inhibition have been left unexplored. Since neuronal protein synthesis is influenced by protein kinases and phosphatases (Morley and Thomas, 1991), a defect in the signaling chain may be responsible for the persistent inhibition of protein synthesis in the CA1 region. For example, pre-ischemic hypothermia, which prevents the down-regulation of PKC and CaMKII, also prevents the persistent inhibition of protein synthesis in the CA1 region (Bergstedt and Wieloch, 1991). Furthermore, administration of staurosporine, a protein kinase inhibitor, into the hippocampus prior to the ischemic insult, mitigates the inhibition of protein synthesis (Hossmann, this volume).

Regulation of the reinitiation of protein synthesis following ischemia

Cellular protein synthesis is commonly divided into an initiation, an elongation and a termination step. Post-ischemic protein synthesis could be inhibited at the elongation step by CaMKII phosphorylation of the elongation factor 2 (Clemens, 1989). However, inhibition of elongation would not lead to the observed post-ischemic ribosomal disaggregation. Also, the decrease in CaMKII activity in the post-ischemic brain would favor an increase rather than a decrease in elongation rate (Ryazanov et al., 1988).

The initiation step of protein synthesis is generally considered to be rate-limiting (Hershey, 1991). The regulation of the initiation is accomplished by the eukaryotic initiation factors (eIFs), out of which eIF-2 and eIF-4 are considered to be the most important. Initiation factor 2 modulates the overall protein synthesis rate, while eIF-4 is believed to regulate the selection and translational efficiency of different mRNA species (Morley and Thomas, 1991). The initiation of protein synthesis starts with the formation of a complex between GTP and eIF-2 which then binds the initiator Met-tRNA, Met-tRNAi, to form a ternary complex [eIF-2·GTP·Met-tRNAi] (Ochoa, 1983; Clemens, 1989). The ternary complex formation is also defined

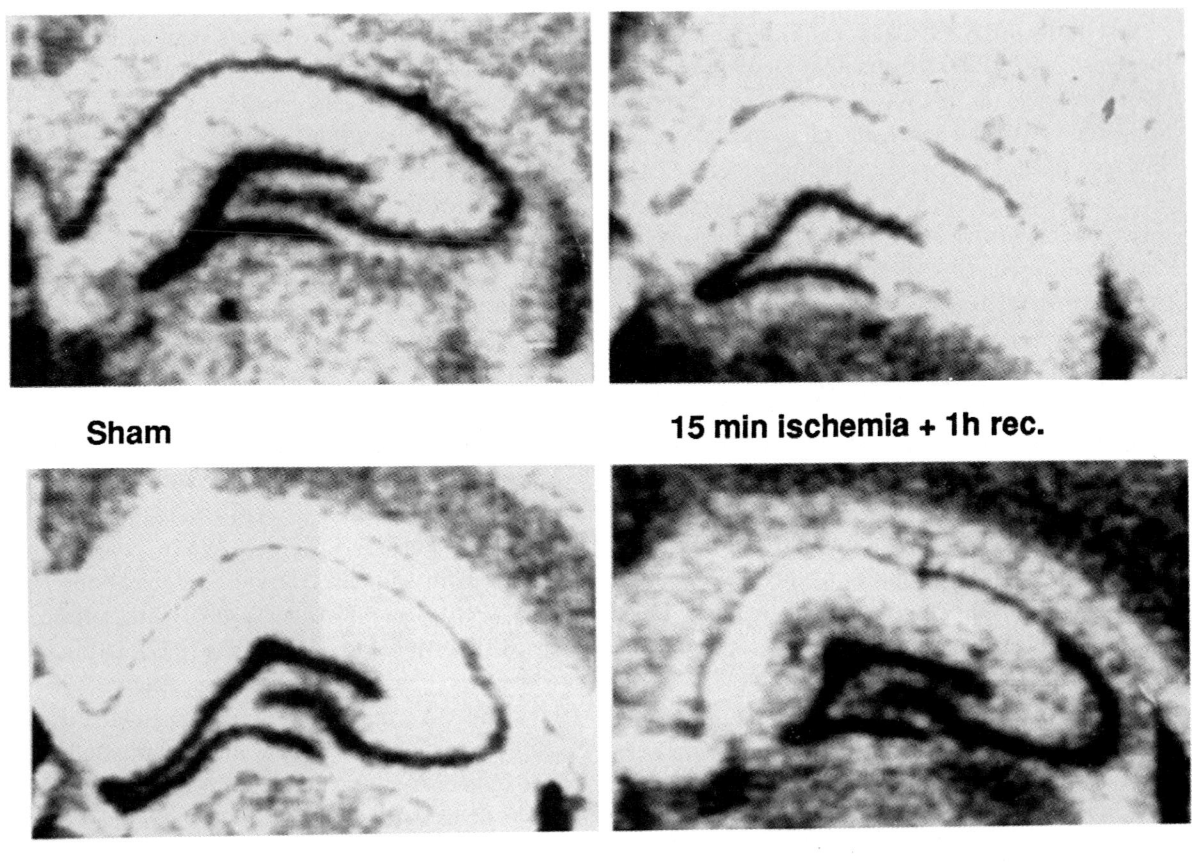

Fig. 1. Autoradiograms of the rat hippocampus (20 μm sections), demonstrating the incorporation of [^{14}C]leucine into brain proteins (TCA precipitate) of control animal, rat subjected to 15 min of ischemia and 1 h of recirculation, 24 h of recirculation, and 48 h of recirculation.

as eIF-2 activity. This ternary complex associates with the 40S ribosomal subunit, to form a pre-initiation complex. Together with additional eIFs and the mRNA to be translated, a 80S · mRNA initiation complex is formed, concomitant with GTP hydrolysis and release of eIF-2 · GDP. The GDP bound to eIF-2 is exchanged for GTP in order to regenerate eIF-2 · GTP for another round of initiation. Since eIF-2 has higher affinity for GDP than for GTP, the exchange process is catalyzed by the guanine nucleotide exchange factor (GEF) (Proud, 1986; Rowlands et al., 1988). Recycling of eIF-2 is a prerequisite for a continued protein synthesis, and the exchange of GDP for GTP is thus a rate-limiting step. Two mechanisms that may regulate the GDP-GTP exchange have been proposed. One mechanism includes the phosphorylation of the α-subunit of eIF-2 which in its phosphorylated state will bind GEF in a stable complex with GDP (Proud, 1986), while the other mechanism involves the phosphorylation of GEF (Tuazon and Traugh, 1991).

The activity of eIF-4 regulates the binding of the 40S pre-initiation complex to the cap region of the 5′ end of the mRNA (Kozak, 1983). Following the formation of the 80S · mRNA complex, the ribosome scans the mRNA until it reaches its initiation codon (AUG) where translation starts. Depending on the phosphorylation state of eIF-4, the nucleotide sequence in the 5′ non-coding region and the secondary structure of the mRNA, the mRNAs may be differentially selected for translation and translated at different rates. During heat shock, which depresses normal protein synthesis and leads to a preferential translation of hsp mRNA, the eIF-4 step is inhibited (Duncan et al., 1987; Lamphear and Panniers, 1991; Rhoads, 1991), presumably due to a decrease in PKC-mediated phosphorylation of eIF-4 (Morley et al., 1991). Heat-shock protein mRNA may still be translated by direct binding of the 40S pre-initiation complex to the AUG region, omitting the cap-binding process (Hultmark et al., 1986). Since protein kinase C is down-regulated after ischemia, a decrease in the activity of eIF-4 would be expected, which may explain the preferential translation of hsp 70 mRNA in the vulnerable CA1 region 24 h post-ischemia (Gonzales et al., 1991; Deshpande et al., 1992).

The effects of intra-ischemic hypothermia on protein synthesis further support the notion of an involvement of protein kinases in the post-ischemic depression of protein synthesis. Intra-ischemic hypothermia prevents the persistent inhibition of [^{14}C]leucine incorporation observed during late reperfusion phases (Bergstedt and Wieloch, 1991). As mentioned above hypothermia prevents the post-ischemic translocation and down-regulation of PKC (Cardell et al., 1991), and thus possibly the inhibition of eIF-4 activity.

Post-ischemic eIF-2 activity

The eIF-2 activity, measured as ternary complex formation, varies during and following transient cerebral ischemia in different brain areas (Hu and Wieloch, 1993a). At the end of an ischemic episode eIF-2 activity does not decrease indicating that the brain has a normal capacity to synthesize proteins, in agreement with electron-microscopical observations (Petito and Pulsinelli, 1984) and ultracentrifugation studies (Cooper et al., 1977). During the reperfusion phase the eIF-2 activity decreases in the CA1 and CA3 regions 1 h post-ischemia (Fig. 2). The eIF-2 activity recovers in the CA3 region by 6 h post-ischemia but remains depressed in the CA1 region. This strongly suggest that the post-ischemic

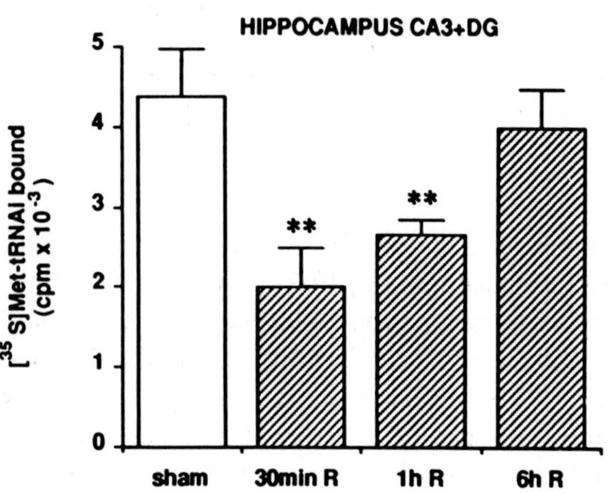

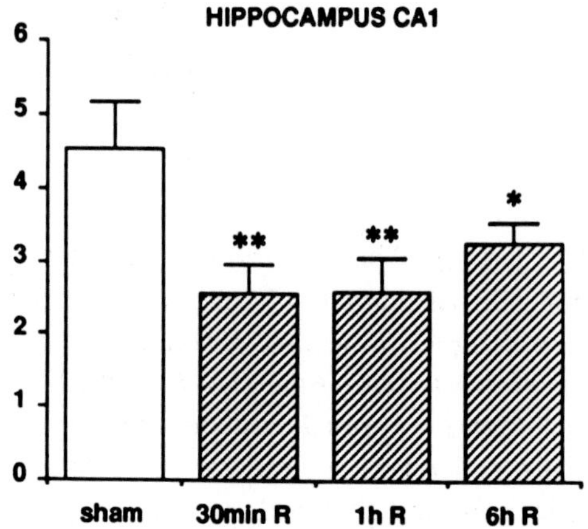

Fig. 2. Ternary complex formation in post-mitochondrial supernatant from the CA1 and CA3 regions of the rat hippocampus exposed to 15 min ischemia and 30 min, 1 h and 6 h of recirculation (* $P < 0.05$; ** $P < 0.01$; vs. sham-operated control, Dunetts test). (From Hu and Wieloch, 1993a.)

depression of protein synthesis is due to a decrease in the eIF-2 activity. A similar depression of ternary complex formation has been observed during conditions where initiation of protein synthesis is depressed such as serum deprivation (Montine and Henshaw, 1989), heat shock (Duncan and Hershey, 1984) and viral infection (Duncan, 1990). The data also imply that factors affecting post-ischemic ternary complex formation in vulnerable neurons exert their inhibitory effect late into the recirculation phase.

Regulation of post-ischemic ternary complex formation

How is ternary complex formation regulated in the post-ischemic brain? Two out of the three subunits constituting initiation factor 2, the α- and β-subunits, can be phosphorylated. The α-subunit is phosphorylated by a specific kinase, eIF-2 kinase (Alcazar et al., 1990), while the β-subunit is phosphorylated among others by PKC and casein kinase II (CKII) (Alcazar et al., 1988). The phosphorylation of the β-subunit does not affect the efficiency of eIF-2 to form the ternary complex formation and thus the initiation rate of protein synthesis, but may affect the binding of the ribosome to the AUG initiation codon on the mRNA and may thus affect the selection of the translated message (Morley and Thomas, 1991). The phosphorylation of the α-subunit on the other hand regulates ternary complex formation and protein synthesis rate in some cell types. For example, heme or double stranded RNA stimulate the eIF-2 kinases to phosphorylate eIF-2α in reticulocytes and HeLa cells, respectively (Panniers and Henshaw, 1983; Rowlands et al., 1988; Sarre et al., 1989). The phosphorylated eIF-2α binds to GEF with a higher affinity than to the unphosphorylated eIF-2α, thereby inhibiting the exchange of GDP for GTP on eIF-2 (Panniers and Henshaw, 1983; Proud, 1986; Rowlands et al., 1988). However, in the post-ischemic brain eIF-2α phosphorylation does not seem to play a regulatory role in the inhibition of ternary complex formation. For example, when post-mitochondrial supernatant (PMS) from rat cortex exposed to ischemia and 1 h recovery was treated with alkaline phosphatase, which dephosphorylates eIF-2α(P), the ternary complex formation in the homogenates was still depressed (Hu and Wieloch, 1993a). On the contrary, recent data indicate that the activation of a phosphatase may be responsible for inhibition of eIF-2 activity (Hu and Wieloch, 1993a). By mixing control PMS with post-ischemic PMS a decrease in eIF-2 activity was observed instead of the expected sum of the eIF-2 activities. (Table I). This suggests that an inhibitor is present in the post-ischemic PMS that is able to diminish the activity of eIF-2 in control PMS. Addition of vanadate, a phosphatase inhibitor, abolishes the inhibition, implying that the inhibitor is a protein tyrosine phosphatase (Lau et al., 1989). Apparently, in the post-ischemic brain a phosphatase is activated leading to a net dephosphorylation of a regulatory protein involved in ternary complex formation. This protein could be GEF.

The activity of GEF, measured as the dissociation rate of a performed eIF-2 · [^{3}H]GDP complex, is persistently depressed in the vulnerable striatum but only transiently depressed in cortex (Fig. 3; Hu and Wieloch, 1993a). The depressed GEF activity, i.e., the decrease in the GDP-GTP exchange, thus most probably is responsible for the decreased eIF-2 ac-

TABLE I

The effect of phosphatase inhibitors on ternary complex formation in cortical post-mitochondrial supernatant from rats exposed to 15 min 2-vessel occlusion ischemia and 30 min recovery

Experimental group	[^{35}S]Met-tRNAi bound[a]
Sham	3.8 ± 0.6
15 Min ischemia + 30 min reperfusion	2.0 ± 0.3
Mix[b]	3.1 ± 0.2
Mix + vanadate[c]	5.1 ± 0.4

[a] Values are given as cpm $\times 10^{-3}$ ± S.D.
[b] Equal volumes of post-mitochondrial supernatant from sham-operated rat neocortex and PMS from rats exposed to 15 min ischemia and 30 min reperfusion were mixed.
[c] 100 μM.

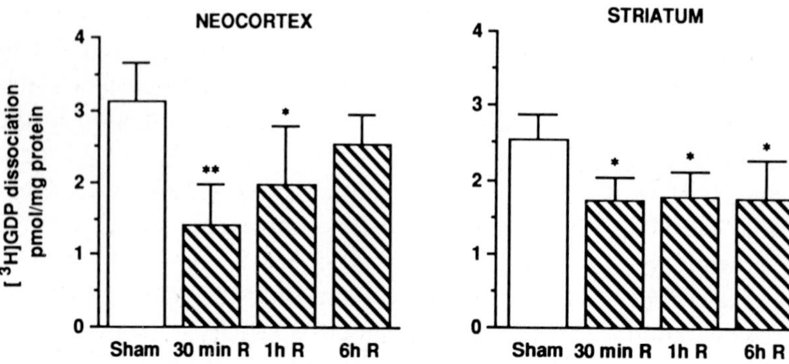

Fig. 3. The guanine exchange factor activity measured as the dissociation rate of preformed [^{3}H]GDP · eIF-2 in the presence of excess GDP, in post-mitochondrial supernatant from cortex and striatum of sham-operated rats and rats exposed to 15 min ischemia and 30 min, 1 h and 6 h recirculation. (** $P < 0.01$ vs. sham-operated control group, Dunett's test). (From Hu and Wieloch, 1993a.)

tivity. The mechanisms by which GEF activity is modulated are not fully elucidated, but purified GEF can be phosphorylated by CKII (Tuazon and Traugh, 1991) which increases the GEF activity five-fold (Dholakia and Wahba, 1988). The post-ischemic activation of a phosphatase during ischemia may dephosphorylate GEF, which explains the observed depression of post-ischemic GEF activity. Since growth factors stimulate protein synthesis (Heidenreich and Toledo, 1989; Montine and Henshaw, 1989), GEF may be activated directly by a growth factor-linked tyrosine kinase (Sommercorn et al., 1987; Klarlund and Czech, 1988) or indirectly through a protein kinase cascade, including CKII.

Modulation of post-ischemic CKII activity

Casein kinase II is a ser/thr protein kinase that is not dependent on cyclic nucleotides, and that is insensitive to calcium/calmodulin (Hathaway and Traugh, 1982). The regulation of CKII is not fully understood, but growth factors activate the enzyme (Klarlund and Czech, 1988). Casein kinase II usually phosphorylates proteins involved in regulating gene expression and protein synthesis (Tuazon and Traugh, 1991). The enzyme is involved in processes related to cell survival, since the deletion of the CKII gene in *Saccharomyces cerevisiae* decreases cell survival (Padmanabha et al., 1990). The CKII activity is also reduced in Alzheimer's disease (Imoto et al., 1989) and in cortex from schizophrenic patients (Aksenova et al., 1991).

The CKII activity in the cytosol from hippocampal homogenates, obtained from brains exposed to ischemia and various periods of recovery, increases in the CA3 region but decreases in the CA1 region (Fig. 4; Hu and Wieloch, 1993b). These changes persist up to 6 h post-ischemia, and are not due to increased levels of the known activators of CKII, spermine or spermidine, since the concentrations of these polyamines are at control or below control levels (Paschen et al., 1988). The regional differences in CKII activity most probably are due to changes in its phosphorylation state. This is supported by several recent investigations. For example, the M-phase-specific cdc2 (cell division control) protein kinase activates CKII 1.5 – 5-fold in vitro (Mulner-Lorillon et al., 1990). Insulin and epidermal growth factor activate CKII in 3T3-L1 mouse adipocytes and H4-IIE rat hepatoma cells by 30 – 150%, by phosphorylating the enzyme (Sommercorn et al., 1987; Ackerman et al., 1990). The mechanisms involved in CKII phosphorylation are not elucidated (Hathaway and Traugh, 1982; Tuazon and Traugh, 1991). Growth factors are sofar the only extracellular signals known to stimulate CKII activity (Sommercorn et al., 1987; Klarlund and Czech, 1988; Ackerman et al., 1990). Casein kinase II is not phosphorylated on a tyrosine

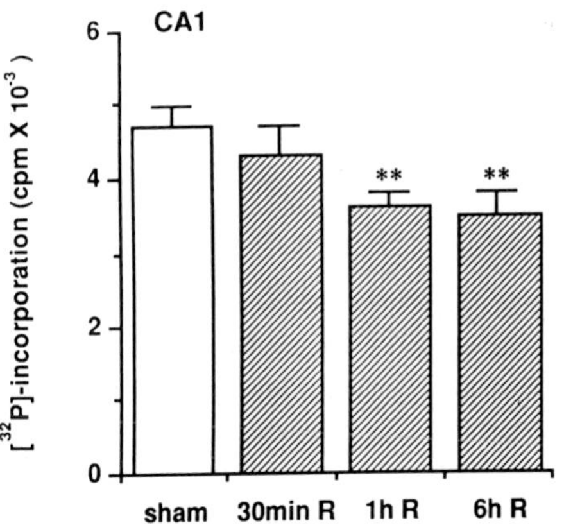

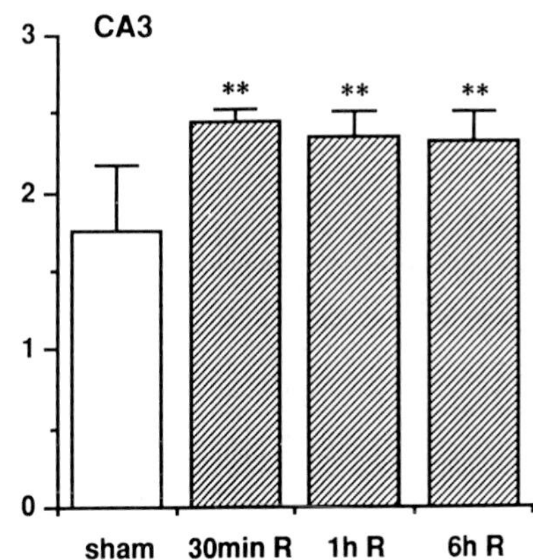

Fig. 4. Casein kinase II activity ([^{32}P] incorporation into β-casein) in the CA1 and CA3 regions of the hippocampus of sham-operated rats (open bars) and from rats exposed to 15 min ischemia and 30 min, 1 h and 6 h recovery (cross-hatched bars). Data are means ± S.D. (* $P < 0.05$ vs. control group, Dunnett's test). (From Hu and Wieloch, 1993b.)

residue implying that a kinase cascade involving intermediate ser/thr kinases are involved in regulating CKII activity.

The post-ischemic increase of CKII activity in the CA3 region and the decrease in the CA1 region of the hippocampus may thus reflect a change in the phosphorylation state of the enzyme due to changes in growth factor receptor activity. The functional implication of CKII modulation after an ischemic insult can only be speculated upon (Hu and Wieloch, 1993b). Cooperative phosphorylation by CKII (Tuazon and Traugh, 1991) may be an important event in the post-ischemic brain, i.e., phosphorylation of proteins by CKII may enhance and facilitate phosphorylation by other protein kinases. As mentioned earlier PKC and CaMKII are partially down-regulated or inhibited in the post-ischemic brain, both in vulnerable and resistant areas. The increased CKII activity in the resistant neurons may enhance phosphorylation of proteins by the down-regulated PKC and CaMKII, while in vulnerable regions, where CKII activity is decreased, a depressed protein phosphorylation by PKC and CaMKII may be augmented. Since growth factors activate CKII, it is tempting to suggest that in vulnerable neurons ischemia causes a defect in the growth factor receptor-mediated signal transduction chain, leading to a decrease in CKII activity and consequently to a depression of GEF and protein synthesis (Fig. 5). It is of interest to note that spermine and spermidine, which are activators of CKII, when given intravenously decrease ischemic damage following transient cerebral ischemia in the rat (Gilad and Gilad, 1991).

Conclusions

In conclusion, transient cerebral ischemia seems to

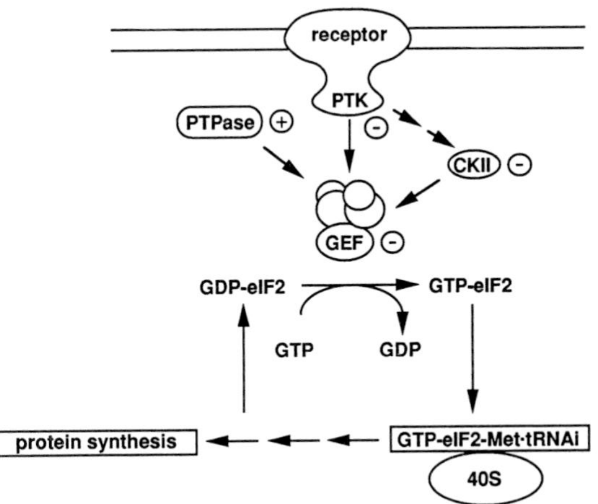

Fig. 5. A schematic and simplified picture of some regulatory events of protein synthesis initiation following cerebral ischemia. PTK, protein tyrosine kinase; PTPase, phosphotyrosine phosphatase; CKII, casein kinase II; GEF, guanine nucleotide exchange factor; eIF-2, eukaryotic exchange factor 2; 40S, 40S ribosomal subunit. The + and − signs denote effects of ischemia on the activities of the particular enzymes.

induce a post-ischemic imbalance between protein kinase and protein phosphatase activities, leading to a net dephosphorylation of proteins in the vulnerable neurons. This imbalance may lead to the persistent changes in processes crucial for neuronal survival such as post-ischemic protein synthesis. The depression of protein synthesis after an ischemic insult most probably is due to a decreased GEF activity, leading to a limited availability of eIF-2 for initiation complex formation. The inhibition of GEF activity in the vulnerable regions could in turn be due to dephosphorylation of GEF, possibly as a consequence of a tyrosine phosphatase activation and a decreased CKII activity. Post-ischemic inhibition of PKC and CaMKII may in addition depress eIF-4 activity leading to a selective translation of mRNA such as heat shock mRNA.

Evidently, if post-ischemic inhibition of protein synthesis is of importance in the pathogenetic process leading to cell death, then the phosphorylation-dephosphorylation processes regulating the intracellular cytokine and growth factor signals may be targets for future therapeutical interventions.

Acknowledgements

This work was supported by the United States Public Health Services (Grant NS 25302), the Swedish Medical Research Council (Grant 8644), The Laerdal Foundation, The Segerfalk Foundation and The Crafoord Foundation.

References

Ackerman, P., Glover, C.V.C. and Osheroff, N. (1990) Stimulation of casein kinase II by epidermal growth factor: relationship between the physiological activity of the kinase and the phosphorylation state of its β-subunit. *Proc. Natl. Acad. Sci. U.S.A.*, 87: 821 – 825.

Aksenova, M.V., Burbaeva, G.Sh., Kandror, K.V., Kapkov, D.V. and Stepanov, A.S. (1991) The decreased level of casein kinase-2 in brain cortex of schizophrenic and Alzheimer's disease patients. *FEBS Lett.*, 279: 55 – 57.

Alcazar, A., Mendez, E., Fando, J.L. and Salinas, M. (1988) Specific phosphorylation of eIF-2 factor from brain by three different protein kinases. *Biochem. Biophys. Res. Commun.*, 153: 313 – 320.

Alcazar, A., Mendez, E., Martin, M.E. and Salinas M. (1990) Purification of a novel eIF-2α protein kinase from calf brain. *Biochem. Biophys. Res. Commun.*, 166: 1237 – 1244.

Alkon, D.L. and Rasmussen, H. (1988) A spatial-temporal model of cell activation. *Science*, 239: 998 – 1005.

Araki, S., Simada, Y., Kaji, K. and Hayashi, H. (1990a) Role of protein kinase C in the inhibition by fibroblast growth factor of apoptosis in serum-depleted endothelial cells. *Biochem. Biophys. Res. Commun.*, 172: 1081 – 1085.

Araki, T., Kato, H. and Kogure, K. (1990b) Regional impairment of protein synthesis following brief cerebral ischemia in the gerbil. *Acta Neuropathol. (Berl.)*, 79: 501 – 505.

Bergstedt, K. and Wieloch, T. (1991) Effect of hypothermia and postischemic NBQX administration on ^{14}C-leucine incorporation into proteins in the rat brain following 15 minute transient 2-VO ischemia. *J. Cereb. Blood Flow Metab.*, 11 (Suppl. 2): S188.

Bodsch, W., Takahashi, K., Barbier, A., Grosse Ophoff, B. and Hossmann, K.A. (1985) Cerebral protein synthesis and ischemia. *Prog. Brain Res.*, 63: 197 – 210.

Boris-Möller, F., Smith, M.-L. and Siesjö, B.K. (1989) Effects of hypothermia on ischemic brain damage: a comparison between preischemic and postischemic cooling. *Neurosci. Res. Commun.*, 5: 87 – 94.

Buchan, A.M., Li, H., Cho, C. and Pulsinelli, W.A. (1991a) Blockade of the AMPA receptor prevents CA1 hippocampal injury following severe but transient forebrain ischemia in the adult rat. *Neurosci. Lett.*, 132: 255 – 258.

Buchan, A.M., Xue, D., Huang, Z.-G., Smith, K.H. and Lesiuk, H. (1991b) Delayed AMPA receptor blockade reduces cerebral infarction induced by focal ischemia. *Neuroreport*, 2: 473 – 476.

Busto, R., Dietrich, W.D., Globus, M.Y.-T., Valdés, I., Scheinberg, P. and Ginsberg, M. (1987) Small differences in intraischemic brain temperature critically determine the extent of ischemic neuronal injury. *J. Cereb. Blood Flow Metab.*, 7: 729 – 738.

Buszaki, G., Freund, T.F., Bayardo, F. and Somogyi, P. (1989) Ischemia-induced changes in the electrical activity of the hippocampus. *Exp. Brain Res.*, 78: 268 – 278.

Cardell, M., Bingren, H., Wieloch, T., Zivin, J. and Saitoh, T. (1990) Protein kinase C is translocated to cell membranes during cerebral ischemia. *Neurosci. Lett.*, 119: 228 – 232.

Cardell, M., Boris-Möller, F. and Wieloch, T. (1991) Hypothermia prevents the ischemia-induced translocation and inhibition of protein kinase C in the rat striatum. *J. Neurochem.*, 57: 1814 – 1817.

Chopp, H.S., Sasaki, T. and Kassell, N.F. (1989) Hippocampal unit activity after transient cerebral ischemia in rats. *Stroke*, 20: 1051 – 1058.

Churn, S.B., Taft, W.C., Billingsley, M.L., Blair, R.E. and De Lorenzo, R.J. (1990) Temperature modulation of ischemia-induced neuronal death and ischemia-induced inhibition of calcium/calmodulin dependent protein kinase II in gerbils.

Stroke, 21: 1715 – 1721.

Clemens, M.J. (1989) Regulatory mechanisms in translational control. *Curr. Opinion Cell Biol.,* 1: 1160 – 1197.

Cooper, H.K., Zalewski, T., Kawakami, S., Hossmann, K.-A. and Kleihues, P. (1977) The effect of ischemia and recirculation on protein synthesis in the rat brain. *J. Neurochem.,* 28: 929 – 934.

DeLeo, J., Toth, L., Schubert, P., Rudolphi, K. and Kreutzberg, G.W. (1987) Ischemia-induced neuronal cell death, calcium accumulation, and glial response in the hippocampus of the Mongolian gerbil and protection by propentofylline. (HWA 285). *J. Cereb. Blood Flow Metab.,* 7: 745 – 751.

Desphande, J., Bergstedt, K., Lindén, T., Kalimo, H. and Wieloch, T. (1992) Ultrastructural changes in the hippocampal CA1 region following transient cerebral ischemia: evidence against programmed cell death. *Exp. Brain Res.,* 88: 91 – 105.

Dholakia, J.N. and Wahba, A.J. (1988) Phosphorylation of the guanine nucleotide exchange factor from rabbit reticulocytes regulates its activity in polypeptide chain initiation. *Proc. Natl. Acad. Sci. U.S.A.,* 85: 51 – 54.

Dienel, G.A., Pulsinelli, W.A. and Duffy, T.E. (1980) Regional protein synthesis in rat brain following acute hemispheric ischemia. *J. Neurochem.,* 35: 1216 – 1226.

Dienel, G.A., Cruz, N.F. and Rosenfeld, S.J. (1985) Temporal profiles of proteins responsive to transient ischemia. *J. Neurochem.,* 44: 600 – 610.

Dumuis, A., Pin, J.P., Oomagari, K., Sebben, M. and Bockaert, J. (1990) Arachidonic acid released from striatal neurons by joint stimulation of ionotropic and metabotropic quisqualate receptors. *Nature,* 347: 182 – 183.

Duncan, R. (1990) Protein synthesis initiation factor modifications during viral infection: implication for translational control. *Electrophoresis,* 11: 219 – 227.

Duncan, R. and Hershey, J. (1984) Heat shock-induced translational alterations in HeLa cells. *J. Biol. Chem.,* 259: 11882 – 11889.

Duncan, R. and Hershey, J. (1985) Regulation of initiation factors during translational repression caused by serum depletion. *J. Biol. Chem.,* 260: 5493 – 5497.

Duncan, R., Milburn, S.C. and Hershey, J.W.B. (1987) Regulated phosphorylation and low abundance of HeLa cell initiation factor eIF-4F suggests a role in translational control. *J. Biol. Chem.,* 262: 380 – 388.

Edelman, A.M., Blumenthal, D.K. and Krebs, E.G. (1987) Protein serine/threonine kinases. *Annu. Rev. Biochem.,* 56: 567 – 613.

Gage, F.H., Batchelor, P., Chen, K.S., Chin, D., Higgins, G.A., Koh, S., Deputy, S., Rosenberg, M.B., Fischer, W. and Björklund, A. (1989) NGF receptor reexpression and NGF-mediated cholinergic neuronal hypertrophy in the damaged adult neostriatum. *Neuron,* 2: 1177 – 1184.

Gilad, G. and Gilad, V.H. (1991) Polyamines can protect against ischemia-induced nerve cell death in gerbil forebrain. *Exp. Neurol.,* 111: 349 – 355.

Gill, R. and Lodge, D. (1991) The neuroprotective action of 2,3-dihydoxy-6-nitro-7-sulfamoyl-benzo(F)quinnoxaline (NBQX) in a rat focal ischemia model. *J. Cereb. Blood Flow Metab.,* 11 (Suppl. 2): S224.

Gonzalez, M.F., Lowenstein, D., Fernyak, S., Hisanaga, K., Simon, R. and Sharp, F. (1991) Induction of heat shock protein 72-like immunoreactivity in the hippocampal formation following transient global ischemia. *Brain Res. Bull.,* 26: 241 – 250.

Gustafson, I., Miyauchi, Y. and Wieloch, T. (1989) Postischemic administration of Idazoxan, an α-2 adrenergic receptor antagonist, decreases neuronal damage in the rat brain. *J. Cereb. Blood Flow Metab.,* 9: 171 – 174.

Hama, T., Huang, K-P. and Guroff, G. (1986) Protein kinase C as a component of nerve growth factor sensitive phosphorylation system in PC 12 cells. *Proc. Natl. Acad. Sci. U.S.A.,* 83: 2353 – 2357.

Hansen, A.J. (1985) Effects of anoxia on ionic distribution in the brain. *Physiol Rev.,* 65: 101 – 135.

Hathaway, G.M. and Traugh, J.A. (1982) Casein kinases – multipotential protein kinases. In: E. Stadtman and B. Horecker (Eds.), *Current Topics in Cellular Regulation,* Academic Press, New York, pp. 101 – 127.

Heidenreich, K.A. and Toledo, S.P. (1989) Insulin receptors mediate growth effects in cultured neurons. I. Rapid stimulation of protein synthesis. *Endocrinology,* 125: 1451 – 1457.

Hershey, J.W. (1991) Translation control in mammalian cells. *Annu. Rev. Biochem.,* 60: 717 – 755.

Houslay, M.D. (1991) "Crosstalk": a pivotal role for protein kinase C in modulating relationships between signal transduction pathways. *Eur. J. Biochem.,* 195: 9 – 27.

Hu, B.G. and Wieloch, T. (1993a) Stress-induced inhibition of protein synthesis initiation. Modulation of initiation factor 2 and guanine exchange factor activities following transient cerebral ischemia in the rat. *J. Neurosci.,* in press.

Hu, B.G. and Wieloch, T. (1993b) Casein kinase II activity in the postischemic rat brain increases in brain regions resistant to ischemia but decreases in vulnerable areas. *J. Neurochem.,* in press.

Huang, K.-P. (1989) The mechanism of protein kinase C activation. *Trends Neurosci.,* 12: 425 – 432.

Hultmark, D., Klemenz, R. and Gehring, W.J. (1986) Translational and transcriptional control elements in the untranslated leader of the heat-shock gene *hsp 22. Cell,* 44: 429 – 438.

Hunter, T. (1989) Protein modification: phosphorylation on tyrosine residues. *Curr. Opinion Cell Biol.,* 1: 1168 – 1181.

Hunter, T. and Cooper, J. (1985) Protein-tyrosine kinases. *Annu. Rev. Biochem.,* 54: 897 – 930.

Imoto, D.S., Masliah, E., DeTeresa, R., Terry, R.D. and Saitoh, T. (1989) Aberrant casein kinase II in Alzheimer's disease. *Brain Res.,* 507: 273 – 280.

Kirino, T. and Sano, K. (1984) Selective vulnerability in the gerbil hippocampus following transient ischemia. *Acta Neuropathol. (Berl.),* 62: 201 – 208.

Kirino, T., Robinson, H.P.C., Miwa, A., Tamura, A. and Kawai, N. (1992) Disturbances of membrane function preceding ischemic delayed neuronal death in the gerbil hippocampus. *J. Cereb. Blood Flow Metab.,* 12: 408 – 418.

Klarlund, J. and Czech, M.P. (1988) Insulin-like growth factor I and insulin rapidly increase casein kinase II activity in BALB/c 3T3 fibroblasts. *J. Biol. Chem.,* 263: 15872 – 15877.

Kochhar, A., Saitoh, T. and Zivin, J. (1989) Reduced protein kinase C activity in ischemic spinal cord. *J. Neurochem.,* 53: 946 – 952.

Kozak, M. (1983) Comparison of initiation of protein synthesis in procaryotes, eucaryotes and organelles. *Microbiol. Rev.,* 47: 1 – 49.

Kozuka, M., Smith, M.-L. and Siesjö, B.K. (1989) Preischemic hyperglycemia enhances postischemic depression of cerebral metabolic rate. *J. Cereb. Blood Flow Metab.,* 9: 478 – 490.

Kromer, L. (1987) Nerve growth factor treatment after brain injury prevents neuronal death. *Science,* 235: 214 – 216.

Lamphear, B.J. and Panniers, R. (1991) Heat shock impairs the interaction of cap-binding protein complex with 5′ mRNA cap. *J. Biol. Chem.,* 266: 2789 – 2794.

Lau, K.-H.W., Farley, J. and Baylink, D. (1989) Phosphotyrosyl protein phosphatases. *Biochem. J.,* 257: 23 – 36.

Le Peillet, E., Arvin, B., Moncada, C. and Meldrum, B.S. (1992) The non-NMDA antagonists, NBQX and GYKI 53466, protect against cortical and striatal cell loss following transient global ischemia in the rat. *Brain Res.,* 571: 115 – 120.

Llinás, R., McGuinness, T.L., Leonard, C.S., Sugimori, M. and Greengard, P. (1985) Intraterminal injection of synapsin I or calcium/calmodulin-dependent protein kinase II alters neurotransmitter release at the squid giant synapse. *Proc. Natl. Acad. Sci. U.S.A.,* 82: 3035 – 3039.

Louis, J.-C., Magal, E. and Yavin, E. (1988) Protein kinase C alterations in the fetal rat brain after global ischemia. *J. Biol. Chem.,* 263: 19282 – 19285.

Mattson, M.P., Murrain, M., Guthrie, P.B. and Kater, S.B. (1989) Fibroblast growth factor and glutamate: opposing roles in the generation and degeneration of hippocampal neuroarchitecture. *J. Neurosci.,* 9: 3728 – 3740.

Minamisawa, H., Nordström, C.-H., Smith, M.-L. and Siesjö, B.K. (1990) The influence of mild body and brain hypothermia on ischemic brain damage. *J. Cereb. Blood Flow Metab.,* 10: 365 – 374.

Montine, K.S. and Henshaw, E.C. (1989) Serum growth factors cause rapid stimulation of protein synthesis and dephosphorylation of eIF-2 in serum deprived Ehrlich cells. *Biochim. Biophys. Acta,* 1014: 282 – 288.

Morley, S.J. and Thomas, G. (1991) Intracellular messengers and the control of protein synthesis. *Pharmacol. Ther.,* 50: 291 – 319.

Morley, S.J., Dever, T.E., Etchison, D. and Traugh, J.A. (1991) Phosphorylation of eIF-4F by protein kinase C or multipotential S6 kinase stimulates protein synthesis at initiation. *J. Biol. Chem.,* 266: 4669 – 4672.

Mulner-Lorillon, O., Cormier, P., Labbé, J.-C., Dorée, M., Poulhe, R., Osborn, H. and Bellé, R. (1990) M-phase-specific cdc2 protein kinase phosphorylates the β-subunit of casien kinase II and increases kinase II activity. *Eur. J. Biochem.,* 193: 529 – 534.

Munekata, K., Hossmann, K.A., Xie, Y., Seo, K. and Oschlies, U. (1987) Selective vulnerability of hippocampus: ribosomal aggregation, protein synthesis, and tissue pH. In: *Cerebrovascular Disease,* Raven Press, New York, pp. 107 – 117.

Nellgård, B. and Wieloch, T. (1992) Postischemia blockade of AMPA but not NMDA receptors mitigates neuronal damage in the rat brain following transient cerebral ischemia. *J. Cereb. Blood Flow Metab.,* 11: 1 – 12.

Nishizuka, Y. (1986) Studies and perspectives of protein kinase C. *Science,* 233: 305 – 312.

Ochoa, S. (1983) Regulation of protein synthesis initiation in eurocaryotes. *Arch. Biochem. Biophys.,* 223: 325 – 349.

Onodera, H., Hara, H., Kogure, K., Fukunaga, K., Ohta, Y. and Miyamoto, K. (1990) Ca^{2+}/calmodulin-dependent protein kinase II immunoreactivity in the rat hippocampus after forebrain ischemia. *Neurosci. Lett.,* 113: 134 – 138.

Padmanabha, R., Chen-Wu, J.L.P., Hanna, D.E. and Glover, C.V.C. (1990) Isolation, sequencing and distribution of the yeast *CKA2* gene: casein kinase II is essential for viability in *Saccharomyces cerevisiae. Mol. Cell. Biol.,* 10: 4089 – 4099.

Panniers, R. and Henshaw, E.C. (1983) A GDP/GTP exchange factor essential for eukaryotic initiation factor 2 cycling in Ehrlich ascites tumor cells and its regulation by eukarotic initiation factor 2 phosphorylation. *J. Biol. Chem.,* 258(13): 7928 – 7934.

Paschen, W., Hallmayer, J. and Röhn, G. (1988) Regional changes of polyamine profiles after reversible cerebral ischemia in mongolian gerbils: effects of nimodipine and barbiturate. *Neurochem. Pathol.,* 8: 27 – 41.

Petito, C. and Pulsinelli, W. (1984) Delayed neuronal recovery and neuronal death in rat hippocampus following severe cerebral ischemia: possible relationship to abnormalities in neuronal processes. *J. Cereb. Blood Flow Metab.,* 4: 194 – 205.

Proud, C.G. (1986) Guanine nucleotides, protein phosphorylation and the control of translation. *Trends Biochem. Sci.,* 11: 73 – 77.

Pulsinelli, W.A. and Duffy, T.E. (1983) Regional energy balance in rat brain after transient forebrain ischemia. *J. Neurochem.,* 40: 1500 – 1503.

Pulsinelli, W.A., Levy, D.E. and Duffy, T.E. (1982) Regional cerebral blood flow and glucose metabolism following transient forebrain ischemia. *Ann. Neurol.,* 11: 499 – 509.

Rhoads, R.E. (1991) Protein synthesis, cell growth and oncogenesis. *Curr. Opinion Cell Biol.,* 3: 1019 – 1024.

Rostas, J.A.P., Weinberger, R.P. and Dunkley, P.R. (1986) Multiple pools and multiple forms of calmodulin-stimulated protein kinase during development: relationship to postsynaptic densities. *Prog. Brain Res.,* 69: 355 – 371.

Rowlands, A.G., Panniers, R. and Henshaw, E.C. (1988) The catalytic mechanism of guanine nucleotide exchange factor action and competitive inhibition by phosphorylated eukaryotic initiation factor 2. *J. Biol. Chem.,* 263: 5526 – 5533.

Ryazanov, A.G., Shestakova, E.A. and Natapov, P.G. (1988) Phosphorylation of elongation factor 2 by EF-2 kinase effects rate of translation. *Nature,* 334: 170 – 173.

Saitoh, T., Masliah, E., Jin, L.W., Cole, G.M., Wieloch, T. and Shapiro, I.P. (1991) Biology of disease. Protein kinases and phosphorylation in neurological disorders and cell death. *Lab. Invest.,* 64: 596 – 616.

Sarre, T.F., Hermann, M. and Bader, M. (1989) Differential effect of hemin-controlled eIF-2α kinases from mouse erythroleukemia cells on protein synthesis. *Eur. J. Biochem.,* 183: 137 – 143.

Scorsone, K.A., Panniers, R., Rowlands, A.G. and Henshaw, E.C. (1987) Phosphorylation of eukaryotic initiation factor 2 during physiological stresses which affect protein synthesis. *J. Biol. Chem.,* 262: 14538 – 14543.

Sheardown, M.J., Nielsen, E.Ø., Hansen, A.J., Jacobsen, P. and Honoré, T. (1990) 2,3-Dihydroxy-6-nitro-7-sulfamoyl-benzo(F)quinoxaline: a neuroprotectant for cerebral ischemia. *Science,* 247: 571 – 574.

Shenolikar, S. and Nairn, A. (1991) Protein phosphatases: recent progress. In: P. Greengard and G. Robinson (Eds.), *Advances in Second Messenger and Phosphoprotein Research,* Raven Press, New York, pp. 1 – 119.

Shigeno, T., Mima, T., Takakura, K., Graham, D.I., Kato, G., Hashimoto, Y. and Furukawa, S. (1991) Amelioration of delayed neuronal death in the hippocampus by nerve growth factor. *J. Neurosci.,* 11: 2914 – 2919.

Siesjö, B.K. (1988) Mechanisms of ischemic brain damage. *Crit. Care Med.,* 16: 954 – 963.

Sommercorn, J., Mulligan, J.A., Lozeman, F. and Krebs, E.G. (1987) Activation of casein kinase II in response to insulin and to epidermal growth factor. *Proc. Natl. Acad. Sci. U.S.A.,* 84: 8834 – 8838.

Thilmann, R., Xie, Y., Kleihues, P. and Kiessling, M. (1987) Persistent inhibition of protein synthesis precedes delayed neuronal death in postischemic gerbil hippocampus. *Acta Neuropathol. (Berl.),* 71: 88 – 93.

Thomas, N.S.B., Matts, R.L., Petryshyn, R. and London, I.M. (1984) Distribution of reversing factor in reticulocyte lysates during active protein synthesis and on inhibition by heme deprivation or double stranded RNA. *Proc. Natl. Acad. Sci. U.S.A.,* 81: 6998 – 7002.

Tuazon, P.T. and Traugh, J.A. (1991) Casein kinase I and II. Multipotential serine protein kinases: structure, function and regulation. *Adv. Second Messengers Phosphoprotein Res.,* 23: 124 – 164.

Tuazon, P., Merrick, W. and Traugh, J. (1989) Comparative analysis of phosphorylation of translational initiation and elongation factors by seven protein kinases. *J. Biol. Chem.,* 264: 2773 – 2777.

Widmann, R., Kuroiwa, T., Bonnekoh, P. and Hossmann, K.-A. (1991) [^{14}C]Leucine incorporation into brain proteins in gerbils after transient ischemia: relationship to selective vulnerability of hippocampus. *J. Neurochem.,* 56: 789 – 796.

Wieloch, T. (1985) Neurochemical correlates to selective neuronal vulnerability. *Prog. Brain Res.,* 63: 69 – 85.

Wieloch, T., Koide, T. and Westerberg, E. (1986) Inhibitory neurotransmitters and neuromodulators as protective agents against ischemic brain damage. In: K. Krieglstein (Ed.), *The Pharmacology of Ischemic Brain Damage,* Elsevier, Amsterdam, pp. 191 – 197.

Wieloch, T., Cardell, M., Bingren, H., Zivin, J. and Saitoh, T. (1991) Changes in the activity of protein kinase C and the subcellular redistribution of its isozymes during and following forebrain ischemia. *J. Neurochem.,* 56: 1227 – 1235.

Yamamoto, H., Fukunaga, K., Lee, K. and Soderling, T. (1992) Ischemia-induced loss of brain calcium/calmodulin dependent protein kinase II. *J. Neurochem.,* 58: 1110 – 1117.

Yoshida, S., Inoh, S., Asano, T., Sano, K., Kubota, M., Shimazaki, H. and Ueta, N. (1980) Effect of transient ischemia on free fatty acids and phospholipids in gerbil brain. Lipid peroxidation as possible cause of postischemic injury. *J. Neurosurg.,* 53: 232 – 331.

SECTION IV

Selective Gene Expression

K. Kogure, K.-A. Hossmann and B.K. Siesjö (Eds.)
Progress in Brain Research, Vol. 96

CHAPTER 13

Stress protein and proto-oncogene expression as indicators of neuronal pathophysiology after ischemia

Thaddeus S. Nowak Jr.[1], Olive C. Osborne and Sadao Suga[2]

Laboratory of Neuropathology and Neuroanatomical Sciences, National Institute of Neurological Disorders and Stroke, National Institutes of Health, Bethesda, MD 20892, U.S.A.

Introduction

In recent years considerable information has accumulated regarding the induced expression of specific gene products in brain following ischemia and other insults, and the possibility has emerged that such effects could be useful in the mapping of physiological and pathological aspects of neuronal activity. Primary attention has centered on the 70 kDa heat shock/stress protein, hsp70, and on the proto-oncogene, c-*fos*, both of which show striking and often overlapping induction after ischemia (Nowak, 1990; Nowak et al., 1990b).

The mRNA encoded by the c-*fos* gene, and its protein product, Fos, appear to provide an index of physiologically relevant cellular activation (Sagar et al., 1988). Together with Jun and other related proteins Fos functions as a transcription factor, coupling diverse stimuli to widespread changes in the expression of other genes (Morgan and Curran, 1991). Activation of several signal transduction cascades can potentially result in depolarization- or receptor-mediated increases in Fos expression (Sheng and Greenberg, 1990). As observed under many stimulus conditions, post-ischemic c-*fos* induction is largely neuronal (Nowak et al., 1990b). Still to be resolved are the precise signals responsible for Fos induction after ischemia and the long term functional consequences of its expression.

The 70 kDa stress/heat shock protein, hsp70, is a component of a cellular response to environmental challenges that has been highly conserved during evolution (Schlesinger et al., 1982; Morimoto et al., 1990). Hsp70 fails to be induced by many of the moderate stimuli such as brief seizures or spreading depression that induce c-*fos*, suggesting that its appearance is only elicited under more pathological conditions. However, like c-*fos*, hsp70 mRNA and protein expression show a neuronal localization following transient ischemia, with magnitude and time course that vary in different cell populations according to the severity of the ischemic insult (Vass et al., 1988; Nowak, 1991; Simon et al., 1991).

Studies of changes in overall protein synthesis activity in brain after ischemia have consistently demonstrated that its recovery lags behind that of energy metabolism (Kleihues and Hossmann, 1971; Hartmann and Becker, 1973; Cooper et al., 1977; Dienel et al., 1980; Morimoto and Yanagihara, 1981; Nowak et al., 1985), and suggest a relationship between the duration of translational deficits and the relative vulnerability of individual neuron

[1] Present address: T.S. Nowak Jr., Department of Neurology, University of Tennessee College of Medicine, 855 Monroe Ave., Link Building, Room 415, Memphis, TN 38163, U.S.A.

[2] Permanent address: Department of Neurosurgery, Keio University School of Medicine, 35 Shinanomachi, Shinjuku-ku, Tokyo 160, Japan.

populations (Dienel et al., 1980; Kirino and Sano, 1984; Thilmann et al., 1986; Widmann et al., 1991). Such deficits would be expected to limit the accumulation of functional proteins encoded by transiently expressed mRNAs. This consideration has further practical implications in view of recent studies indicating that moderate ischemic or hyperthermic stress may confer protection against subsequent more severe ischemic insults (Kitagawa et al., 1990, 1991; Kirino et al., 1991), with the working hypothesis that induced changes in gene expression contribute to the observed effect.

The present overview will focus on results obtained in studies of the expression of hsp70 as well as the transcription factors Fos and Jun following transient global ischemia, examining both the induction of the mRNAs and the synthesis of the encoded proteins. Current results obtained in the gerbil bilateral carotid artery occlusion model are consistent with the suggestion that translational recovery plays an important role in determining the accumulation of proteins encoded by induced mRNAs in specific neuron populations. These studies begin to define conditions of prior stress that can give rise to a given functional response, and thereby provide basic information necessary for a rational approach to studies of induced ischemic tolerance. The demonstrated increase of Jun-like immunoreactivity in CA1 neurons following brief ischemia suggests that complex cascades of altered gene expression initiated by priming insults are likely to contribute to any observed protection.

Hsp70 expression after ischemia

An adequate summary of the heat shock/stess response is beyond the scope of this presentation, but has been provided in a number of comprehensive reviews (Lindquist, 1986; Lindquist and Craig, 1988; Morimoto et al., 1990), and the literature regarding stress protein induction in brain has been recently summarized (Brown, 1990; Nowak, 1990). Frequently studied components of this response include the closely related 70 kDa molecules of the hsp70 family, some of which are normally abundant in brain (Whatley et al., 1986; Vass et al., 1988; Green and Liem, 1989), that function in the intracellular processing and trafficking of other proteins (Ungewickel, 1985; Chappell et al., 1986; Munro and Pelham, 1986; Chirico et al., 1988; Deshaies et al., 1988; Flynn et al., 1989). In rodents it is possible to distinguish a strictly inducible species that is expressed in neurons and glia only under pathological conditions (Vass et al., 1988; Marini et al., 1990), and the term "hsp70" will here refer to this protein and its mRNA. A specific function for this induced protein remains to be identified.

Hsp70 protein and mRNA are expressed in brain after ischemia (Nowak, 1985; Dienel et al., 1986; Jacewicz et al., 1986; Kiessling et al., 1986; Dwyer et al., 1989) and display a strictly neuronal induction subsequent to brief transient global insults (Vass et al., 1988; Nowak, 1991; Simon et al., 1991). Hyperthermic stress in vivo also induces hsp70 in brain (Heikkila et al., 1981; Brown, 1983; Cosgrove and Brown, 1983; Nowak, 1988), with a generalized localization in glia and cerebral vasculature but in select neuron populations only (Sprang and Brown, 1987; Marini et al., 1990; Blake et al., 1990). Hsp70 is expressed in diverse cell types after focal ischemia and traumatic injury (Brown et al., 1989; Gonzalez et al., 1989; Gower et al., 1989), after neonatal hypoxia-ischemia (Ferriero et al., 1990) or after more severe global ischemic insults (Gonzalez et al., 1991). Such observations suggest that cell populations may differ in their intrinsic thresholds for responsiveness to various stimuli, or that hsp70 induction may occur by several distinct mechanisms. Recent studies have identified multiple heat shock factors, proteins that recognize the heat shock element upstream of heat shock genes and thus are involved in transcriptional regulation of the heat shock response (Scharf et al., 1990; Rabindran et al., 1991; Schuetz et al., 1991); these could conceivably allow activation by different signal transduction pathways. Ubiquitin and proteins of other size classes characteristic of the heat shock response are known to be induced after ischemia (Dienel et al., 1986; Jacewicz et al., 1986; Kiessling et al., 1986; Magnusson and Wieloch, 1989; Nowak et al., 1990b), but the general absence of hsp70 in control tissues and its striking accumulation following stress make it an ideal marker for responsive cells.

An increasingly clear understanding of the relationship between post-ischemic hsp70 induction and the progression of neuronal injury has evolved from studies in global ischemia models. As shown in Fig. 1, ischemia of 5 – 10 min duration in the gerbil results in hsp70 mRNA expression in all major hippocampal neuron populations (Nowak, 1991), although minimal hsp70 immunoreactivity is subsequently detected in CA1 neurons destined to be lost (Vass et al., 1988). Conversely, recent observations following very short periods of four-vessel occlusion in the rat demonstrate that hsp70 immunoreactivity can be preferentially expressed in vulnerable dentate hilus and CA1 neurons after modest insults

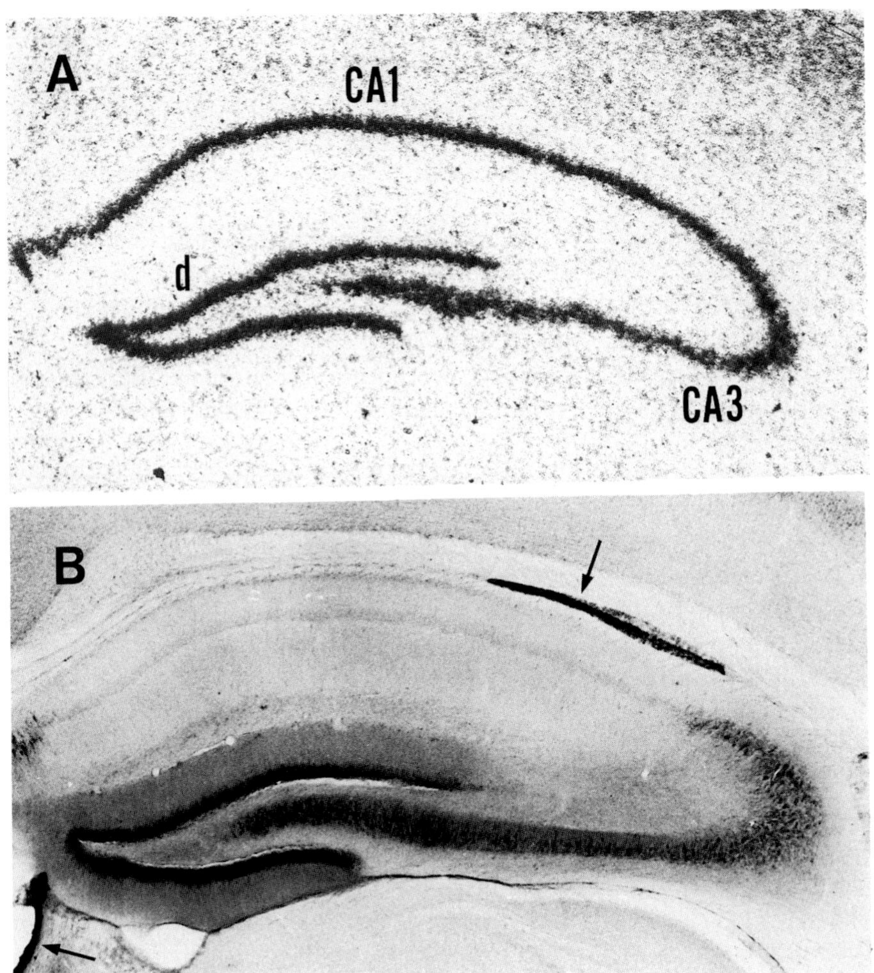

Fig. 1. Comparison between hsp70 mRNA expression and hsp70 protein immunoreactivity following 5 min ischemia in the gerbil. *A*. In situ hybridization with a ^{35}S-labeled oligonucleotide probe (Nowak, 1991) detects hsp70 mRNA throughout major hippocampal neuron populations at 6 h recirculation. *B*. Detection of hsp70 with a selective monoclonal antibody (Vass et al., 1988) demonstrates strong immunoreactivity in dentate granule cells and CA3 neurons at 24 h recirculation, with the absence of positive cells in CA1. Strong staining of ependyma (arrow) is always evident in brains of control as well as post-ischemic gerbils, while in situ hybridization only occasionally detects hsp70 mRNA in these cells (Nowak, 1991).

that allow cell survival (Simon et al., 1991). Taken together these findings suggest that transcriptional induction of hsp70 should provide a sensitive indicator of neuron populations at risk following ischemia and other insults. The extent to which immunoreactive hsp70 is then expressed in a given cell would depend on multiple factors such as the magnitude and duration of hsp70 mRNA expression, the coincident recovery of substantial protein synthesis activity, as well as other factors that may affect detectability of the protein, which are likely to vary among experimental models.

Findings in the gerbil model illustrate the potential complexity of such interactions. Comparison of the time course of hsp70 mRNA expression evaluated by in situ hybridization (Nowak, 1991) with that of hsp70 immunoreactivity (Vass et al., 1988) suggests a coupled inverse relationship, in that the sequential disappearance of mRNA in dentate granule cells and CA3 neurons coincides with the detection of immunoreactivity, while hybridization persists in CA1 neurons that apparently fail to express the protein. Detection of the immunoreactive protein is considerably delayed relative to the expected recovery of protein synthesis activity in dentate and CA3 (Thilmann et al., 1986), indicating that newly synthesized hsp70 may not always be accessible to the monoclonal antibody used in these studies, and raising the possibility that such factors could also contribute to the absence of hsp70 immunoreactivity in CA1. Significant, though transient, protein synthesis recovery has been described after 5 min ischemia in the gerbil (Thilmann et al., 1986; Widmann et al., 1991) and accumulation of ornithine decarboxylase has been detected in CA1 neurons in this model (Müller et al., 1991; Paschen, this volume), further supporting the argument that hsp70 may be present but undetected in vulnerable neurons. Studies of more classical heat shock in cultured cells have demonstrated a preferential nucleolar concentration of hsp70 during the period of stress (Welch and Suhan, 1986), with a cytoplasmic localization during recovery. Hsp70 immunoreactivity is clearly distributed throughout neuronal cytoplasm in all reported ischemia studies, suggesting that the protein may be available to detection in perfused brain only under conditions of "relaxation" subsequent to the active stress. The prolonged expression of hsp70 mRNA, in proportion to the relative vulnerability of individual neuron populations after ischemia, may reflect impairment of feedback mechanisms under conditions of limited hsp70 accumulation (DiDomenico et al., 1982) or stabilization of hsp70 mRNA in association with a persistent stress (Petersen and Lindquist, 1988). It may be speculated that the consistent observation of hsp70-positive ependyma in control gerbils (Vass et al., 1988; Kirino et al.,1991) reflects the response to an unrecognized prior stimulus condition, with transient transcriptional induction that is not routinely detected by in situ hybridization (Nowak, 1991).

In contrast to the gerbil, significant immunoreactive hsp70 has been detected in CA1 neurons of the rat following moderate ischemic insults (Simon et al., 1991). Hsp70 immunoreactivity showed a biphasic dependence on ischemic duration in vulnerable neurons such as dentate hilus and CA1, with diminished hsp70 detection after longer insults that resulted in a higher proportion of injured cells as judged by positive staining with acid fuchsin. Nevertheless, marked hsp70 expression was evident in CA1 over a range of ischemic insults in the rat that typically result in the loss of a significant proportion of this neuron population, suggesting that many hsp70 positive cells may go on to die in this model. These observations are consistent with other rat studies (Magnusson et al., 1989; Chopp et al., 1991), implying that there may be relatively better recovery of CA1 protein synthesis activity following moderate ischemia in the rat, or perhaps greater accessibility of hsp70 to immunological detection, and raise the possibility that successful expression of hsp70 protein may not be strictly interpreted as an indicator of neuronal survival. Careful quantitative evaluations of amino acid incorporation, in situ hybridization and immunocytochemistry in sections from the same animal may help to resolve this issue.

Ischemia of 2 min is an apparent threshold insult required for induction of hsp70 mRNA in the gerbil

(Nowak and Osborne, 1991; Nowak et al., 1992), with an initial distribution in hippocampus comparable to that seen after longer occlusions. The duration of hsp70 mRNA expression in CA1 neurons is relatively prolonged following 2 min ischemic insults, suggesting that this may already be a relatively severe insult in the gerbil. Consistent differences can be noted, however, in comparison with hsp70 mRNA expression after 5 min insults (Fig. 2). Hsp70 hybridization remains intense throughout CA1 at 24 h recirculation after 2 min ischemia, but by 48 h tends to disappear from all but the more medial regions, where some cell damage can occur after even this mild challenge. In contrast, hsp70 hybridization after 5 min ischemia persists throughout the pyramidal layer at 48 h, with a diminished signal sometimes observed in medial CA1 due to early cell loss. These observations provide further support for the correlation between lasting hsp70 mRNA expression and the severity of the insult experienced by a given cell population. They also emphasize the need for parallel histological characterizations for accurate interpretation of hybridization data, since loss of the hsp70 signal occurs with either cell recovery or cell death.

As in the rat, short ischemic insults in the gerbil that do not produce severe CA1 damage result in detectable expression of hsp70 immunoreactivity in these neurons (Kirino et al., 1991), and appear to induce a condition of tolerance to more severe ischemia (Kitagawa et al., 1990; Kirino et al., 1991).

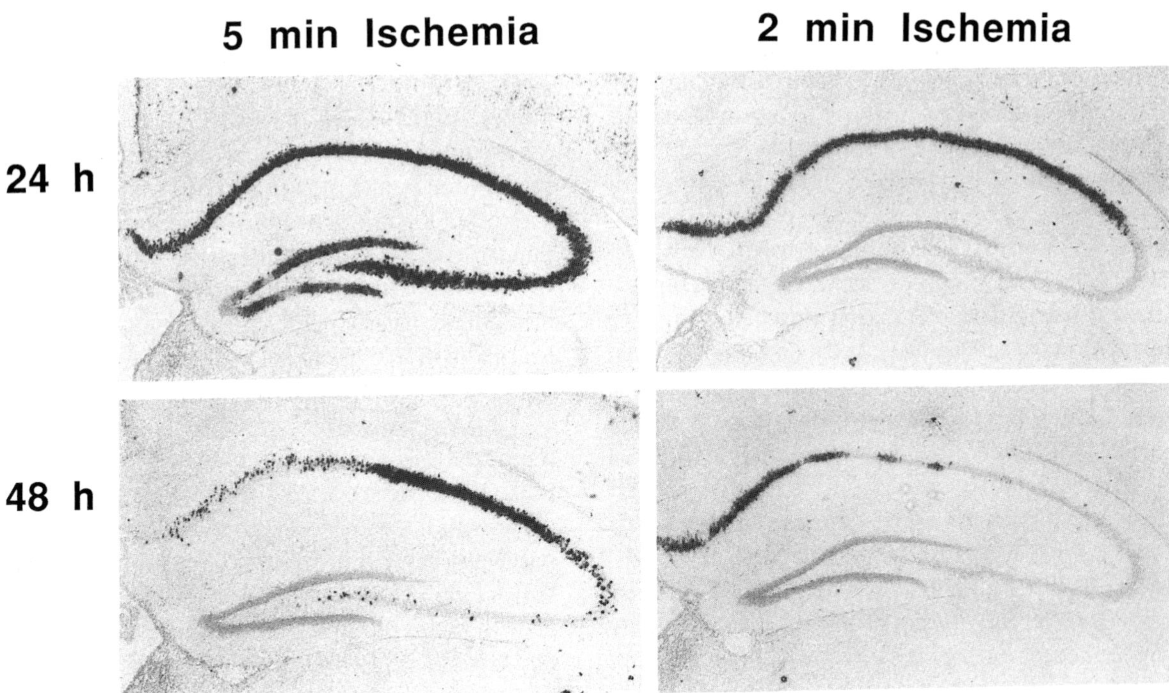

Fig. 2. Persistent hsp70 hybridization in hippocampus following 2 min and 5 min ischemic insults in the gerbil. Sections were hybridized with the ^{35}S-labeled probe, coated with emulsion, exposed and lightly counterstained after development. Brightfield photomicrographs illustrate dark clusters of silver grains overlying individual cells. After 5 min ischemia and 24 h recirculation a severely affected animal shows hybridization in all major cell fields; the lasting signal in dentate granule cells is unusual at this time point. Substantial hybridization is evident throughout CA1 at 24 h following even a short 2 min insult. At 48 h recirculation hsp70 hybridization persists in CA1 of animal subjected to 5 min ischemia, with early loss of neurons in the medial CA1 accounting for decreased signal at this time, while scattered cells of CA3 remain positive. Only the most vulnerable medial CA1 neurons show sustained hsp70 mRNA expression at 48 h after brief 2 min ischemia.

In view of studies demonstrating tolerance phenomena following moderate stresses that induce a heat shock response (Li and Werb, 1982; Widelitz et al., 1986; Mizzen and Welch, 1988) it is attractive to consider that hsp70 expression may be a component of a similar mechamism responsible for the observed ischemic protection. Brief hyperthermia has also been suggested to result in later ischemic tolerance (Chopp et al., 1989; Kitagawa et al., 1991), although available evidence indicates that expression of hsp70 mRNA or protein is minimal in the neurons that are protected (Sprang and Brown, 1987; Blake et al., 1990; Marini et al., 1990). Recent studies have shown that hyperthermia inducing a detectable stress response in neurons in vitro also results in protection against subsequent glutamate toxicity (Lowenstein et al., 1991; Rordorf et al., 1991), further supporting the possibility of a role for this response in ischemic tolerance in vivo.

The 2 min ischemic insult required for hsp70 induction is apparently equivalent to the threshold for energy depletion and loss of ion homeostasis (Yamaguchi et al., 1986). Since brief periods of calcium influx, e.g., following spreading depression, are not sufficient to induce hsp70 (Nowak et al., 1991), other signals activated subsequent to more prolonged depolarization must be required for activation of the response. Based on the anatomical data, and by analogy with results obtained for c-*fos* (see below), it is intriguing to suggest a correlation between hsp70 induction and proposed excitotoxic mechanisms of post-ischemic neuronal injury. Hsp70 induction following administration of kainic acid in vivo has been demonstrated (Uney et al., 1988; Vass et al., 1989; Gonzalez et al., 1989). Alternatively, recent studies indicate that moderate hyperthermia during the early hours of recirculation may play a critical role in hippocampal injury (Kuroiwa et al., 1990). While temperatures reached under these conditions are usually below the threshold for protein synthesis disruption and induction of the stress response by acute, transient temperature elevation (Nowak, 1988; Nowak et al., 1990a), moderate hyperthermia of longer duration may contribute to the selective neuronal stress response after ischemia. The observed attenuation of hsp70 expression by the *N*-methyl-D-aspartate (NMDA) receptor antagonist, MK-801 (Nowak, 1989, 1991), appears to be mediated in part by the hypothermia that can accompany administration of the drug (Buchan and Pulsinelli, 1990), Finally, glutamate has been shown to precipitate oxidative stress under some in vitro conditions (Murphy et al., 1989), which in any case is a demonstrated feature of post-ischemic recirculation (Oliver et al., 1990). Further studies are required to clarify the roles of such factors in the stress response after ischemia.

Fos expression after ischemia

Fos protein and the corresponding c-*fos* mRNA are detected in scattered neurons under control conditions and show striking increases in neuronal expression following seizures (Dragunow and Robertson, 1987a,b; Morgan et al., 1987) and after other more modest stimuli such as sensory nerve stimulation (Hunt et al., 1987) or even behavioral stresses (Nakajima et al., 1989). Such observations have supported the utility of c-*fos* induction in the mapping of functional neuronal activity (Sagar et al., 1988). Increased c-*fos* expression is also observed in brain under clearly pathological conditions such as traumatic injury (Dragunow and Robertson, 1988; Sharp et al., 1989) and hyperthermia (Dragunow et al., 1989), and after global or focal ischemia (Onodera et al., 1989; Jørgensen et al., 1989; Gunn et al., 1990; Nowak et al., 1990b; Welsh et al., 1992).

Activation of several signal transduction pathways can result in c-*fos* induction, mediated either via calcium/cyclic AMP-dependent or growth factor-stimulated response elements (Sheng and Greenberg, 1990). Increased c-*fos* expression in response to complex stimuli such as ischemia may potentially arise from a composite of contributions involving several distinct mechanisms; current evidence supports this suggestion. Under many stimulus conditions there are striking parallels in c-*fos* and hsp70 induction (Andrews et al., 1987; Gubits and Fairhurst, 1988), with predominantly neuronal expression following global ischemia

(Nowak et al., 1990b), or status epilepticus subsequent to kainic acid administration (compare Le Gal La Salle, 1988, with Vass et al., 1989; Gonzalez et al., 1989), but prominent glial and vascular expression following hyperthermia (Dragunow et al., 1989 vs. Marini et al., 1990), focal ischemia or infarction (Gonzalez et al., 1989 vs. Gunn et al., 1990) or brain injury (Dragunow and Robertson, 1988 vs. Brown et al., 1989). The threshold ischemic insult for c-*fos* induction in the gerbil model is comparable to that required for hsp70 induction (see above), and shows an identical initial distribution (Nowak and Osborne, 1991; Nowak et al., 1992). On the other hand there is a striking, generalized c-*fos* induction in neurons throughout an injured hemisphere (Dragunow and Robertson, 1988; Herrera and Robertson, 1989), apparently mediated by the transient depolarization associated with spreading depression (Herrera and Robertson, 1990), that is not associated with hsp70 expression (Nowak et al., 1991). This presumably accounts for widespread c-*fos* induction ipsilateral to a focal ischemic insult (Welsh et al., 1992), and may constitute a pathophysiological correlate to the NMDA receptor-mediated c-*fos* induction that has been demonstrated in vitro (Szekely et al., 1989). Kainic acid induces a more prolonged expression of Fos and related antigens than is observed following administration of NMDA, perhaps by a distinct mechanism (Sonnenberg et al., 1989a). As noted above for the heat shock response, antagonism of NMDA receptors can attenuate post-ischemic Fos protein expression in a gerbil ischemia model (Uemura et al., 1991), but the detailed mechanisms responsible for c-*fos* induction after transient global ischemia remain to be fully identified.

The consequence of c-*fos* mRNA induction and the expression of functional Fos protein is a coordinated activation and repression of other genes at the level of mRNA transcription. This is mediated by the dimerization of Fos, Jun and other closely related proteins to form functional transcription factor complexes that interact with identified "AP-1" and other regulatory sequences located in the upstream regions of target genes (Curran and Franza, 1988). The composition of these complexes varies with time after a given stimulus as the expression of Fos and Fos-related antigens (Fra) sequentially rise and fall (Sonnenberg et al., 1989a; Dragunow, 1990; Szekely et al., 1990), and complexes may be formed having different functional activities (Ivashkiv et al., 1990). Stimuli may have dissociated effects on induction of Fos and Jun (Bartel et al., 1989; Gubits et al., 1990; Wisden et al., 1990), proteins and mRNAs of the Jun family may be differentially expressed (Bartel et al., 1989; Wisden et al., 1990), and dimers with repressor activity have been identified (Nakabeppu and Nathans, 1991), so that complex and varied reprogramming of gene expression may be expected in response to various inducing stimuli. There is strong evidence supporting the regulation of specific genes in brain by Fos/Jun mechanisms, including stimulus-induced changes in the expression of opioid peptides (Draisci and Iadarola, 1989; Sonnenberg et al., 1989b; Gall et al., 1990) or nerve growth factor (Gall and Isackson, 1989; Hengerer et al., 1990), but a functionally integrated response arising from the spectrum of changes that may be initiated by any given stimulus has yet to be recognized.

We have recently evaluated the expression of Fos- and Jun-like immunoreactivities in gerbil brain after ischemia, with particular emphasis on their time course and distribution in hippocampus after ischemia of varied duration (Suga and Nowak, 1991). Representative sections illustrating the main findings of this study are shown in Fig. 3. Fos immunoreactivity is detected in scattered neurons of control gerbil brain. Ischemia of 5 min duration results in prominent Fos expression in dentate granule cells and CA3 neurons at 2 – 3 h recirculation. After 2 min ischemia Fos expression in granule cells is present at 2 h but is already reduced by 3 h, suggesting that more rapid down-regulation of Fos expression may occur after the shorter insult. Staining of CA3 neurons is also more pronounced after 2 min than after 5 min occlusions. Prominent positive neurons are evident in dentate hilus at 3 – 4 h following 2 min ischemia but are much less

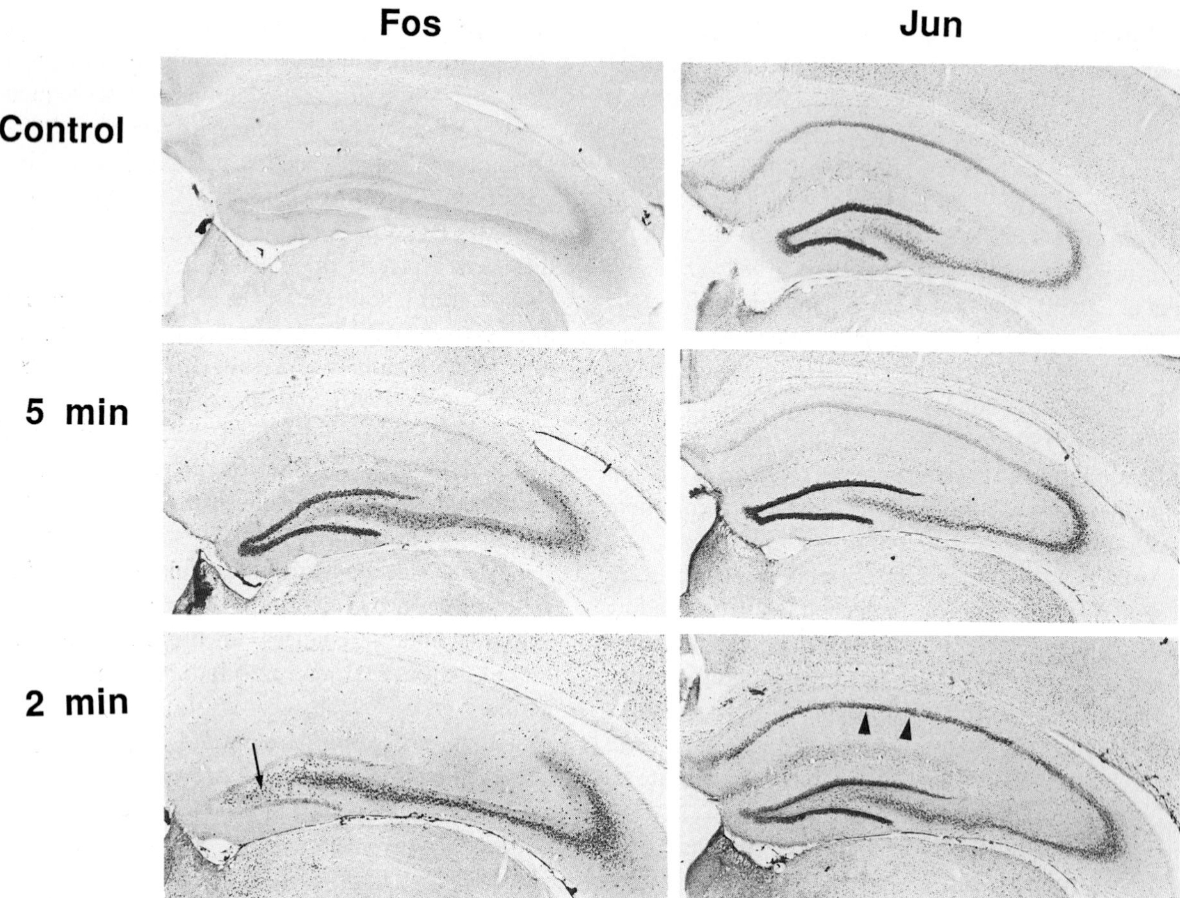

Fig. 3. Fos- and Jun-like immunoreactivities in gerbil hippocampus after 5 min and 2 min ischemia. Animals were subjected to the indicated ischemic interval or to sham procedures and were perfused with buffered 4% paraformaldehyde at recirculation intervals of 3 h (Fos) and 6 h (Jun). Vibratome sections (50μm) were prepared and incubated with rabbit polyclonal antibodies directed against Fos and Jun peptides (products PC05 and PC06, Oncogene Science, Inc., Manhasset, NY), and immunoreactivity was visualized with a peroxidase-coupled detection system using diaminobenzidine as substrate. Notable differences include the more transient expression of Fos immunoreactivity in dentate granule cells after 2 min ischemia, which is already diminished at the 3 h time point illustrated, but the more prominent staining of neurons in dentate hilus (small arrow) and CA3 after the shorter insult. Jun-like immunoreactivity in CA1 is prominent at 6 h in animals subjected to 2 min but not 5 min ischemia (arrowheads).

noticeable after 5 min occlusions, consistent with the interpretation that the early vulnerability of this cell population (Johansen et al., 1987) may be reflected in protein synthesis deficits that impair Fos accumulation. No significant increase in Fos-positive neurons is detected in CA1 after either 2 min or 5 min ischemia, in keeping with the known deficits in protein synthesis in these cells during early recirculation (Thilmann et al., 1986; Widmann et al., 1991). These observations generally agree with those of other recent studies that also failed to detect Fos-positive CA1 neurons in the gerbil after 5 or 15 min ischemia (Uemura et al., 1991; Takemoto et al., 1991). Some in situ hybridization results suggest that c-*fos* mRNA may show a longer time course of expression in a rat ischemia model, with preferential expression in vulnerable neurons (Jørgensen et al., 1989), but these findings remain to be confirmed.

Jun-like immunoreactivity is prominent in CA3 neurons and dentate granule cells of control hippocampus and becomes more intense after both 2 min and 5 min ischemia. This distribution is consistent with the reported constitutive expression of c-*jun* mRNA in control rat brain (Wisden et al., 1990). In the present context, the most interesting feature of Jun staining is its striking localization in CA1 neurons at recirculation intervals of 6 – 24 h after 2 min but not after 5 min ischemia. We have not yet evaluated the time course and distribution of c-*jun* and related mRNAs so it is not known whether there are differences in the expression of these mRNAs in CA1 after ischemic insults of graded intensity. It also remains to be determined which of the Jun-like proteins that may be detected by the antibody are responsible for the staining that is observed. Nevertheless, this result does demonstrate that an mRNA encoding a protein of the Jun family is expressed in these cells after 2 min ischemia and that sufficient recovery of protein synthesis has occurred to allow the accumulation of Jun-like immunoreactivity at recirculation intervals beyond 6 h. A delayed component of c-*jun* mRNA induction has also been demonstrated following glutamate stimulation of cerebellar granule cell neurons in vitro (Szekely et al., 1990). The present observation complements studies demonstrating hsp70 expression in CA1 neurons after 2 min ischemia (Kirino et al., 1991), and identifies a protein of known function that is expressed in vulnerable neurons after mild insults suggested to produce subsequent ischemic tolerance. Given the role of Jun and related proteins in transcriptional regulation, this finding allows the prediction that many additional changes in gene expression will eventually be identified under such priming conditions.

Induction of at least one other transcription factor mRNA has also been demonstrated after focal ischemia (Abe et al., 1991), although expression of the encoded protein and its response to global ischemic insults remain to be characterized. The *zif/268* sequence (also known as Krox 24, Egr-1 or NGFI-A) encodes a "zinc finger" protein that acts at yet another class of regulatory sites (Milbrandt, 1987; Lemaire et al., 1988; Sukhatme et al., 1988; Christy and Nathans, 1989). This mRNA and the encoded protein are expressed at significant levels in control brain (Milbrandt, 1987; Herdegen et al., 1990; Wisden et al., 1990; Abe et al., 1991) and the factor presumably functions in the physiological regulation of neuronal gene expression. Hippocampal *zif/268* mRNA is induced following high frequency perforant path stimulation by a mechanism that appears to be sensitive to inhibition by NMDA receptor antagonists, while seizure-induced expression is less sensitive to such agents (Cole et al., 1989). NMDA receptor-mediated induction of *zif/268* has been demonstrated in cultured cerebellar granule cells (Szekely et al., 1990), but growth factors are more potent than membrane depolarization in the induction of *zif/268* in PC12 cells (Bartel et al., 1989). The signal transduction mechanisms responsible for post-ischemic induction of *zif/268* and its potential contributions to long-term cellular responses to such insults will undoubtedly be subjects of future investigations.

Summary and conclusions

Induction of hsp70 mRNA and protein appear to provide useful markers for delineating stages in the progression of neuronal pathophysiology after ischemia. Detection of hsp70 encoded by the induced mRNA is dependent on complex interactions between the time course of mRNA expression and recovery of protein synthesis in a given neuron population, and perhaps other factors relating to specific aspects of hsp70 physiology, during recirculation intervals of hours to days. Transient mRNA expression and subsequent detection of immunoreactive hsp70 protein appear to identify neurons more likely to survive ischemia and other insults, while prolonged expression of hsp70 mRNA is associated with more severe neuronal injury.

Fos and Jun immunoreactivities are also increased after ischemia, and provide indexes of functional gene expression during earlier recirculation periods. The accumulation of Fos immunoreactivity in particular designates neurons in which rapid recovery of protein synthesis during 1 – 3 h recirculation has allowed translation of the very transiently expressed c-*fos* mRNA. Jun-like immunoreactivity allows an evaluation of events at later recirculation intervals, and provides a clear demonstration of synthesis and accumulation of induced protein in CA1 neurons at 6 h following 2 min ischemia.

Detailed understanding of the significance of such interactions between transcriptional and translational events will continue to evolve as information accumulates regarding the expression of additional mRNAs and proteins after ischemia. The present demonstration that Jun-like immunoreactivity accumulates in CA1 neurons after brief ischemia indicates that widespread changes in gene expression, expected as a consequence of such primary effects on transcription factor activity, are likely to contribute to the phenomenon of induced ischemic tolerance and to other persistent changes in the brain following diverse insults.

References

Abe, K., Kawagoe, J., Sato, S., Sahara, M. and Kogure, K. (1991) Induction of the "zinc finger" gene after transient focal ischemia in rat cerebral cortex. *Neurosci. Lett.,* 123: 248 – 250.

Andrews, G.K., Harding, M.A., Calvet, J.P. and Adamson, E.D. (1987) The heat shock response in HeLa cells is accompanied by elevated expression of the c-*fos* proto-oncogene. *Moll. Cell. Biol.,* 7: 3452 – 3458.

Bartel, D.B., Sheng, M., Lau, L.F. and Greenberg, M.E. (1989) Growth factors and membrane depolarization activate distinct programs of early response gene expression: dissociation of *fos* and *jun* induction. *Genes Dev.,* 3: 304 – 313.

Blake, M.J., Nowak Jr., T.S. and Holbrook, N.J. (1990) In vivo hyperthermia induces expression of hsp70 mRNA in brain regions controlling the neuroendocrine response to stress. *Mol. Brain Res.,* 8: 89 – 92.

Brown, I.R. (1983) Hyperthermia induces the synthesis of a heat shock protein by polysomes isolated from the fetal and neonatal mammalian brain. *J. Neurochem.,* 40: 1490 – 1493.

Brown, I.R. (1990) Induction of heat shock (stress) genes in the mammalian brain by hyperthermia and other traumatic events: a current perspective. *J. Neurosci. Res.,* 27: 247 – 255.

Brown, I.R., Rush, S. and Ivy, G.O. (1989) Induction of a heat shock gene at the site of tissue injury in the rat brain. *Neuron,* 2: 1559 – 1564.

Buchan, A. and Pulsinelli, W.A. (1990) Hypothermia but not the *N*-methyl-D-aspartate antagonist, MK-801, attenuates neuronal damage in gerbils subjected to transient global ischemia. *J. Neurosci.,* 10: 311 – 316.

Chappell, T.G., Welch, W.J., Schlossman, D.M., Palter, K.B., Schlesinger, M.J. and Rothman, J.E. (1986) Uncoating ATPase is a member of the 70 kilodalton family of stress proteins. *Cell,* 45: 3 – 13.

Chirico, W.J., Waters, M.G. and Blobel, G. (1988) 70 kDa heat shock-related proteins stimulate protein translocation into microsomes. *Nature,* 332: 805 – 810.

Chopp, M., Chen, H., Ho, K.-L., Dereski, M.O., Brown, E., Hetzel, F.W. and Welch, K.M.A. (1989) Transient hyperthermia protects against subsequent forebrain ischemic cell damage in the rat. *Neurology,* 39: 1396 – 1398.

Chopp, M., Li, Y., Dereski, M.O., Levine, S.R., Yoshida, Y. and Garcia, J.H. (1991) Neuronal injury and expression of 72-kDa heat-shock protein after forebrain ischemia in the rat. *Acta Neuropathol. (Berl.),* 83: 66 – 71.

Christy, B. and Nathans, D. (1989) DNA binding site of the growth factor-inducible protein Zif268. *Proc. Natl. Acad. Sci. U.S.A.,* 86: 8737 – 8741.

Cole, A.J., Saffen, D.W., Baraban, J.M. and Worley, P.F. (1989) Rapid increase of an immediate early gene messenger RNA in hippocampal neurons by synaptic NMDA receptor activation. *Nature,* 340: 474 – 476.

Cooper, H.K., Zalewska, T., Hossmann, K.-A. and Kleihues, P. (1977) The effect of ischemia and recirculation on protein synthesis in the rat brain. *J. Neurochem.,* 28: 929 – 934.

Cosgrove, J.W. and Brown, I.R. (1983) Heat shock protein in mammalian brain and other organs after a physiologically relevant increase in body temperature induced by D-lysergic acid diethylamide. *Proc. Natl. Acad. Sci. U.S.A.,* 80: 569 – 573.

Curran, T. and Franza Jr., B.R. (1988) Fos and Jun: the AP-1 connection. *Cell,* 55: 395 – 397.

Deshaies, R.J., Koch, B.D., Werner-Washburne, M., Craig, E.A. and Schekman, R. (1988) A subfamily of stress proteins facilitates translocation of secretory and mitochondrial precursor polypeptides. *Nature,* 332: 800 – 805.

DiDomenico, B.J., Bugaisky, G.E. and Lindquist, S. (1982) The heat shock response is self-regulated at both the transcriptional and posttranscriptional levels. *Cell,* 31: 593 – 603.

Dienel, G.A., Pulsinelli, W.A. and Duffy, T.E. (1980) Regional protein synthesis in rat brain following acute hemispheric ischemia. *J. Neurochem.,* 35: 1216 – 1226.

Dienel, G.A., Kiessling, M., Jacewicz, M. and Pulsinelli, W.A. (1986) Synthesis of heat shock proteins in rat brain cortex after transient ischemia. *J. Cereb. Blood Flow Metab.,* 6: 505 – 510.

Dragunow, M. (1990) Presence and induction of Fos B-like immunoreactivity in neural, but not non-neural, cells in adult rat brain. *Brain Res.,* 533: 324 – 328.

Dragunow, M. and Robertson, H.A. (1987a) Generalized seizures induce c-fos protein(s) in mammalian neurons. *Neurosci. Lett.,* 82: 157 – 161.

Dragunow, M. and Robertson, H.A. (1987b) Kindling stimulation induces c-fos protein(s) in granule cells of the dentate gyrus. *Nature,* 329: 441 – 442.

Dragunow, M. and Robertson, H.A. (1988) Brain injury induces c-fos protein(s) in nerve and glial-like cells in adult mammalian brain. *Brain Res.*, 455: 295 – 299.

Dragunow, M., Currie, R.W., Robertson, H.A. and Faull, R.L.M. (1989) Heat shock induces c-fos protein-like immunoreactivity in glial cells in adult rat brain. *Exp. Neurol.*, 106: 105 – 109.

Draisci, G. and Iadarola, M.J. (1989) Temporal analysis of increases in c-*fos*, preprodynorphin and preproenkephalin mRNAs in rat spinal cord. *Mol. Brain Res.*, 6: 31 – 37.

Dwyer, B.E., Nishimura, R.N. and Brown, I.R. (1989) Synthesis of the major inducible heat shock protein in rat hippocampus after neonatal hypoxia-ischemia. *Exp. Neurol.*, 104: 28 – 31.

Ferriero, D.M., Soberano, H.Q., Simon, R.P. and Sharp, F.R. (1990) Hypoxia-ischemia induces heat shock protein-like (hsp72) immunoreactivity in neonatal rat brain. *Dev. Brain Res.*, 53: 145 – 150.

Flynn, G.C., Chappell, T.G. and Rothman, J.R. (1989) Peptide binding and release by proteins implicated as catalysts of protein assembly. *Science*, 245: 385 – 390.

Gall, C.M. and Isackson, P.J. (1989) Limbic seizures increase neuronal production of messenger RNA for nerve growth factor. *Science*, 245: 758 – 761.

Gall, C.M., Lauterborn, J., Isackson, P. and White, J. (1990) Seizures, neuropeptide regulation, and mRNA expression in the hippocampus. In: J. Storm-Mathisen, J. Zimmer and O.P. Ottersen (Eds.), *Understanding the Brain Through the Hippocampus. The Hippocampal Region as a Model for Studying Brain Structure and Function – Progress in Brain Research, Vol. 83*, Elsevier Science Publishers, Amsterdam, pp. 371 – 390.

Gonzalez, M.F., Shiraishi, K., Hisanaga, K., Sagar, S.M., Mandabach, M. and Sharp, F.R. (1989) Heat shock proteins as markers of neural injury. *Mol. Brain Res.*, 6: 93 – 100.

Gonzalez, M.F., Lowenstein, D., Fernyak, S., Hisanaga, K., Simon, R. and Sharp, F.R. (1991) Induction of heat shock protein 72-like immunoreactivity in the hippocampal formation following transient global ischemia. *Brain Res. Bull.*, 26: 241 – 250.

Gower, D.J., Hollman, C., Lee, S. and Tytell, M. (1989) Spinal cord injury and the stress protein response. *J. Neurosurg.*, 70: 605 – 611.

Green, L.A.D. and Liem, R.K.H. (1989) β-Internexin is a microtubule-associated protein identical to the 70-kDa heat-shock cognate protein and the clathrin uncoating ATPase. *J. Biol. Chem.*, 264: 15210 – 15215.

Gubits, R.M. and Fairhurst, J.L. (1988) c-*fos* mRNA levels are increased by the cellular stressors, heat shock and sodium arsenite. *Oncogene*, 3: 163 – 168.

Gubits, R.M., Wollack, J.B., Yu, H. and Liu, W.-K. (1990) Activation of adenosine receptors induces c-*fos*, but not c-*jun*, expression in neuron-glia hybrids and fibroblasts. *Mol. Brain Res.*, 8: 275 – 281.

Gunn, A.J., Dragunow, M., Faull, R.L.M. and Gluckman, P.D. (1990) Effects of hypoxia-ischemia and seizures on neuronal and glial-like c-fos protein levels in the infant rat. *Brain Res.*, 531: 105 – 116.

Hartmann, J.F. and Becker, R.A. (1973) Disaggregation of polyribosomes in intact gerbils following ischemia. An ultrastructural study. *Stroke*, 4: 964 – 968.

Heikkila, J.J., Cosgrove, J.W. and Brown, I.R. (1981) Cell-free translation of free and membrane-bound polysomes and polyadenylated mRNA from rabbit brain following administration of D-lysergic acid diethylamide in vivo. *J. Neurochem.*, 36: 1229 – 1238.

Hengerer, B., Lindholm, D., Heumann, R., Rüther, U., Wagner, E.F. and Thoenen, H. (1990) Lesion-induced increase in nerve growth factor mRNA is mediated by c-*fos*. *Proc. Natl. Acad. Sci. U.S.A.*, 87: 3899 – 3903.

Herdegen, T., Walker, T., Leah, J.D., Bravo, R. and Zimmermann, M. (1990) The Krox 24 protein, a new transcription regulating factor: expression in the rat central nervous system following afferent somatosensory stimulation. *Neurosci. Lett.*, 120: 21 – 24.

Herrera, D.G. and Robertson, H.A. (1989) Unilateral induction of c-fos protein in cortex following cortical devascularization. *Brain Res.*, 503: 205 – 213.

Herrera, D.G. and Robertson, H.A. (1990) Application of potassium chloride to the brain surface induces the c-*fos* proto-oncogene: reversal by MK-801. *Brain Res.*, 510: 166 – 170.

Hunt, S.P., Pini, A. and Evans, G. (1987) Induction of c-fos-like protein in spinal cord neurons following sensory stimulation. *Nature*, 328: 632 – 634.

Ivashkiv, L.B., Liou, H.-C., Kara, C.J., Lamph, W.W., Verma, I.R. and Glimcher, L.H. (1990) mXBP/CRE-BP2 and c-*jun* form a complex which binds to cyclic AMP, but not to the 12-*O*-tetradecanoylphorbol-13-acetate response element. *Mol. Cell. Biol.*, 10: 1609 – 1621.

Jacewicz, M., Kiessling, M. and Pulsinelli, W.A. (1986) Selective gene expression in focal cerebral ischemia. *J. Cereb. Blood Flow Metab.*, 6: 263 – 272.

Johansen, F.F., Zimmer, J. and Diemer, N.H. (1987) Early loss of somatostatin neurons in dentate hilus after cerebral ischemia in the rat precedes CA1 pyramidal loss. *Acta Neuropathol. (Berl.)*, 73: 110 – 114.

Jørgensen, M.B., Deckert, J., Wright, D.C. and Gehlert, D.R. (1989) Delayed c-*fos* proto-oncogene expression in the rat hippocampus induced by transient global cerebral ischemia: an in situ hybridization study. *Brain Res.*, 484: 393 – 398.

Kiessling, M., Dienel, G.A., Jacewicz, M. and Pulsinelli, W.A. (1986) Protein synthesis in postischemic rat brain: a two-dimensional electrophoretic analysis. *J. Cereb. Blood Flow Metab.*, 6: 642 – 649.

Kirino, T. and Sano, K. (1984) Fine structural nature of delayed neuronal death following ischemia in the gerbil hippocampus. *Acta Neuropathol. (Berl.)*, 62: 209 – 218.

Kirino, T., Tsujita, Y. and Tamura, A. (1991) Induced tolerance to ischemia in gerbil hippocampal neurons. *J. Cereb. Blood Flow Metab.,* 11: 299 – 307.

Kitagawa, K.,Matsumoto, M., Tagaya, M., Hata, R., Ueda, H., Niinobe, M., Handa, N., Fukunaga, R., Kimura, K., Mikoshiba, K., and Kamada, T. (1990) "Ischemic tolerance" phenomenon found in brain. *Brain Res.,* 528: 21 – 24.

Kitagawa, K., Matsumoto, M., Tagaya, M., Kuwabara, K., Hata, R., Handa, N., Fukunaga, R., Kimura, K. and Kamada, T. (1991) Hyperthermia-induced neuronal protection against ischemic injury in gerbils. *J. Cereb. Blood Flow Metab.,* 11: 449 – 452.

Kleihues, P. and Hossmann, K.-A. (1971) Protein synthesis in the cat brain after prolonged cerebral ischemia. *Brain Res.,* 35: 409 – 418.

Kuroiwa, T., Bonnekoh, P. and Hossmann, K.-A. (1990) Prevention of postischemic hyperthermia prevents ischemic injury of CA1 neurons in gerbils. *J. Cereb. Blood Flow Metab.,* 10: 550 – 556.

Le Gal La Salle, G. (1988) Long-lasting and sequential increase of c-fos oncoprotein expression in kainic acid-induced status epilepticus. *Neurosci. Lett.,* 88: 127 – 130.

Lemaire, P., Relevant, O., Bravo, R. and Charnay, P. (1988) Two mouse genes encoding potential transcription factors with identical DNA-binding domains are activated by growth factors in cultured cells. *Proc. Natl. Acad. Sci. U.S.A.,* 85: 4691 – 4695.

Li, G.C. and Werb, Z. (1982) Correlation between synthesis of heat shock proteins and development of thermotolerance in Chinese hamster fibroblasts. *Proc. Natl. Acad. Sci. U.S.A.,* 79: 3218 – 3222.

Lindquist, S. (1986) The heat-shock response. *Annu. Rev. Biochem.,* 55: 1151 – 1191.

Lindquist, S. and Craig, E.A. (1988) The heat-shock proteins. *Annu. Rev. Genet.,* 22: 631 – 677.

Lowenstein, D.H., Chan, P.H. and Miles, M.F. (1991) The stress protein response in cultured neurons: characterization and evidence for a protective role in excitotoxicity. *Neuron,* 7: 1053 – 1060.

Magnusson, K. and Wieloch, T. (1989) Impairment of protein ubiquitination may cause delayed neuronal death. *Neurosci. Lett.,* 96: 264 – 270.

Magnusson, K., Deshpande, J., Linden, T., Kalimo, H. and Wieloch, T. (1989) Delayed neuronal death in the rat hippocampus is preceded by heat shock protein synthesis and loss of protein ubiquitination (abstract). *J. Cereb. Blood Flow Metab.,* 9 (Suppl. 1): S11.

Marini, A.M., Kozuka, M., Lipsky, R.L. and Nowak Jr., T.S. (1990) 70-Kilodalton heat shock protein induction in cerebellar astrocytes and cerebellar granule cells in vitro: comparison with immunocytochemical localization after hyperthermia in vivo. *J. Neurochem.,* 54: 1509 – 1516.

Milbrandt, J. (1987) A nerve growth factor-induced gene encodes a possible transcriptional regulatory factor. *Science,* 238: 797 – 799.

Mizzen, L.A. and Welch, W.J. (1988) Characterization of the thermotolerant cell. I. Effects on protein synthesis activity and the regulation of heat-shock protein 70 expression. *J. Cell Biol.,* 106: 1105 – 1116.

Morgan, J.I. and Curran, T. (1991) Stimulus-transcription coupling in the nervous system: Involvement of the inducible proto-oncogenes *fos* and *jun*. *Annu. Rev. Neurosci.,* 14: 421 – 451.

Morgan, J.I., Cohen, D.R., Hempstead, J.L. and Curran, T. (1987) Mapping patterns of c-*fos* expression in the central nervous system after seizure. *Science,* 237: 192 – 197.

Morimoto, K. and Yanagihara, T. (1981) Cerebral ischemia in gerbils: polyribosomal function during progression and recovery. *Stroke,* 12: 105 – 110.

Morimoto, R., Tissieres, A. and Georgopoulos, C. (1990) *Stress Proteins in Biology and Medicine,* Cold Spring Harbor Laboratory, Cold Spring Harbor, NY.

Müller, M., Cleef, M., Röhn, G., Bonnekoh, P., Pajunen, A.E.I., Bernstein, H.-G. and Paschen, W. (1991) Ornithine decarboxylase in reversible cerebral ischemia: an immunohistochemical study. *Acta Neuropathol. (Berl.),* 83: 39 – 45.

Munro, S. and Pelham, H.R.B. (1986) An hsp70-like protein in the ER: identity with the 78 kDa glucose-regulated protein and immunoglobulin heavy chain binding protein. *Cell,* 46: 291 – 300.

Murphy, T.H., Miyamoto, M., Sastre, A., Schnaar, R.L. and Coyle, J.T. (1989) Glutamate toxicity in a neuronal cell line involves inhibition of cystine transport leading to oxidative stress. *Neuron,* 2: 1547 – 1558.

Nakabeppu, Y. and Nathans, D. (1991) A naturally occurring truncated form of FosB that inhibits Fos/Jun transcriptional activity. *Cell,* 64: 751 – 759.

Nakajima, T., Daval, J.-L., Gleiter, C.H., Deckert, J., Post, R.M. and Marangos, P.J. (1989) C-fos mRNA expression following electrical-induced seizure and acute nociceptive stress in mouse brain. *Epilepsy Res.,* 4: 156 – 159.

Nowak Jr., T.S. (1985) Synthesis of a stress protein following transient ischemia in the gerbil. *J. Neurochem.,* 45: 1635 – 1641.

Nowak, Jr., T.S. (1988) Effects of amphetamine on protein synthesis and energy metabolism in mouse brain: role of drug-induced hyperthermia. *J. Neurochem.,* 50: 285 – 294.

Nowak Jr., T.S. (1989) MK-801 prevents 70 kDa stress protein induction in gerbil brain after ischemia: the heat shock response as a marker for excitotoxic pathology. In: J. Krieglstein (Ed.), *Pharmacology of Cerebral Ischemia 1988: Proceedings of the Second International Symposium on the Pharmacology of Cerebral Ischemia,* CRC Press, Boca Raton, FL, pp. 229 – 234.

Nowak Jr., T.S. (1990) Protein synthesis and the heat shock/stress response after ischemia. *Cerebrovasc. Brain Metab. Rev.,* 2: 345 – 366.

Nowak Jr., T.S. (1991) Localization of 70 kDa stress protein mRNA induction in gerbil brain after ischemia. *J. Cereb. Blood Flow Metab.,* 11: 432 – 439.

Nowak Jr., T.S. and Osborne, O.C. (1991) Threshold ischemic duration for stress protein induction in gerbil brain (abstract). *Stroke,* 22: 131.

Nowak Jr., T.S., Fried, R.L., Lust, W.D. and Passonneau, J.V. (1985) Changes in brain energy metabolism and protein synthesis following transient bilateral ischemia in the gerbil. *J. Neurochem.,* 44: 487 – 494.

Nowak Jr., T.S., Bond, U. and Schlesinger, M.J. (1990a) Heat shock RNA levels in brain and other tissues after hyperthermia and transient ischemia. *J. Neurochem.,* 54: 451 – 458.

Nowak Jr., T.S., Ikeda, J. and Nakajima, T. (1990b) 70 Kilodalton heat shock protein and *c-fos* gene expression following transient ischemia. *Stroke,* 21 (Suppl. III): 107 – 111.

Nowak Jr., T.S., Osborne, O.C. and Mies, G. (1991) Cortical spreading depression induces the proto-oncogene, *c-fos*, but not the stress protein, hsp70 (abstract). *J. Cereb. Blood Flow Metab.,* 11: S215.

Nowak Jr., T.S., Osborne, O.C. and Ikeda, J. (1992) Role of altered gene expression in development of neuronal changes after ischemia. In: U. Ito, T. Kirino, T. Kuroiwa and I. Klatzo (Eds.), *Maturation Phenomenon in Cerebral Ischemia,* Springer-Verlag, Berlin, pp. 121 – 128.

Oliver, C.N., Starke-Reed, P.E., Stadtman, E.R., Liu, G.J., Carney, J.M. and Floyd, R.A. (1990) Oxidative damage to brain proteins, loss of glutamine synthetase activity, and production of free radicals during ischemia/reperfusion-induced injury to gerbil brain. *Proc. Natl. Acad. Sci. U.S.A.,* 87: 5144 – 5147.

Onodera, H., Kogure, K., Ono, Y., Igarashi, K., Kiyota, Y. and Nagaoka, A. (1989) Proto-oncogene *c-fos* is transiently induced in the rat cerebral cortex after forebrain ischemia. *Neurosci. Lett.,* 98: 101 – 104.

Petersen, R. and Lindquist, S. (1988) The *Drosophila hsp70* message is rapidly degraded at normal temperatures and stabilized by heat shock. *Gene,* 72: 161 – 168.

Rabindran, S.K., Giorgi, G., Clos, J. and Wu, C. (1991) Molecular cloning and expression of a human heat shock factor, hsf1. *Proc. Natl. Acad. Sci. U.S.A.,* 88: 6906 – 6910.

Rordorf, G., Koroshetz, W.J. and Bonventre, J.V. (1991) Heat shock protects cultured neurons from glutamate toxicity. *Neuron,* 7: 1043 – 1051.

Sagar, S.M., Sharp, F.R. and Curran, T. (1988) Expression of c-fos protein in brain: metabolic mapping at the cellular level. *Science,* 240: 1328 – 1331.

Scharf, K.-D., Rose, S., Zott, W., Schöff, F. and Nover, L. (1990) Three tomato genes code for heat stress transcription factors with a region of remarkable homology to the DNA-binding domain of the yeast hsf. *EMBO J.,* 9: 4495 – 4501.

Schlesinger, M.J., Ashburner, M. and Tissieres, A. (1982) *Heat Shock from Bacteria to Man,* Cold Spring Harbor Laboratory, Cold Spring Harbor, NY.

Schuetz, T.J., Gallo, G.J., Sheldon, L., Tempst, P. and Kingston, R.E. (1991) Isolation of a cDNA for hsf2: evidence for two heat shock factor genes in humans. *Proc. Natl. Acad. Sci. U.S.A.,* 88: 6911 – 6915.

Sharp, F.R., Gonzalez, M.F., Hisanaga, K., Mobley, W.C. and Sagar, S.M. (1989) Induction of the *c-fos* gene product in rat forebrain following cortical lesions and NGF injections. *Neurosci. Lett.,* 100: 117 – 122.

Sheng, M. and Greenberg, M.E. (1990) The regulation and function of *c-fos* and other immediate early genes in the nervous system. *Neuron,* 4: 477 – 485.

Simon, R.P., Cho, H., Gwinn, R. and Lowenstein, D.H. (1991) The temporal profile of 72-kDa heat-shock protein expression following global ischemia. *J. Neurosci.,* 11: 881 – 889.

Sonnenberg, J.L., Mitchelmore, C., Macgregor-Leon, P.F., Hempstead, J., Morgan, J.I. and Curran, T. (1989a) Glutamate receptor agonists increase the expression of Fos, Fra, and AP-1 DNA binding activity in the mammalian brain. *J. Neurosci. Res.,* 24: 72 – 80.

Sonnenberg, J.L., Rauscher III, F.J., Morgan, J.I. and Curran, T. (1989b) Regulation of proenkephalin by Fos and Jun. *Science,* 246: 1622 – 1625.

Sprang, G.K. and Brown, I.R. (1987) Selective induction of a heat shock gene in fiber tracts and cerebellar neurons of the rabbit brain detected by in situ hybridization. *Mol. Brain Res.,* 3: 89 – 93.

Suga, S. and Nowak Jr., T.S. (1991) Localization of immunoreactive Fos and Jun proteins in gerbil brain: effect of transient ischemia (abstract). *J. Cereb. Blood Flow Metab.,* 11: S352.

Sukhatme, V.P., Cao, X., Chang, L.C., Tsai-Morris, C.H., Stamenkovich, D., Ferreira, P.C.P., Cohen, D.R., Edwards, S.A., Shows, T.B., Curran, T., Le Beau, M.M. and Adamson, E.D. (1988) A zinc finger-encoding gene coregulated with *c-fos* during growth and differentiation, and after cellular depolarization. *Cell,* 53: 37 – 43.

Szekely, A.M., Barbaccia, M.L., Alho, H. and Costa, E. (1989) In primary cultures of cerebellar granule cells the activation of *N*-methyl-D-aspartate-sensitive glutamate receptors induces *c-fos* mRNA expression. *Mol. Pharmacol.,* 35: 401 – 408.

Szekely, A.M., Costa, E. and Grayson, D.R. (1990) Transcriptional program coordination by *N*-methyl-D-aspartate-sensitive glutamate receptor stimulation in primary cultures of cerebellar neurons. *Mol. Pharmacol.,* 38: 624 – 633.

Takemoto, O., Tomimoto, H. and Yanagihara, T. (1991) Induction of *c-fos* and *c-jun* gene products and heat shock protein after transient cerebral ischemia in gerbils (abstract). *Stroke,* 22: 131.

Thilmann, R., Xie, Y., Kleihues, P. and Kiessling, M. (1986) Persistent inhibition of protein synthesis precedes delayed neuronal death in postischemic gerbil hippocampus. *Acta Neuropathol. (Berl.),* 71: 88 – 93.

Uemura, Y., Kowall, N.W. and Beal, M.F. (1991) Global ischemia induces NMDA receptor-mediated *c-fos* expression in neurons resistant to injury in gerbil hippocampus. *Brain Res.,* 542: 343 – 347.

Uney, J.B., Leigh, P.N., Marsden, C.D., Lees, A. and Anderton, B.H. (1988) Stereotaxic injection of kainic acid into the striatum of rats induces synthesis of mRNA for heat shock protein 70. *FEBS Lett.,* 235: 215 – 218.

Ungewickel, E. (1985) The 70 kDa mammalian heat shock proteins are structurally and functionally related to the uncoating protein that releases triskelion from coated vesicles. *EMBO J.,* 4: 3385 – 3391.

Vass, K., Welch, W.J. and Nowak Jr., T.S. (1988) Localization of 70 kDa stress protein induction in gerbil brain after ischemia. *Acta Neuropathol. (Berl.),* 77: 128 – 135.

Vass, K., Berger, M.L., Nowak Jr., T.S., Welch, W.J. and Lassmann, H. (1989) Induction of stress protein hsp70 in nerve cells after status epilepticus in the rat. *Neurosci. Lett.,* 100: 259 – 264.

Welch, W.J. and Suhan, J.P. (1986) Cellular and biochemical events in mammalian cells during and after recovery from physiological stress. *J. Cell Biol.,* 103: 2035 – 2052.

Welsh, F.A., Moyer, D.J. and Harris, V.A. (1992) Regional expression of heat shock protein-70 mRNA and c-*fos* mRNA following focal ischemia in rat brain. *J. Cereb. Blood Flow Metab.,* 12: 204 – 212.

Whatley, S.A., Leung, T., Hall, C. and Lim, L. (1986) The brain 68-kilodalton microtubule-associated protein is the cognate form of the 70-kilodalton mammalian heat-shock protein and is present as a specific isoform in synaptosomal membranes. *J. Neurochem.,* 47: 1576 – 1583.

Widelitz, R.B., Magun, B.E. and Gerner, E.W. (1986) Effects of cycloheximide on thermotolerance expression, heat shock protein synthesis, and heat shock protein mRNA accumulation in rat fibroblasts. *Mol. Cell. Biol.,* 6: 1088 – 1094.

Widmann, R., Kuroiwa, T., Bonnekoh, P. and Hossmann, K.A. (1991) [^{14}]Leucine incorporation into brain proteins in gerbils after transient ischemia: relationship to selective vulnerability of hippocampus. *J. Neurochem.,* 56: 789 – 796.

Wisden, W., Errington, M.L., Williams, S., Dunnett, S.B., Waters, C., Hitchcock, D., Evan, G., Bliss, T.V.P. and Hunt, S.P. (1990) Differential expression of immediate early genes in the hippocampus and spinal cord. *Neuron,* 4: 603 – 614.

Yamaguchi, T., Wagner, H.G. and Klatzo, I. (1986) Postischemic pathophysiology in the gerbil brain – changes of extracellular K^+ and Ca^{2+}. In: A. Baethmann, K.G. Go and A. Unterberg (Eds.), *Mechanisms of Secondary Brain Damage,* Plenum, New York, pp. 249 – 258.

K. Kogure, K.-A. Hossmann and B.K. Siesjö (Eds.)
Progress in Brain Research, Vol. 96

CHAPTER 14

Possible involvement of c-*fos* translational regulation in the interaction between glutamate and neurotrophic factors in brain ischemia

Kinya Hisanaga[1,2] and Kyuya Kogure[2]

[1] *Department of Neurology, University of California at San Francisco, and Veterans Affairs Medical Center, San Francisco, CA, U.S.A. and* [2] *Department of Neurology, Institute of Brain Diseases, Tohoku University School of Medicine, Sendai, Japan*

Glutamate and neurotrophic factors in brain ischemia

The development of cerebral infarction is a complex process that involves initiation and subsequent maturation. There are now convincing data showing that glutamate is involved in the initiating neuroexcitatory mechanism which leads to neuronal death (Rothman, 1983, 1984; Benveniste et al., 1984). Among several kinds of glutamate receptors *N*-methyl-D-aspartate (NMDA) receptor is believed to play the most important role in the neurotoxicity by inducing the Ca^{2+} influx via a receptor-gated Ca^{2+} channel (Simon et al., 1984; Choi, 1988). The steep rise in intracellular Ca^{2+} induced by glutamate may activate Ca^{2+}-dependent proteases and may cause the generation of free radicals, which in turn, leads to the breakdown of the cytoskeleton and membranes (Kogure et al., 1985; Siman and Noszek, 1988). NMDA antagonists have been reported to attenuate delayed hippocampal neuronal death which is produced by transient forebrain ischemia in rodents (Gill et al., 1987).

Neurotrophic factors, such as nerve growth factor (NGF) and fibroblast growth factor (FGF), constitute another class of intercellular signaling molecules which may play important roles in neurodegeneration. Target-derived neurotrophic factors are known to promote the survival of the projecting neurons after axotomy in vivo and in vitro (Barde, 1989), and the deficiency has been implicated to the cause of some neurodegenerative diseases (Appel, 1981).

In previous studies we showed that the extract of hippocampus obtained from rats, which had been subjected to transient forebrain ischemia two weeks before, maintained choline acetyltransferase activity of cultured septal neurons to some extent for several days, indicating that neurotrophic factor(s) for septal cholinergic neurons might be released in the hippocampus after ischemic injury (Hisanaga et al., 1989). Increased production of neurotrophic factors might also constitute a protective mechanism ameliorating brain damage after ischemia, particularly neuronal necrosis of the delayed type (Schmidt-Kastner and Freund, 1991), which develops over several days after the insult. NGF content has been reported to be increased in the hippocampus five days after hypoxic injury (Lorez et al., 1989). Shigeno et al. (1991) showed that intraventricular injection of NGF either before or after 5 min forebrain ischemia in the Mongolian gerbil significantly reduced the occurrence of delayed neuronal death. A neurotrophic factor, basic FGF (Morrison et al., 1986; Walicke et al., 1986), is also known to increase in brain after ischemic injury (Kiyota et al., 1991) and to promote the survival of thalamic neurons after cortical ischemic injury

(Yamada et al., 1991).

Excitatory amino acid neurotransmitters and neurotrophic factors have frequently been suggested independently to play roles in neurodegenerative processes. Recently, considerable attention has focused on the interaction between glutamate and neurotrophic factors. Aloe (1988) showed that damage to the striatum and hippocampus caused by glutamate agonists can be prevented by intracerebral injection of NGF. Mattson et al. (1989) showed that pretreatment of cultured hippocampal neurons with FGF reduces glutamate-induced increases in intracellular Ca^{2+} levels and attenuates the subsequent neuronal death. They also showed that pretreatment with the RNA synthesis inhibitor actinomycin D or the protein synthesis inhibitor cycloheximide prevents the action of FGF on glutamate-induced increases in intracellular calcium or neurodegeneration. These findings implicate that both ongoing transcription and translation might be required in order for FGF to protect against glutamate neurotoxicity. Imbalances in these systems, i.e., excitatory amino acid neurotransmitters and neurotrophic factors, may lead to neurodegeneration. Cellular calcium-regulating systems may be a common focus of neurotransmitter and neurotrophic factor actions.

Immediate early genes as third messengers

The trophic actions of neurotrophic factors are believed to be mediated, at least in part, by changes in gene and/or protein expression, which generally require periods of hours to days to be accomplished (Greene and Shooter, 1980). Recently, cellular immediate early genes have been vigorously investigated because of their action as third messengers in intracellular signal transduction systems (Morgan and Curran, 1991).

The best characterized immediate early gene, c-*fos*, is rapidly induced by a variety of extracellular stimuli. c-*fos* encodes the Fos protein which forms heterodimers with Jun, the protein product of c-*jun*. The Fos-Jun heterodimer binds to regulatory sequences of the target genes and regulates their expression.

Multiple signaling pathways have been implicated in immediate early gene expression. These include calcium-calmodulin kinase, cyclic AMP-protein kinase A and phosphatidylinositol-protein kinase C (Morgan and Curran, 1991).

c-*fos* mRNA and/or Fos protein expression are induced in brain in response to a variety of stimuli, including ischemia (Jørgensen et al., 1989; Onodera et al., 1989), generalized seizures, electrical stimulation and dehydration (Morgan and Curran, 1991). Activation of NMDA glutamate receptors seems to be important for c-*fos* expression in some populations of neurons (Szekely et al., 1987, 1989; Cole et al., 1989; Sonnenberg et al., 1989; Sharp et al., 1990).

To better understand the role that NMDA receptor activation plays during neuronal *fos* expression, we have used primary cortical neuronal cultures. Recently, we found that c-*fos* mRNA and Fos-like protein were induced in cultured cortical neurons after treatment with glutamate, basic FGF or other substances, and that blockade of NMDA receptors by the antagonists seemed to inhibit basic FGF-induced Fos-like protein expression without inhibiting c-*fos* mRNA expression (Hisanaga et al., 1992). These findings suggest that c-*fos* translational regulation may be involved in the interaction between glutamate and basic FGF in the physiological conditions, and possibly in the pathophysiological conditions such as brain ischemia.

c-*fos* mRNA and Fos protein expression in cultured neurons

Primary cortical neuronal cultures

Dissociated cortical cells were prepared from 16 – 17-day-old Sprague-Dawley rat fetuses as described previously (Hisanaga and Sharp, 1990; Hisanaga et al., 1992). Cells were suspended in Eagle's medium (MEM) containing 10% fetal calf serum, and plated on poly-D-lysine-coated multiwell plates at a density of $1 \times 10^6/cm^2$. The medium was changed to serum-free and Mg^{2+}-free

MEM 4 – 5 h after seeding (Mg^{2+} can act as an antagonist of the NMDA receptor). After culturing in serum-free MEM for three days, neurons were treated with the agents described below.

c-fos mRNA expression

c-*fos* mRNA was analyzed using Northern blotting as described previously (Hisanaga et al., 1990). The RNA was extracted from the neuronal cultures after 30 min incubations with each agent. Total cellular RNA (10 μg) was loaded onto a 1.5% agarose/2.2 M formaldehyde gel. Following electrophoresis, the RNA was transferred to a nylon membrane (Schleicher and Schuell) by capillary blotting. The rRNA on the membrane was stained with 0.02% methylene blue and 0.3 M sodium acetate to monitor whether RNA transfer had been done evenly and to locate the position of RNA species (not shown). c-*fos* riboprobe was prepared from full length c-*fos* cDNA (generously provided by Dr. T. Curran, Roche Research Center) using SP6 RNA polymerase and ^{32}P-CTP. Radiolabeled RNA was purified over a Nensorb column (DuPont). The nylon membranes were hybridized with the riboprobe and exposed to Kodak XAR film at −70°C with an intensifying screen.

L-Glutamate (10 μM) and PKC activator, 12-*O*-tetra-decanoylphorbol-13-acetate (TPA, 50 nM) induces c-*fos* mRNA, in agreement with previous reports in cultured cerebellar neurons (Szekely et al., 1987, 1989) (Fig. 1). Basic FGF (5 ng/ml, Fig. 1) (generously provided by Dr. P.A. Walicke, UCSD), KCl (46 mM with the osmolarity adjusted by the addition of water), $ZnCl_2$ (100 μM) and vasoactive intestinal peptide (VIP, 1 μM) (not shown) also induced c-*fos* mRNA. NGF (100 ng/ml) and epidermal growth factor (20 ng/ml) did not induce c-*fos* mRNA (not shown).

Fifteen minutes pretreatment with a non-competitive NMDA antatonist, MK-801 ((+)-5-methyl-10,11-dihydro-5H-dibenzo[a,d]cyclohepten-5,10-imine maleate, Merck Sharp and Dohme, 0.1 μM) completely blocked glutamate induction of c-*fos* mRNA. Pretreatment with competitive antagonists, CPP (4-(3-phosphonopropyl)piperazin-2-carboxylic acid, Research Biochemicals, 10 μM) and APH (2-amino-7-phosphonoheptanoate, Cambridge Research Biochemicals, 30 – 100 μM), substantially, but not completely, blocked glutamate induction of c-*fos* mRNA (Fig. 1). These antagonists only partially blocked c-*fos* mRNA expression induced by TPA (Fig. 1), high K^+, Zn^{2+} and VIP (not shown), while they had little or no effect on basic FGF-induced c-*fos* mRNA expression (Fig. 1).

These findings suggest that NMDA receptor activation is required for glutamate-induced c-*fos* expression in cortical neurons, and that TPA, basic FGF, high K^+, Zn^{2+} and VIP induce the c-*fos* gene via non-NMDA receptor-mediated mechanisms. Possible mediators for c-*fos* induction by these latter agents are phosphatidylinositol/protein kinase C (by TPA: Castagna et al., 1982; by VIP: Malhotra

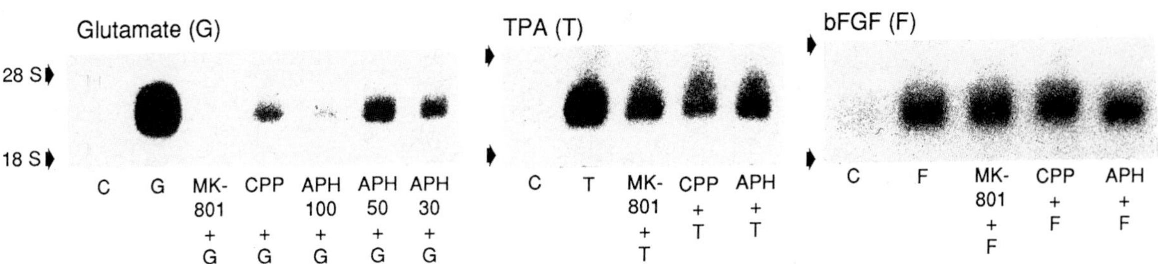

Fig. 1. Northern blots showing induction of c-*fos* mRNA. Cells were treated for 30 min with glutamate (10 μM), TPA (50 nM), and basic FGF (bFGF, 5 ng/ml) 15 min after the addition of MK-801 (0.1 μM), CPP (10 μM) or APH (30, 50 and 100 μM for glutamate, 30 μM for the others). Glutamate induction of c-*fos* mRNA is completely blocked by the non-competitive antagonist MK-801 but is only partially blocked by the competitive antagonists CPP and APH. NMDA antagonists partially reduce TPA-induced c-*fos* mRNA, and have little or no effect on basic FGF-induced c-*fos* mRNA.

et al., 1989) and tyrosine kinase (by FGF: Coughlin et al., 1988).

Fos-like protein expression

Immunostaining for Fos-like protein was carried out as described previously (Hisanaga et al., 1990). Some antibodies against synthetic peptides of Fos recognize Fos and a set of Fos-related antigens, which are proteins that are also induced by extracellular stimuli and have antigenic, structural and DNA binding properties in common with Fos (Morgan and Curran, 1991). We used an affinity-purified polyclonal rabbit antibody that was raised in our laboratory to the M2 peptide (Fos 132 – 154; Sagar et al., 1988; Sharp et al., 1989a,b,c, 1991; Sagar and Sharp, 1990; Hisanaga et al., 1990). This antibody recognizes Fos and two lower molecular weight Fos-related antigens on Western blots of

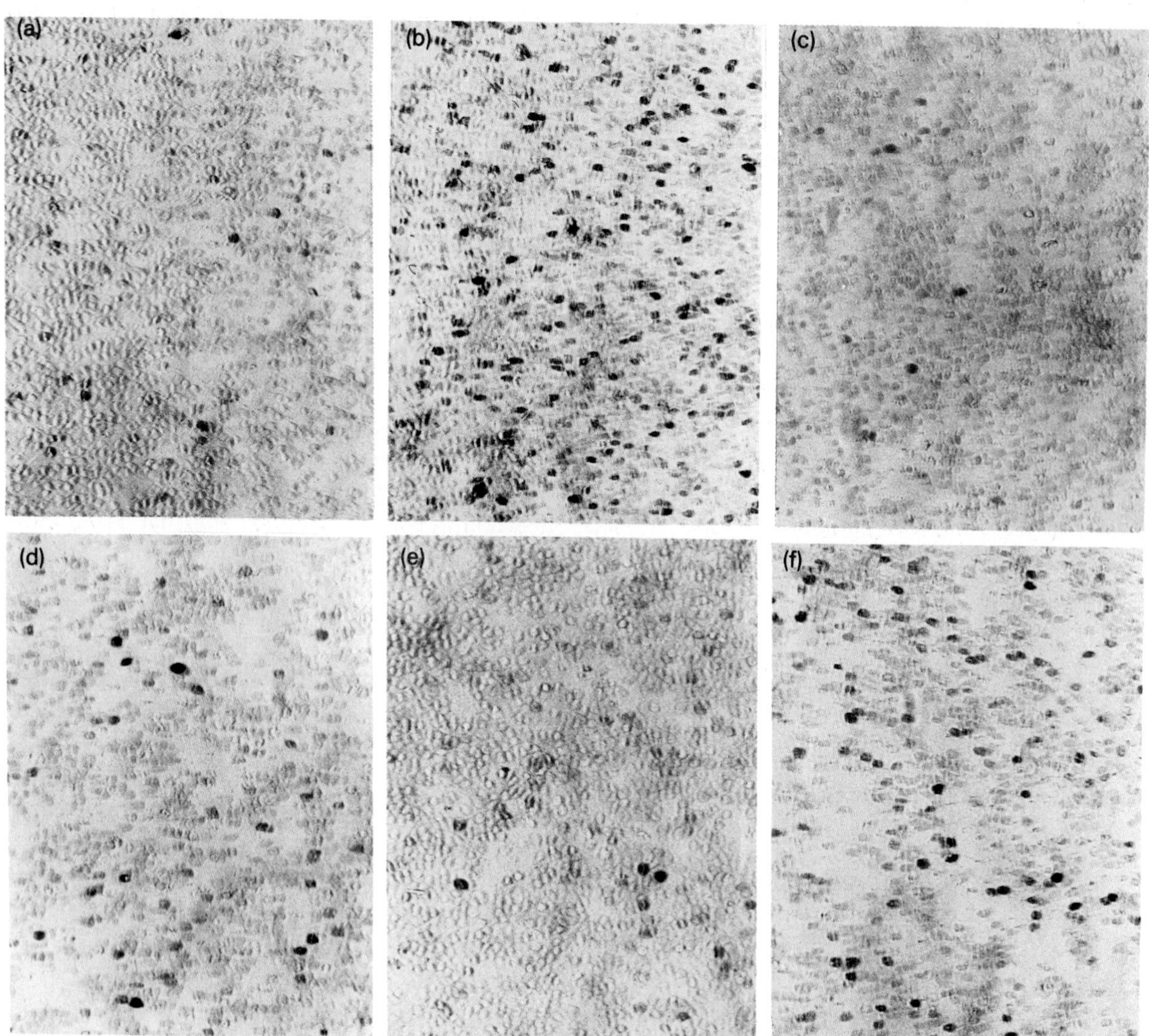

Fig. 2. FLP induced by glutamate (10 μM for 2 h) and the effects of NMDA antagonists. Cells were treated for 2 h with glutamate as described in Fig. 1. *a*, Control; *b*, glutamate; *c*, MK-801 (0.1 μM/glutamate; *d*, CPP (10 μM)/glutamate; *e*, APH (100 μM)/glutamate; *f*, APH (30 μM)/glutamate. Note that MK-801 reduces the number of FLP-immunoreactive cells to control level, whereas inhibition by CPP and APH is incomplete.

serum-stimulated HeLa cells (Aronin et al., 1990).

Neurons were fixed after 2 h incubations with each agent and stained with the polyclonal antibody to Fos-like protein. The bound antibodies were visualized using the avidin-biotin-peroxidase method, as previously described (Hisanaga et al., 1990). The specificity of the immunochemical reaction was shown by the reduction of immunostaining following pre-absorption of the antibody with the synthetic M2 peptide antigen (1 μg/ml).

Only a few neurons (0.5 – 1.5% of the total neurons) in control cultures exhibited nuclear Fos-like protein immunoreactivity (Figs. 2*a*, 3*a*, 4*a*). A marked increase of Fos-like protein immunoreac-

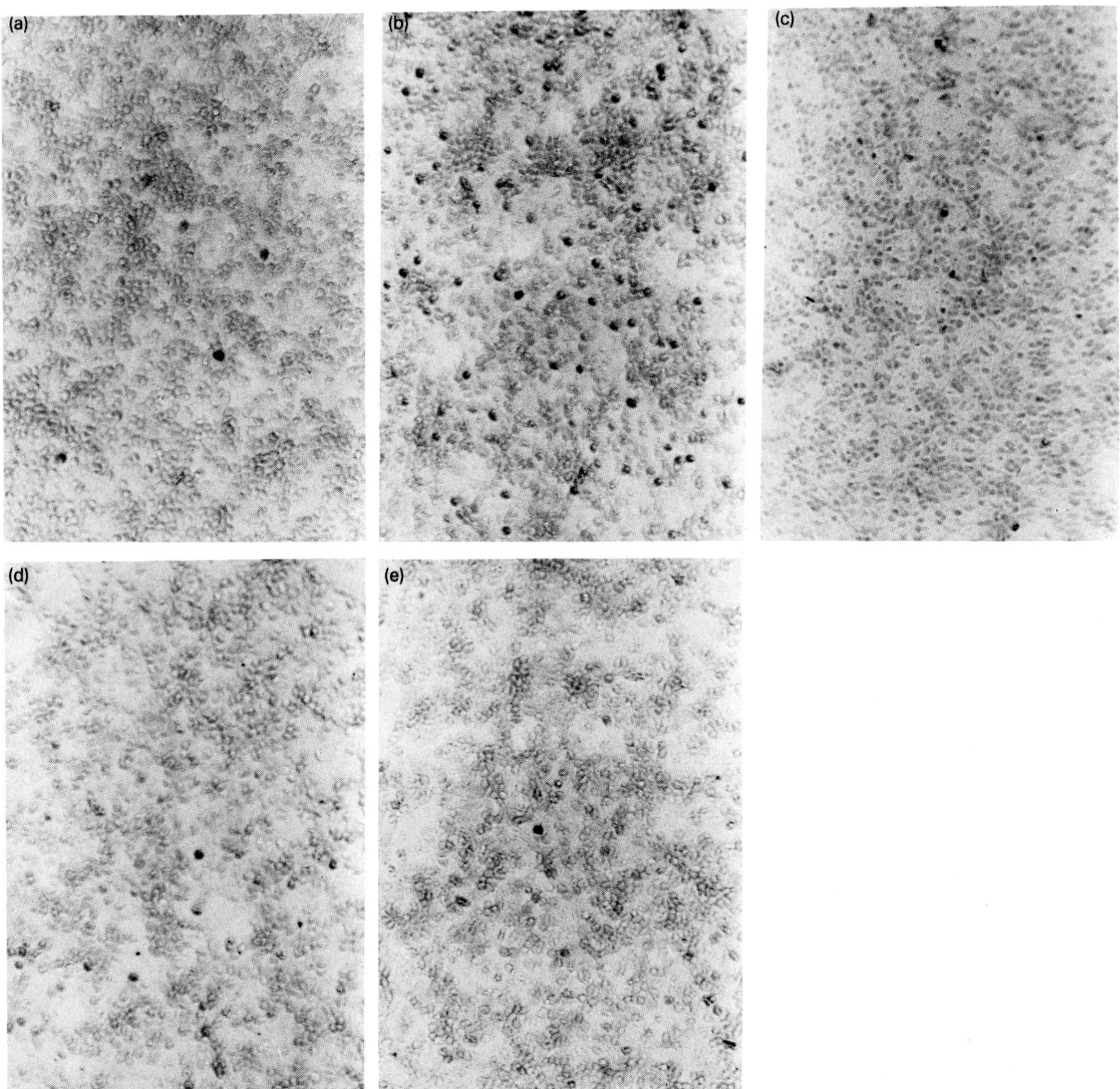

Fig. 3. FLP induced by TPA (50 nM) and the effects of NMDA antagonists. Cells were treated as described in Figs. 1 and 2. *a*, Control; *b*, TPA; *c*, MK-801 (0.1 μM)/TPA; *d*, CPP (10 μM)/TPA; *e*, APH (30 μM)/TPA. Note that NMDA antagonists completely block FLP expression.

tivity occurred in the nuclei of 4 – 13% of neurons present in a culture dish after treatment with glutamate (Fig. 2*b*), TPA (Fig. 3*b*), basic FGF (Fig. 4*b*), high K^+, Zn^{2+} and VIP (not shown). NGF, epidermal growth factor, platelet-derived growth factor (1 unit/ml), somatostatin (1 μM), neuropeptide Y (1 μM) and carbachol (1, 10 and 50 mM) did not induce Fos-like protein in cultured neurons (not shown). Though MK-801 has been reported to induce c-*fos* in cortex in vivo (Dragunow and Faull, 1990), it did not induce c-*fos* in cultured cortical neurons.

The glutamate induction of Fos-like protein was completely blocked by pretreatment with MK-801, and substantially, but not completely, blocked by CPP and APH (Fig. 2). Unexpectedly, all of the NMDA antagonists completely blocked Fos-like protein expression by TPA, basic FGF (Figs. 3, 4), high K^+, Zn^{2+} and VIP (not shown).

Treatment of the cultures with NMDA an-

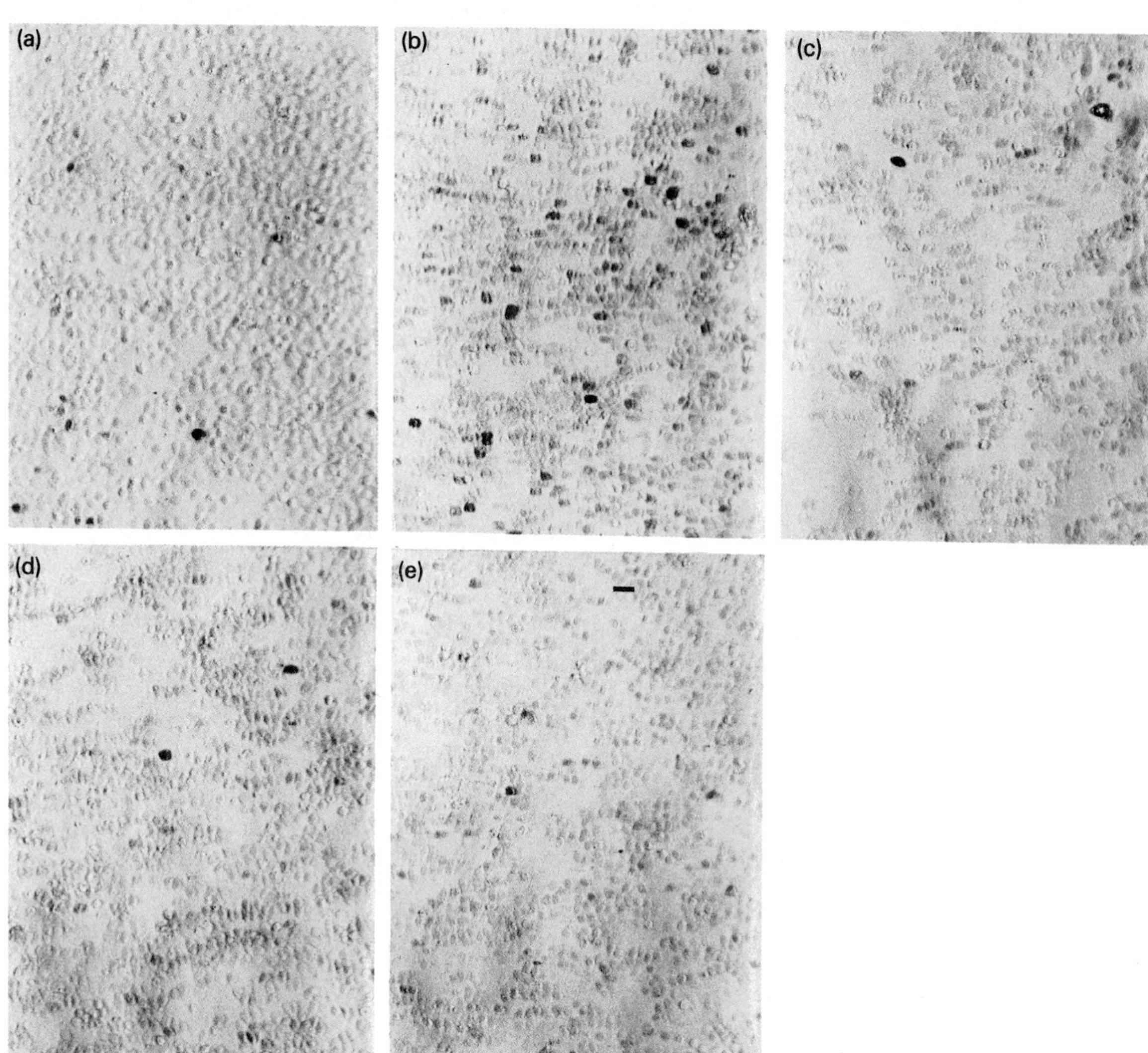

Fig. 4. FLP induced by basic FGF (5 ng/ml) and the effects of NMDA antagonists. Cells were treated as described in Figs. 1 and 2. *a*, Control; *b*, basic FGF; *c*, MK-801 (0.1 μM)/basic FGF; *d*, CPP (10 μM)/basic FGF; *e*, APH (30 μM)/basic FGF. Note that NMDA antagonists completely block FLP expression.

tagonists had no effect on total protein synthesis as measured by [^{3}H]leucine incorporation into trichloroacetic acid-precipitable material (Hisanaga et al., 1992).

NMDA antagonists block Fos translation?

These studies show that c-*fos* mRNA and Fos-like protein are induced by glutamate, TPA, basic FGF, high K^+, Zn^{2+} and VIP in cultured cortical neurons.

VIP acts on VIP receptors on target neurons and stimulates the cAMP-protein kinase A and phosphatidylinositol-protein kinase C systems (Malhotra et al., 1989; Magistretti, 1990). VIP modulates mitosis, neurite elaboration and survival of neuroblasts (Pincus et al., 1990).

Synaptic vesicles contain Zn^{2+} and release it into the synaptic cleft during excitation. Zn^{2+} concentrations in the extracellular space can rise to 300 μM after K^+ depolarization of hippocampal slices (Assaf and Chung, 1984; Howell et al., 1984). Though Zn^{2+} attenuates the neurotoxic effects of NMDA agonists on cortical neurons in a non-competitive fashion, it increases the neurotoxic effects of quisqualate agonists (Peters et al., 1987; Westbrook and Mayer, 1987; Koh and Choi, 1988). Though Zn^{2+} may modulate the postsynaptic response to the co-released transmitter glutamate, it can also kill neurons in high (250 μM) concentrations (Yokoyama et al., 1986).

Although NMDA receptor antagonists only partially block c-*fos* mRNA expression by these agents, NMDA antagonists block Fos-like protein expression by all of these agents. From these results we hypothesize that many extracellular signals induce c-*fos* transcription, but that Fos protein translation by all signals requires concurrent activation of the NMDA receptors in cortical neurons.

The mechanism by which NMDA antagonists prevent the induction of Fos protein via multiple signaling pathways is unknown. There are several possibilities. First, the Fos protein could be synthesized but rapidly degraded so that it is not detected immunocytochemically. Since NMDA receptor activation can modify protease activity (Choi, 1988), NMDA antagonists might activate enzymes responsible for Fos protein catabolism. Secondly, NMDA receptor activation may be required to translate the Fos protein from c-*fos* mRNA. Similar regulation of translation occurs in other systems. Expression of yeast transcription activator GCN4 (the DNA binding site of which is related to the Fos-Jun binding site) is regulated mainly at the translational level. The activation of a protein kinase following extracellular stimulation appears to mediate the translational regulation of GCN4 mRNA (Hinnebusch, 1990). In addition, one known Ca^{2+}/calmodulin kinase modulates translation by phosphorylating the elongation factor 2 (Ryazanov et al., 1988). Further studies are required to prove whether NMDA receptor activation regulates Fos translation.

Possible mechanisms concerning the interaction between glutamate and neurotrophic factors in brain ischemic injury

Neurotrophic factors may be involved in adaptive mechanisms, such as sprouting, that occur in response to alterations in activity or injury in the adult CNS (Crutcher, 1987). In other words, these factors could induce plastic responses in specific neuronal systems leading to synaptic reorganization. For example, NGF is known to stimulate sprouting of cholinergic axons in the adult rat cerebral cortex and hippocampus (Ernfors et al., 1990). Roles for neurotrophic factors in age-related neuronal losses and in specific neurodegenerative disorders, including Alzheimer's disease, have also been suggested (Appel, 1981). It is likely that neurotrophic factors play an important role in neuronal reorganization or neuronal plasticity after ischemic injury.

The cellular mechanisms by which neurotrophic factors influence neuronal cell survival and neuronal plasticity are not yet clear. The survival-promoting effects of NGF apparently require its retrograde transport from axonal endings to the cell soma (Barde, 1989). Protein synthesis seems to be required for the outgrowth-promoting effects of NGF (Greene and Shooter, 1980). These data are consistent with the hypothesis that NGF influences the expression of mRNAs and proteins which promote neuronal survival and neurite outgrowth. FGF also appears to require mRNA and protein synthesis for its neurotrophic action (Mattson et al., 1989). It is possible that Fos is one of the proteins which are required for the action of neurotrophic factors.

Neurotransmitters also have developmental roles as regulators of neurite outgrowth and synaptogenesis. Stimulation of NMDA receptors is believed to play a critical role in neuronal plasticity. In situ studies demonstrated that blockade of NMDA receptors in the vertebrate visual system results in a disruption of the normal segregation of synapses in the tectum (Cline et al., 1987). In addition, there is very strong evidence that glutamate mediates the synaptic plasticity associated with long-term potentiation in the mammalian hippocampus (Lynch, 1986). NMDA antagonists cause learning impairment (Morris et al., 1986) and prevent plasticity in the cortex and other brain regions (McDonald and Johnston, 1990). Fos could play a role in NMDA-mediated- as well as neurotrophic factor-mediated plasticity, by producing long-term changes in gene expression. Many proteins may be required for neuronal plasticity, and Fos may be a common protein which both glutamate and neurotrophic factors require for their action on plasticity.

Our results suggest that if neurotrophic factors such as FGF, and neurotransmitters/neuromodulators such as VIP and Zn^{2+}, mediate plasticity by induction of c-*fos* mRNA, the expression of Fos protein by these agents requires concurrent activation of the NMDA receptor. Therefore, it is possible that NMDA antagonists prevent cortical plasticity by blocking induction of the Fos protein that would otherwise be induced by neurotrophic factors, neurotransmitters and neuromodulators.

The interaction between glutamate and neurotrophic factors seems to be important in both the acute stage and the chronic stage of brain ischemia. The increase of glutamate release causes neuronal damage in the acute stage, and neurotrophic factors may struggle to attenuate the neurotoxicity. Ishikawa et al. (1991) showed a steep increase in cortical NGF content following a cavity lesioning as early as 16 h, in contrast to FGF, which became elevated more than ten days later. Messenger RNA for brain-derived neurotrophic factor (BDNF), a member of the NGF family, also has been shown to increase immediately after brain ischemia, while mRNA for neurotrophin-3, another member of the NGF family, decreases after the insult (Lindvall et al., 1992; Takeda et al., 1992). Glutamate release seems to stimulate NGF and BDNF synthesis via NMDA receptors and non-NMDA receptors (Ernfors et al., 1991; Zafra et al., 1991; Lindvall et al., 1992). In the chronic stage of brain ischemia, glutamate seems to help neurotrophic factors to promote neuronal reorganization by influencing intracellular signals such as c-*fos* expression as shown in the present study.

Neurotrophic factors have received much interest because of their potency as future therapeutics for brain diseases, including brain ischemia and degenerative disorders. It may prove more important to investigate signal transduction systems for neurotrophic factors and their interaction with other environmental signals like neurotransmitters.

Acknowledgements

We thank Dr. Frank R. Sharp and Dr. Stephen M. Sagar, University of California at San Franscisco, for their kind suggestions.

References

Aloe, L. (1988) Intracerebral pretreatment with nerve growth factor prevents irreversible brain lesions in neonatal rats injected with ibotenic acid. *Biotechniques,* 5: 1085 – 1086.

Appel, S.H. (1981) A unifying hypothesis for the cause of amyotrophic lateral sclerosis, Parkinsonism and Alzheimer disease. *Ann. Neurol.,* 10: 499 – 505.

Aronin, N., Sagar, S.M., Sharp, F.R. and Schwartz, W.J. (1990) Light regulates expression of a Fos-related protein in rat suprachiasmatic nuclei. *Proc. Natl. Acad. Sci. U.S.A.,* 87: 5959 – 5962.

Assaf, S.Y. and Chung, S.H. (1984) Release of endogenous Zn^{2+} from brain tissue during activity. *Nature,* 308:

734 – 736.

Barde, Y-A. (1989) Trophic factors and neuronal survival. *Neuron,* 2: 1525 – 1534.

Benveniste, H., Drejer, J., Schousboe, A. and Diemer, N.H. (1984) Elevation of the extracellular concentrations of glutamate and aspartate in rat hippocampus during transient cerebral ischemia monitored by intracerebral microdialysis. *J. Neurochem.,* 43: 1369 – 1374.

Castagna, M., Takai, Y., Kaibuchi, K., Sano, K., Kikkawa, U. and Nishizuka, Y. (1982) Direct activation of calcium-activated, phospholipid-dependent protein kinase by tumor-promoting phorbol esters. *J. Biol. Chem.,* 257: 7847 – 7851.

Choi, D.W. (1988) Glutamate neurotoxicity and diseases of the nervous system. *Neuron,* 1: 623 – 634.

Cline, H.T., Debski, E.A. and Constantine-Paton, M. (1987) *N*-methyl-D-aspartate receptor antagonist desegregates eye-specific stripes. *Proc. Natl. Acad. Sci. U.S.A.,* 84: 4342 – 4345.

Cole, A.J., Saffen, D.W., Baraban, J.M. and Worley, P.F. (1989) Rapid increase of an immediate early gene messenger RNA in hippocampal neurons by synaptic NMDA receptor activation. *Nature,* 340: 474 – 476.

Coughlin, S.R., Barr, P.J., Cousens, L.S., Fretto, L.J. and Williams, L.T. (1988) Acidic and basic fibroblast growth factors stimulate tyrosine kinase activity in vivo. *J. Biol. Chem.,* 263: 988 – 993.

Crutcher, K.A. (1987) Sympathetic sprouting in the central nervous system: a model for studies of axonal growth in the mature mammalian brain. *Brain Res. Rev.,* 12: 203 – 233.

Dragunow, M. and Faull, R.L.M. (1990) MK-801 induces c-*fos* protein in thalamic and neocortical neurons of rat brain. *Neurosci. Lett.,* 111: 39 – 45.

Ernfors, P., Ibanez, C.F., Ebendal, T., Olson, L. and Persson, H. (1990) Molecular cloning and neurotrophic activities of a protein with structural similarities to nerve growth factor: developmental and topographical expression in the brain. *Proc. Natl. Acad. Sci. U.S.A.,* 87: 5454 – 5458.

Ernfors, P., Bengzon, J., Kokaia, Z., Persson, H. and Lindvall, O. (1991) Increased levels of messenger RNAs for neurotrophic factors in the brain during kindling epileptogenesis. *Neuron,* 7: 165 – 176.

Gill, R., Foster, A.C. and Woodruff, G.N. (1987) Systemic administration of MK-801 protects against ischemia-induced hippocampal neurodegeneration in the gerbil. *J. Neurosci.,* 7: 3343 – 3349.

Greene, L.A. and Shooter, E.M. (1980) The nerve growth factor: biochemistry, synthesis, and mechanism of action. *Annu. Rev. Neurosci.,* 3: 353 – 402.

Hinnebusch, A.G. (1990) Involvement of an initiation factor and protein phosphorylation in translational control of GCN4 mRNA. *Trends Biochem. Sci.,* 15: 148 – 152.

Hisanaga, K. and Sharp, F.R. (1990) Marked neurotrophic effects of diffusible substances released from non-target cerebellar cells on thalamic neurons in culture. *Dev. Brain Res.,* 54: 151 – 160.

Hisanaga, K., Kogure, K., Tsukui, H., Takei, N., Nishio, C. and Hatanaka, H. (1989) Increase in choline acetyltransferase activity in septum of rats after transient forebrain ischemia: a possible role of factors released in the hippocampus. *Neurosci. Lett.,* 105: 321 – 325.

Hisanaga, K., Sagar, S.M., Hicks, K.J., Swanson, R.A. and Sharp, F.R. (1990) c-*fos* proto-oncogene expression in astrocytes associated with differentiation or proliferation but not depolarization. *Mol. Brain Res.,* 8: 69 – 75.

Hisanaga, K., Sagar, S.M. and Sharp, F.R. (1992) *N*-methyl-D-aspartate antagonists block Fos-like protein expression induced via multiple signalling pathways in cultured cortical neurons. *J. Neurochem.,* 58: 1836 – 1844.

Howell, G.A., Welch, M.G. and Frederickson, C.J. (1984) Stimulation-induced uptake and release of zinc in hippocampal slices. *Nature,* 308: 736 – 738.

Ishikawa, R., Nishikiori, K. and Furukawa, S. (1991) Appearance of nerve growth factor and acidic fibroblast growth factor with different time courses in the cavity-lesioned cortex of the rat brain. *Neurosci. Lett.,* 127: 70 – 72.

Jørgensen, M.B., Deckert, J., Wright, D.C. and Gehlert, D.R. (1989) Delayed c-*fos* proto-oncogene expression in the rat hippocampus induced by transient global cerebral ischemia: an in situ hybridization study. *Brain Res.,* 484: 393 – 398.

Kiyota, Y., Takami, K., Iwane, M., Shino, A., Miyamoto, M., Tsukuda, R. and Nagaoka, A. (1991) Increase in basic fibroblast growth factor-like immunoreactivity in rat brain after forebrain ischemia. *Brain Res.,* 545: 322 – 328.

Kogure, K., Arai, H., Abe, K. and Nakano, M. (1985) Free radical damage of the brain following ischemia. In: K. Kogure, K.A. Hossmann, B.K. Siesjö and F.A. Welsh (Eds.), *Progress in Brain Res. Vol. 63,* Elsevier, Amsterdam, pp. 237 – 259.

Koh, J.-Y. and Choi, D.W. (1988) Zinc alters excitatory amino acid neurotoxicity on cortical neurons. *J. Neurosci.,* 8: 2164 – 2171.

Lindvall, O., Ernfors, P., Bengzon, J., Kokaia, Z., Smith, M-J., Siesjö, B.K. and Persson, H. (1992) Differential regulation of mRNAs for nerve growth factor, brain-derived neurotrophic factor, and neurotrophin 3 in the adult rat brain following cerebral ischemia and hypoglycemic coma. *Proc. Natl. Acad. Sci. U.S.A.,* 89: 648 – 652.

Lorez, H., Keller, F., Ruess, G. and Otten, U. (1989) Nerve growth factor increases in adult rat brain after hypoxic injury. *Neurosci. Lett.,* 98: 339 – 344.

Lynch, G. (1986) *Synapse, Circuits, and the Beginnings of Memory,* MIT press, Cambridge, MA.

Magistretti, P.J. (1990) VIP neurons in the cerebral cortex. *Trends Pharmacol. Sci.,* 11: 250 – 254.

Malhotra, R.K., Wakade, T.D. and Wakade, A.R. (1989) Cross-communication between acetylcholine and VIP in controlling catecholamine secretion by affecting cAMP, inositol triphosphate, protein kinase C, and calcium in rat adrenal medulla. *J. Neurosci.,* 9: 4150 – 4157.

Mattson, M.P., Murrain, M., Guthrie, P.B. and Kater, S.B. (1989) Fibroblast growth factor and glutamate: opposing roles in the generation and degeneration of hippocampal neuroarchitecture. *J. Neurosci.,* 9: 3728 – 3740.

McDonald, J.W. and Johnston, M.V. (1990) Physiological and pathophysiological roles of excitatory amino acids during central nervous system development. *Brain Res. Rev.,* 15: 41 – 70.

Morgan, J.I. and Curran, T. (1991) Stimulus-transcription coupling in the nervous system: involvement of the inducible proto-oncogenes *fos* and *jun. Annu. Rev. Neurosci.,* 14: 421 – 451.

Morris, R.G.M., Anderson, E., Lynch, G.S. and Baudry, M. (1986) Selective impairment of learning and blockade of long-term potentiation by an *N*-methyl-D-aspartate receptor antagonist AP5. *Nature,* 319: 774 – 776.

Morrison, R.S., Sharma, A., deVellis, J. and Bradshaw, R.A. (1986) Basic fibroblast growth factor supports the survival of cerebral cortical neurons in primary culture. *Proc. Natl. Acad. Sci. U.S.A.,* 83: 7537 – 7541.

Onodera, H., Kogure, K., Ono, Y., Igarashi, K., Kiyota, Y. and Nagaoka, A. (1989) Proto-oncogene c-*fos* is transiently induced in the rat cerebral cortex after forebrain ischemia. *Neurosci. Lett.,* 98: 101 – 104.

Peters, S., Koh, J. and Choi, D.W. (1987) Zinc selectively blocks the action of *N*-methyl-D-aspartate on cortical neurons. *Science,* 236: 589 – 593.

Pincus, D.W., DiCicco-Bloom, E.M. and Black, I.B. (1990) Vasoactive intestinal peptide regulates mitosis, differentiation and survival of cultured sympathetic neuroblasts. *Nature,* 343: 564 – 567.

Rothman, S.M. (1983) Synaptic activity mediates death of hypoxic neurons. *Science,* 220: 536 – 537.

Rothman, S.M. (1984) Synaptic release of excitatory amino acid neurotransmitter mediates anoxic neuronal death. *J. Neurosci.,* 4: 1884 – 1891.

Ryazanov, A.G., Shestakova, E.A. and Natapov, P.G. (1988) Phosphorylation of elongation factor 2 by EF-2 kinase affects rate of translation. *Nature,* 334: 170 – 173.

Sagar, S.M. and Sharp, F.R. (1990) Light induces a Fos-like nuclear antigen in retinal neurons. *Mol. Brain Res.,* 7: 17 – 21.

Sagar, S.M., Sharp, F.R. and Curran, T. (1988) Expression of c-*fos* protein in brain: metabolic mapping at the cellular level. *Science,* 240: 1328 – 1331.

Schmidt-Kastner, R. and Freund, T.F. (1991) Selective vulnerability of the hippocampus in brain ischemia. *Neuroscience,* 40: 599 – 636.

Sharp, F.R., Gonzalez, M.F., Hisanaga, K., Mobley, W.C. and Sagar, S.M. (1989a) Induction of the c-*fos* gene product in rat forebrain following cortical lesions and NGF injections. *Neurosci. Lett.,* 100: 117 – 122.

Sharp, F.R., Gonzalez, M.F., Sharp, J.W. and Sagar, S.M. (1989b) C-*fos* expression and [^{14}C] 2-deoxyglucose uptake in the caudal cerebellum of the rat during motor/sensory cortex stimulation. *J. Comp. Neurol.,* 284: 621 – 636.

Sharp, F.R., Griffith, J., Gonzalez, M.F. and Sagar, S.M. (1989c) Trigeminal nerve section induces Fos-like immunoreactivity (FLI) in brain-stem and decreases FLI in sensory cortex. *Mol. Brain Res.,* 6: 217 – 220.

Sharp, F.R., Sagar, S.M., Hicks, K., Lowenstein, D. and Hisanaga, K. (1991) c-*fos* mRNA, Fos, and Fos-related antigen induction by hypertonic saline and stress. *J. Neurosci.,* 11: 2321 – 2331.

Sharp, J.W., Sagar, S.M., Hisanaga, K., Jasper, P. and Sharp, F.R. (1990) The NMDA receptor mediates cortical induction of *fos* and *fos*-related antigens following cortical injury. *Exp. Neurol.,* 109: 323 – 332.

Shigeno, T., Mima, T., Takakura, K., Graham, D.I., Kato, G., Hashimoto, Y. and Furukawa, S. (1991) Amelioration of delayed neuronal death in the hippocampus by nerve growth factor. *J. Neurosci.,* 11: 2914 – 2919.

Siman, R. and Noszek, J.C. (1988) Excitatory amino acids activate calpain I and induce structural protein breakdown in vivo. *Neuron,* 1: 279 – 287.

Simon, R.P., Swan, J.H., Griffiths, T. and Meldrum, B.S. (1984) Blockade of *N*-methyl-D-aspartate receptors may protect against ischemic damage in the brain. *Science,* 226: 850 – 852.

Sonnenberg, J.L., Mitchelmore, C., Macgregor-Leon, P.F., Hempstead, J., Morgan, J.I. and Curran, T. (1989) Glutamate receptor agonists increase the expression of Fos, Fra, and AP-1 DNA binding activity in the mammalian brain. *J. Neurosci. Res.,* 24: 72 – 80.

Szekely, A.M., Barbaccia, M.L. and Costa, E. (1987) Activation of specific glutamate receptor subtypes increases c-*fos* proto-oncogene expression in primary cultures of neonatal rat cerebellar granule cells. *Neuropharmacology,* 26: 1779 – 1782.

Szekely, A.M., Barbaccia, M.L., Alho, H. and Costa, E. (1989) In primary cultures of cerebellar granule cells the activation of *N*-methyl-D-aspartate-sensitive glutamate receptors induces c-*fos* mRNA expression. *Mol. Pharmacol.,* 35: 401 – 408.

Takeda, A., Onodera, H., Yamasaki, Y., Furukawa, K., Kogure, K., Obinata, M. and Shibahara, S. (1992) Decreased expression of neurotrophin-3 mRNA in the rat hippocampus following transient forebrain ischemia. *Brain Res.,* 569: 177 – 180.

Walicke, P., Cowan, W.M., Ueno, N., Baird, A. and Guillemin, R. (1986) Fibroblast growth factor promotes survival of dissociated hippocampal neurons and enhances neurite extension. *Proc. Natl. Acad. Sci. U.S.A.,* 83: 3012 – 3016.

Westbrook, G.L. and Mayer, M.L. (1987) Micromolar concentrations of Zn^{2+} antagonize NMDA and GABA responses of hippocampal neurons. *Nature,* 328: 640 – 643.

Yamada, K., Kinoshita, A., Kohmura, E., Sakaguchi, T., Taguchi, J., Kataoka, K. and Hayakawa, T. (1991) Basic fibroblast growth factor prevents thalamic degeneration after cortical infarction. *J. Cereb. Blood Flow Metab.,* 11: 472 – 478.

Yokoyama, M., Koh, J. and Choi, D.W. (1986) Brief exposure

to zinc is toxic to cortical neurons. *Neurosci. Lett.*, 71: 351 – 355.

Zafra, F., Castrén, E., Thoenen, H. and Lindholm, D. (1991) Interplay between glutamate and γ-aminobutyric acid transmitter systems in the physiological regulation of brain-derived neurotrophic factor and nerve growth factor synthesis in hippocampal neurons. *Proc. Natl. Acad. Sci. U.S.A.*, 88: 10037 – 10041.

K. Kogure, K.-A. Hossmann and B.K. Siesjö (Eds.)
Progress in Brain Research, Vol. 96

CHAPTER 15

Selective gene expression after brain ischemia

Koji Abe and Kyuya Kogure

Department of Neurology, Institute of Brain Diseases, Tohoku University School of Medicine, Sendai, Japan

Introduction

Eukaryotic genes are regulated differentially in response to a complex set of environmental and developmental conditions (Struhl, 1989). An essential part of gene expression is the binding of a regulatory protein (transcription factor) to the recognition sequence of the appropriate gene (Klug and Rhodes, 1987). A novel protein motif for nucleic acid recognition (called "zinc finger") has been recognized as one such transcription factor, which is induced in response to a mitogenic stimulus in cultured cells and an electrical stimulation in rat hippocampus (Klug and Rhodes, 1987; Sukhatme et al., 1987; Struhl, 1989; Wisden et al., 1990). A recent study suggests a possible relationship between induction of a transcription factor gene and heat shock protein (HSP) 70 gene (Kingston et al., 1984).

HSP70 is induced by stress such as with heat shock, ischemia, trauma or surgical wounding (Nowak, 1985; Kiessling et al., 1986; Fujino et al., 1987; Lindquist, 1988; Parde, 1988; Abe et al., 1991c). HSP70 may afford cytoprotection (Pelham, 1989) and its induction precedes the recovery of normal protein synthesis (Nowak, 1985). Cells injected with an antibody against HSP70 become more susceptible to the lethal effects of heat shock treatment (Riabowl et al., 1988). COS cells recover from heat shock more rapidly than usual when cells are transfected with a plasmid that constitutively expresses HSP70, even when synthesis of other heat shock proteins is blocked (Pelham, 1984). Moreover, hyperthermia increases the production of heat shock protein and attenuates the susceptibility of rat retinal photoreceptor cells to light-induced damage (Barbe et al., 1988).

Amyloid β-protein is a core component of senile plaques in Alzheimer's disease brain, and is derived from a larger precursor protein (amyloid precursor protein, APP) (Kang et al., 1987; Kitaguchi et al., 1988; Ponte et al., 1988; Tanzi et al., 1988). It is well known that messenger RNA (mRNA) for APP is distributed ubiquitously in human organs with some preferential distribution between three different sizes of APP mRNA (Neve et al., 1988), namely APP695, APP751 and APP770 mRNAs, encoding 695, 751 and 770 amino acid precursors, respectively. APP751 and APP770 differ from APP695 by a 56 amino acid residue domain which exhibits 50% homology with the Kunitz family of serine protease inhibitor (KPI). These different types of APP mRNAs are produced by alternative splicing of the premature APP gene transcripts (Kitaguchi et al., 1988). Regional differences in the amount between APP695 mRNA and APP751/770 mRNA within brain and non-neuronal tissues have been indicated (Lewis et al., 1987; Higgins et al., 1988; Neve et al., 1988; Weidermann et al., 1989). APPs which have the KPI domain, i.e., APP751 and APP770, have been shown to be protease nexin-II involving a regulation of a chymotrypsin-like protease (Van Nostrand et al., 1987). However, the exact role of

Abbreviations: APP, amyloid precursor protein; HSC, heat shock cognate protein; HSP, heat shock protein; KPI, Kunitz-type serine protease inhibitor.

each APP species has not been fully understood (Neve, 1989; Whitson et al., 1989; Yanker et al., 1989).

Brief periods of global ischemia (even for 5 min) causes cell death in hippocampal CA1 pyramidal neurons days after reperfusion. Other neurons such as parietal cortical neurons or hippocampal CA3 neurons are much less vulnerable (Kirino, 1982; Pulsinelli et al., 1982). The cause of delayed neuronal damage is not fully elucidated although many putative mechanisms have been proposed (Wieloch, 1985; Imdall and Hossmann, 1986; Rothman and Olney, 1986; Westerberg et al., 1987; Vass et al., 1988; Xie et al., 1989). Energy metabolism recovers rapidly (Arai et al., 1982), whereas protein synthesis does not (Bodsch et al., 1985). The disaggregation of polysomes in CA1 cells is among the earliest pathological findings (Petito and Pulsinelli, 1984; Nowak, 1985; Dwyer et al., 1986). An immunohistochemical examination recently showed that HSP70 protein staining is much lower in the CA1 than in the CA3 neurons or cortical neurons following transient ischemia (Vass et al., 1988).

Expression of immunoreactive APP has recently been reported in reactive astrocytes following neuronal damage by an intraventricular injection of kainic acid in rats (Siman et al., 1989). However, it is not known whether certain species of APP were induced selectively by neuronal damage (Siman et al., 1989). The promotor area of APP gene has been cloned (Salbaum et al., 1988), and a role of heat shock response was suggested in an induction of APP.

Cerebral ischemia is a simple model to give a stress to the nervous system and to change signal transduction, growth regulation and neuronal differentiation (Kogure, 1988), which should activate some transcription factors and induce HSP70 (Nowak, 1985; Dienel et al., 1986; Sukhatme et al., 1987; Kogure, 1988; Jørgensen et al., 1989; Abe et al., 1991b), or APP gene expression (Siman et al., 1989; Abe et al., 1991d). Therefore, we attempted to examine possible inductions of the "zinc finger" gene and HSP70 gene after transient focal ischemia in rat cerebral cortex, of APP mRNA with a treatment of heat shock in human lymphoblastoid cell lines, and of specific APP mRNA species in relation to the induction of HSP70 in a persistent occlusion model of middle cerebral artery (MCA) of rats.

Materials and methods

Rat experiments

For the analysis of a transient focal ischemia, a model of MCA occlusion using a microembolus of nylon thread was used (Abe et al., 1988a,b). During the surgical preparation for MCA occlusion, male rats of Wistar strain, weighing 250 – 280 g, were lightly anesthetized by inhalation of a nitrous oxide/oxygen/halothane (69%: 30%: 1%) mixture. When the animals began to awake after discontinuing the anesthesia, the origin of the right MCA was occluded for 30 min by insertion of a nylon thread via the common carotid artery. After 30 min of ischemia, the nylon thread was removed and the animals recovered for 1, 3 and 8 h or 1, 2 and 7 days until decapitation. Sham control animals were treated with cervical surgery, but without the following insertion of nylon thread. Body temperature was monitored in all animals, and was maintained at 37°C using a heat pad during the surgical preparation, and the occlusion of MCA. After reperfusion, no attempt was made to maintain body temperature constant. The animals recovered in the room at 22 – 25°C. At the end of the reperfusion, rats were decapitated and the center of the cortex of the occluded MCA area was dissected for Northern analysis. After the dissection, the brains were quickly frozen in liquid nitrogen, and stored at – 80°C until extraction of RNA. Samples from five animals were combined in each time point to yield about 800 mg of each group. The amounts of "zinc finger" coding mRNA, HSP70 mRNA, and tubulin mRNA were examined in the above brains.

Total RNA was extracted by the modified method of Chomczynski and Sacchi (1987) (the RNA isolation kit by Stratagene, CA, U.S.A.) using guanidine isothiocyanate. Northern blot analyses for hybridization were performed by the method of

Maniatis et al. (1982). RNAs were separated in a denaturing agarose gel (1.2%, W/V) containing 0.5 M formaldehyde. Three probes for zinc finger, HSP70 (pH2.3, Wu et al., 1985), and tubulin (Lemishka et al., 1981) mRNAs were used against Northern blot. An oligonucleotide probe of unique sequence for the detection of zinc finger mRNA was synthesized on a MilliGen DNA synthesizer (Cyclon Plus). The probe sequence for zinc finger was 45 mer which is complimentary to nucleotides spanning amino acids 2–16 (Milbrandt, 1987) 5′-CCGTTGCTCAGCAGCATCATCTCCTCCAG TTTGGGGTAGTTGTCC-3′. This probe was 3′ end-labeled using terminal deoxynucleotidyl transferase (Pharmacia LKB) and a 30:1 molar ratio of radiolabeled ATP:oligonucleotide. The synthetic oligonucleotide was radiolabeled with [a-^{32}P] dATP (6000 Ci/mmol, Amersham). The blot was hybridized with the oligonucleotide (10 pg/μl) at 42°C for 20 h in a buffer containing formamide (50% formamide, 5 × SSC, 5 × Denhardt's solution, 100 μg/ml fish sperm DNA, 50 mM KPO_4 and 0.2% SDS). The membrane was washed to a final stringency of 1 × SSC (1 × SSC = 150 mM NaCl + 15 mM Na_3-citrate) + 0.2% SDS (sodium dodecyl sulfate) at 55°C. The filter was exposed to Kodak X-ray film for 20 h at −80°C. The filter was then stripped off the radiolabeled oligonucleotide by an incubation with 0.2% SDS solution at 65°C to then hybridize with the probe for HSP70. The human genomic DNA probe for HSP70 was radiolabeled with ^{32}P by a random primer labeling using Klenow fragment of *E. coli* DNA polymerase I, and hybridized against Northern blot (total counts = 6 × 10^6 cpm/ml) at 42°C for 20 h in the same hybridizing solution as above. After hybridization, the filter was washed with 2 × SSC + 0.2% SDS at room temperature, then washed again with 0.1 × SSC + 0.2% SDS at 65°C. The filter was exposed to X-ray film, and then hybridized with radiolabeled cDNA probe for tubulin. The amount of tubulin mRNA was measured as an internal standard.

For the analysis of a persistent focal ischemia, Long Evans rats (male, 250–300 g) were anesthetized by intraperitoneal injection of ketamine (80 mg/kg) and intramuscular injection of xylazine (6 mg/kg). Body temperature was monitored by a rectal probe and maintained at 37 ± 0.5°C using a homothermic blanket control unit. Focal ischemia was produced using the method of Chen et al. (1986). The right MCA was exposed and ligated at two points, and then cut between them. Just after the ligation of MCA, bilateral common carotid arteries were occluded with small aneurysmal clips for 1 h. After the removal of the clips, the animals recovered until decapitation without any attempt to maintain body temperature constant. Three animals each were sacrificed at 0 (sham control), 1, 2, 4 and 8 h and 1, 2, 4, 7 and 21 days after the MCA ligation. Immediately after decapitation, the rat brains were cut on ice, and the ipsilateral sensorimotor cortex was carefully dissected to avoid contamination of adjacent structures such as ependymal cells. The cerebellar hemispheres were also dissected for the control. The dissections were completed within 3 min, the tissue samples were then quickly frozen in liquid nitrogen, and stored at −80°C until extraction of RNA. Samples from the three animals were combined to yield 100–200 mg cortex and 300–400 mg cerebellum at each time point.

Total RNA was extracted in the same way as above. A part of cDNA encoding the KPI domain of APP was excised from the original cDNA clone (HL124, Tanzi et al., 1988), and was cloned into a plasmid vector Bluescript SK$^-$ (Stratagene, CA, U.S.A.) as a 122 bp insert with *Hae* III arms. This cDNA insert was cut from the vector by *BamH* I/*Pst* I digestion as a 137 bp insert (pKunBS) in a low melt agarose gel, radiolabeled with ^{32}P and hybridized. After hybridization, the filter was washed with 2 × SSC + 0.1% SDS at room temperature, then washed again with 1 × SSC + 0.1% SDS at room temperature in the case of the KunBS probe. The filter was exposed to Kodak X-ray film for 20 h at −80°C. The filter was then stripped of the radiolabeled KunBS probe by incubation with 0.2% SDS solution at 65°C for hybridization with the probes against FB68L (for total APP, Tanzi et al.,

1988), HSP70 and tubulin (Lemishka et al., 1981) in that order. In the cases of FB68L, HSP70 and tubulin probes, the filter was finally washed with 0.5 × SSC + 0.1% SDS at 65°C. The FB68L probe recognizes all three APP mRNAs, while the KunBS probe recognizes only APP751/770 mRNAs which have a sequence coding the KPI domain.

Gerbil experiments

Mongolian gerbils (*Meriones unguiculatus*), aged 8 – 10 weeks and weighing 60 – 80 g, were lightly anesthetized by inhalation of a nitrous oxide/oxygen/halothane (69%: 30%: 1%) mixture (Abe et al., 1989) or ether. As the animal began to awake from anesthesia, both common carotid arteries were occluded for 10 min using surgical clips. The animals were maintained at room temperature (22 – 23°C) during the 10 min common carotid occlusion. The clips were then removed and the animals recovered for 1, 4 and 8 h and 1, 2, 7 or 21 days until decapitation. Sham animals were sacrificed just after exposing the carotid arteries without clamping the vessels. Animals were excluded if they developed seizures or neurological findings. Immediately after decapitation, the gerbil brains were cut on ice while being careful to avoid contamination by adjacent structures reported to normally produce HSP70 protein such as ependyma (Vass et al., 1988). The brains were cut in the coronal plane (2 mm thickness) through the hippocampal formation. The cortex and overlying ependymal layer were removed. The hippocampus was then divided in the sagittal plane just medial to the junction of CA1 and CA2. The CA1 sector was isolated by horizontal section. The sample containing CA2 and CA3 was divided horizontally into a superior (CA2) and an inferior (CA3) segment. The tissues containing parietal cortex, area CA3 or area CA1 were pooled from the two hemispheres. The dissections were completed within 3 min, and the tissue samples were quickly frozen in liquid nitrogen, and stored at – 80°C until extraction of RNA. Samples from ten animals were combined (cortex 300 – 500 mg; CA1 area 40 – 80 mg; CA3 area 20 – 40 mg, at each time point). The amounts of HSP70, APP and tubulin mRNAs were examined in the above brains and brains of unanesthetized normal gerbils.

Total RNA was extracted in the same way as above. Four probes, HSP70 gene (pH2.3), FB68L (for total APP), pKunBS (for KPI) andα-tubulin gene (Lemishka et al., 1981), were used against the Northern blot. The HSP70 probe (pH2.3) can hybridize both HSP70 mRNA and HS cognate protein (HSC) 70 mRNA (Dworniczak and Mirault, 1987) under these hybridizing and washing conditions (Abe et al., 1991b,c). Filters were exposed to Kodak X-ray film for 20 h at – 80°C.

Human lymphoblastoid cells

Human lymphoblastoid cell lines were established by EB virus transformation from lymphocytes of twelve individuals (age-matched, six males and six females, 57.8 ± 3.2 and 55.0 ± 4.7 (mean age ± S.D.) respectively) who do not have neurological or other major disorders. Cell lines were cultured in RPMI1640 medium with 20% fetal calf serum (Gibco, MD, U.S.A.) supplemented with ampicillin (100 IU/ml) and streptomycin (100 μg/ml) in a CO_2 incubator (5% CO_2) at 37°C. Once the cells became confluent (about 10^6 cells/ml) in 200 ml media in a large flask, the medium was exchanged for new medium. The cell suspension was thoroughly mixed by pipeting, and was divided into 30 ml aliquots in six small flasks (50 ml). The cells in small flasks were kept at 37°C in the CO_2 incubator overnight before the treatment with heat shock. On the next day, five of the six small flasks were taken out of the CO_2 incubator to be treated with heat shock (one flask was left for the control study). The caps of the flasks were quickly closed tight to avoid losing CO_2 during the heat shock treatment, and were then put in an iron cage which was pre-heated in a water bath at 42°C. The cage containing the culture flasks was immersed in the water bath at 42°C for 30 min. No shaking was performed during the incubation. A pilot study showed that it takes 5 – 6 min for the temperature of the culture media to increase from 37°C to 42°C. After the heat shock treatment, the cage was lifted from the water bath. The caps of the flasks were made loose again, and the flasks were quickly returned to the CO_2 incubator. The cells recovered in the incubator at 37°C for 1, 3, 8, 24 and 48 h after the heat shock treatment. An examination by trypan blue staining showed no significant loss of cell viability until two days after the treatment (data not shown). At the end of recovery, the flask was removed from the incubator, and the cell suspension was transferred into a 50 ml conical bottom tube (Falcon nr. 2070), and cells were collected by centrifugation at 1000 × *g* for 5 min at 4°C. The supernatant was aspirated off and the tube was quickly immersed in liquid nitrogen to freeze the cells inside the tube. The frozen cells in the tubes were kept at −80°C until extraction of RNA. Cells for the control were collected and frozen simultaneously without heat shock treatment.

Total RNA was extracted in the same way as above. Three probes for APP gene (FB68L), HSP70 gene (pH2.3) and actin gene (American Type Culture Collection nr. 57059; Gunning et al., 1984), were used against the Northern blot. The cDNA probe for APP (1.1 Kb *Eco* RI insert of FB68L plasmid) was radiolabeled with ^{32}P. After hybridization, the filter was washed with 2 × SSC + 0.1% SDS at room temperature, then washed again with 0.5 × SSC + 0.1% SDS at 65°C. Filters were exposed to Kodak X-ray film for 20 h at −80°C. The filter was then stripped of the radiolabeled APP probe by incubation with a 0.2% SDS solution (containing 5 mM Tris-HCl, pH 8.0, 2 mM Na_2EDTA, and 0.1 × Denhardt's solution as recommended by Amersham) at 65°C and hybridized with the probes for HSP70 and actin in that order.

Densitometric analysis was performed by Ultroscan Laser XL (Pharmacia LKB, NJ, U.S.A.). Comparisons of experimental and control values of densitometric analyses of autoradiograms were made with a non-parametrical test such as the Wilcoxon rank-sum (Wilcoxon's *U*) test.

Results

Rat experiments

As shown in Fig. 1, the zinc finger mRNA is present in the cerebral cortex of sham control rats. It is induced by transient ischemia with a maximum at 1 h after the reperfusion. For 8−48 h after the reperfusion, the amount of the zinc finger mRNA decreased as compared with the amount in the sham control. However, the amount recovered by seven days after the reperfusion. The experiment of zinc finger gene expression was repeated using an additional five animals, and the result was reproducible (data not shown). The level of mRNA in cells is regulated by the balance of its synthesis and degradation. The transient increase of zinc finger-coding mRNA shown in this experiment may be due to an increasing synthesis or a result of post-transcriptional regulation (decreased degradation), or both. Even though our results did not show which mechanism contributed to the transient increase of this mRNA, it is still of interest that the level of this mRNA transiently increased at 1 h and decreased for a long time (from 8 h to at least two days of reperfusion). In contrast, HSP70 mRNA is not pres-

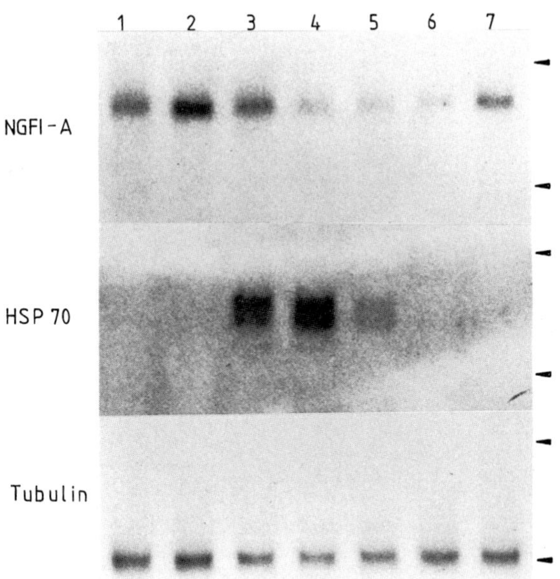

Fig. 1. Autoradiograms of Northern blot analyses show changes of gene expressions of zinc finger (NGFI-A), HSP70 and tubulin. 1, 2, 3, 4, 5, 6 and 7 represent the case of sham control, 1, 3 and 8 h, 1, 2 and 7 days of reperfusion, respectively, after 30 min of transient focal ischemia of rat cerebral cortex. Each lane contains 15 μg of total RNA, and arrowheads indicate 28s and 18s ribosomal RNAs.

ent in the group of sham control (Fig. 1). However, it is also induced by a transient ischemia with a maximum at 8 h after the reperfusion. The amount of HSP70 mRNA became undetectable by two days after the reperfusion. Although the probe for HSP70 mRNA used in this experiment (pH2.3) detects only one size of mRNA which codes inducible HSP70 species in humans (Wu et al., 1985; Abe et al., 1991a), the same probe detects two different sizes of mRNA for HSP70 (2.8 Kb and 3.0 Kb) in rats using the hybridization and washing conditions applied in this experiment (Abe et al., 1991c). A synthetic oligonucleotide which selectively detects inducible species of the HSP70 family mRNA also detected two closely spaced doublets of inducible mRNA in rats (Marini et al., 1990). The two sizes of mRNA for HSP70 changed almost in the same manner after ischemia. The level of tubulin mRNA showed a small decrease at 3 – 24 h.

As shown in Fig. 2, both HSP70 mRNA and APP mRNA which encodes the KPI domain ("KPI" in the figure) were induced, while the total amount of APP ("Total APP" in the figure) did not change. APP mRNA which encodes the KPI domain began to increase after one day, reaching a maximum at four days, and then decreased but remained elevated for as long as 21 days. Because the amount of APP695 mRNA is much higher than that of APP751/770 mRNA, the induction of APP751/770 mRNAs does not contribute significantly to the change of total APP mRNA. The amount of total APP and KPI-containing APP mRNAs did not shown significant changes in the cerebellum (Fig. 2). Induction was not observed in the level of tubulin mRNA in the cerebral cortex and the cerebellum.

The ^{32}P-labeled HSP70 probe hybridized to three different sizes of mRNA corresponding to 3.0 Kb, 2.8 Kb and 2.4 Kb. The 3.0 Kb and 2.8 Kb mRNAs correspond to HSP70 mRNA which is the major inducible species among the HSP70 family, while the smallest message corresponds to HS cognate protein (HSC) 70 mRNA which is constitutively expressed

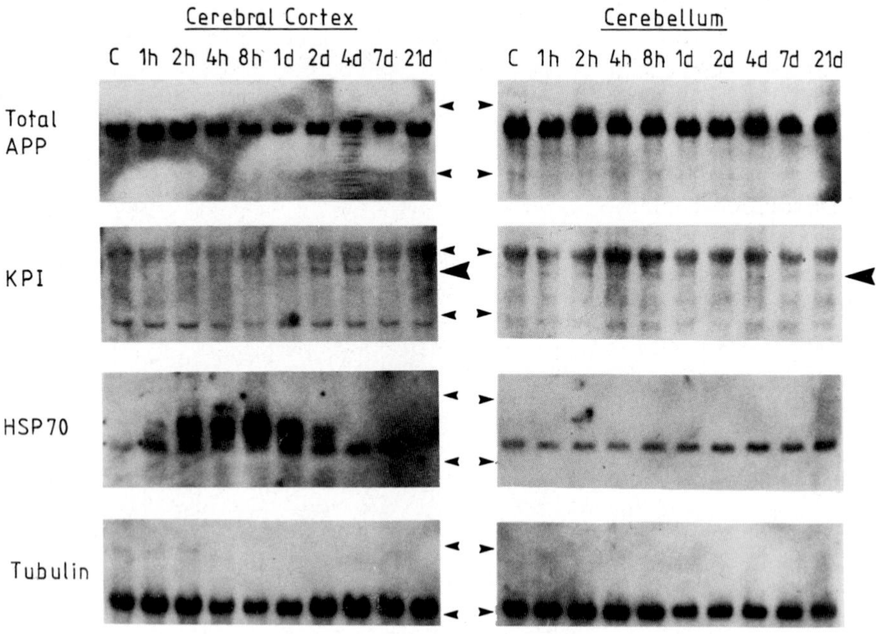

Fig. 2. Northern blot analyses of APP, HSP70 and tubulin mRNAs in rat cerebral cortex (the territory of the occluded MCA) and cerebellum at 1 – 8 h and 1 – 21 days after the occlusion of unilateral middle cerebral artery. C represents the sham control. Small arrowheads represent ribosomal RNAs. The large arrowheads represent APP mRNAs which have the KPI domain. The weak signals just below the 18s ribosomal RNA in KPI are the remaining signals of a former probe.

(Dworniczak and Mirault, 1987). In order to visualize changes more clearly, optical densities (OD) were determined from autoradiograms (Ultroscan XL Laser Densitometer, Pharmacia LKB, N.J., U.S.A.). After subtracting background, ODs were expressed as a ratio against the control value (Fig. 3). Optical densities of two different sizes of HSP70 mRNAs were combined because bands were sometimes too close to analyze individually by densitometry. Messenger RNAs for HSP70 reached a maximum at 8 h and then decreased. On the other hand, APP mRNA which encodes the KPI domain began to increase just after the peak of the induction of HSP70 mRNA, reaching a maximum at four days, and remained elevated for as long as 21 days.

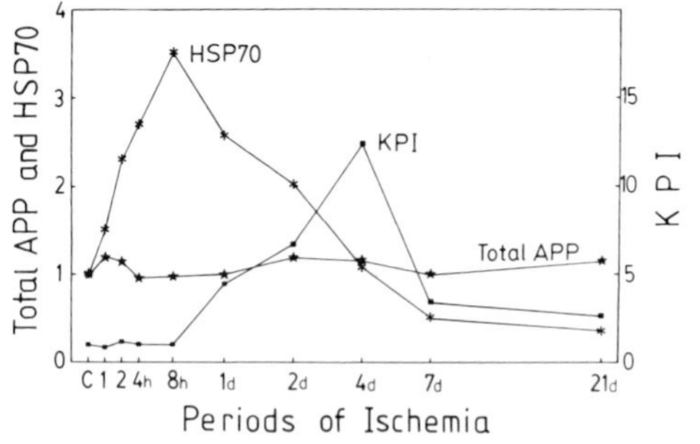

Fig. 3. Densitometric analysis of the change of optical densities expressed as ratio with the value of the sham control. Stars, asterisks and squares represent the changes of total APP mRNA, HSP70 mRNA or APP mRNA which encode the KPI domain, respectively.

Gerbil experiments

Analysis of Northern blots revealed hybridization of the ^{32}P-labeled HSP70 probe to two sizes of mRNA corresponding to 2.8 Kb and 2.4 Kb (Fig. 4). Based on the nature of the probe and the hybridizing conditions in this experiment (Wu et al., 1985; Abe et al., 1991b,c), the 2.8 Kb mRNA represents HSP70 mRNA, and the 2.4 Kb mRNA may correspond to HSC70 mRNA. In the control condition, CA1 cells had the highest amounts of HSP70 and HSC70 mRNAs, but the lowest amounts of APP and tubulin mRNAs, as compared with cortical cells or CA3 cells. With reperfusion, both HSP70 mRNA and HSC70 mRNA were induced. The levels of both HSP70 and HSC70 mRNAs reached a maximum at 8 h and then declined. The increase of HSP70 mRNA was relatively smaller in the CA1 cells than in the parietal cortical cells and CA3 cells at 8 h after reperfusion. After seven days, HSP70 expression in the CA1 and CA3 regions was below control levels.

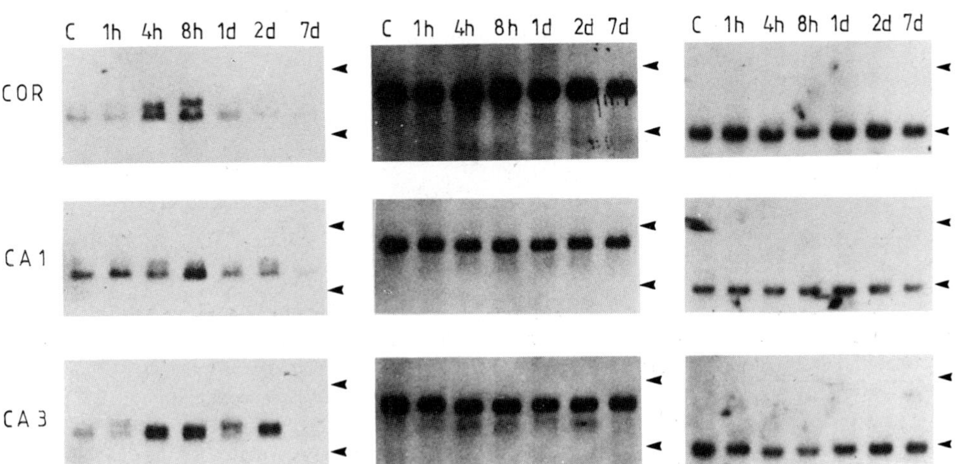

Fig. 4. Northern blot analyses of HSP70, APP and tubulin in the parietal cortex (COR), hippocampal CA1 (CA1), or CA3 (CA3) sectors at 1 – 8 h and 1 – 7 days of reperfusion after 10 min of ischemia. Each lane contains 15 μg of total RNA. C represents the sham control, and arrowheads represent 28s and 18s ribosomal RNAs.

The increase of HSP70 mRNA in the CA3 region occurred earlier, was larger and sustained longer than that in the parietal cortex. A careful examination of the results shows that the induction of HSP70 mRNA continued up to two days in CA1 cells, when the amount of the message in cortical cells already decreased below the level in CA1 cells. No significant induction was observed in the amount of APP mRNA or tubulin mRNA after ischemia.

As shown in Fig. 5, the amounts of total APP and KPI-containing APP mRNA did not change during 21 days of reperfusion after 10 min of transient forebrain ischemia, even though HSP70 mRNA was induced with a maximum at 8 h.

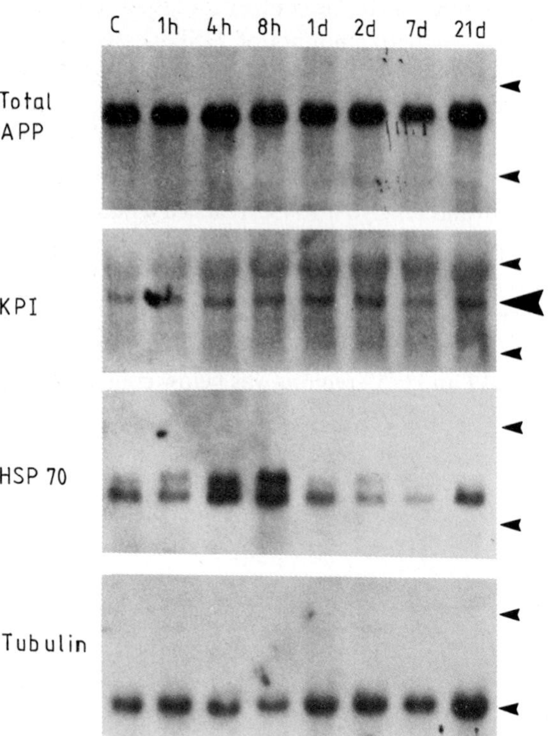

Fig. 5. Northern blot analyses of APP, HSP70 and tubulin in gerbil cerebral cortex after 10 min of transient forebrain ischemia. The probe FB68L recognizes total amount of APP mRNA (Total APP). The KunBS probe recognizes APP751/770 mRNAs (KPI). Each lane contained 15 μg of total RNA. C represents the sham control. Small arrowheads represent ribosomal RNAs. The large arrow head represents APP mRNAs which have KPI domain. Amounts of messages at 21 days look relatively greater than control level, probably because of greater amount of loading of RNA.

Human lymphoblastoid cells

APP and actin mRNAs are expressed in the control condition (Fig. 6). However, HSP70 mRNA is not present in a detectable level in the control condition. HSP70 mRNA was induced at 1 h and 3 h after the heat shock treatment, which again became undetectable at 8 h. APP mRNA level also increased after the heat shock treatment at 3 and 8 h. Statistical analyses indicate an increase of about 40 – 60% of this mRNA level, and there was no significant difference in the induction between males and females (Table I). The level of APP mRNA transiently decreased by a small amount at 24 h, then recovered to the steady level at 48 h (Table I).

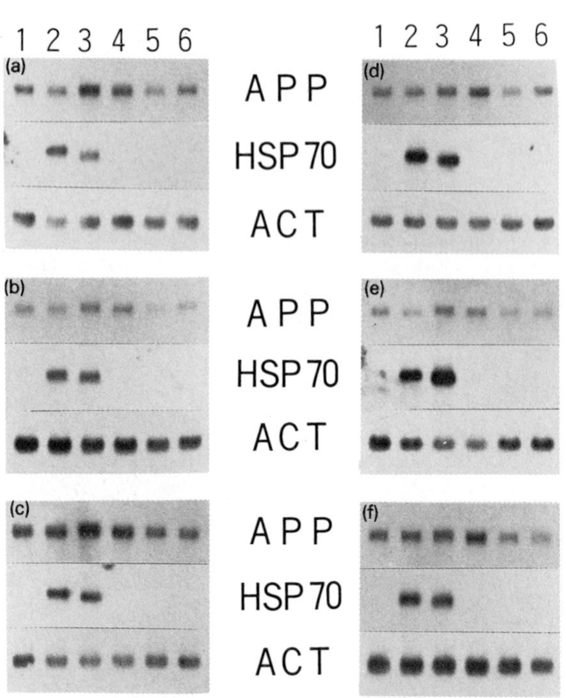

Fig. 6. Autoradiograms of Northern blots for APP, HSP70 and actin (ACT) in cultured lymphoblastoid cells show inductions of APP mRNA and HSP70 mRNA after 30 min of heat shock treatment at 42° C. The results of six individuals out of 12 are shown in this figure. a, b, c, d, e and f represent the cases of each individual. Densitometric analyses of all the individuals (12 cases) are summarized in the Table I. 1, 2, 3, 4, 5 and 6 represent the case of control, and the cases of 1, 3, 8, 24, and 48 h after the heat shock treatment, respectively. Each lane contained 15 μg of total RNA.

TABLE I

Changes of gene expression of APP mRNA in lymphoblastoid cells after heat shock treatment

Period	Male (n = 6)	Female (n = 6)
Control	100.0 ± 0.0	100.0 ± 0.0
1 h	104.9 ± 17.1	90.4 ± 9.7
3 h	161.2 ± 30.3*	144.6 ± 17.2*
8 h	149.3 ± 12.6*	162.6 ± 32.4*
24 h	85.9 ± 4.8*	85.8 ± 11.3*
48 h	92.9 ± 9.0	98.5 ± 9.8

Subjects were age-matched: six males (57.8 ± 3.2, mean age ± S.D.) and six females (55.0 ± 4.7). Optical densities (O.D.) were measured using a densitometer. Data are expressed as mean ± S.D. of % O.D. of the control. 1, 3, 8, 24 and 48 h represent the hours after 30 min of the heat shock treatment.
* $P < 0.05$ against the control.

Discussion

Zinc finger gene expression

A new protein motif for binding DNA and RNA has emerged, conveniently called the "zinc finger". It was originally discovered to be present in tandem in the *Xenopus* transcription factor IIIA (TFIIIA), but it is now known that it is ubiquitous among species and cells (Klug and Rhodes, 1987). Milbrandt first found that the zinc finger gene is induced by nerve growth factor (so called NGFI-A; nerve growth factor inducible protein-A), and it may serve as a possible transcriptional regulatory factor (Milbrandt, 1987). It is now recognized that the zinc finger gene is one of several transcription factors, and it utilizes the "zinc finger" motif to bind nucleic acid, just as in the case of jun/fos/myc oncoproteins which utilize the "leucine zipper" motif for DNA binding (Struhl, 1989). Recent important findings on the role of the zinc finger gene are that deregulated expression of this gene contributes to retroviral-mediated malignant transformation of cells (Wright et al., 1990) and that this gene is homozygously deleted in Wilms tumor which is an autosomal recessive childhood nephroblastoma (Gessler et al., 1990). These data suggest a crucial role of this gene in cell growth regulation and differentiation. Neuronal cells may require changes of gene expression in the recovery process from a transient ischemic stress (Kogure, 1988; Abe et al., 1989, 1991b) to adapt metabolic responses of neuronal cells after ischemia or to achieve a specific neuronal plasticity to integrate a post-ischemic neuronal network (Sheng and Greenberg, 1990). The transient increase of zinc finger-coding mRNA after ischemia observed in this study may reflect one aspect of such rearrangement of gene expression of neuronal cells in the brain.

A recent study suggests that c-*myc* gene products enhance HSP70 gene expression (Kingston et al., 1984). c-*fos* proto-oncogene was transiently induced in the hippocampus or cerebral cortex after transient ischemia of rat forebrain (Jørgensen et al., 1989; Onodera et al., 1989). Both c-*myc* and c-*fos* proteins are part of transcription factors which utilize the "leucine zipper" for DNA binding. However, no report has shown whether the zinc finger gene, another type of transcription factor, may regulate HSP70 gene expression. Of course, our results are not direct evidence of this putative relationship. However, it can be said that the expression of zinc finger gene occurred earlier than the induction of HSP70 after ischemia. Further studies are required to clarify the possible relationship.

Our results suggest that an early nuclear response occurs before HSP70 induction begins after transient focal ischemia in rat brain.

HSP70 gene expression

The relatively high level of HSC70 mRNA expression found normally in the hippocampal CA1 region suggests an active turnover of clathrin in this area. HSC70 gene is constitutively expressed in normal development and differentiation in cells (Dwornicзak and Mirault, 1987). Clathrin forms a coat of pinocytotic vesicle in the cell (Flaherty et al., 1990). HSC70 participates in the disassembly of the clathrin cage and involves intracellular transportation. The induction of HSC70 mRNA found in this experiment may relate to the induction of immunoreactive clathrin in this area (Yoshimi et al.,

1990), suggesting a role for clathrin in the selective neuronal damage of CA1 cells.

Reperfusion is associated with large increases in HSP70 mRNA expression in cortex and CA3 whereas a less dramatic increase developed in CA1. It is presumed that the observed changes occurred principally within neurons since immunohistochemical staining for HSP70 following ischemia failed to show significantly the presence of this protein in glia or vascular elements (Vass et al., 1988). The continuous elevation of HSP70 mRNA in CA1 cells suggests that CA1 cells are under continuous stressful conditions after reperfusion (Wieloch, 1985). However, the lower mRNA levels at 4 and 8 h in CA1 cells than in cortical cells suggest a limitation of the induction of the mRNA in these cells (Theodorakis and Morimoto, 1987). An impairment of protein ubiquitination has been shown immunohistochemically in rat hippocampal CA1 neurons after an ischemic insult (Magnusson and Wieloch, 1989). Taken together with our results, this is of interest because CA1 cells do not produce enough HSP70 mRNA and ubiquitin after ischemia although both are essential in stress response. The relatively high levels of HSP70 mRNA expression found normally in the hippocampal CA1 region may relate to the existence of a dense glutamatergic innervation (Lynch and Baudry, 1984; Wieloch, 1985) and tonic activation of NMDA receptors by ambient glutamate (Sah et al., 1989). In fact, a close relationship between excitotoxic stress and HSP70 induction has been indicated (Uney et al., 1988; Vass et al., 1989).

Recent studies indicate that activation of HSP70 gene is limited by the release of an initiated RNA polymerase transcription complex into productive elongation (McClure, 1985; McKnight and Tjian, 1986; Roberts, 1988; Rougvie and Lis, 1989). RNA polymerase II itself could be the target of transcription factors such as heat shock factor (HSF) or the target of hypothetical proteins which inhibit RNA polymerase II activity (Zimario and Wu, 1986). The recent identification of a heat-labile protein which stabilizes HSP70 mRNA in human cells (Theodorakis and Morimoto, 1987) suggests the possibility that posttranscriptional mechanisms regulate heat shock gene expression as well.

An overload of calcium has been reported in CA1 neurons after brief ischemia (Dienel, 1984; Sakamoto et al., 1986; Deshpande et al., 1987). Although treatment with calcium ionophore induces transcription of HSP70 gene, a massive calcium influx to the cell may also inhibit transcription of this gene (Roos et al., 1986; Lee, 1987; Laverriere et al., 1988). However, low transcription in CA1 cells begins far earlier (already at 3 h, Fig. 4) than the start of a massive influx of extracellular calcium into the CA1 cells (at 8 h, Sakamoto et al., 1986). This suggests that the initial exposure to a light calcium overload which recovers within 2 h of reperfusion (Tsuda et al., 1989) may prevent a sufficient production of transcripts long after the reperfusion in CA1 cells in contrast to the other cells.

Heat shock induces such changes in cells as: loss of DNA polymerase a and b activities, blockade of RNA splicing, loss of translational activity, movement of HSP70 into and out of the nucleus, and changes in nucleolar morphology (Parde, 1988). Similar changes have also been reported in cerebral ischemia (Kirino, 1982; Bodsch et al., 1985; Nowak, 1985; Dwyer et al., 1986; Kiessling et al., 1986). HSP70 is essential for the restoration of normal ribosome assembly, promotes the synthesis of new ribosome and accelerates the recovery of nucleolar morphology after heat shock (Pelham, 1984, 1989; Lowe and Moran, 1986) by an ATP-dependent mechanism (Lewis and Pelham, 1985). Therefore, if HSP70 is produced in sufficient amounts within CA1 cells after ischemia, this protein could potentially protect against cell death. Further study is necessary to clarify the exact mechanism why CA1 cells can not produce enough HSP70 mRNA, and this may reveal the reason of at least one aspect of the vulnerability of CA1 cells after brief ischemia.

A sustained induction of HSP70 mRNA has been reported in gerbil hippocampal CA1 sector after 5 min of transient forebrain ischemia using a synthetic oligonucleotide as probe in an in situ hybridization study (Nowak, 1991). The data seem to be different from our result. In general, Northern blot analysis shows a relative amount of a message in total mRNA pool size. Therefore, signal intensity depends on the ratio of the hybridizing mRNA/total mRNA. On the other hand, in situ hybridization detects an absolute amount of a message which should not be affected by the size of the total mRNA pool. Therefore, if the size of the total mRNA pool changes significantly after ischemia, the results of Northern blot and in situ hybridization analyses could be different. The CA1 cells are under the most stressful condition and have a structural failure of polysomes (Kirino, 1982; Petito and Pulsinelli, 1984; Dwyer et al., 1986) after a transient ischemia, a condition in which total mRNA pool could be increasing by a posttranscriptional mechanism while total protein synthesis decreases (Bodsch et al., 1985; Theodorakis and Morimoto, 1987).

APP gene expression

The level of mRNA is determined by a balance of new synthesis and degradation in a cell. In the study of human lymphoblastoid cells, the change of APP mRNA may be the result of change in the synthesis or degradation or both. As compared with the non-induction of actin mRNA, the increase in APP mRNA level should be a specific change in these cells. A preliminary report (Sasaki et al., 1990) suggested a very small induction (1.2-fold) of APP mRNA in an established human cell line (Hela cells) 90 min after heat shock treatment (43°C), thus at a time before the evident induction of APP mRNA seen in this experiment.

Our in vitro study gives no direct evidence of the role of heat shock response in an induction of APP. Another technique such as transfection of HSP gene into cells to constitutively express HSP mRNA in cells may serve as direct evidence of the relationship. However, it can be said that the induction of HSP70 mRNA preceded that of APP mRNA, suggesting the role of heat shock response in the induction of APP. APP695 mRNA does not contain KPI domain, and is much more abundant in brain than in other tissues (Neve et al., 1988; Tanzi et al., 1988). On the other hand, both APP751 and APP770 mRNAs (containing KPI domain) are ubiquitously expressed in almost all tissues including peripheral blood cells (Kitaguchi et al., 1988; Ponte et al., 1988; Tanzi et al., 1988). Because the cDNA probe used in this experiment for APP mRNA (FB68L) detects all APP mRNA species (Tanzi et al., 1988), our results did not show which type of APP mRNA was induced in the peripheral blood cell-derived lymphoblastoid cells. Further studies such as polymerase chain reaction analysis (Golde et al., 1990) or Northern blot analysis using synthetic oligonucleotides (Neve et al., 1988), which can detect each mRNA species may resolve this question. It would be of interest to compare the APP induction in lymphoblastoid cells lines between normal subjects and Alzheimer's disease patients of the familial type (a deficit which is evidently of genetic origin). Changes in gene expression of APP might be different after stress such as heat shock.

A recent work suggests an induction of immunoreactive APP in reactive astrocytes in rat hippocampus after neuronal damage by kainate injection (Siman et al., 1989), suggesting a role of APP in an integration of the tissue after neuronal damage. An overexpression of APP may not directly result in the formation of senile plaques. However, it may be possible that APP can be induced in response to a stress in vitro (our result) and in vivo (Siman et al., 1989), which may relate in part to the normal and/or pathological functions of APP.

However, the gerbil experiment showed that no species of APP mRNA changed even though HSP70 mRNA was greatly induced (Fig. 5). Although the promotor area of the APP gene has the sequence of heat shock consensus elements (Salbaum et al., 1988), the results indicate that APP gene may not simply be regulated by heat shock response. In fact, the APP gene promotor sequence showed that at least four mechanisms could regulate the APP gene expression: the stress response; Jun/Fos response; the putative protein binding at the GC-rich element; and the possible methylation of the CpG region (Salbaum et al., 1988). APP is not a homogeneous single molecule, but is composed of several isoforms (Golde et al., 1990). APPs with the Kunitz type protease inhibitor (KPI) domain (APP770, APP751, and APP563, encoding 770, 751 or 563 amino acid precursors, respectively) may have biological functions different from APP without the KPI domain (APP695). Thus, no change in the level of APP mRNA in the cortex of gerbils suggests that further investigations will be required on the role of heat shock response in an induction of APP gene in this model.

On the other hand, the study of persistent focal ischemia in rats showed that the KPI-containing APP mRNA was induced after the induction of HSP70 mRNA, while mRNA for APP695 was not. HSP70 immunoreactivity was found in many neurons in the cortex involved from 4 h to two days, but was not seen at four days (data not shown). Our results did not show whether this induction of APP mRNA was of neuronal, astroglial or other origin. A further study such as in situ hybridization technique may be necessary to answer this question. However, a morphological study by light microscopy showed that numbers of reactive astrocytes and microglia began to increase with neuronal loss one day after the insult in the territory involved (Chen et al., 1986), suggesting that APP mRNA may be induced in the reactive astrocytes or microglia. This phenomenon is of interest in light of the fact that the amount of APP increases in the specific areas of hippocampus in the Alzheimer's disease brain predominantly due to the APP751/770 mRNAs (Neve et al., 1988; Neve, 1989), where both neuronal loss and formation of senile plaques are prominent (Lewis et al., 1987). Induction of APP mRNA may not directly result in senile plaque formation. However, because of the close relationship between senile plaque formation and neuronal death (Lewis et al., 1987; Neve et al., 1988; Tanzi et al., 1988), our results suggest that neuronal death could change β-amyloid generation. The induction of APP mRNA was accompanied by neuronal death and reactive astrocytosis.

A recent study showed that APP751 and/or APP770 is protease nexin-II (PN-II), a protease inhibitor that is synthesized and secreted by cells (Van Nostrand et al., 1989). It forms SDS-resistant complexes with the epidermal growth factor (EGF)-binding protein, the γ-subunit of nerve growth factor and trypsin; the complexes then bind back to the cells and are rapidly internalized and degraded (Van Nostrand and Cunningham, 1987). It is now suggested that the physiological function of PN-II/APP, a potent anti-chymotrypsin, is the regulation of a chymotrypsin-like protease, which could generate amyloid β-protein and other peptides that contribute to the formation of neuritic plaques (Van Nostrand et al., 1989). Thus APP may have a role in the regulation of certain proteases in the extracellular environment. Cerebral infarction involves activation of various proteases (Siesjö, 1981). Therefore, our results suggest a selective role of APP species containing the KPI domain, which may be involved in the regulation of chymotrypsin-like protease in the integrative process of rat brain cells after cerebral ischemia.

Conclusions

An essential part of gene expression and regulation is the binding of a regulatory protein (transcription factor) to the recognition sequence of the appropriate gene. A novel protein motif for nucleic acid recognition (called "zinc finger") is one such transcription factor. A relationship between gene expressions of a transcription factor and heat shock protein (HSP) 70 has been suggested. Zinc finger gene is normally expressed in rat cerebral cortex, and is induced by transient ischemia with a maximum at 1 h after the 30 min of transient occlusion of MCA. In contrast, HSP70 mRNA is not expressed in normal condition, but is greatly induced by transient ischemia with a maximum at 8 h of reperfusion.

In an attempt to examine a possible relationship between heat shock stress and an induction of amyloid precursor protein, cultured lymphoblastoid cells established from twelve human subjects were treated with heat shock. HSP70 mRNA was induced at 1 and 3 h, and returned to an undetectable level by 8 h. APP mRNA was also induced at 3 and 8 h, and recovered to the steady level by 48 h. No induction was observed in actin mRNA which was measured as an internal standard.

Induction of APP mRNA was examined in a persistent MCA occlusion model of rats in relation to an induction of HSP70 mRNA. A strong induction of HSP70 mRNA was observed with a maximum at 8 h after the beginning of the insult. APP mRNA species which contain the KPI domain were induced from 24 h to 21 days after the insult with a maximum at four days, while total amounts of APP mRNA did not change. A transient forebrain ischemia in gerbil did not induce APP gene expression while it induced HSP70 gene expression.

These results indicate that the gene expression for a transcription factor changes in the early stage of reperfusion after cerebral ischemia before HSP70 induction begins; that APP mRNA is induced by heat shock treatment after the induction of HSP70 mRNA in vitro, suggesting a role of heat shock response in an induction of APP; and that a certain species of APP which contains the KPI domain has a specific role in the integrative process of rat focal cerebral ischemia.

Acknowledgements

This work was partly supported by Monbusho Grant 01044018.

References

Abe, K., Araki, T. and Kogure, K. (1988a) Recovery from edema and of protein synthesis differs between the cortex and caudate following transient focal ischemia in rats. *J. Neurochem.*, 51: 1470 – 1476.

Abe, K., Yuki, S. and Kogure, K. (1988b) Strong attenuation of ischemic and postischemic brain edema in rats by a novel free radical scavenger. *Stroke*, 19: 480 – 485.

Abe, K., Yoshidomi, M. and Kogure, K. (1989) Arachidonic acid metabolism in ischemic neuronal damage. *Ann. N.Y. Acad. Sci.*, 559: 259 – 268.

Abe, K., St. George-Hyslop, P.H., Tanzi, R.E. and Kogure, K. (1991a) Induction of amyloid precursor protein mRNA after heat shock in cultured human lymphoblastoid cells. *Neurosci. Lett.*, 125: 169 – 171.

Abe, K., Kawagoe, J., Sato, S., Sahara, M. and Kogure, K. (1991b) Induction of the "zinc finger" gene after transient focal ischemia in rat cerebral cortex. *Neurosci. Lett.*, 123: 248 – 250.

Abe, K., Tanzi, R.E. and Kogure, K. (1991c) Induction of HSP70 mRNA after transient ischemia in gerbil brain. *Neurosci. Lett.*, 125: 166 – 168.

Abe, K., Tanzi, R.E. and Kogure, K. (1991d) Selective induction of Kunitz-type protease inhibitor domain-containing amyloid precursor protein mRNA after persistent focal ischemia in rat cerebral cortex. *Neurosci. Lett.*, 125: 172 – 174.

Arai, H., Lust, W.D. and Passonneau, J.V. (1982) Delayed metabolic changes-induced 5 min ischemia in gerbil brain. *Trans. Am. Soc. Neurochem.*, 13: s177.

Barbe, M.F., Tytell, M., Gower, D.J. and Welch, W.J. (1988) Hyperthermia protects against light damage in the rat retina. *Science*, 243: 1817 – 1820.

Bodsch, W., Takahashi, K., Barbier, B., Ophoff, G. and Hossmann, K.A. (1985) Cerebral proteins and ischemia. *Prog. Brain Res.*, 63: 197 – 210.

Chen, S.T., Hsu, C.Y., Hogan, E.L., Maricq, H. and Balentine, J.D. (1986) A model of focal ischemic stroke in the rats: reproducible extensive cortical infarction. *Stroke*, 17: 738 – 743.

Chomczynski, P. and Sacchi, N. (1987) Single step method of RNA isolation by acid guanidine thiocyanate-phenol-chloroform extraction. *Anal. Biochem.*, 162: 156 – 159.

Deshpande, J.K., Siesjö, B.K. and Wieloch, T. (1987) Calcium accumulation and neuronal damage in the rat hippocampus following cerebral ischemia. *J. Cereb. Blood Flow Metab.*, 7: 89 – 95.

Dienel, G.A. (1984) Regional accumulation of calcium in postischemic rat brain. *J. Neurochem.*, 43: 913 – 915.

Dienel, G.A., Kiessling, M., Jacewicz, M. and Pulsinelli, W.A. (1986) Synthesis of heat shock proteins in rat brain cortex after transient ischemia. *J. Cereb. Blood Flow Metab.*, 6: 505 – 510.

Dworniczak, B. and Mirault, M.E. (1987) Structure and expression of a human gene coding for a 71 Kd heat shock "cognate" protein. *Nucleic Acid Res.*, 15: 5181 – 5197.

Dwyer, B.E., Wasterlain, C.G., Fujikawa, D.G. and Yamada, L. (1986) Brain protein metabolism in epilepsy. In: A.V. Delgado-Escueta, A.A. Wand, D.M. Woodbury and R.J. Porter (Eds.), *Advance in Neurology, Vol. 44*, Raven Press, New York, pp. 903 – 918.

Flaherty, K.M., DeLuca-Flaherty, C. and McKay, D.B. (1990) Three dimensional structure of the ATPase fragment of a 70 K heat shock cognate protein. *Nature*, 346: 623 – 628.

Fujino, N., Hatayama, T., Kinoshita, H. and Yukioka, M. (1987) Induction of mRNAs for heat shock proteins in livers of rats after ischemia and partial hepaterectomy. *Mol. Cell. Biol.*, 77: 173 – 177.

Gessler, M., Poustka, A., Cavenee, W., Neve, R.L., Orkin, S.H. and Bruns, G.A.P. (1990) Homozygous deletion in Wilms tumors of a zinc-finger gene identified by chromosome jumping. *Nature*, 343: 774 – 778.

Golde, T.E., Estus, S., Usiak, M., Younkin, L.H. and Younkin, S.G. (1990) Expression of β amyloid protein precursor mRNAs: recognition of a novel alternatively spliced form and quantitation in Alzheimer's disease using PCR. *Neuron,* 4: 253 – 267.

Gunning, P., Ponte, P., Kedes, L., Eddy, R. and Shows, T. (1984) Chromosomal location of the co-expressed human skeletal and cardiac actin gene. *Proc. Natl. Acad. Sci. U.S.A.,* 81: 1813 – 1817.

Higgins, G.A., Dawes, L.R. and Neve, R.L. (1988) Expression of APP mRNA transcripts in Down syndrome and Alzheimer's disease. *Soc. Neurosci. Abstr.,* 14: s637.

Imdall, A. and Hossmann, K.A. (1986) Morphometric evaluation of postischemic capillary perfusion in selectively vulnerable areas of gerbil brain. *Acta Neuropathol. (Berl.),* 69: 267 – 271.

Jørgensen, M.B., Deckert, J., Wright, D.C. and Gehlert, D.R. (1989) Delayed c-*fos* proto-oncogene expression in the rat hippocampus induced by transient global ischemia: an in situ hybridization study. *Brain Res.,* 484: 393 – 398.

Kang, J., Lamaire, H.-G., Unterbeck, A., Salbaum, J.M., Masters, C., Grezeschik, K.-H., Multhaup, G., Beyreuther, K. and Müller-Hill, B. (1987) The precursor of Alzheimer's disease amyloid A4 protein resembles a cell-surface receptor. *Nature,* 325: 733 – 736.

Kiessling, M., Dienel, G.A., Jacewicz, M. and Pulsinelli, W.A. (1986) Protein synthesis in postischemic rat brain: a two-dimensional electrophoretic analysis. *J. Cereb. Blood Flow Metab.,* 6: 642 – 649.

Kingston, R.E., Baldwin Jr., A.S. and Sharp, P.A. (1984) Regulation of heat shock protein 70 gene expression by c-*myc*. *Nature,* 312: 280 – 282.

Kirino, T. (1982) Delayed neuronal death in the gerbil hippocampus following ischemia. *Brain Res.,* 239: 57 – 69.

Kitaguchi, N., Takahashi, Y., Tokushima, Y., Shiojiri, S. and Ito, H. (1988) Novel precursor of Alzheimer's disease amyloid protein shows protease inhibitor activity. *Nature,* 331: 530 – 532.

Klug, A. and Rhodes, D. (1987) "Zinc fingers": a novel protein motif for nucleic acid recognition. *Trends Biol. Sci.,* 12: 464 – 469.

Kogure, K. (1988) Signal transducing system in postischemic death of selectively vulnerable brain cells. In: *Excepta Medica International Congress Series,* 856: 95 – 114.

Laverriere, J.N., Tixier-Vidal, A., Buisson, N., Morrin, A., Martial, J.A. and Gourdji, D. (1988) Preferential role of calcium in the regulation of prolactin gene transcription by thyrotropin-releasing hormones in GH3 pituitary cells. *Endocrinology,* 122: 333 – 340.

Lee, A.S. (1987) Coordinated regulation of a set of genes by glucose and calcium ionophores in mammalian cells. *Trends Neurosci.,* 16: 376 – 379.

Lemishka, I.R., Farmer, S., Racaniello, V.R. and Sharp, P.A. (1981) Nucleotide sequence and evolution of mammalian a-tubulin messenger RNA. *J. Mol. Biol.,* 151: 101 – 120.

Lewis, D.A., Campbell, M.J., Terry, R.D. and Morrison, J.H. (1987) Laminar and regional distributions of neurofibrillary tangles and neuritic plaques in Alzheimer's disease: a quantitative study of visual and auditory cortices. *J. Neurosci.,* 7: 1799 – 1808.

Lewis, M.T. and Pelham, H.R.B. (1985) Involvement of ATP in the nucleolar functions of the 70 kd heat shock protein. *EMBO J.,* 4: 3137 – 3143.

Lindquist, S. (1988) The heat-shock proteins. *Annu. Rev. Genet.,* 22: 631 – 677.

Lowe, D.G. and Moran, L.A. (1986) Molecular cloning and analysis of DNA complementary to three mouse Mr. = 68,000 heat shock protein mRNA. *J. Biol. Chem.,* 261: 2102 – 2112.

Lynch, G. and Baudry, M. (1984) The biochemistry of memory: a new and specific hypothesis. *Science,* 224: 1057 – 1063.

Magnusson, K.G. and Wieloch, T.W. (1989) Impairment of protein ubiquitination may cause delayed neuronal death. *Neurosci. Lett.,* 96: 264 – 270.

Maniatis, T., Fritsch, E.F. and Sanbrook, J. (1982) *Molecular Cloning,* Cold Spring Harbor Laboratory, Cold Spring Harbor, NY, pp. 187 – 206.

Marini, A.M., Kozuka, M., Lipsky, R.H. and Nowak Jr., T.S. (1990) 70-Kilodalton heat shock protein induction in cerebellar astrocytes and cerebellar granule cells in vitro: comparison with immunocytochemical location after hyperthermia in vivo. *J. Neurochem.,* 54: 1509 – 1516.

McClure, W.R. (1985) Mechanism and control of transcription initiation in prokaryotes. *Annu. Rev. Biochem.,* 54: 171 – 204.

Mcknight, S. and Tjian, R. (1986) Transcriptional selectivity of viral genes in mamamalian cells. *Cell,* 46: 795 – 805.

Milbrandt, J. (1987) A nerve growth factor-induced gene encodes a possible transcriptional regulatory factor. *Science,* 238: 797 – 799.

Neve, R.L. (1989) Genetic studies support a neuronal origin for the beta amyloid polypeptide. *Neurobiol. Aging,* 10: 400 – 402.

Neve, R.L., Finch, E.A. and Dawes, L.R. (1988) Expression of the Alzheimer's amyloid precursor gene transcripts in the human brain. *Neuron,* 1: 669 – 677.

Nowak Jr., T.S. (1985) Synthesis of a stress protein following transient ischemia in the gerbil. *J. Neurochem.,* 45: 1635 – 1641.

Nowak Jr., T.S. (1991) Localization of 70 kDa stress protein mRNA induction in gerbil brain after ischemia. *J. Cereb. Blood Flow Metab.,* 11: 432 – 439.

Onodera, H., Kogure, K., Ono, Y., Igarashi, K., Kiyota, Y. and Nagaoka, A. (1989) Proto-oncogene c-*fos* is transiently induced in the rat cerebral cortex after forebrain ischemia. *Neurosci. Lett.,* 98: 101 – 104.

Parde, M.L. (1988) The heat shock response in biology and human disease: a meeting review. *Genes Dev.,* 2: 83 – 85.

Pelham, H.R.B. (1984) HSP70 accerelates the recovery of nucleolar morphology after heat shock. *EMBO J.,* 3: 3095 – 3100.

Pelham, H.R.B. (1989) Heat shock and the sorting of luminal ER proteins. *EMBO J.,* 8: 3171 – 3176.

Petito, C.K. and Pulsinelli, W.A. (1984) Delayed neuronal recovery and neuronal death in rat hippocampus following severe cerebral ischemia: possible relationship to abnormality in neuronal process. *J. Cereb. Blood Flow Metab.,* 4: 194 – 205.

Ponte, P., Gonzalez-Dewitt, P., Scilling, J., Hsu, D., Wallace, W., Fuller, F. and Cordell, B. (1988) A new A4 amyloid mRNA contains a domain homologous to serine protease inhibitors. *Nature,* 331: 525 – 527.

Pulsinelli, W.A., Brieley, L.B. and Plum, F.C. (1982) Temporal profile of neuronal damage in a model of transient ischemia. *Ann. Neurol.,* 11: 491 – 498.

Riabowl, K.L., Mizzen, L.A. and Welch, W.J. (1988) Heat shock is lethal to fibroblasts microinjected with antibodies against hsp70. *Science,* 242: 433 – 436.

Roberts, J.W. (1988) Phage lambda and the regulation of transcription termination. *Cell,* 52: 5 – 6.

Roos, B.A., Fisher, J.A., Pignat, W., Alander, C.B. and Raisz, L.G. (1986) Evaluation of the in vivo and in vitro calcitonin-regulating actions of non-calcitonin peptides produced via calcitonin gene expression. *Endocrinology,* 118: 46 – 51.

Rothman, S.M. and Olney, J.W. (1986) Glutamate and pathophysiology of hypoxic brain damage. *Ann. Neurol.,* 19: 105 – 111.

Rougvie, A.E. and Lis, J.T. (1989) The RNA polymerase II molecule at the 5′ end of the uninduced hsp70 gene of *D. Melanogaster* is transcriptionally engaged. *Cell,* 54: 795 – 804.

Sah, R., Hestin, S. and Nicoll, R.A. (1989) Tonic activation of NMDA receptors by ambient glutamate enhances excitability of neurons. *Science,* 246: 815 – 818.

Sakamoto, N., Kogure, K., Kato, H. and Ohtomo, H.G. (1986) Disturbed Ca^{2+} homeostasis in the gerbil hippocampus following brief transient ischemia. *Brain Res.,* 364: 372 – 376.

Salbaum, J.M., Weidermann, A., Lemaire, H.-G., Masters, C.L. and Beyreuther, K. (1988) The promotor of Alzheimer's disease amyloid A4 precursor gene. *EMBO J.,* 7: 2807 – 2819.

Sasaki, H., Yoshikai, S., Izumi, R. and Sakaki, Y. (1990) Structure and expression of Alzheimer's amyloid beta-protein precursor gene. In: T. Miyatake, D.J. Selkoe and Y. Ihara (Eds.), *Molecular Biology and Genetics of Alzheimer's Disease – Excepta Medica International Congress Series,* 884: 105 – 112.

Sheng, M. and Greenberg, M.E. (1990) The regulation and function of c-*fos* and other immediate early genes in the nervous system. *Neuron,* 4: 477 – 485.

Siesjö, B.K. (1981) Cell damage in the brain: a speculative synthesis. *J. Cereb. Blood Flow Metab.,* 1: 155 – 185.

Siman, R., Card, J.P., Nelson, R.B. and Davis, L.G. (1989) Expression of β-amyloid precursor protein in reactive astrocytes following neuronal damage. *Neuron,* 3: 275 – 285.

Struhl, K. (1989) Helix-turn-helix, zinc-finger, and leucine-zipper motifs for eukaryotic transcriptional regulatory proteins. *Trends Biol. Sci.,* 14: 137 – 140.

Sukhatme, V.P., Kartha, S., Toback, F.G., Taub, R., Hoober, R.G. and Tsai-Morris, C-H. (1987) A novel early growth response gene rapidly induced by fibroblast, epithelial cells and lymphocyte mitogens. *Oncogene Res.,* 1: 343 – 355.

Tanzi, R.E., McClatchey, A.I., Lamperti, E.D., Gusella, J.F. and Neve, R.L. (1988) Protease inhibitor domain encoded by an amyloid protein precursor mRNA associated with Alzheimer's disease. *Nature,* 331: 528 – 530.

Theodorakis, N.G. and Morimoto, R.I. (1987) Posttranscriptional regulation of HSP70 expression in human cells. *Mol. Cell. Biol.,* 7: 4357 – 4368.

Tsuda, T., Kogure, K., Ishii, K. and Orihara, H. (1989) Postischemic changes of calcium and endogenous antagonist in the rat hippocampus studied by proton-induced X-ray emission analysis. *Brain Res.,* 484: 228 – 233.

Uney, J.B., Leigh, P.N., Marsden, C.D., Lees, A. and Anderson, B.H. (1988) Stereotaxic injection of kainic acid into the striatum of rats induces synthesis of mRNA for heat shock protein 70. *FEBS Lett.,* 235: 215 – 218.

Van Nostrand, W.E. and Cunningham, D.D. (1987) Purification of protease nexin II from human fibroblasts. *J. Biol. Chem.,* 262: 8508 – 8514.

Van Nostrand, W.E., Wagner, S.L., Suzuki, M., Choi, B.H., Farrow, J.S. and Cunningham, D.D. (1989) Protease nexin-II, a potent anti-chymotrypsin, shows identity to amyloid-protein precursor. *Nature,* 341: 546 – 549.

Vass, K. Welch, W.J. and Nowak Jr., T.S. (1988) Localization of 70 kDa stress protein induction in gerbil brain after ischemia. *Acta Neuropathol. (Berl.),* 77: 128 – 135.

Vass, K., Berger, M.L. and Lassman, H. (1989) Kainic acid-induced expression of stress protein HSP70 in nerve cells. *J. Cereb. Blood Flow Metab.,* 9 (Suppl. 1): s228.

Weidermann, A., Konig, G., Burke, D., Fisher, P., Salbaum, J.M., Masters, C.L. and Beyreuther, K. (1989) Identification, biogenesis, and localization of precursors of Alzheimer's disease A4 amyloid protein. *Cell,* 57: 115 – 126.

Westerberg, E., Deshpande, J.K. and Wieloch, T. (1987) Regional differences in arachidonic release in rat hippocampal CA1 and CA3 regions during cerebral ischemia. *J. Cereb. Blood Flow Metab.,* 7: 189 – 192.

Whitson, J.S., Selkoe, D.J. and Cotman, C.W. (1989) Amyloid β-protein enhances the survival of hippocampal neurons in vitro. *Science,* 243: 1488 – 1490.

Wieloch, T. (1985) Neurochemical correlates to selective neuronal vulnerability. *Prog. Brain Res.,* 63: 69 – 85.

Wisden, W., Errington, M.L., Williams, S., Dunnett, S.B., Waters, C., Hitchcock, D., Evan, G., Bliss, T.V.P. and Hunt, S.P. (1990) Differential expression of immediate early genes in the hippocampus and spinal cord. *Neuron,* 4: 603 – 614.

Wright, J.J., Gunter, K.C., Mitsuya, H., Irving, S.G., Kelly, K. and Siebenlist, U. (1990) Expression of a zinc finger gene in HTLV-I- and HTLV-II-transformed cells. *Science,* 248: 588 – 591.

Wu, B., Hunt, C. and Morimoto, R.I. (1985) Structure and expression of the human gene encoding major heat shock protein HSP70. *Mol. Cell. Biol.,* 5: 330 – 341.

Xie, Y., Herget, T., Starzinski-Powitz, J. and Hossmann, K.A. (1989) Regional evaluation of RNA content in post-ischemic gerbil brain by in situ hybridization. *J. Cereb. Blood Flow Metab.,* 9 (Suppl. 1): s1.

Yanker, B.A., Dawes, L.R., Fisher, S., Villa-Komaroff, L., Oster-Granite, M.L. and Neve, R.L. (1989) Neurotoxicity of a fragment of the amyloid precursor associated with Alzheimer's disease. *Science,* 245: 417 – 420.

Yoshimi, K., Kudo, T., Iwata, N. and Nishimura, K. (1990) Change of clathrin precedes delayed neuronal death of CA1 cells after ischemia. *Jpn. J. Neurochem.,* 29: 456 – 457.

Zimario, V. and Wu, C. (1986) Induction of sequence specific binding of *Drosophila* heat shock activator protein without protein synthesis. *Nature,* 327: 727 – 730.

K. Kogure, K.-A. Hossmann and B.K. Siesjö (Eds.)
Progress in Brain Research, Vol. 96

CHAPTER 16

Molecular pathology of head trauma: altered βAPP metabolism and the aetiology of Alzheimer's disease

Stephen M. Gentleman, David I. Graham[1] and Gareth W. Roberts

Serious Mental Afflictions Research Team, Department of Anatomy and Cell Biology, St Mary's Medical School, Imperial College, London, W2 1PG, and [1]Department of Neuropathology, Institute of Neurological Sciences, Southern General Hospital, Glasgow, G51 4TF, Great Britain

Background

Alzheimer's disease (AD) is the commonest neurodegenerative disease of old age and affects millions of people over the age of 65 in the western world. It has long been thought that Alzheimer's disease could be caused by many different factors both environmental and genetic. This belief has been given additional veracity by linkage studies which indicate aetiological heterogeneity (St. George-Hyslop et al., 1990). Yet each of the causal factors conspire to produce a condition with a characteristic clinical syndrome and neuropathological stigmata.

Considerable progress has been made in determining the identity of the proteins and molecular events involved in the molecular pathology of Alzheimer's disease, the most widely known of which are the inevitability of Alzheimer's disease in Downs syndrome patients with trisomy of chromosome 21 (Tomlinson, 1992) and the point mutations at codon 717 within exon 17 of the β-amyloid precursor protein gene on chromosome 21 (Goate et al., 1991). However, these genetic causes of Alzheimer's disease account for a vanishingly small proportion of patients who suffer from the disease (< 0.01%, Gentleman and Roberts, 1991). It is probable that the overwhelming majority of cases are caused by a variety of environmental factors which may be either sufficient to trigger disease by themselves or sufficient when acting synergistically with the patients genotype (Roberts et al., 1991; Royston et al., 1992).

One of the best documented environmental precipitants of Alzheimer's disease is a previous history of head trauma. However, the question arises: how does a head injury and its attendant acute pathology relate to the metabolism of the β-amyloid precursor protein and the chronic neurodegenerative process observed in Alzheimer's disease?

Recent studies have begun to fill in the gaps which will link these two neuropathological processes. Below we have undertaken the first tentative synthesis of these data in an attempt to produce a more complete understanding of the dynamics of the molecular neuropathology of Alzheimer's disease.

Link between Alzheimer's disease and head trauma: epidemiology

AD can be caused by a variety of factors. Approximately 20% of AD cases are thought to be familial with almost 5% exhibiting an autosomal dominant pattern of inheritance (Van Duijn et al., 1991). Screening of the amyloid precursor protein (βAPP) gene on chromosome 21 (Goldgaber et al., 1987; Kang et al., 1987), which gives rise to the β-amyloid protein (β-AP) found in plaques (Glenner and Wong, 1984; Masters et al., 1985), has revealed a mutation in some AD families (Goate et al., 1991; Naruse et al., 1991). This missense mutation at codon 717 (βAPP 717) causes a valine to isoleucine change which segregates with AD in separate pedigrees from the U.K., U.S.A. and Japan.

However, other early onset families do not show this mutation and linkage analysis indicates a heterogeneity in the genetic causes of AD with the probability that other genes, possibly on other chromosomes, are also involved (St George-Hyslop et al., 1990). Thus, only a minor proportion of AD cases are thought to be directly related to gene abnormalities. Another genetically determined form of AD is that due to a partial duplication of chromosome 21 as seen in Down's syndrome. It is now well established that persons with trisomy 21 show the neuropathological changes of AD commensurate with a decline in cognitive functioning by their fourth decade (Tomlinson, 1992).

Epidemiological studies suggest that familial AD and Down's syndrome account for only about 20% of all cases of AD. It is thought that a large proportion of the remaining 80% of cases are due to environmental factors or to an interaction between genetic and environmental factors. Pertinent environmental factors include head injury, acute infections, excessive use of alcohol or drugs and exposure to toxic agents such as aluminium and neurotoxic amino acids (Gautrin and Gauthier, 1989).

Head injury is the environmental factor most consistently associated with AD (Corsellis et al., 1973; Roberts, 1988; Van Duijn et al., 1991). The evidence linking head injury to a subsequent Alzheimer-like degeneration has been largely derived from epidemiological studies (e.g., French et al., 1991). Of nine studies which have addressed head injury as a risk factor in AD three have found a statistically significant association and a further four have found a positive association (Mortimer et al., 1991). Difficulties in interpreting the epidemiological data have stemmed from the small size of individual studies. To overcome this a meta analysis of the pooled studies (EURODEM) has been performed and has reconfirmed the significant association between head injury and AD (Mortimer et al., 1991). Neuropathological studies also provide support for such an association (Rudelli et al., 1982). From the results of epidemiological studies it has been variously estimated to play a role in 2 – 20% of AD cases (Mortimer et al., 1991).

However, these data are essentially circumstantial, although certainly suggestive. A more direct link between head injury and Alzheimer-type pathology can only be established by direct neuropathological observation.

Link between head trauma and Alzheimer's disease: neuropathology

The repeated blows to the head experienced by boxers (particularly professionals) are associated with a dementing syndrome, dementia pugilistica, the clinical symptoms and course of which are progressive and have been well described (Roberts, 1969). The disease is characterised neuropathologically by a cavum septum, neuronal loss, cerebellar scarring and intense neurofibrillary tangle formation in the cortex (Corsellis et al., 1973).

Until recently, dementia pugilistica was regarded as a separate diagnostic entity from the most common form of dementia, Alzheimer's disease. Although their clinical pictures were similar, the cerebral cortex of the boxers showed no appreciable neuritic plaque formation, as defined by silver and Congo red histochemistry (Corsellis et al., 1973). However, in the mid 1980's the main constituent protein of AD plaques and angiopathic deposits (β-amyloid protein or β-AP) was isolated (Glenner and Wong, 1984). Subsequently antibodies to β-amyloid protein have been produced (Allsop et al., 1986) which are more sensitive and specific than routine histochemical techniques (Gentleman et al., 1989). Using these antibodies we were able to show that the brains of boxers with dementia pugilistica contain large numbers of diffuse plaques composed of β-AP (Roberts et al., 1990a). Furthermore we have also shown that the tangles in dementia pugilistica are ubiquitinated (Dale et al., 1991), occasionally decorated with β-AP (Allsop et al., 1990) and that they are immunologically indistinguishable from those seen in AD (Roberts, 1988).

Within our society there are social situations where head injury and concussion are likely; contact sports such as boxing are examples of this. However, these types of events could be viewed as exceptional. We were aware of this and have attempted to broaden our neuropathological perspective. Repeated head injury occurs in more mundane social situations, wife beating being one such unfortunate example. Recently (Roberts et al., 1990b), we described the similarities between the molecular pathology seen in the brain of an elderly woman repeatedly battered by her husband over a period of decades and that found in the brains of boxers suffering from dementia pugilistica (essentially, tangles and multiple diffuse β-protein plaques in the cortex).

The presence of large numbers of diffuse β-protein deposits has also been described in the cerebral cortex of other long-term survivors of head trauma. In particular, they have been observed in a 33-year-old man who died demented some years after a single incidence of trauma to the head (Clinton et al., 1991).

Therefore it is likely that head injury can trigger β-protein deposition in the brains of certain susceptible individuals. We have argued that a preponderance of diffuse plaques such as that seen in the cortex in dementia pugilistica might indicate a long-term consequence of head injury (Clinton et al., 1991). By extrapolation it has also been suggested that a large ratio of diffuse to classic plaque types might indicate an environmental trigger to the Alzheimer disease process (Clinton et al., 1991).

Our studies have shown that careful examination of the neuropathology of well documented cases generates a considerable amount of data to support a causal link between the neuronal trauma generated by head injury and the subsequent initiation of a neurodegenerative process.

Despite this progress, the cases and situations described above still represent relatively rare events and as such their aetiological linkage to Alzheimer's disease (a very common disorder) could be viewed as tenuous.

Molecular pathology of head trauma

Head injury is a common life event. Over 2,500,000 people per year are admitted to accident and emergency clinics as a result of head injury in the U.K. and U.S.A. Of these approximately 10% die and 30% have a persisting psychological or neurological problem (Anon, 1990). To test our hypothesis that head injury could trigger an Alzheimer-type pathological process we have examined the brains from patients who died as a result of head trauma with varying survival intervals. We have determined the presence and extent of such Alzheimer-type pathology (principally diffuse β-amyloid protein deposits) and compared this with the extent of such pathology found in aging controls.

The primary objective of the project was to determine whether there is more Alzheimer-type pathology in the brains of head-injured patients than in age- and sex-related controls.

Methodological details and preliminary findings were published on 16 cases with ages ranging from 10 to 63 years, and post-traumatic survival times ranging from six to 18 days (Roberts et al., 1992). Of these, six (38%) were found to have β-AP deposits in the cortex (Fig. 1). Our initial findings of the deposition of β-protein in the brains of patients dying within 15 days of head injury had never been described before.

It has been suggested that some of the β-protein deposits we observed could have been due to the age of the patients (mean age of initial sample: 50 years) or to us detecting cases who were suffering from preclinical Alzheimer's disease. Substantial numbers of β-AP deposits in the cortex are most often associated with Alzheimer's disease (Yamaguchi et al., 1988). Alzheimer's disease affects some 5% of the population aged 65 years or more and 20% of those aged over 85 years (Anon, 1990). In the U.K. alone some 300,000 citizens are affected. It could be argued that the cases examined by us already had a dementing process which contributed to their head injury. However, we feel that it is highly unlikely that 30% should be suffering from preclinical AD when the prevalence rate for AD in this age group (most were under 65) is less than 0.01% (Anon, 1990). The difficulties of disentangling the age-related phenomenon of β-protein deposition from the trauma-related phenomena could only be answered satisfactorily by increasing our sample size.

We have since greatly expanded our investigation and we have now examined a total of 152 head injury cases (109 males, 43 females, age range: eight weeks to 85 years) with survival times ranging from 4 h to 2.5 years (manuscript in preparation). The majority of the injuries were attributable to road traffic accidents or to falls. Comprehensive histological studies were undertaken and each case was analysed to assess the amount of contusional injury (Adams et al., 1985), the severity and distribution of any ischaemic damage (Graham et al., 1989), the presence and severity of any diffuse axonal injury (Adams et al., 1989) and whether the intracranial pressure had been high during life as a result of supratentorial expanding lesions (Adams and Graham, 1976; Adams, 1992).

When examined microscopically, 30% (46 of 152) of the cases showed evidence of substantial β-AP deposition. The amount of β-AP deposited varied from isolated foci to extensive deposits throughout the cortical ribbon. The nature and amount of β-protein deposits was different from and more extensive than that seen in a large series of controls of the same age without head injury (n = 65, age range: 14–99 years) (Fig. 2).

We have replicated and extended our original findings that 30% of the cases of severe head injury exhibit diffuse β-protein deposition. Our control data demonstrate that, although there is an effect of

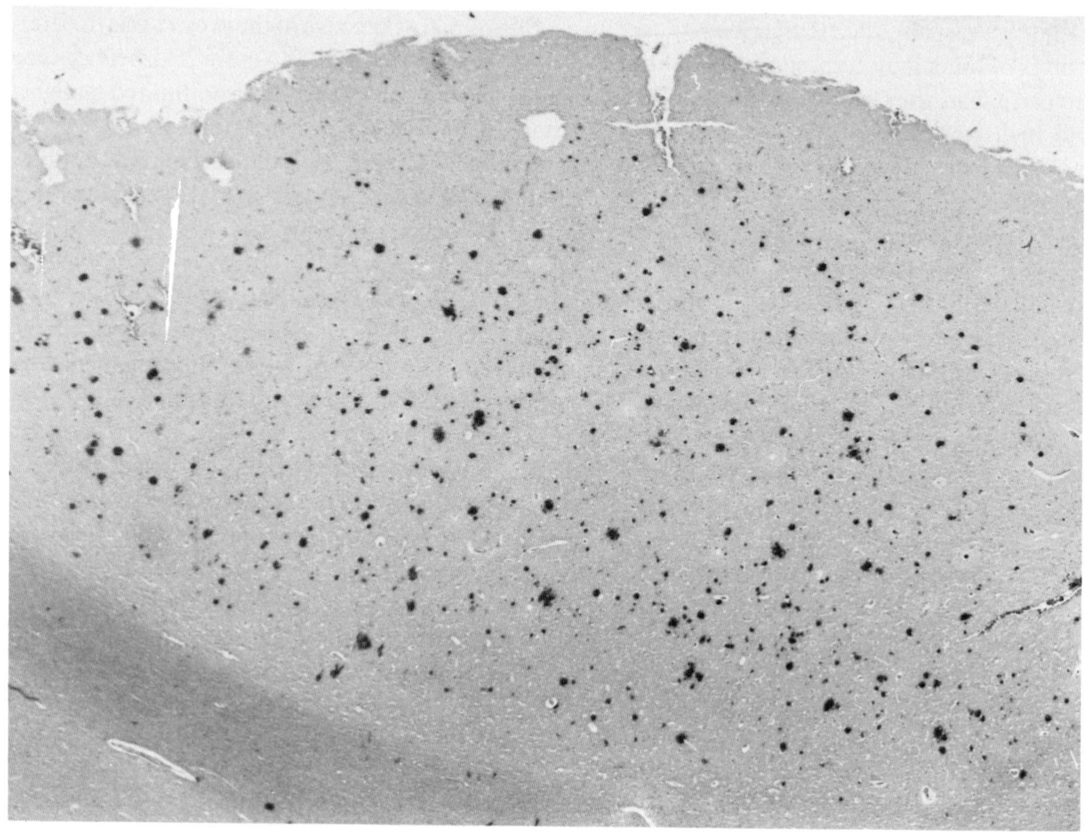

Fig. 1. Multiple diffuse β-AP immunoreactive deposits in the insula of a 46-year-old male who survived for ten days.

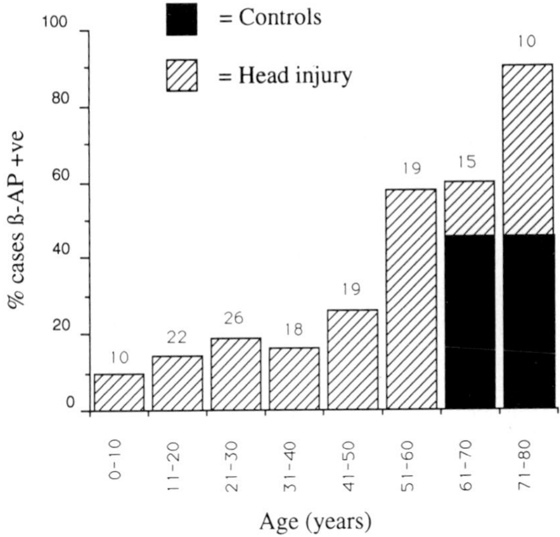

Fig. 2. Histograms detailing the percentage of positive cases in each decade. Column numbers represent total number of *head injury* cases in each decade. Controls: $n = 65$, ages ranged from 14 to 99 years. Using the same methodology no controls under 60 were positive.

age, this merely serves to accentuate the phenomenon. These data are consistent with our proposal that head injury can trigger an Alzheimer-type pathological response.

A direct correlation between the multiple pathologies observed in these patients and the β-protein deposition found in some is not possible at present. However, it is conceivable that the force of the blow which caused the injury somehow determines the extent of β-protein deposition. This inference is supported by the focal nature of the β-protein deposition. One interpretation of the data is that deposition occurs in or around a nidus of neuronal, dendritic or axonal damage, possibly related to ischaemia. This type of damage is widespread in the brains of head-injured patients (Adams, 1992) and would be consistent with the multiple foci of β-protein deposition throughout the cortical ribbon.

Molecular pathology: βAPP expression is an acute phase response

The particularly surprising feature arising from the data is the short delay between head injury and the appearance of β-AP deposits. Alzheimer's disease has a mean time course of seven years (Lishman, 1987). The process of β-AP deposition and subsequent plaque and tangle formation is assumed to be a gradual one where the accretion of protein to form plaques and the subsequent appearance of tangles occurs over months or years (see Clinton et al., 1991, for discussion). Our observations demonstrate that this need not necessarily be so and that β-AP deposition can occur within days of the trigger event.

This evidence from direct observation of the human brain is supported by inference from the data derived from animal studies. Expression of βAPP mRNA has been reported in reactive astrocytes following neuronal damage caused by intraventricular injection of kainic acid (Siman et al., 1989; Kawarabayashi et al., 1991). βAPP immunoreactivity is deposited around the site of ibotenic acid lesions and was still present 100 days after the lesion (Nakamura et al., 1992). Furthermore, it appears that there is a selective induction of the βAPP mRNA which contains the Kunitz protease inhibitor domain (βAPP 751/770) in the cortex of rats which have undergone middle cerebral artery occlusion to produce focal ischaemia (Abe et al., 1991). The dominant βAPP mRNA species (βAPP 695) remained unchanged. The induction of βAPP 751/770 was observed after one day, reached a maximum at four days and remained elevated at 21 days. In axotomised animals βAPP expression is increased and the βAPP 751 transcript expression remains elevated (Scott et al., 1991); βAPP immunoreactivity also accumulates within axonal swelling around infarcts in the human brain (Ohgami et al., 1992). Recently it has been shown that transgenic mice which overexpress the human βAPP 751 transcript spontaneously develop β-protein deposit plaques (Quon et al., 1991).

Our results together with the data from animal studies suggest that the induction of βAPP 751/770 in the brain is a normal response to neuronal stress (Roberts et al., 1991) and that this response is analogous to the induction of heat shock proteins (Lowe and Mayer, 1990).

However, in humans it is clear that this normal, possibly protective, induction can metamorphose into a pathological process in certain susceptible individuals. The basis of this susceptibility is unknown, although it seems reasonable to suppose that its molecular roots might lie in some common polymorphism of the controlling elements of the βAPP gene which causes overexpression of the βAPP 751 transcript or its processing enzymes. This putative mechanism might explain the pathological phenomena we have observed and perhaps more importantly link our observations to the proposal that head trauma might cause AD.

Functions of βAPP

The physiological consequences of the pathological observations described above become more pertinent when considered against the background of the latest data on the normal cellular functions of βAPP. Confocal microscopy has shown that βAPP is localised at synaptic sites and that the amount of βAPP present within a neurone might be related to its level of synaptic activity (Schubert et al., 1991). βAPP expression appears to be regulated at the level of the neurone (Scott et al., 1991; Schubert et al., 1991). On the basis of these data it has been proposed that βAPP turnover is related to synaptic turnover and plasticity. These functions are critically involved in the acute and chronic phases of neuronal injury. Alterations in βAPP metabolism might be expected to have profound effects on synaptic transmission.

Trauma βAPP, acute phase response and Alzheimer's disease: a hypothesis

Following the initial identification of the β-AP in neuritic plaques and as the main constituent of the vascular deposits, there was debate as to whether the mis-metabolism of βAPP and subsequent deposition of β-AP triggered the neuronal degeneration, i.e., played a causal role, or was merely the end result of neuronal degeneration or vascular damage. These scenarios must now be regarded as unlikely in the light of the discovery of the mutations in the βAPP gene (Hardy and Allsop, 1991).

The results of the studies described and discussed above have substantially altered our understanding of the molecular pathology of Alzheimer's disease. Both the genetic and the head injury studies reinforce the point that, whatever the cause of Alzheimer's disease, the overexpression, abnormal metabolism of βAPP and consequent deposition of β-protein is a central event in the pathogenesis and evolution of AD (Roberts et al., 1991; Royston et al., 1992).

These observations can be related to one another. The resulting synthesis demonstrates how several phenomena, each well described in isolation, can illuminate the full panorama of the molecular pathology which underlies the neurodegenerative processes observed in Alzheimer's disease (Fig. 3).

Genetic defects may exert a direct effect on βAPP synthesis or metabolism thereby initiating a slowly evolving accumulation of β-protein. In the case of Down's syndrome, the extra chromosome 21 may result in increased transcription of βAPP leading to a relative excess of β-protein production, whereas the βAPP 717 mutation may influence βAPP proteolysis resulting in its inappropriate degradation and leading to subsequent β-AP deposition.

Environmental precipitants of Alzheimer's disease may also act through a variety of mechanisms with the common end-point of β-AP deposition. There is now evidence from a wide range of animal studies demonstrating that procedures which cause neuronal trauma within the CNS (stab wounds, administration of excitatory amino acids, ischaemia and axotomy) result in increased expression of the 751 form of βAPP. We have demonstrated an analogous situation in the brains of humans. Thus, the overexpression of βAPP is part of the acute phase response.

Head injury is almost invariably accompanied by a degree of ischaemia. The pathophysiology of ischaemia is well known (e.g., Siesjö et al., 1991) and the molecular cascade which follows this kind of damage is now known to trigger the overexpression of βAPP (Fig. 3).

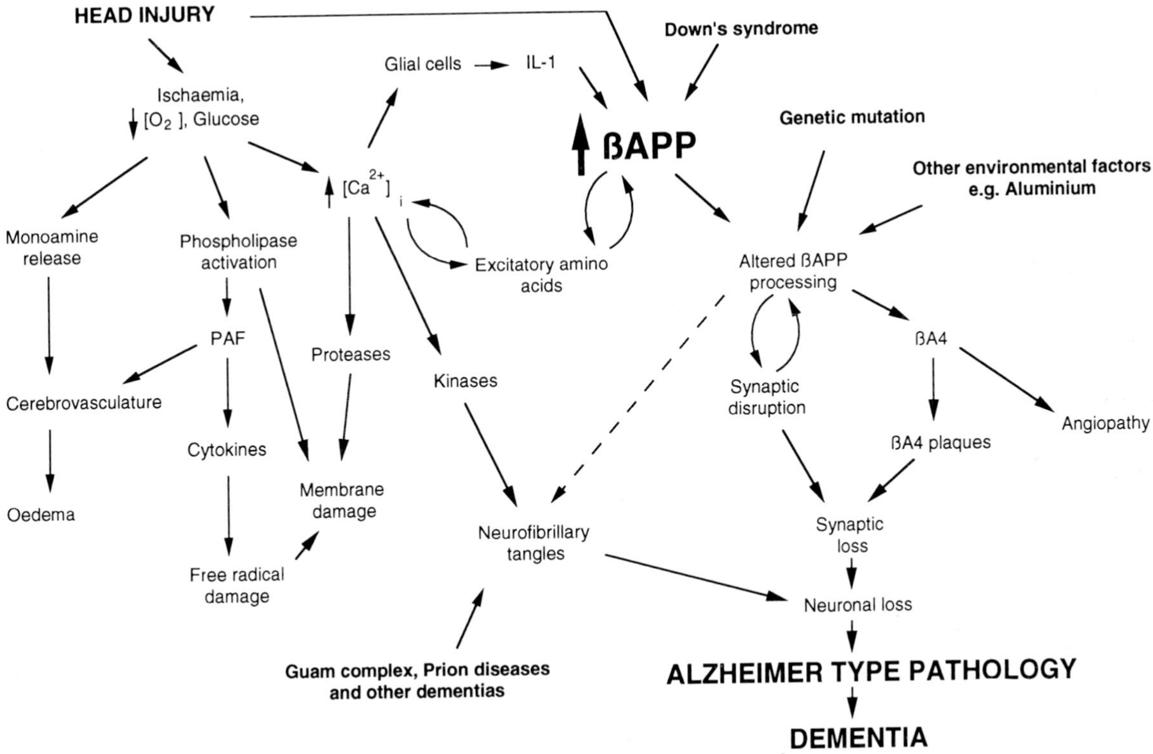

Fig. 3. Flow diagram showing potential areas of interaction between the pathological processes underlying head injury and Alzheimer's disease. The scheme focuses particularly on the central role of the β-amyloid precursor protein (βAPP). PAF, platelet activating factor; IL-1, interleukin 1; β-AP, β-amyloid protein.

βAPP overexpression is also mediated indirectly by other components of the acute phase protein response and might augment the toxicity of excitatory amino acids (Mattson et al., 1991). In a recent study the promoter region of the βAPP gene was isolated and found to be induced by the cytokine interleukin-1 (IL-1) in vitro. IL-1 immunoreactivity is increased in AD, and recent observations indicate that there is overexpression of IL-1 mRNA in Alzheimer's disease. It has also been suggested that IL-1, possibly acting via induction of IL-6, may induce an acute phase response within the brain leading to increased synthesis of α_1-antichymotrypsin and βAPP. Both of these proteins, which are overexpressed in Alzheimer's disease contain promoter sequences on the gene which may be responsive to IL-6 (see Royston et al., 1992, for review).

IL-1 is present in normal brain where it exerts a diverse range of activities on immune function, and coordination of many aspects of the acute phase response to trauma and infection (see Rothwell, 1991, for review). Brain IL-1 expression is rapidly induced following brain injury and recent interest has focused on its modulation of the brain response to injury, e.g., astrogliosis and neuronal sprouting – neuropathological processes strongly associated with the AD neurodegenerative process. It has been demonstrated that IL-1 regulates nerve growth factor (NGF), and an IL-1-NGF cascade has been postulated in AD. The neurotrophic effects of the stimulated NGF may underlie the axonal and dendritic sprouting associated with the degenerative process in Alzheimer's disease.

Together these pieces make a coherent hypothesis

wherein the neuronal trauma and ischaemia which accompany head trauma cause a cascade of molecular events which result in βAPP 751 overexpression. Extended periods of βAPP overexpression (as in trisomy of chromosome 21) increase the likelihood of the mis-metabolism of βAPP (as do βAPP mutations) and the subsequent deposition of β-AP. From this event unfold the full neurodegenerative phenomena of Alzheimer's disease. We propose (Fig. 3):

– that neuronal trauma leads directly to the increased expression of βAPP 751;

– that the other regulatory elements of the acute phase response can and do contribute and modulate the expression of βAPP 751;

– that local overexpression of βAPP for an extended period of time overloads the neurones capacity to metabolize βAPP 751;

– that mis-metabolised βAPP 751 is deposited as β-AP at synaptic sites;

– that the presence of β-AP at synaptic sites disrupts synaptic transmission, thus causing neuronal dysfunction;

– that the neurone's attempt to remedy this dysfunction leads to aberrant sprouting of neurites and synaptic pathology in and around β-AP deposits (localised acute phase response);

– that this phenomenon stresses synaptically linked neurones and causes them to overexpress βAPP (spreading disease);

– that aberrant neurites, axons and subsequently neurones develop paired helical filaments and degenerate;

– that once this process has involved a threshold quantity of neuronal circuitry the clinical symptoms of dementia are observed.

From molecular pathology to therapy

At present there is no effective treatment to prevent or arrest the progression of Alzheimer's disease.

Together, the data on the molecular pathology of Alzheimer's disease and the conceptualisation of the pathological processes as a series of anatomically linked acute phase responses distributed over time suggest a rational and direct approach to therapy. The identification of βAPP mis-metabolism (including excess synthesis) as the critical event in the pathogenesis of AD leads to the proposition that manipulating the factors which regulate βAPP may help control its overexpression, thereby offering the potential to slow or even prevent the cascade of events which culminate in the final common pathway of amyloid deposition and the formation of Alzheimer-type pathology.

We have suggested (Royston et al., 1992) that one possible "route" to mis-metabolism of βAPP is a consequence of the acute response of the brain following injury or ischaemia. Several studies show that focal ischaemia in the rat results in the cellular accumulation of βAPP in the area immediately around the lesion. Administration of recombinant IL-1 receptor antagonist significantly inhibits (> 50%) ischaemic damage in the rat. This provides the first direct evidence of a causal link between IL-1 and neural damage. Using this paradigm, pretreatment of a parallel group of animals with an IL-1 receptor antagonist results in a marked reduction in the extent and degree of immunostaining to βAPP.

Whilst such results are of course preliminary they offer the intriguing possibility that the vast amount of work which has documented the pathophysiology of the acute phase response and ischaemia may lay the foundation for a new generation of treatments which will finally address the therapeutic challenge presented by chronic neurodegenerative disorders.

Acknowledgements

This work was supported by the Medical Research Council (U.K.).

References

Abe, K., Tanzi, R.E. and Kogure, K. (1991) Selective induction of Kunitz-type protease inhibitor domain-containing amyloid precursor protein mRNA after persistent focal ischaemia in rat cerebral cortex. *Neurosci. Lett.*, 125: 172 – 174.

Adams, J.H. (1992) Head injury. In: J.H. Adams and L.W. Duchen (Eds.), *Greenfield's Neuropathology*, 5th edition, Edward Arnold, London, Melbourne, Auckland.

Adams, J.H. and Graham, D.I. (1976) The relationship between ventricular fluid pressure and the neuropathology of raised intracranial pressure. *Neuropathol. Appl. Neurobiol.,* 2: 323 – 332.

Adams, J.H., Doyle, D., Graham, D.I., McLellan, D.R., Genarelli, T.A., Pastuszko, M. and Sakamoto, T. (1985) The contusion index: a reappraisal in human and experimental non-missile head injury. *Neuropathol. Appl. Neurobiol.,* 11: 299 – 308.

Adams, J.H., Doyle, D., Ford, I., Genarelli, T.A., Graham, D.I. and McLellan, D.R. (1989) Diffuse axonal injury in head injury: definitions, diagnosis and grading. *Histopathology.* 15: 49 – 59.

Allsop, D., Laudon, M., Kidd, M., Lowe, J.S., Reynolds, G.P. and Gardener, A. (1986) Monoclonal antibodies raised against a subsequence of plaque core proteins react with plaque cores, plaque periphery and cerebrovascular amyloid in Alzheimer's disease. *Neurosci. Lett.,* 68: 253 – 256.

Allsop, D., Haga, S., Bruton, C., Ishii, T. and Roberts, G.W. (1990) Neurofibrillary tangles in some cases of dementia pugilistica share antigens with amyloid beta protein of Alzheimer's disease. *Am. J. Pathol.,* 136: 255 – 260.

Anon editorial (1990) Head trauma victims in the UK: undeservedly underserved. *Lancet,* 335: 886 – 887.

Clinton, J., Ambler, M.W. and Roberts, G.W. (1991) Post-traumatic Alzheimer's disease: preponderance of a single plaque type. *Neuropathol. Appl. Neurobiol.,* 17: 69 – 74.

Corsellis, J.A.N., Bruton, C.J. and Freeman-Browne, D. (1973) The aftermath of boxing. *Psychol. Med.,* 3: 270 – 273.

Cras, P., Kawai, M., Lowery, D., Gonzalez-DeWhitt, P., Greenberg, B. and Perry, G. (1991) Senile plaque neurites in Alzheimer's disease accumulate amyloid precursor protein. *Proc. Natl. Acad. Sci. U.S.A.,* 88: 7552 – 7556.

Dale, G.E., Leigh, P.N., Luthert, P., Anderton, B.H. and Roberts, G.W. (1991) Neurofibrillary tangles in dementia pugilistica are ubiquitinated. *J. Neurol. Neurosurg. Psychiatry,* 54: 116 – 118.

French, L.R., Schuman, L.M. and Mortimer, J.A. (1991) A case-control study of dementia of the Alzheimer type. *Am. J. Epidemiol.,* 121: 414 – 421.

Gautrin, D. and Gauthier, S. (1989) Alzheimer's disease: environmental factors and etiologic hypotheses. *Can. J. Neurol. Sci.,* 16: 375 – 387.

Gentleman, S.M. and Roberts, G.W. (1991) Risk factors in Alzheimer's disease. *Br. Med. J.,* 304: 118 – 119.

Gentleman, S.M., Bruton, C.J., Allsop, D., Lewis, S.J., Polak, J.M. and Roberts, G.W. (1989) A demonstration of the advantages of immunostaining in the quantification of amyloid plaque deposits. *Histochemistry,* 92: 355 – 358.

Glenner, G.G. and Wong, C.W. (1984) Alzheimer's disease: initial report of the purification and characterization of a novel cerebrovascular amyloid protein. *Biochem. Biophys. Res. Commun.,* 120: 885 – 890.

Goate, A., Chartier-Harlin, M-C. and Mullan, M. (1991) Segregation of a missense mutation in the amyloid precursor protein gene with familial Alzheimer's disease. *Nature,* 349: 704 – 706.

Goldgaber, D., Lerman, M.I., McBride, O.W., Saffiotti, U. and Gajdusek, D.C. (1987) Characterization and chromosomal localization of a cDNA encoding brain amyloid of Alzheimer's disease. *Science,* 235: 877 – 880.

Graham, D.I., Ford, I., Adams, J.H., Doyle, D., Teasdale, G.M. and Lawrence, A.E. (1989) Ischaemic brain damage is still common in fatal non-missile head injury. *J. Neurol. Neurosurg. Psychiatry,* 52: 346 – 350.

Hardy, J. and Allsop, D. (1991) Amyloid deposition as the central event in the aetiology of Alzheimer's disease. *Trends Pharmacol. Sci.,* 12: 383 – 388.

Johnson, S.A., McNeill, T., Cordell, B. and Finch, C.E. (1990) Relation of neuronal APP-751/APP-695 mRNA ratio and neuritic plaque density in Alzheimer's disease. *Science,* 248: 854 – 857.

Kang, J., Lemaire, H.-G., Unterbeck, A., Salbaum, J.M., Masters, C.L., Grzeschik, K.H., Multhaup, G., Beyreuther, K. and Muller-Hill, B. (1987) The precursor of Alzheimer's disease amyloid A4 protein resembles a cell-surface receptor. *Nature,* 325: 733 – 736.

Kawarabayashi, T., Shoji, M., Harigaya, Y., Yamaguchi, H. and Hirai, S. (1991) Expression of APP in the early stages of brain damage. *Brain Res.,* 563: 334 – 338.

Kennedy, H., Kametani, F. and Allsop, D. (1992) Only Kunitz inhibitor-containing isoforms of secreted Alzheimer amyloid precursor protein show amyloid immunoreactivity in normal cerebrospinal fluid. *Neurodegeneration,* 1: 59 – 64.

Lishman, W.A. (1987) Senile dementias, presenile dementias and pseudodementias. In: *Organic Psychiatry,* 2nd edition, Blackwell Scientific, London, Oxford.

Lowe, J. and Mayer, R.J. (1990) Ubiquitin, cell stress and diseases of the nervous system. *Neuropathol. Appl. Neurobiol.,* 16: 281 – 291.

Masters, C.L., Simms, G., Weinmon, N.A., Beyreuther, K., Multhaup, G. and MacDonald, B.L. (1985) Amyloid plaque core proteins in Alzheimer's disease and Down's syndrome. *Proc. Natl. Acad. Sci. U.S.A.,* 82: 4245 – 4249.

Mattson, M.P., Cheng, B., Davis, D., Bryant, K., Lieberburg, I. and Rydel, R.E. (1992) β-Amyloid peptides destabilize calcium homeostasis and render human cortical neurons vulnerable to excitotoxicity. *J. Neurosci.,* 12: 376 – 389.

McGeer, P.L. and Rogers, J. (1992) Anti-inflammatory agents as a therapeutic approach to Alzheimer's disease. *Neurology,* 42: 447 – 449.

Mortimer, J.A., Van Duijn, C.M. and Chandra, V. (1991) Head trauma as a risk factor for Alzheimer's disease: a collaborative re-analysis of case-control studies. *Int. J. Epidemiol.,* 20: S28.

Nakamura, Y., Takeda, M., Niigawa, H., Hariguchi, S. and Nishimura, T. (1992) Amyloid β-protein precursor deposition in rat hippocampus lesioned by ibotenic acid injection.

Neurosci. Lett., 136: 95 – 98.

Naruse, S., Igarashi, S. and Kobayashi, H. (1991) Mis-sense mutation Val-Ile in exon 17 of amyloid precursor protein gene in Japanese familial Alzheimer's disease. *Lancet,* 337(8747): 978 – 979.

Ohgami, T., Kitamoto, T. and Tateishi, J. (1992) Alzheimer's amyloid precursor protein accumulates within axonal swellings in human brain lesions. *Neurosci. Lett.,* 136: 75 – 78.

Quon, C., Wang, Y., Catalano, R., Marian Scardina, J., Murakami, K. and Cordell, B. (1991) Formation of β-amyloid protein deposits in brains of transgenic mice. *Nature,* 352: 239 – 241.

Roberts, A.J. (1969) *Brain Damage in Boxers,* Pitman, London.

Roberts, G.W. (1988) Immunocytochemistry of neurofibrillary tangles in dementia pugilistica and Alzheimer's disease: evidence for common genesis. *Lancet,* 2(8626 – 8627): 1456 – 1458.

Roberts, G.W., Allsop, D. and Bruton, C.J. (1990a) The occult aftermath of boxing. *J. Neurol. Neurosurg. Psychiatry,* 53: 373 – 378.

Roberts, G.W., Whitwell, H.L., Acland, P.R. and Bruton, C.J. (1990b) Dementia in a punch-drunk wife. *Lancet,* 335(8694): 918 – 919.

Roberts, G.W., Gentleman, S.M., Lynch, A. and Graham, D.I. (1991) βA4 amyloid protein deposition in brain after head trauma. *Lancet,* 338: 1422 – 1423.

Rothwell, N.J. (1991) Functions and mechanisms of interleukin 1 in the brain. *Trends Pharmacol. Sci.,* 12: 430 – 436.

Royston, M.C., Rothwell, N.J. and Roberts, G.W. (1992) Alzheimer's disease: pathology to potential treatments? *Trends Pharmacol. Sci.,* 13: 131 – 133.

Rudelli, R., Strom, J.O. and Welch, P.T. (1982) Post-traumatic premature Alzheimer's disease: neuropathologic findings and pathogenetic considerations. *Arch. Neurol.,* 39: 570 – 575.

Scott, J.N., Parhad, I.M. and Clark, A.W. (1991) β-Amyloid precursor protein gene is differentially expressed in axotomized sensory and motor systems. *Mol. Brain. Res.,* 10: 315 – 325.

Schubert, W., Prior, R., Weidemann, A., Dircksen, H., Multhaup, G., Masters, C.L. and Beyreuther, K. (1991) Localization of Alzheimer's βA4 amyloid precursor protein at central and peripheral synaptic sites. *Brain Res.,* 563: 184 – 194.

Siesjö, B.K., Memezawa, H. and Smith, M.L. (1991) Neurocytotoxicity: pharmacological implications. *Fundam. Clin. Pharmacol.,* 5: 755 – 767.

Siman, R., Card, J.P., Nelson, R.B. and Davis, L.G. (1989) Expression of β-amyloid precursor protein in reactive astrocytes following neuronal damage. *Neuron,* 3: 275 – 285.

St. George-Hyslop, P.H., Haines, J.L., Farrer, L.A., Polinsky, R., Van-Broeckhoven, C., Goate, A., McLachlan, D.R., Orr, H., Bruni, A.C. and Sorbi, S. (1990) Genetic linkage studies suggest that Alzheimer's disease is not a single homogeneous disorder. *Nature,* 347: 194 – 197.

Sumi, S.M., Bird, T.D., Nochlin, D. and Raskind, M.A. (1992) Familial presenile dementia with psychosis associated with cortical neurofibrillary tangles and degeneration of the amygdala. *Neurology,* 42: 120 – 127.

Tomlinson, B.E. (1992) Ageing and the dementias. In: J.H. Adams and L.W. Duchen (Eds.), *Greenfield's Neuropathology,* 5th edition, Edward Arnold, London, pp. 1284 – 1410.

Van Duijn, C.M., Hofman, A. and Kay, D.W.K. (1991) Risk factors for Alzheimer's disease: a collaborative analysis of case-control studies. *Int. J. Epidemiol.,* 20: S4.

Van Nostrand, W.E., Farrow, J.S., Wagner, S.L., Bhasin, R., Goldgaber, D., Cotman, C.W. and Cunningham, D. (1991) The predominant form of the amyloid β-protein precursor in human brain is protease nexin 2. *Proc. Natl. Acad. Sci. U.S.A.,* 88: 10302 – 10306.

Yamaguchi, H., Hirai, S., Morimatsu, M., Shoji, M. and Ihora, Y. (1988) A variety of cerebral amyloid deposits in the brains of Alzheimer-type dementia demonstrated by β-protein immunostaining. *Acta Neuropathol. (Berl.),* 76: 541 – 549.

K. Kogure, K.-A. Hossmann and B.K. Siesjö (Eds.)
Progress in Brain Research, Vol. 96

CHAPTER 17

Role of phospholipase A_2 and membrane-derived lipid second messengers in membrane function and transcriptional activation of genes: implications in cerebral ischemia and neuronal excitability

Nicolas G. Bazan, Geoffrey Allan and Elena B. Rodriguez de Turco

LSU Eye Center and Neuroscience Center, Louisiana State University Medical Center School of Medicine, New Orleans, LA 70112, U.S.A.

Introduction

Pathways which generate membrane phospholipid-derived second messengers in brain are rapidly activated by neuronal stimuli or ischemia. Synapses are particularly enriched in phospholipid-degrading and modifying enzymes (e.g., phospholipases A_2; Bazan, 1971) which have important roles in the signal transduction of neurotransmitters and neurotrophic factors. Moreover, the metabolism of specific pools of phospholipids in excitable membranes is acutely sensitive to cerebral ischemia and convulsions (Bazan et al., 1970; Birkle and Bazan, 1987). The physiological mechanisms through which extracellular signals are translated into long-term phenotypic changes of neural cells are poorly understood. Studying the mechanisms and consequences of the changes in membrane phospholipid metabolism induced by cerebral ischemia and convulsions is essential to understand how these conditions can bring about brain damage. Also, similar pathways may be involved in normal neuronal development and adaptation.

The mechanisms which lead to the rapid activation of brain phospholipases during ischemia and seizures are of major importance in understanding the neurochemical consequences of these conditions. The membrane phospholipids of brain and retina are highly enriched in polyunsaturated fatty acids (PUFA), especially arachidonate (20:4ω3) and docosahexaenoate (22:6ω3) (Cotman et al., 1967; Sun and Sun, 1972; Aveldaño and Bazan, 1975). Release of free arachidonic acid is the rate-limiting step in the cascade that results in the formation of the biologically active eicosanoids. Furthermore, phospholipase A_2 (PLA_2) also leads to the synthesis of platelet-activating factor (PAF) (Ramesha and Pickett, 1986; Suga et al., 1990; Bazan 1990; Bazan et al., 1991), an alkyl-ether phospholipid which is a potent mediator of inflammatory and immune processes (Braquet et al., 1987). Here we summarize the nature of the changes in membrane phospholipid-derived second messenger generation elicited by ischemia and convulsions; address synaptosome-specific activation of phospholipases A_2, A_1 and C and the arachidonic acid cascade; and examine a hypothesis on how PAF might, in addition to its short-term effects, be involved in long-term changes in neuronal phenotype via activation of nuclear proto-oncogenes. These latter effects may link selective membrane phospholipid hydrolysis with synaptic remodeling and plasticity changes through the modulation of gene expression.

Changes in second-messenger synthesis during cerebral ischemia and convulsions

Cerebral ischemia and convulsions lead to many changes in the activities of second-messenger systems in the brain. Some of the pathways depicted in Fig. 1 are activated at an early stage under these conditions. The energy deficit resulting from oxygen deprivation during cerebral ischemia results in a failure of energy-dependent systems, including ion channels. The resulting depolarization has neurochemical consequences similar to that observed by overstimulation of neurotransmitter signaling systems, for instance during potassium depolarization (Birkle and Bazan, 1987). Furthermore, depolarization enhances neurotransmitter release that in turn augments stimulation of receptor-mediated second-messenger systems. One consequence of these events is a net influx of free calcium from the extracellular milieu. There are also localized changes in intracellular pH through down-regulation of the sodium-proton antiport. Initial activation of phospholipase C results in degradation of polyphosphoinositides (PPI) and transient accumulation of diacylglycerol and IP_3. The former activates protein kinase C (PKC) and the latter stimulates mobilization of calcium from endoplasmic reticulum (Berridge, 1984; Nishizuka, 1984). A raise in intracellular calcium levels, in turn, activates PLA_2, resulting in the release of free fatty acids, including arachidonic acid, from phosphatidylcholine (PC). A recent cloning study shows that a PLA_2 which specifically releases arachidonic acid from the sn-2 position of phospholipids is distinct from the secreted forms of PLA_2 found in digestive secretions and venoms (Clark et al., 1991). It contains, however, a sequence similar to the calcium-dependent membrane translocation domains of phospholipase C, protein kinase C gamma, GTPase activator proteins (GAP), and the p65 synaptic vesicle protein. Depolarization of localized cytoplasmic areas adjacent to the plasma membranes activates PLA_2 in platelets (Siffert et al., 1990). Therefore, failure of the sodium-proton antiport in brain during ischemia and convulsions might also contribute to PLA_2 activation. The consequences of arachidonic acid release include subsequent formation of biologically active prostaglandins and hydroxyeicosatetraenoic acids (HETEs) (Birkle and Bazan, 1987).

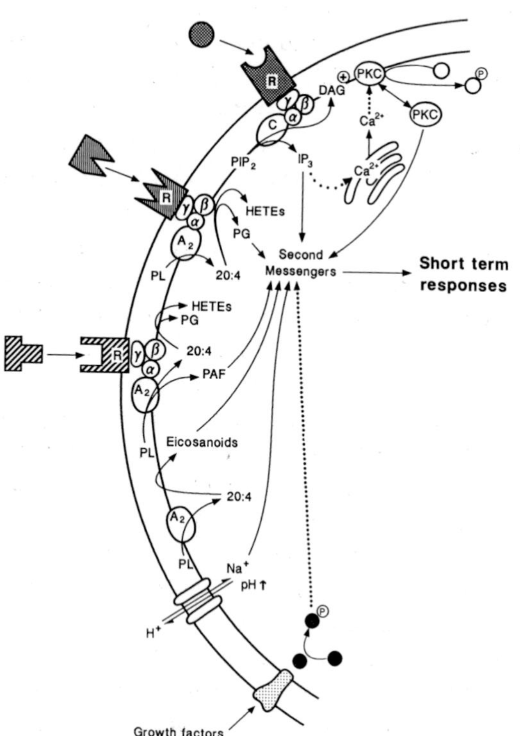

Fig. 1. Schematic representation of the second-messenger systems which can be perturbed in the brain as a result of seizures and ischemia.

A fraction of the phosphatidylcholines (PC) from brain membrane phospholipids contains a small, but metabolically very active, 1-O-alkyl-2-arachidonoyl-glycerophosphorylcholine component. PLA_2-catalyzed release of arachidonic acid from this lipid gives rise to 1-O-alkyl-*lyso*-GPC (*lyso*-PAF), the direct precursor of PAF. Free polyunsaturated fatty acids (PUFAs) and PAF accumulated during the oxygen deprivation phase of cerebral ischemia can, upon reperfusion, be two of the main causes of brain damage. Free PUFA levels in normal brain are normally negligible, their amounts are tightly regulated and they are protected by efficient anti-oxidation mechanisms. During the reperfusion phase following cerebral ischemia, enzyme-mediated oxygenation of arachidonic acid results in the synthesis of eicosanoids. However, the sudden increase in oxygen tension in affected areas of the brain can also lead to non-enzymatic oxygenation of the unsaturated lipids and free radical generation, and consequently to cell damage and death (Bazan and Rodriguez de Turco, 1980).

The long-term responses of neural cells to ischemia-induced damage may lead to one of the following: cell death, cell recovery or phenotypic modification to take over the functions of dead or damaged neurons. The latter two presumably include the linking of short-term biochemical events in the cytoplasm and extranuclear membranes with long-term changes in gene expression. Such changes could involve the actions of neurotrophic factors and include participation of non-neuronal cells such as glia, the endothelial cells of the microvasculature and components of the circulatory system.

A single seizure induces a transient degradation of polyphosphoinositides and accumulation of free fatty acids and diacylglycerols in rat brain

Acute neurotransmitter release in the adult CNS, such as that produced by electroconvulsive shock (ECS), induces a transient accumulation of free fatty acids (FFA) and diacylglycerol (DAG) (Bazan, 1970; Bazan et al., 1971). A similar accumulation of FFA and DAG occurs during cerebral ischemia (Bazan, 1970; Aveldaño and Bazan, 1975), when a shortage of ATP leads to membrane depolarization and neurotransmitter release. The FFA and DAG pools produced under these conditions exhibit a net enrichment in arachidonic acid (20:4) and stearic acid (18:0). This indicates receptor-mediated activation of phospholipase subtypes which preferentially utilize membrane-derived PPI, which in brain is enriched with 20:4 and 18:0 acyl chains (Bazan et al., 1981). During brain trauma both A and C type phospholipases are activated: accumulation of FFA and DAG concomitant with degradation of PPI occurs in the brain during cerebral ischemia (Yoshida et al., 1986; Sun et al., 1990) and after one ECS

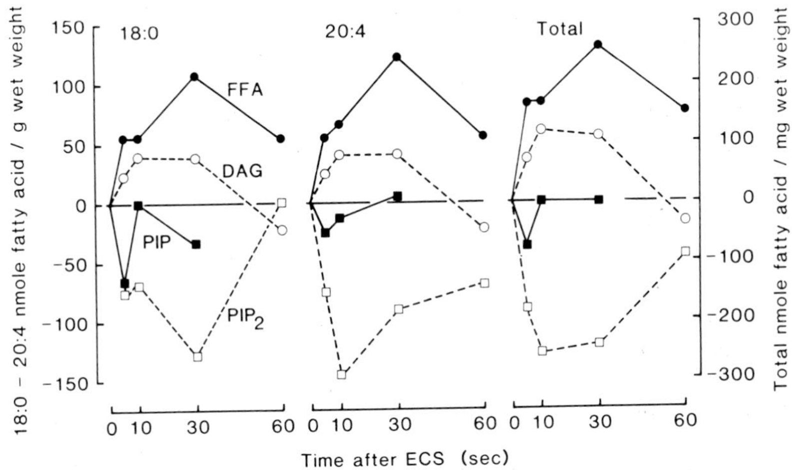

Fig. 2. Transient degradation of polyphosphoinositides and accumulation of free fatty acids and diacylglycerols in rat brain after ECS. Plotted values in nmoles of fatty acids per mg of wet weight are net changes obtained by subtracting basal values from experimental ones. Original values published by Reddy and Bazan (1987).

(Reddy and Bazan, 1987).

In experiments to study levels of both ECS-induced phospholipase A_1 and A_2 and phospholipase C reaction products (Reddy and Bazan, 1987) rats were given a single ECS (750 msec, 130 V, 150 p.p.s.), and brain was rapidly fixed by high-energy head-focused microwave irradiation at different times. These ECS conditions lead to a tonic-clonic seizure lasting 8 – 10 sec with full behavioral recovery within 1 min. A 30% decrease in phosphatidylinositol 4,5-bisphosphate (PIP_2) occurs during the first 10 sec, followed by a stationary phase up to 30 sec and a return to basal levels shortly after (Fig. 2). DAG levels show a similar profile. However, FFA accumulates in a biphasic manner, a rapid accumulation within the first 5 sec is followed by a slower increase between 10 and 30 sec. Changes in levels of phosphatidylinositol 4-phosphate (PIP) are small. This may result either from its phosphodiesteratic degradation or its further phosphorylation to replenish PIP_2. Moreover, activation of PI kinase is necessary to increase the availability of PIP for further phosphorylation to PIP_2. A net decrease of 20:4 acyl chains in PIP_2 and PIP within the first 5 – 10 sec is accompanied by an increase of similar magnitude in 20:4 in FFA and DAG. This suggests that PPI is the primary membrane lipid involved in these early events. FFA levels 2 – 5 sec after ECS are greater than that which could be derived solely from the released DAG, suggesting that PLA_2 and PLA_1 are activated at the same time as PLC. The later increase in FFA levels (10 – 30 sec) could derive from further metabolism of released 20:4-DAG via diacylglycerol lipase and/or via Ca^{2+}-mediated activation of PLA_2 which targets phospholipid pools enriched in 20:4. A soluble PLA_2, found in CNS, that translocates to membranes when intracellular Ca^{2+} levels rise (Yoshihara and Watanabe, 1990) could be responsible for the release of unsaturated fatty acids after IP_3-induced Ca^{2+} mobilization. In addition, a smaller increase in levels of other acyl groups such as palmitic acid (16:0) and oleic acid (18:1) in both DAG and FFA indicates some metabolism of phosphatidylcholine (PC). This also occurs during cerebral ischemia (Bazan, 1970; Lee and Hajra, 1991). Simultaneous release of choline and FFA has been reported to occur in the brain during seizures (Flynn and Wecker, 1987). Degradation of PC could contribute to the enlargement of the DAG pool, resulting in a prolonged stimulation of PKC and/or modulation of its activity at a different subcellular level. Alternatively, stimulation of this PC/DAG pathway could increase the availability of the precursor DAG for inositol lipid resynthesis. Of interest is that analysis of the acyl chains of DAG and inositol lipids in rat brain shows that, besides the main PPI-derived species containing 18:0 and 20:4, species characteristic of PC-derived lipids are also prevalent (i.e., 16:0 – 18:1, 16:0 – 16:0, 16:0 – 20:4) (Lee and Hajra, 1991). In summary, analysis of early changes in membrane phospholipid metabolism triggered by a single ECS demonstrates a direct precursor-product relationship between degraded PPI and released DAG and FFA.

Seizures induce activation of the arachidonic acid cascade in nerve terminals

Bicuculline-induced status epilepticus triggers a sustained accumulation of FFA and DAG in the brain (Bazan et al., 1982; Siesjö et al., 1982; Rodriguez de Turco et al., 1983). Seventeen-fold and 6.5-fold increases in levels of free 20:4 and 20:4-DAG, respectively, are observed 3 – 4 min post-injection. This coincides with the first major tonic-clonic seizure. Synaptic membrane phospholipids, which are

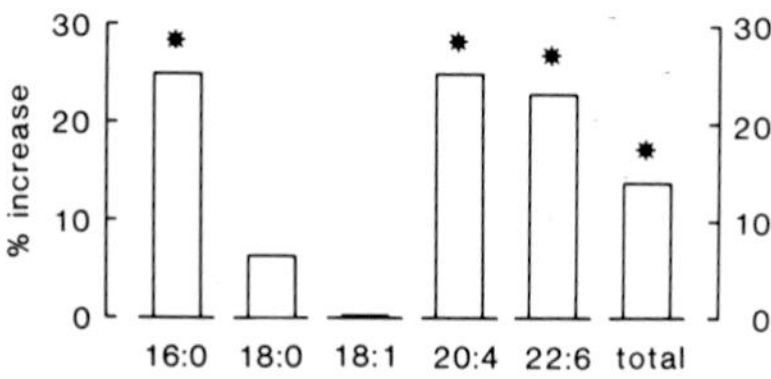

Fig. 3. Accumulation of free fatty acids in brain synaptosomes from bicuculline-treated rats. Rats were killed 4 min after their treatment with bicuculline (10 mg/kg, i.p.). Synaptosomes from untreated and bicuculline-treated rats were isolated, lipid extracted and FFA analyzed by GLC. Values were recalculated from Birkle and Bazan (1987). Asterisks denote statistically significant increases over control.

highly enriched in 20:4 and 22:6 (Cotman et al., 1964; Sun and Sun, 1972), are a particular target of seizure-activated PLA_2. Accumulation of these PUFAs occurs in synaptosomes isolated from the brains of bicuculline-treated rats (Fig. 3), but not in microsomes (Birkle and Bazan, 1987). This suggests that the PLA_2 responsive to elevated neuronal activity resides in a specific subcellular compartment.

The release of 20:4 from synaptosomal lipids and its subsequent metabolism via the lipoxygenase and cyclooxygenase pathways were followed during bicuculline-induced seizures (Birkle and Bazan, 1987). Rat brains were prelabeled "in vivo" by bilateral intraventricular injection of [1-^{14}C]20:4 sodium salt (1 μCi per hemisphere) 30 min prior to administration of bicuculline (10 mg/kg, i.p.). Compared with untreated animals, 30% less label is recovered from synaptosomal lipids and there is a 30% increase in labeling of free fatty acids (Fig. 4).

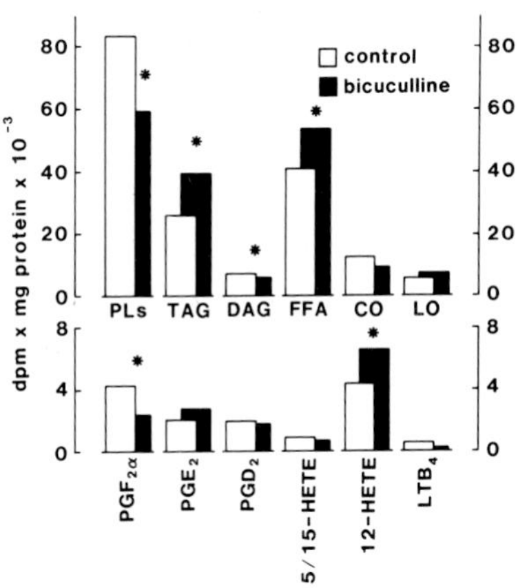

Fig. 4. Activation of arachidonic acid cascade in nerve terminals during bicuculline-induced seizure. Rats were labeled in vivo by intraventricular injection of [1-^{14}C]20:4 (1 μCi in each ventricle). After 30 min, bicuculline (10 mg/kg) was injected i.p. and rats killed 4 min later. Synaptosomes were isolated by density gradient centrifugation, and lipids were extracted, isolated by thin layer chromatography and quantified by liquid scintillation counting (Marcheselli and Bazan, 1990). Cycloxygenase (CO) and lipoxygenase (LO) products of [1-^{14}C]20:4 were isolated and quantified by high performance liquid chromatography (Birkle and Bazan, 1987). Asterisks denote statistically significant differences between control and bicuculline-treated rats. Values were recalculated from those published by Birkle and Bazan (1987).

PC and PI, followed by PE release most 20:4 (Birkle and Bazan, 1987). A significant proportion of released [^{14}C]20:4 is esterified into triacylglycerol (TAG). This suggests an active role of TAG as a transient reservoir of 20:4 to prevent this essential fatty acid from escaping through the circulation or from being oxidized. A similar transient accumulation of 20:4-TAG has been shown to take place during early transient cerebral ischemia (Yoshida et al., 1986). A small proportion of free [^{14}C]20:4 is metabolized via the cyclooxygenase and lipoxygenase pathways. The lipoxygenase pathway, but not the cyclooxygenase pathway, is stimulated in the synaptosomes of bicuculline-treated rats. A significantly higher accumulation of 12-HETE is observed as a consequence of in vivo convulsions in synaptic, but not in microsomal membranes (Birkle and Bazan, 1987). This indicates that not only the release of 20:4 but also its further metabolism via lipoxygenation is selectively stimulated in the synapses during seizures.

Seizures trigger prolonged changes in synaptosomal arachidonate metabolism with a priming effect on the lipoxygenase pathway

The prolonged effect on 20:4 metabolism of a single bicuculline-induced tonic-clonic seizure was assessed using "in vitro" manipulations of [1-^{14}C]20:4 labeled synaptosomes (Birkle and Bazan, 1987). When synaptosomes isolated from the brains of untreated rats are incubated under normal (5 mM K^+) and depolarizing (45 mM K^+) conditions for 30 min, [1-^{14}C]20:4 is released mainly from PC (44% of total released label), PI (21%) and TAG (21%) (Fig. 5). Only PI degradation is significantly increased by depolarization. The released [1-^{14}C]20:4 is further metabolized mainly via the cyclooxygenase pathway. Depolarization stimulates the synthesis of prostaglandins 6 keto-$F_{1\alpha}$ and D_2 while it decreases the labeling recovered in thromboxane B_2. Lipoxygenation of 20:4 is very low under normal conditions (3.9% of total radioactivity). However, depolarization stimulates these pathways: the labels in 5-HETE, 15-HETE, 12-

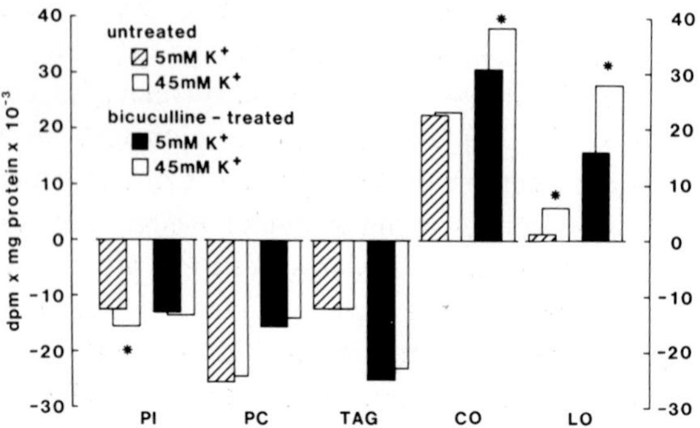

Fig. 5. Loss of arachidonoyl chains from membrane lipids and triacylglycerides in synaptosomes from control and bicuculline-treated rats. Synaptosomes were incubated for 30 min in buffer containing 5 mM K^+ or 45 mM K^+. Lipids were extracted from untreated and incubated synaptosomes obtained from control and bicuculline-treated rats. Values represent the difference between samples incubated in medium containing 45 mM K^+ or 5 mM K^+. All differences between basal and incubated samples are statistically significant. Values were recalculated from Birkle and Bazan (1977). Other details as in Fig. 4.

HETE and leukotriene B_4 account for 7.7% of the total radioactivity recovered.

In synaptosomes from bicuculline-treated rats, changes in lipid labeling and metabolism of [1-^{14}C]-20:4 induced by in vitro incubations differ from those in untreated rats. Triacylgycerols show the highest decrease of label (40% of total released [1-^{14}C]20:4) followed by PC (25%) and PI (21%) (Fig. 5). Interestingly, [1-^{14}C]20:4, incorporated during in vivo seizures into synaptosomal TAG (Fig. 4), is actively released during in vitro incubation. At the same time, phospholipids such as PC and phosphatidylserine (PS) (not shown) release less label. This is a consequence of in vivo release of labeled 20:4 resulting form PLA_2 activation during seizures. In contrast to control animals, no further accumulation of labeling is observed in the FFA pool. There is, however, active metabolism of 20:4 both through the lipoxygenase and cyclooxygenase pathways. Seizures increase lipoxygenation of 20:4. 12-HETE, then 15-HETE and 5-HETE are the main labeled lipoxygenase products in synaptosomes incubated with 5 mM K^+, accounting for 7.6% and 4.6% of total label recovered. This compares with 2% and 1.5%, respectively, in synaptosomes from control animals. Depolarization raises levels of lipoxygenase products to 4.7 times those in control synaptosomes. The accumulation of cyclooxygenase products in synaptosomes from bicuculline-treated rats shows similar values compared to controls when incubated with 5 mM and 45 mM K^+. However, levels of individual products differ. In bicuculline-treated samples, prostaglandins E_2, D_2 and $F_{2\alpha}$ are the main components while in prostaglandins 6 keto $F_{1\alpha}$ and D_2 predominate in controls. These results indicate that seizure activity results in the specific activation in synapses of selected branches of the arachidonic acid cascade. Furthermore, the high levels of lipoxygenase products observed when synaptosomal metabolism is activated by depolarization demonstrate the priming effect of seizures at this level.

Dissociation between PLA_2- and PLC-mediated 20:4 and 20:4-DAG release in the immature brain during anoxia and convulsions

In contrast to the rapid membrane phospholipid degradation in the brains of mature mammals undergoing ischemia or convulsions, the brains of infant mammals and poikilotherms display much less rapid and extensive lipid degradation activity (Bazan, 1970, 1971; Aveldaño and Bazan, 1975). This correlates with the higher vulnerability of mature brain to some pathophysiological conditions and suggests that overstimulation of membrane lipid degradation processes may contribute to the development of irreversible brain damage. Newborn mouse pups can withstand 40 min of anoxia under nitrogen (Rodriguez de Turco and Bazan, 1983). Strikingly, no 20:4 accumulation is observed during this long period of anoxia (Fig. 6). A slow release of 20:4, compared with that observed in adult brain during oxygen deprivation, is observed after 45 – 60 min of anoxia. Also, no 20:4-DAG accumulates during 60 min of anoxia. This suggests that the enzymatic mechanisms involved in 20:4 and 20:4-DAG release in the brain utilize distinct pathways, such as the simultaneous activity of

PLA_2 and PLC, rather than the sequential activity of PLC and DAG lipase. The absence of a metabolically active pool of PPI in synaptic membranes from newborn brain (Uma and Ramakrishna, 1983) also suggests a precursor-product relationship with the 20:4-DAG released in mature brain during ischemia. 20:4-containing membrane phospholipid is also highly preserved in the brains of infant rats undergoing seizures (Morelli de Liberti et al., 1985). In five-day-old rats, pentylenetetrazol-induced seizures result in accumulation of FFA and DAG derived from lipids other than those containing 20:4 (Fig. 7). In summary, in the brains of infant mammals, the absence or low activity of receptor-mediated pathways with PLA_2 an/or PLC activity targeted at 20:4-phospholipids, contribute to preserve neuronal membrane structure and function.

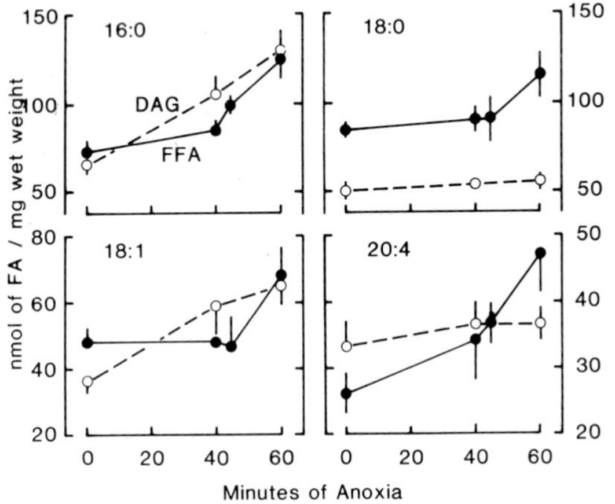

Fig. 6. Changes in free fatty acid and diacylglycerol-acyl groups in the newborn brain during anoxia. Mouse pups were kept under nitrogen for different periods of time. Open symbols: DAG acyl-groups. Closed symbols: individual FFA.

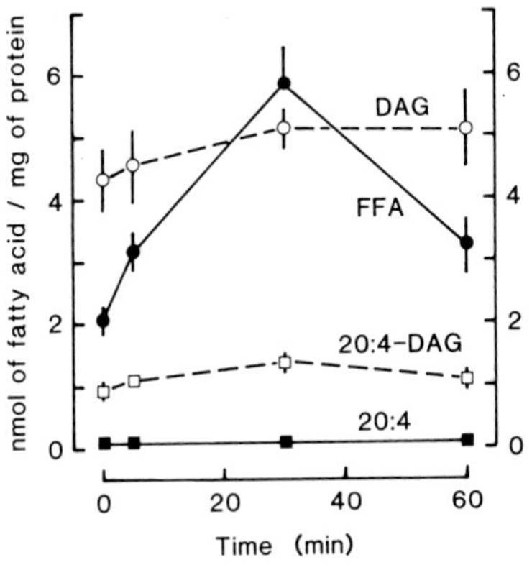

Fig. 7. Pentylenetetrazol-induced seizures do not mobilize arachidonate from membrane phospholipids in the immature animal brain. Five-day-old rat pups were treated with PTZ (Morelli de Liberti et al., 1985) and killed at different times during the convulsive phase. Closed circles: total free fatty acid; closed squares: free arachidonic acid (20:4); open circles: total diacylglycerol; open squares: arachidonoyl-diacylglycerol.

PAF-mediated effects on transcriptional activity of neuronal genes

Of the reaction products generated by PLA_2 activation during cerebral ischemia and convulsions, only PAF has so far been shown potentially to mediate long-term changes in neuronal phenotype via

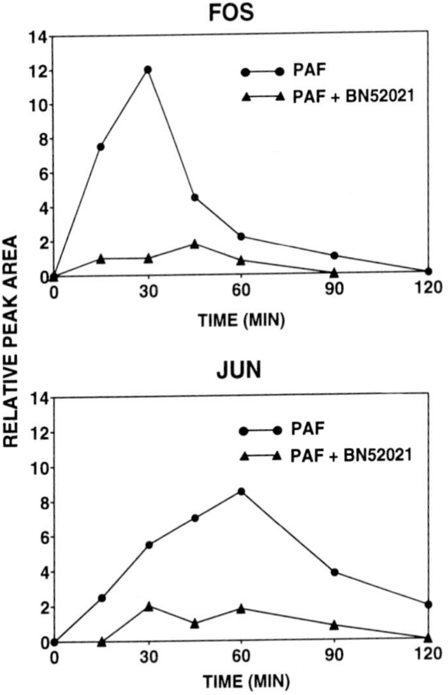

Fig. 8. PAF transiently induces c-*fos* and c-*jun* in SH-SY5Y cells. Cells were treated with 1 μM PAF for the times indicated, total cellular RNA isolated, and c-*fos* and c-*jun* mRNA levels determined by slot-blot hybridization densitometry (Squinto et al., 1989). When the PAF antagonist BN 52021 (1 μM) was used, this was added 1 h before PAF addition.

transcriptional activation of nuclear proto-oncogenes. Administration of 1 μM PAF to the human neuroblastoma cell line SH-SY5Y transiently activates transcription of the c-*fos* and c-*jun* proto-oncogenes (Squinto et al., 1989; 1990). The kinetics of induction (c-*fos* mRNA levels peak at 30 min and c-*jun* mRNA levels peak at 60 min (Fig. 8)) are characteristic of the effects of a number of receptor-mediated neuronal stimuli on these genes. These include the activities of neurotransmitters and neurotrophic factors, neuropathological states induced by cerebral ischemia and chemically and electrically induced seizures (for review, see Doucet et al., 1990). Pretreatment of the cells with the ginkgolide PAF antagonist BN-52021 at 1 μM 1 h before addition of PAF almost totally inhibits activation of the proto-oncogenes. Fos and jun proteins can combine in homo- and heterodimers and act as components of AP-1 transcription factor complexes. These are proposed to bind to consensus *cis*-regulatory sequences (AP-1 sites) in the 5′ non-transcribed regions of target genes and alter their transcriptional activity. PAF induces the formation of an active AP-1 complex. When PAF is administered to SH-SY5Y cells which have been previously transfected with a mammalian expression vector construct which contains four tandem AP-1 sites in its promoter, transcriptional activity is detected from a reporter gene in the construct (Squinto et al., 1989). This activity is completely an-

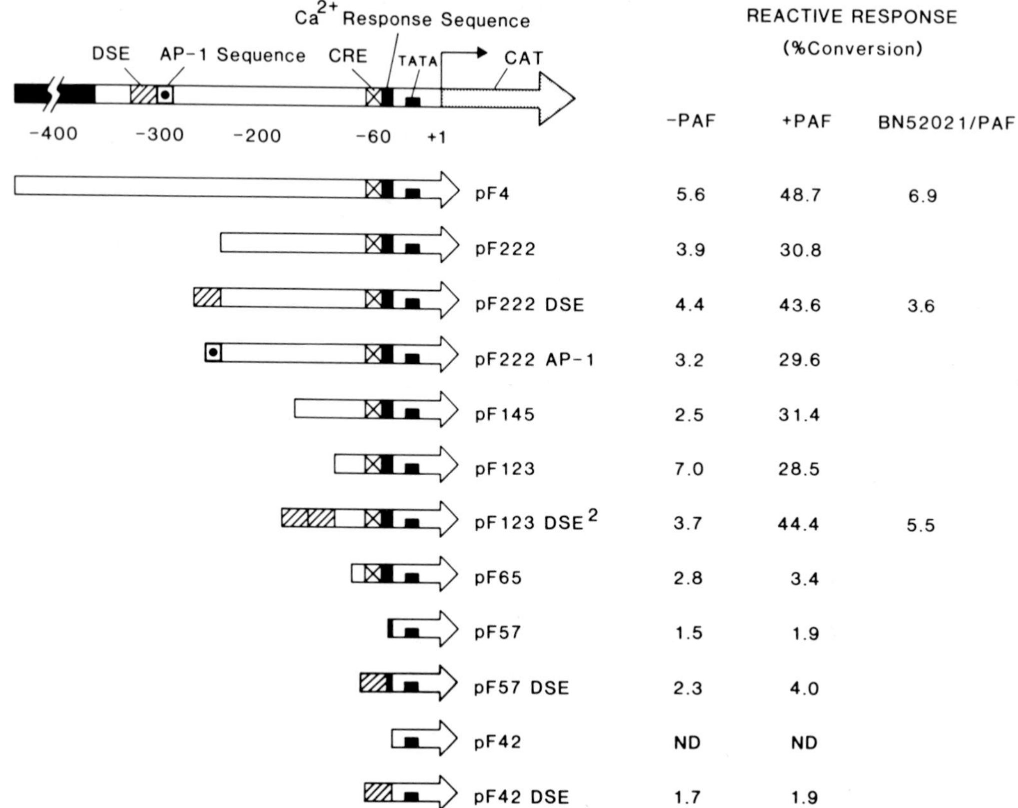

Fig. 9. Analysis of deletion mutants of the *fos* promoter and identification of a region responsible for PAF-indicated transcriptional activation. Recombinant *fos*-promoter deletion mutant chloramphenicol acetyl transferase (CAT) constructs were transfected into SH-SY5Y cells and CAT activity assayed 36 h after exposure to 1 μM PAF. When used, BN 52021 was added 1 h before PAF. The figure shows a schematic representation of the different deletion mutants of the *fos* promoter used and how these affect PAF-inducible CAT activity.

tagonized by pretreatment with BN-52021. Studies of deletion mutants of the *fos* promoter show that the region of the promoter required for PAF to elicit *fos* transcription overlaps regions required for elevated free Ca^{2+} and cyclic AMP to exert similar effects (Fig. 9). There is evidence that PAF is also involved in c-*fos* activation in vivo. A single ECS induces elevated levels of c-*fos* mRNA in the rat hippocampus, and to a lesser extent, in the cortex. Intraperitoneal injection of the triazolobenzodiazepine PAF antagonist BN-50730, 30 min before ECS, decreases both the amplitude and duration of *fos* induction in the hippocampus and, to a lesser extent, in the cortex (Marcheselli et al., 1991). Paradoxically, BN-50730 does not antagonize PAF-induced c-*fos* expression in the SH-SY5Y line (Doucet et al., 1991). This implies either a heterogeneity of PAF receptors between the rat brain and human neuroblastoma cells, or that exogenous and endogenous PAF stimulate c-*fos* expression via distinct receptors. PAF binding studies in rat brain membrane preparations show two distinct types of binding site: two high-affinity microsomal sites and a lower affinity synaptosomal site (Marcheselli et al., 1990). The former are antagonized by BN-50730, but not BN-52021, while the latter shows preferential binding for BN-52021.

Evidence for long-term effects of PAF on neural cells expression has been shown by Kornecki and Ehrlich (1988), who demonstrate that treatment of the mouse/rat neuroblastoma × glioma hybrid cell line NG108-15 with PAF at 50 nM – 2.5 μM induces morphological differentiation after 3 – 4 days. In the SH-SY5Y line, after treatment with 1 μM PAF or 250 nM of the non-hydrolyzable, biologically active PAF analogue N-methylcarbamyl PAF, levels of calcyclin mRNA rise after 8 h and return to basal values by 24 h (Allan and Bazan, 1989; Allan et al., 1990). Under these conditions expression of the mRNA encoding heat shock protein 70 is unaffected, suggesting that the cells are not undergoing a stress response but may be involved in a physiologically relevant process. Calcyclin is a small calmodulin-like calcium-binding protein expressed during the G_1 phase of the cell cycle. The expression of calcyclin is elevated in several cell types in response to some growth factors (Calabretta et al., 1986) and in the differentiation of some neuroblastoma lines (Tonini et al., 1991).

Molecular differentiation of a pure neuronal cell line in response to PAF has not been reported. This suggests that if PAF has a role in the neuroregenerative and remodeling events following cerebral ischemia and convulsions, perhaps other components in the CNS are involved.

References

Allan, G. and Bazan, N.G. (1989) Differential increase in levels of c-*fos* and calcyclin, but not heat-shock protein 24, mRNAs in response to platelet-activating factor in a human neuroblastoma cell line. *Soc. Neurosci. Abstr.,* 15: 842.

Allan, G., Moerschbaecher, III, J.M. and Bazan, N.G. (1990) Elevated levels of expression of GAP-43 and calcyclin mRNAs during TPA-induced differentiation of a human neuroblastoma cell line. *Soc. Neurosci. Abstr.,* 16: 814.

Aveldaño, M.I. and Bazan, N.G. (1975) Rapid production of diacylglycerols enriched in arachidonate and stearate during early brain ischemia. *J. Neurochem.,* 25: 919 – 920.

Bazan, N.G. (1970) Effects of ischemia and electroconvulsive shock on free fatty acid pool in the brain. *Biochim. Biophys. Acta,* 218: 1 – 10.

Bazan, N.G. (1971) Free fatty acid production in cerebral white and grey matter of the squirrel monkey. *Lipids,* 6: 211 – 212.

Bazan, N.G. (1990) Neuronal cell signal transduction and second messengers in cerebral ischemia. In: J. Krieglstein and H. Oberpichler (Eds.), *Pharmacology of Cerebral Ischemia – Proceedings of the Third International Symposium on Pharmacology of Cerebral Ischemia,* Wissenschaftliche Verlagsgesellschaft, Stuttgart, pp. 391 – 398.

Bazan, N.G. and Rakowski, H. (1970) Increased levels of brain free fatty acids after electro-convulsive shock. *Life Sci.,* 9: 501 – 507.

Bazan, N.G. and Rodriguez de Turco, E.B. (1980) Membrane lipids in the pathogenesis of brain edema: phospholipids and arachidonic acid, the earliest membrane components changed at the onset of ischemia. In: J. Cervós-Navarro and R. Ferszt (Eds.), *Advances in Neurology: Brain Edema, Vol. 28,* Raven Press, New York, pp. 197 – 205.

Bazan, N.G., Bazan, H.E.P., Kennedy, W.G. and Joel, C.D. (1971) Regional distribution and rate of production of free fatty acids in rat brain. *J. Neurochem.,* 18: 1387 – 1393.

Bazan, N.G., Aveldaño de Caldironi, M.I. and Rodriguez de Turco, E.B. (1981) Rapid release of free arachidonic acid in the central nervous system due to stimulation. *Prog. Lipid Res.,* 20: 523 – 529.

Bazan, N.G., Morelli de Liberti, S.M. and Rodriguez de Turco, E.B. (1982) Arachidonic acid and arachidonoyl-diglycerides increase in rat cerebrum during bicuculline-induced status epilepticus. *Neurochem. Res.,* 7: 839 – 843.

Bazan, N.G., Squinto, S.P., Braquet, P., Panetta, T. and Marcheselli, V.L. (1991) Platelet-activating factor and polyunsaturated fatty acids in cerebral ischemia or convulsions: intracellular PAF-binding sites and activation of a Fos/Jun/Ap-1 transcriptional signaling system. *Lipids,* 25: 1236 – 1242.

Berridge, M.J. (1984) Inositol trisphosphate and diacylglycerol as second messengers. *Biochem. J.,* 220: 345 – 360.

Birkle, D.L. and Bazan, N.G. (1987) Effect of bicuculline-induced status epilepticus on prostaglandins and hydroxyeicosatetraenoic acids in rat brain subcellular fractions. *J. Neurochem.,* 348: 1768 – 1778.

Braquet, P., Touqui, L., Shen, T.Y. and Vargaftig, B.B. (1987) Perspectives in platelet-activating factor research. *Pharmacol. Rev.,* 39: 97 – 145.

Calabretta, B., Battini, R., Kaczmarek, L., De Riel, J.K. and Baserga, R. (1986) Molecular cloning of the cDNA for a growth factor-inducible gene with strong homology to S-100, a calcium-binding protein. *J. Biol. Chem.,* 261: 12628 – 12632.

Clark, J.D., Lin, L.-L., Kriz, R.W., Ramesha, C.S., Sultzman, L.A., Lin, A.Y., Milona, N. and Knopf, J.L. (1991) A novel arachidonic acid-selective cytosolic PLA_2 contains a Ca^{2+} dependent translocation domain with homology to PKC and GAP. *Cell,* 65: 1043 – 1051.

Cotman, C., Blank, M.L., Moehl, A. and Snyder, F. (1967) Lipid composition of synaptic plasma membranes isolated from rat brain by zonal centrifugation. *Biochemistry,* 3: 4606 – 4611.

Doucet, J.P., Squinto, S.P. and Bazan, N.G. (1990) Fos-Jun and the primary genomic response in the nervous system: physiological role and pathophysiological significance. *Mol. Neurobiol.,* 4: 27 – 55.

Doucet, J.P., Marcheselli, V.L. and Bazan, N.G. (1991) Triazolobenzodiazepine-based antagonism of platelet-activating factor and induction of *fos* expression in human SH-SY5Y neuroblastoma cells. *Soc. Neurosci. Abstr.,* 17: 170.

Flynn, C.J. and Wecker, L. (1987) Concomitant increases in the levels of choline and free fatty acids in rat brain: evidence supporting the seizure-induced hydrolysis of phosphatidylcholine. *J. Neurochem.,* 48: 1178 – 1184.

Kornecki, E. and Ehrlich, Y.H. (1988) Neuroregulatory and neuropathological actions of the ether phospholipid platelet-activating factor. *Science,* 240: 1792 – 1794.

Lee, C. and Hajra, A.K. (1991) Molecular species of diacylglycerols and phosphoglycerides and the postmortem changes in the molecular species of diacylglycerols in rat brain. *J. Neurochem,* 565: 370 – 379.

Marcheselli, V.L. and Bazan, N.G. (1990) Quantitative analysis of fatty acids in phospholipids, diacylglycerols, free fatty acids, and other lipids. *J. Nutr. Biochem.,* 1(7): 382 – 388.

Marcheselli, V.L., Rosskowska, M., Domingo, M.T., Braquet, P. and Bazan, N.G. (1990) Distinct platelet-activating factor binding sites in synaptic endings and in intracellular membranes of rat cerebral cortex. *J. Biol. Chem.,* 265: 9140 – 9145.

Marcheselli, V.L., Doucet, J.P. and Bazan, N.G. (1991) Platelet-activating factor is a mediator of *fos* expression induced by a single seizure in rat hippocampus. *Soc. Neurosci. Abstr.,* 17: 349.

Morelli de Liberti, S.A., Santos de Schub, E.B. and Rodriguez de Turco, E.B. (1985) Circannual rhythm of free acids and diacylglycerols in 5-day-old rat brain during pentylenetetrazol-induced convulsions. *J. Neurochem.,* 45: 1055 – 1061.

Nishizuka, Y. (1984) The role of protein kinase C in cell surface signal transduction and tumor promotion. *Nature,* 308: 693 – 698.

Ramesha, C.S. and Pickett, W.C. (1986) Platelet-activating factor and leukotriene biosynthesis is inhibited in polymorphonuclear leukocytes depleted of arachidonic acid. *J. Biol. Chem.,* 261: 7592 – 7595.

Reddy, T.S. and Bazan, N.G. (1987) Arachidonic acid, stearic acid and diacylglycerol accumulation correlates with the loss of phosphatidylinositol 4,5-bisphosphate in cerebrum 2 seconds after electroconvulsive shock. Complete reversion of changes 5 minutes after stimulation. *J. Neurosci. Res.,* 18: 449 – 455.

Rodriguez de Turco, E.B. and Bazan, N.G. (1983) Changes in free fatty acids and diglycerides in mouse brain at birth and during anoxia. *J. Neurochem.,* 41: 794 – 800.

Rodriguez de Turco, E.B., Morelli de Liberti, S. and Bazan, N.G. (1983) Stimulation of free fatty acid and diacylglycerol accumulation in cerebrum and cerebellum during bicuculline-induced status epilepticus. Effect of pretreatment with alpha-methyl-p-tyrosine and p-chlorophenylalamine. *J. Neurochem.,* 40: 252 – 259.

Siesjö, B.K., Ingvar, M. and Westerberg, Z. (1982) The influence of bicuculline-induced seizures on free fatty acid concentrations in cerebral cortex, hippocampus and cerebellum. *J. Neurochem.,* 39: 796 – 802.

Siffert, W., Siffert, G., Scheid, P. and Akkerman, J.W. (1990) Na^+/H^+ exchange modulates Ca^{2+} mobilization in human platelets stimulated by ADP and a thromboxane mimetic. *J. Biol. Chem.,* 265: 719 – 725.

Squinto, S.P., Block, A.L., Braquet, P. and Bazan, N.G. (1989) Platelet-activating factor stimulates a Fos/Jun AP-1 transcriptional system in human neuroblastoma cells. *J. Neurosci. Res.,* 24: 558 – 566.

Squinto, S.P., Braquet, P., Block, A.L. and Bazan, N.G. (1990) Platelet-activating factor activates HIV promoter in transfected SH-SY5Y neuroblastoma cells and MOLT-4 T lymphocytes. *J. Mol. Neurosci.,* 52: 79 – 84.

Suga, K., Kawasaki, Y., Blank, M.L. and Snyder, F. (1990) An arachidonoyl (polyenoic)-specific phospholipase A_2 activity regulates the synthesis of platelet-activating factor in granulocytic HL-60 cells. *J. Biol. Chem.*, 265: 12363 – 12371.

Sun, G.Y. and Sun, A.Y. (1972) Phospholipids and acyl groups synaptosomal and myelin membranes isolated from the cerebral cortex of squirrel monkey *(Saimiri Sciureus). Biochim. Biophys. Acta,* 280: 306 – 315.

Sun, G.Y., Yoa, F.-G. and Lin, T.-N. (1990) Degradation of poly-phosphoinositides in brain subcellular membranes in response to decapitation insult. *Neurochem. Int.,* 174: 529 – 535.

Tonini, G.F., Casalaro, A., Cara, A. and Di Martino, D. (1991) Inducible expression of calcyclin, a gene with strong homology to S-100 protein, during neuroblastoma cell differentiation, and its prevalent expression in Schwann-like cell lines. *Cancer Res.,* 51: 1733 – 1737.

Uma, S. and Ramakrishna, C.V. (1983) Studies on polyphosphoinositides in developing rat brain. *J. Neurochem.,* 40: 914 – 916.

Yoshida, S., Ikeda, M., Busto, R., Santiso, M., Martinez, E. and Ginsberg, M.D. (1986) Cerebral phosphoinositide, triacylglycerol, and energy metabolism in reversible ischemia; origin and fate of free fatty acids. *J. Neurochem.,* 47: 744 – 757.

Yoshihara, Y. and Watanabe, Y. (1990) Translocation of phospholipase A_2 from cytosol to membranes in rat brain induced by calcium ions. *Biochem. Biophys. Res. Commun.,* 170: 484 – 490.

SECTION V

Maturation Phenomena

K. Kogure, K.-A. Hossmann and B.K. Siesjö (Eds.)
Progress in Brain Research, Vol. 96

CHAPTER 18

Presynaptic terminals in hippocampal gliosis following transient ischemia in the Mongolian gerbil

Takaaki Kirino

Department of Neurosurgery, Teikyo University School of Medicine, Tokyo 173, Japan

Introduction

In the central nervous system, certain groups of neurons are selectively damaged even by a transient, brief ischemic insult. When neurons are selectively destroyed and removed, the injured brain region falls into gliosis. A well-known and classical example of gliosis is encountered in the hippocampal CA1 sector following brief ischemia. This pathological alteration is frequently found in epileptic patients and in victims of transient but profound cerebral ischemia (Brierley and Graham, 1984; Siesjö and Wieloch, 1986). The gliotic change in the hippocampus has aroused interest among pathologists for more than a century. Sommer (1880) first reported that one-third of epileptic patients showed an extensive loss of neurons in a circumscribed portion of the hippocampus. This area is now frequently called Sommer's sector, which corresponds to the CA1 subfield of the hippocampus.

A later pathological study revealed that anoxia/ischemia causes an almost identical lesion in the hippocampus (Brierley and Graham, 1984). The mechanism of this hippocampal damage has been a subject of controversy. Spielmeyer (1925) and his colleagues laid emphasis on the role of local circulatory disturbance. On the contrary, Vogt and Vogt (1922) believed that a difference in physical or chemical characteristics of individual neurons was the major cause of this hippocampal injury. Recently, it has become possible to easily reproduce ischemic hippocampal damage and ensuing gliosis in rodents. Brief ischemia in the Mongolian gerbil (Kirino, 1982) or in the rat (Pulsinelli et al., 1982; Smith et al., 1984) kills most of the neurons in the CA1 sector. Following neuronal death in the CA1 sector, the number of reactive astroglia increases and the area gradually shrinks (Mudrick and Baimbridge, 1989; Kirino et al., 1990). Ultimately, the CA1 subfield becomes a thin, slit-like structure.

During the acute phase after brief ischemia, pyramidal cells in the CA1 sector are selectively injured and destroyed. Most afferent fibers and synaptic terminals remain morphologically unchanged (Kirino, 1982; Johansen et al., 1984). Further morphological studies have shown that these presynaptic structures maintain their structural integrity for an extended period of time. Kirino et al. (1990) observed presynaptic terminals in the CA1 sector where most of the neurons are absent 12 months after ischemia. Bonnekoh et al. (1990) described structurally intact synapses in the CA1 sector ten months following ischemic insult. The study in this communication was conducted to observe the maintenance of presynaptic terminals and to evaluate the survival of terminals by a morphometric method.

Materials and methods

Male Mongolian gerbils (*Meriones unguiculatus*, 60 – 90 g) were subjected to transient ischemia.

The animals were anesthetized with 2% halothane in 30% O_2 and 70% N_2. The carotid arteries were occluded for 5 min with aneurysm clips.

Light microscopy

One month (n = 10), three months (n = 10), six months (n = 13) and 12 months (n = 7) following ischemia, the animals were fixed by transcardiac perfusion with 3.5% formaldehyde in 0.1 M phosphate buffer (pH = 7.4). The brains were embedded in paraffin, and 5 μm thick sections containing the dorsal hippocampi were cut and stained with hematoxylin-eosin or luxol fast blue-cresyl violet. Untreated gerbils (n = 11) were fixed in the same way and used as normal controls. One section which included the dorsal hippocampus 0.5 – 1.0 mm posterior to its most rostral tip (Loskota et al., 1974) was selected from each animal. The area of the CA1 subfield of each hippocampal region and the length of the CA1 stratum pyramidale were measured on enlarged photographs. The width of the CA1 sector was calculated by dividing the area of the CA1 sector by the length of the CA1 stratum pyramidale. The average of the values of right and left sides was used as the value for each animal.

Electron microscopy

Gerbils were subjected to 5 min of forebrain ischemia as described above. One month (n = 4), three months (n = 4), six months (n = 5) and 12 months (n = 7) following the operation, the animals were perfusion-fixed with 2.0% paraformaldehyde and 2.5% glutaraldehyde in 0.1 M cacodylate buffer (pH = 7.4). The specimens containing the dorsal hippocampus, as described above, were post-fixed in 2% OsO_4. Tissue samples were embedded in Epon. Thin sections were cut with a diamond knife, stained with uranyl acetate and lead citrate, and observed using a Hitachi HS-9 or JEOL 100CX electron microscope. The main area of observation was the neuropil in the striatum radiatum of the CA1 sector. Untreated normal gerbils (n = 5) served as normal controls.

For morphometric analysis, the specimens from the one month group (n = 4), three month group (n = 4), six month group (n = 5) and 12 month group (n = 7) were used. Thin sections from each specimen were mounted on slit grids. Consecutive electron microscopic photographs were taken from each specimen. Photographs were taken starting just below the stratum pyramidale (although pyramidal cells were already absent) and a series of ten photographs of the neuropil in the stratum radiatum was obtained perpendicular to the stratum pyramidale at the magnification of 8300. One series of film for each specimen covered a rectangular area which had a width of 12.0 μm and a height of 84.4 μm. Presynaptic terminals were counted on printed pictures and the sum of ten photographs was used as a value for each animal. The density of presynaptic terminals was expressed as a number per mm^2 of the CA1 stratum radiatum. The width of the CA1 subfield was measured on Epon embedded semi-thin sections. The measurement was obtained in the region of CA1 where the electron microscopic specimen was taken.

Results

Light microscopy

Following 5 min of ischemia, all of the gerbils (n = 40) developed neuronal necrosis in the CA1 sector. The pattern of hippocampal damage was identical to that already described (Kirino, 1982; Kirino and Sano, 1984). The average thickness of the CA1 sector in the normal gerbils was 501 ± 19 (S.D.) μm. At one month following ischemia (Fig. 1*a*), the thickness was 505 ± 30 μm and there was no significant difference from the normal animals. At three months after ischemia (Fig. 1*b*), the thickness was 425 ± 23 μm. At six months after ischemia (Fig. 1*c*), the thickness was 387 ± 39 μm and at 12 months (Fig. 1*d*), it was 359 ± 14 μm. Three or more months after ischemia, the thickness of the CA1 sector was significantly lower ($P < 0.001$) than that of normal gerbils.

Electron microscopy

Brief ischemia for 5 min destroyed most of the

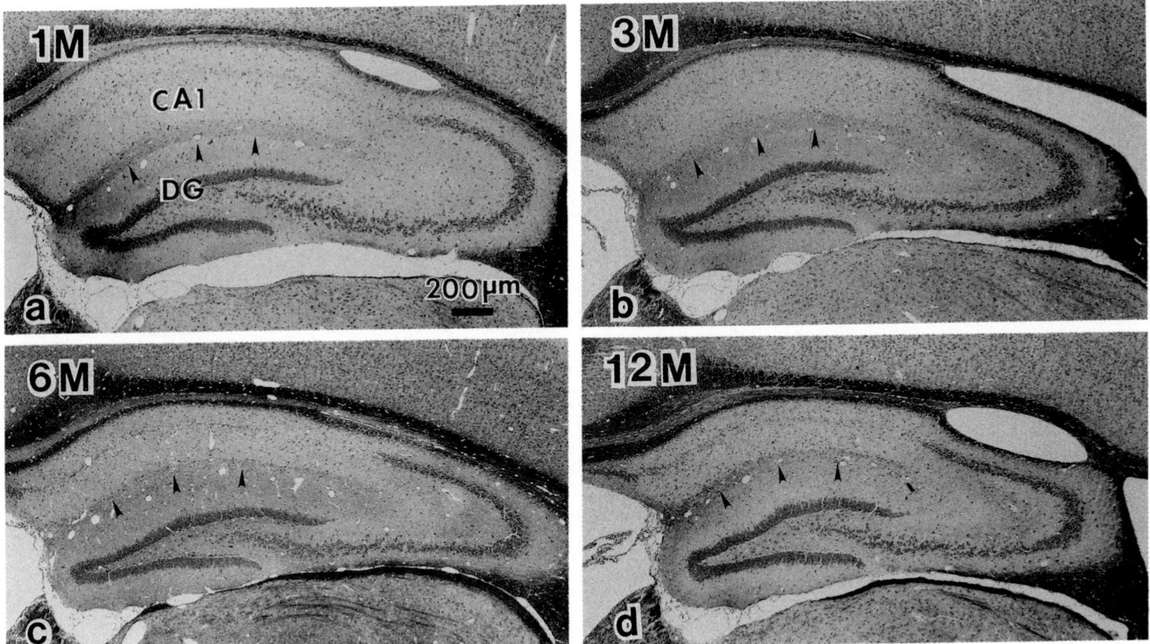

Fig. 1. Gradual shrinkage of the CA1 sector. The fused hippocampal fissure which divides the CA1 sector (CA1) and the dentate gyrus (DG) is indicated by arrowheads. At one month following ischemia (*a*), the thickness of CA1 is similar to that of normal animals. At three months after ischemia (*b*) and thereafter (*c,d*), the thickness progressively decreases. (Paraffin, cresyl violet and luxol fast blue; bar in *a*, 200 μm).

CA1 neurons in all of the gerbils ($n = 20$) examined by electron microscopic observation. At one month following ischemia, most of the pyramidal cells in the CA1 sector had disappeared. In the stratum radiatum, the typical radiating pattern of dendritic shafts had been lost. On the other hand, many terminals containing abundant clear vesicles were seen in the neuropil (Fig. 2). These terminals were frequently apposed to membranous structures containing electron-dense, amorphous material. In the interface between the membranous structure and the vesicle-containing terminals, specialized plasma membrane was observed.

At three months following ischemia (Fig. 3), numerous vesicle-containing terminals were seen in the stratum radiatum. They were associated with a membranous structure, the inside of which was packed with electron-dense, flocculent material. The fine structure of the neuropil was basically similar to that seen one month following ischemia.

At six months after ischemic insult (Fig. 4), the vesicle-containing terminals were still abundant, but they were usually not apposed to membranous structures. Where membrane specialization was observed in the vesicle-containing terminals, degenerative dendritic structures were seen opposite the specialized plasma membrane.

At 12 months after ischemia, many presynaptic terminals were still present and their fine structure was similar to that observed six months after ischemia (Fig. 5). Presynaptic terminals were not evenly distributed. While they were numerous and found as clusters in some regions, a complex network of astrocytic processes was dominant and presynaptic terminals were sparse in other areas.

Morphometric analysis revealed a progressive decrease of presynaptic terminals in the CA1 sector (Fig. 6*a*). At one month following ischemia, the density of presynaptic terminals in the stratum radiatum was $472 \times 10^3 \pm 158 \times 10^3$ (S.D.)/mm^2. At three months after ischemia, the density was $506 \times 10^3 \pm 23 \times 10^3/\text{mm}^2$; at six months it was $261 \times 10^3 \pm 53 \times 10^3/\text{mm}^2$, and at 12 months it was $118 \times 10^3 \pm 26 \times 10^3/\text{mm}^2$. The relatively large variance in the one month group was due to the fact that one specimen in this group showed a very low density value (242×10^3). At the same time, gradual shrinkage of the CA1 sector was noted (Fig. 6*b*). Therefore, the value obtained from serial photographs overestimated the actual population of the presynaptic terminal. The thickness of the CA1 sector was 629 ± 26 (S.D.) μm in normal gerbils. The thickness was 573 ± 45 μm at one month following ischemia. There was a slight difference in the thickness of CA1 between the normal and one month groups ($P < 0.05$). The thickness was 510 ± 13 μm at three months, 424 ± 39 μm at six months and 278 ± 53 μm at 12 months following ischemia. Since Epon-embedded specimens shrink by only a few percent (Weibel, 1969), the rate of tissue shrinkage measured by Epon-embedded hippocampi more correctly delineates the actual atrophy of the CA1 sector. If the shrinkage factor is taken into consideration on the assumption that CA1 shrinkage occurred linearly in the direction perpendicular to the stratum pyramidale, the

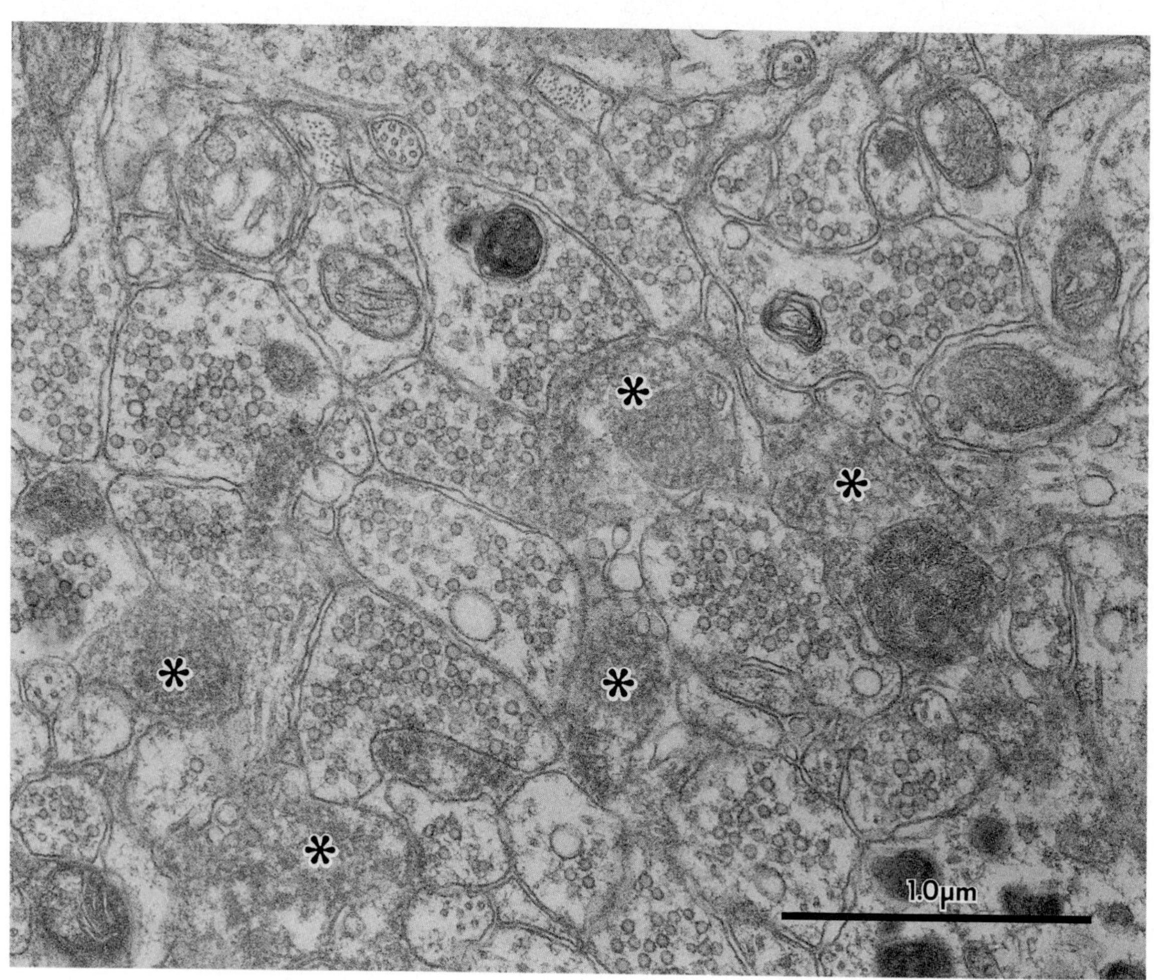

Fig. 2. At one month following ischemia, presynaptic terminals with numerous synaptic vesicles are seen in the CA1 neuropil. These terminals are apposed to degenerative dendritic processes (*). (Stratum radiatum of the CA1 sector; bar, 1 μm).

estimated value indicates a faster decrease of presynaptic terminals (Fig. 6*c*). The average value for the one month group was used for the baseline CA1 thickness. At three months following ischemia, the average-corrected density was $450 \times 10^3 \pm 31 \times 10^3$ (S.D.)/mm^2, and at six months the corrected value was $194 \times 10^3 \pm 45 \times 10^3$/mm^2. At 12 months after ischemia, the corrected density was $57 \times 10^3 \pm 14 \times 10^3$/mm^2. The corrected density value for the three month group was not statistically different from that of the one month group. The corrected densities in the six month and 12 month groups were significantly lower than those in the one month or three month groups (Student's *t*-test, $P < 0.01$).

Discussion

Brief ischemia for 5 min in the Mongolian gerbil, as in the present experiment, causes extensive neuronal destruction of the CA1 sector. Most of the CA1 pyramidal cells were injured and lost within four days

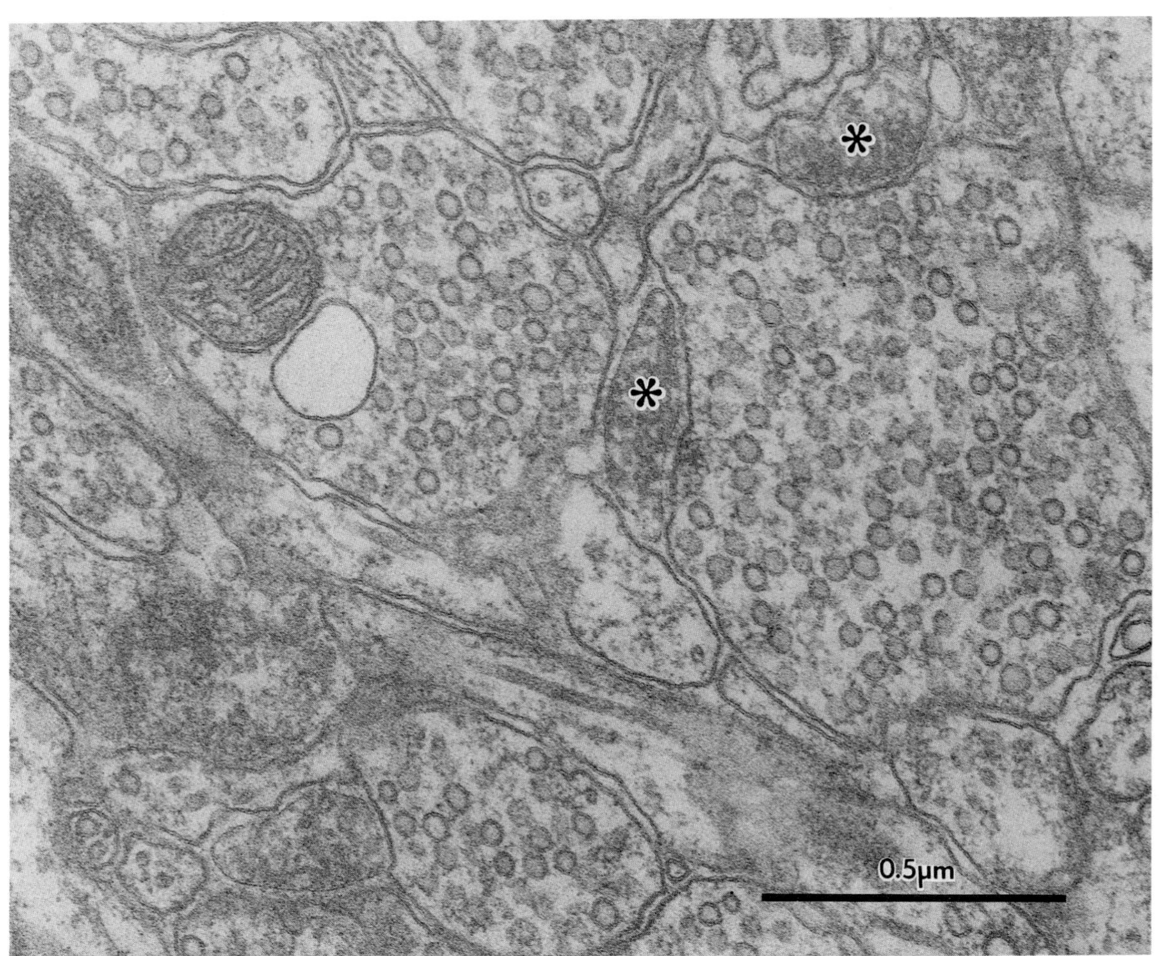

Fig. 3. At three months following ischemia, presynaptic terminals are numerous in the neuropil. They are frequently apposed to degenerative membranous structures (*). The inside of these structures is occupied by flocculent material. (Stratum radiatum of the CA1 sector; bar, 0.5 μm).

following ischemia (Kirino, 1982). Presynaptic terminals, on the other hand, chronically maintained their structure for an extended period of time. The CA1 sector progressively shrank until finally the width became almost half that of the normal CA1. The density of presynaptic terminals progressively decreased. We measured the density of terminals by counting on ten consecutive electron microscopic images. Although this method gave a quantitative estimate of presynaptic terminals in a two-dimensional plane, it did not yield quantitative data in a three-dimensional tissue volume. The counted area covered a ribbon-like region which had a width of 12.0 μm and a height of 84.4 μm. This scanning area was insufficient for evaluating the presynaptic density in the normal animals since the normal stratum radiatum was occupied by thick dendritic shafts of the pyramidal cells. Therefore, we only compared the densities of presynaptic terminals obtained from gerbils, the CA1 sectors of which were damaged and gliotic following ischemia. The synaptic density gradually and continuously decreased and at the same time, the entire CA1 area shrank in the direction perpendicular to the stratum pyramidale. When judged by data corrected by the shrinkage factor, the density of presynaptic ter-

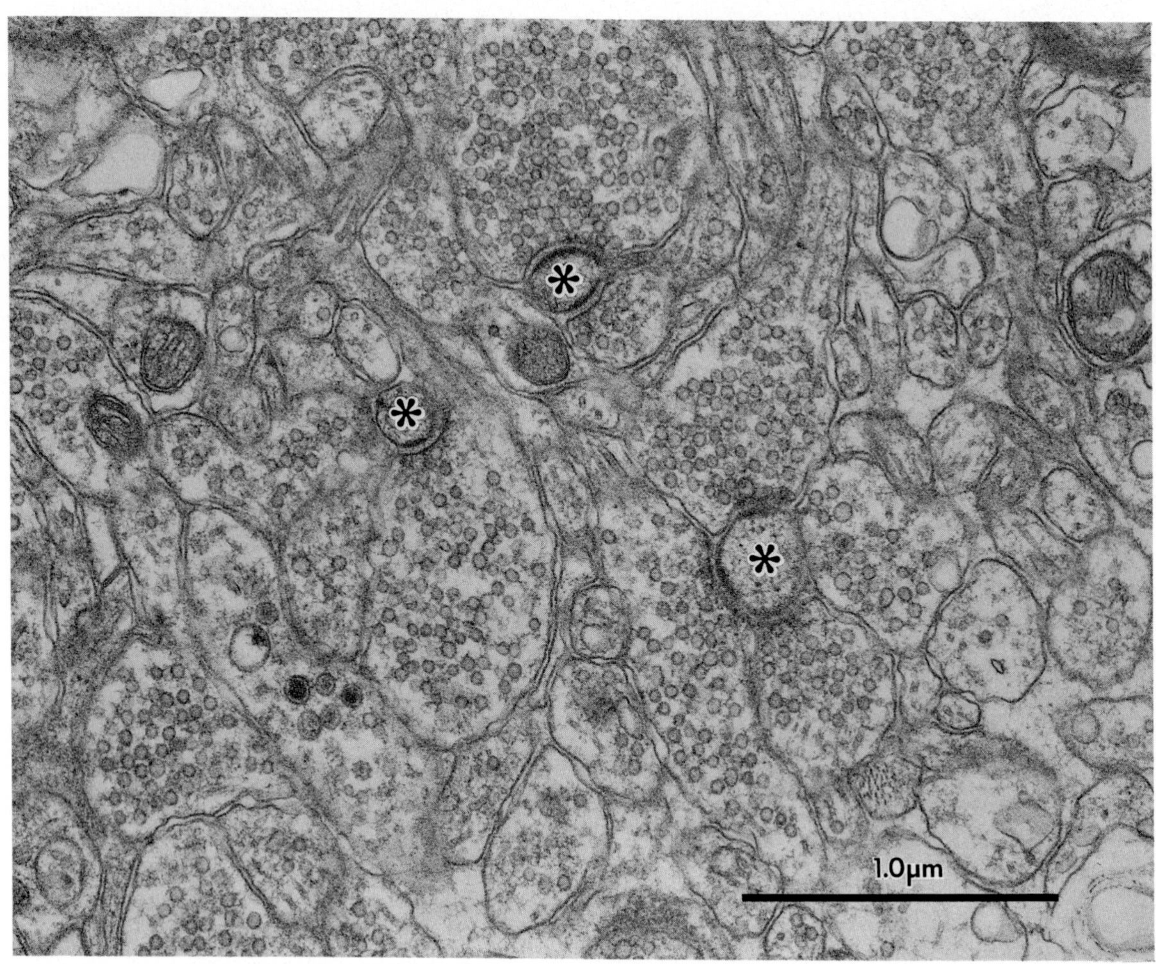

Fig. 4. At six months after ischemia, vesicle-containing terminals are commonly seen. There are extremely shrunken postsynaptic membranous structures (*). (Stratum radiatum of the CA1 sector; bar, 1 μm).

minals was well maintained until three months following ischemia. Then, the density gradually fell until it became about 12% after 12 months following the initial ischemic insult compared with that in the one month group. Presynaptic terminals still remained in considerable numbers 12 months following ischemia, which is about one-third of the gerbil's life span (Arrington et al., 1973).

Presynaptic terminals in the gliotic CA1 region contained numerous clear synaptic vesicles inside. These observations indicate that the ischemic injury to the CA1 sector is almost purely postsynaptic. This result may support the hypothesis that excitotoxins such as glutamate are the major factors which kill CA1 neurons following ischemia. After injection of excitotoxins such as kainic acid, a similar morphological change has been described, in which mainly the postsynaptic structure was damaged and presynaptic terminals and afferent fibers were left undisturbed (Coyle et al., 1978; Olney et al., 1986). Excitotoxic injury to the nervous system is often described as "axon-sparing dendro-somatotoxic". We concluded that the structures which exhibited clear vesicles and membrane thickening were presynaptic terminals. This is reinforced by the fact that synapsin I, a specific marker of presynaptic ter-

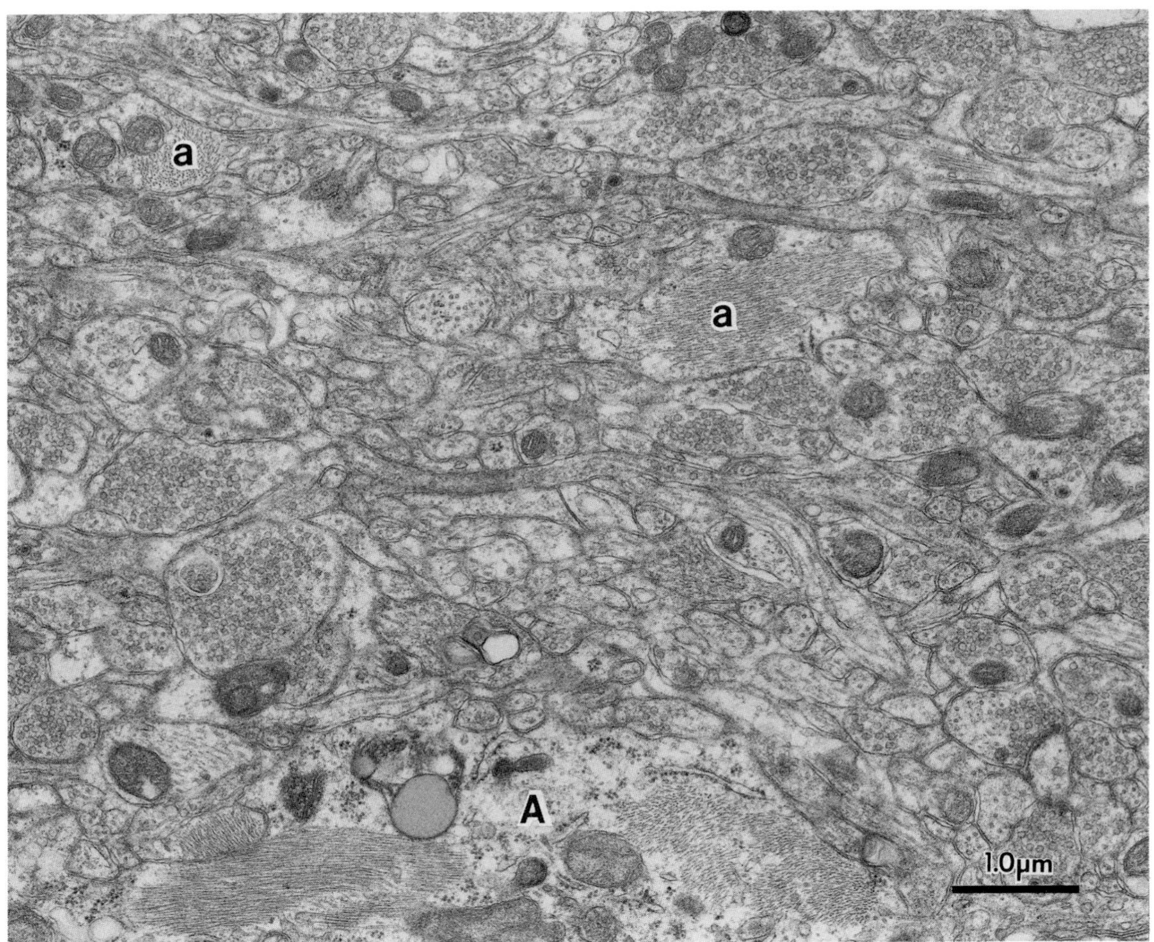

Fig. 5. At 12 months after ischemia, the neuropil is filled with reactive astrocytes (A), astrocytic processes (a) and presynaptic terminals. Astrocytic processes contain intermediate filaments. (Stratum radiatum of the CA1 sector; bar, 1 μm).

minals, was preserved in the chronic stage following ischemia. Kitagawa et al. (1992) examined immunostaining using an antibody against synapsin I and showed that immunoreaction was seen during

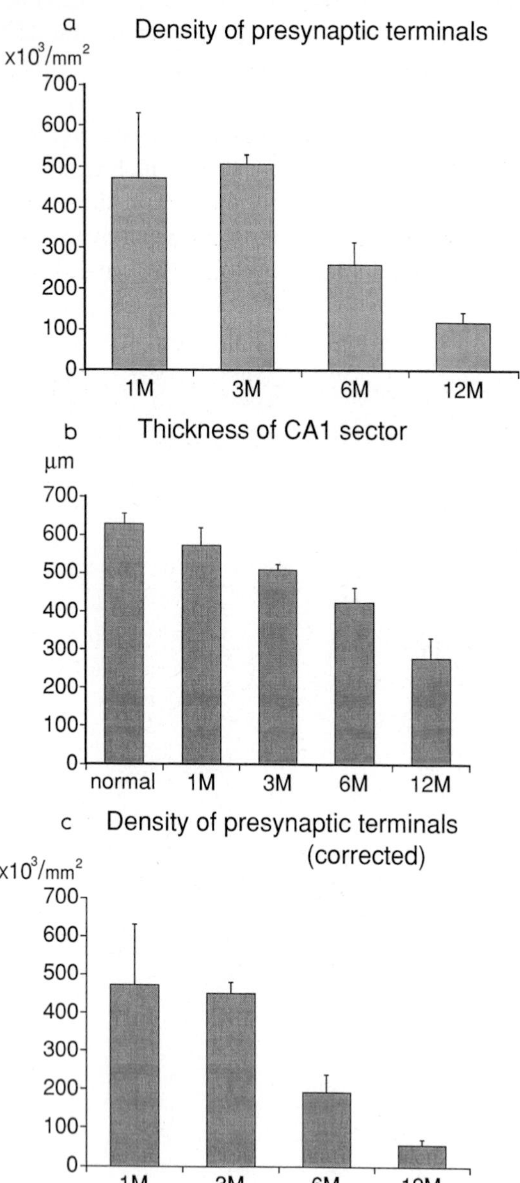

Fig. 6. Progressive decrease of presynaptic terminals in the CA1 sector (*a*). The values are expressed as mean ± S.D. At the same time, the thickness of the CA1 sector decreases (*b*). When the shrinkage factor is taken into account and the values are corrected (*c*), the decrease in the density of presynaptic terminals appears faster than that shown in Fig. 6*a*.

the observation period ranging from seven days to two months following ischemia in the gerbil. In a chronic stage, Kirino et al. (1990) destroyed CA3 neurons by stereotaxic kainate injection to animals whose hippocampal CA1 had been damaged by preceding ischemia. Four days following kainate injection, numerous terminal degenerations were found in the gliotic CA1 sector. This result implied that many, but not all, chronically maintained presynaptic terminals in gliosis of CA1 were from surviving CA3 neurons.

Presynaptic terminals in the gliotic CA1 sector were frequently apposed to membranous structures. The membranous structures were highly degenerative. The inside of this structure lacked normal cellular organelles and was filled with amorphous, flocculent material. These membranous structures seemed to be remnants of dendritic membrane because there was membranous specialization in the interface between the membranous structures and presynaptic terminals. Westerberg et al. (1989) examined dynamic changes of excitatory amino acid receptors in the rat hippocampus following ischemia. They found that, although extensive dendritic degeneration in the stratum radiatum was seen seven days following ischemia, only 25% of the binding of NMDA receptors was lost in CA1. It is possible to speculate that most of the molecules of the NMDA receptor remain in a relatively intact form on the degenerative membranous remnants.

A progressive increase of reactive astroglial cells was observed in the CA1 sector. Immunostaining, using an antibody against glial fibrillary acidic protein, clearly demonstrated this increase (Tønder et al., 1989; Kirino et al., 1990). This astroglial reaction was also observed in the striatum in the rat following transient ischemia (Petito and Rabiak, 1982). Reactive glial cells contained massive intermediate fibers. Beck et al. (1990) observed glucose utilization in rat hippocampus following ischemia. Significant increases in glucose utilization were observed in most layers of the CA1 sector at two and three weeks post-ischemia when most of the neurons were absent. At three months after ischemia, glucose utilization was reduced in all hippocampal areas including CA1. Although the increased glucose metabolism may be a reflection of increased astroglial activity, the authors suggested that the increase in glucose utilization in the CA1 subfield indicates long-lasting presynaptic hyperexcitation. Johansen et al. (1984) have shown that most axons were undamaged four days following ischemia in the rat and that Na^+-dependent glutamate high-affinity uptake was maintained. These data may indicate that presynaptic terminals are structurally intact and also maintain their functional activity. They may release neurotransmitters to surrounding extracellular space and these released transmitter substances may exert an excitatory effect on surviving neurons in or around the damaged CA1 sector. This assumption, however, has not been confirmed electrophysiologically.

The reason why so many presynaptic terminals remain for a long time is not known. Injured brain tissue is reported to produce certain trophic factors (Nieto-Sampedro et al., 1982). If such substances are synthesized in the gliotic CA1 sector, they may facilitate the long-term maintenance of presynaptic terminals or may inhibit their retraction. This hypothesis is supported by the fact that fetal neural tissue grafts could well survive and often became large when transplanted to the hippocampus following ischemia. Tønder et al. (1989) examined the structural and connective interaction of fetal hippocampal neurons grafted to ischemic lesions of the adult rat hippocampus. They confirmed that fetal CA1 neurons grafted to ischemic hippocampal lesions became structurally well incorporated and could establish nerve connections with the host brain. Onifer and Low (1990) have shown that spatial memory deficit due to ischemic hippocampal damage was ameliorated by intra-hippocampal transplants of fetal hippocampal neurons. These experiments have demonstrated that the gliotic hippocampal CA1 sector serves as a good target to examine the interconnection between host and transplanted neural tissue. Katayama et al. (1991) also have demonstrated that, only when ischemia-induced extensive death of CA1 neurons and transplantation was performed one week after the ischemia, did a large number of grafted neurons survive. They postulated that certain trophic factors were involved in the survival of grafted fetal hippocampal neurons. The specific molecules which are active in the gliotic hippocampal CA1 sector, however, have not been identified.

The hippocampus falls into gliosis following loss of neurons due to ischemia/anoxia or epilepsy. Gliotic change has been considered as a passive, regressive tissue reaction. On the other hand, gliotic tissue is frequently associated with active, pathological states such as epileptogenesis. Epilepsy is frequently encountered in patients who suffer selective loss of neurons and long-standing gliosis. Epileptic seizure following focal brain injury develops much later after the onset of initial insult. Such a focal lesion is reported to contain a large amount of excitatory amino acids such as glutamate (Sherwin et al., 1988). We, as well as Bonnekoh et al. (1990), postulate that chronically maintained presynaptic terminals are potentially involved in local epileptogenesis.

Acknowledgements

The author would like to thank Dr.I. Takahashi, Laboratory of Electron Microscopy, Teikyo University School of Medicine for his helpful suggestions. This work was supported by a Grant-in-Aid for Scientific Research on Priority Areas from the Ministry of Education, Science and Culture of Japan.

References

Arrington, L.R., Beaty, Jr., T.C. and Kelley, K.C. (1973) Longevity, and reproductive life of the Mongolian gerbil. *Lab. Animal Sci.,* 23: 262 – 265.

Beck, T., Wree, A. and Schleicher, A. (1990) Glucose utilization in rat hippocampus after long-term recovery from ischemia. *J. Cereb. Blood Flow Metab.,* 10: 542 – 549.

Bonnekoh, P., Barbier, A., Oschlies, U. and Hossmann, K.-A. (1990) Selective vulnerability in the gerbil hippocampus: morphological changes after 5-min ischemia and long survival times. *Acta Neuropathol. (Berl.),* 80: 18 – 25.

Brierley, J.B. and Graham, D.I. (1984) Hypoxia and vascular disorders of the central nervous system. In: J.H. Adams,

J.A.N. Corsellis and L.W. Duchen (Eds.), *Greenfield's Neuropathology,* 4th edition, Edward Anold, London, pp. 125 – 156.

Coyle, J.T., Molliver, M.E. and Kuhar, M.J. (1978) In situ injection of kainic acid: a new method for selectively lesioning neuronal cell bodies while sparing axons of passage. *J. Comp. Neurol.,* 180: 301 – 324.

Johansen, F.F., Jørgensen, M.B., von Lubitz, D.K.J.E. and Diemer, N.H. (1984) Selective dendrite damage in hippocampal CA1 stratum radiatum with unchanged axon ultrastructure and glutamate uptake after transient cerebral ischaemia in the rat. *Brain Res.,* 291: 373 – 377.

Katayama, Y., Tsubokawa, T., Koshinaga, M. and Miyazaki, S. (1991) Temporal pattern of survival and dendritic growth of fetal hippocampal cells transplanted into ischemic lesions of the adult rat hippocampus. *Brain Res.,* 562: 352 – 355.

Kirino, T. (1982) Delayed neuronal death in the gerbil hippocampus following ischemia. *Brain Res.,* 239: 57 – 69.

Kirino, T. and Sano, K. (1984) Selective vulnerability in the gerbil hippocampus following transient ischemia. *Acta Neuropathol. (Berl.),* 62: 201 – 208.

Kirino, T., Tamura, A. and Sano, K. (1990) Chronic maintenance of presynaptic terminals in gliotic hippocampus following ischemia. *Brain Res.,* 510: 17 – 25.

Kitagawa, K., Matsumoto, M., Sobue, K., Tagaya, M., Okabe, T., Niinobe, M., Ohtsuki, T., Handa, N., Kimura, K., Mikoshiba, K. and Kamada, T. (1992) The synapsin I brain distribution in ischemia. *Neuroscience,* 46: 287 – 299.

Loskota, W.J., Lomax, P. and Verity, M.A. (1974) *A Stereotaxic Atlas of the Mongolian Gerbil Brain (Meriones unguiculatus)*, Ann Arbor Science, Ann Arbor, MI.

Mudrick, L.A. and Baimbridge, K.G. (1989) Long-term structural changes in the rat hippocampal formation following cerebral ischemia. *Brain Res.,* 493: 179 – 184.

Nieto-Sampedro, M., Lewis, E.R., Cotman, C.W., Manthorpe, M., Skaper, S.D., Barbin, G., Longo, F.M. and Varon, S. (1982) Brain injury causes a time-dependent increase in neuronotrophic activity at the lesions site. *Science,* 217: 860 – 861.

Olney, J.W., Collins, R.C. and Sloviter, R.S. (1986) Excitotoxic mechanisms of epileptic brain damage. *Adv. Neurol.,* 44: 857 – 877.

Onifer, S.M. and Low, W.C. (1990) Spatial memory deficit resulting from ischemia-induced damage to the hippocampus is ameliorated by intrahippocampal transplants of fetal hippocampal neurons. *Prog. Brain Res.,* 82: 359 – 366.

Petito, C.K. and Rabiak, T. (1982) Early proliferative changes in astrocytes in post-ischemia non-infarcted rat brain. *Ann. Neurol.,* 11: 510 – 518.

Pulsinelli, W.A., Brierley, J.B. and Plum, F. (1982) Temporal profile of neuronal damage in a model of transient forebrain ischemia. *Ann. Neurol.,* 11: 491 – 498.

Sherwin, A., Robitaille, Y., Quesney, F., Olivier, A., Villemure, J., Leblanc, R., Feindel, W., Andermann, E., Gotman, J., Andermann, F., Ethier, R. and Kish, S. (1988) Excitatory amino acids are elevated in human epileptic cerebral cortex. *Neurology,* 38: 920 – 923.

Siesjö, B.K. and Wieloch, T. (1986) Epileptic brain damage: pathophysiology and neurochemical pathology. *Adv. Neurol.,* 44: 813 – 847.

Smith, M-L., Auer, R.N. and Siesjö, B.K. (1984) The density and distribution of ischemic brain injury in the rat following 2 – 10 min of forebrain ischemia. *Acta Neuropathol. (Berl.),* 64: 319 – 332.

Sommer, W. (1880) Erkrankung des Ammonshorns als ätiologisches Moment der Epilepsie. *Arch. Psychiat.,* 10: 631 – 675.

Spielmeyer, W. (1925) Zur Pathogenese der örtlich elektiver Gehirnveränderungen. *Z. Ges. Neurol. Psychiatr.,* 99: 756 – 776.

Tønder, N., Sørensen, T., Zimmer, J., Jørgensen, M.B., Johansen, F.F. and Diemer, N.H. (1989) Neural grafting to ischemic lesions of the adult rat hippocampus. *Exp. Brain Res.,* 74: 512 – 526.

Vogt, C. and Vogt, O. (1922) Erkrankungen der Grosshirnrinde im Lichte der topistik Pathoklise und Pathoarchitektonik. *J. Psychol. Neurol.,* 28: 1 – 171.

Weibel, E.R. (1969) Stereological principles for morphometry in electron microscopic cytology. *Int. Rev. Cytol.,* 26: 235 – 302.

Westerberg, E., Monaghan, D.T., Kalimo, H., Cotman, C.W. and Wieloch T.W. (1989) Dynamic changes of excitatory amino acid receptors in the rat hippocampus following transient cerebral ischemia. *J. Neurosci.,* 9: 798 – 805.

K. Kogure, K.-A. Hossmann and B.K. Siesjö (Eds.)
Progress in Brain Research, Vol. 96

CHAPTER 19

Long-term structural and biochemical events in the hippocampus following transient global ischemia

Hiroshi Onodera, Hiromitsu Aoki and Kyuya Kogure

Department of Neurology, Institute of Brain Diseases, Tohoku University School of Medicine, Sendai 980, Japan

Introduction

The hippocampus is associated with memory processes and numerous studies have been done to investigate synaptic plasticity in this architecture. Moreover, the hippocampus is among the most vulnerable regions in the central nervous system to various deleterious conditions. The CA1 pyramidal cells in the hippocampus are among those neurons highly susceptible to ischemic insult, although neurons in the CA3 and in the dentate gyrus are resistant (Kirino, 1982; Pulsinelli et al., 1982). However, post-ischemic changes in neurotransmitter receptor binding and second messenger systems are not restricted to the ischemic-damaged CA1 subfield. Histologically intact CA3 and dentate gyrus also showed marked modulation in signal transduction systems.

A transneuronal compensatory response to a localized neuronal lesion may involve several directly or indirectly associated neurons. This could involve a reorganization of synaptic inputs to brain areas not directly denervated by the damage. The hippocampus receives inputs from various areas in the central nervous system mainly via the perforant path to dentate granule cells. These neurons in turn project to CA3 pyramidal cells via mossy fibers, and CA3 pyramidal cells project to CA1 pyramidal cells via Schaffer's and commissural fibers. Thus, lesions in these pathways induce synaptic reorganization and alter neuronal excitability. It is of great importance to analyze neuronal circuitry and synaptic transmission long after brain injury. In the present review, we discuss the long-term structural and biochemical events in the hippocampus following transient global ischemia. Moreover, the effect of neuronal transplantation of fetal hippocampus into the ischemic-damaged CA1 subfield on synaptic plasticity is also discussed. This information may also be of value for the treatment of patients suffering from brain damage.

Histopathology

In the present report, we used a rat 20-min transient forebrain ischemia model (four-vessel occlusion method). Histopathological estimation was made 1 – 100 days after ischemic insult (Pulsinelli and Brierley, 1979).

Short-term alteration

Four-vessel occlusion lasting 20 min eliminated the CA1 pyramidal neurons and a small population of hilar neurons was also damaged, although interneurons in the CA1, CA3 pyramidal neurons and dentate granule neurons were resistant. The CA1 pyramidal cells were depleted and GABAergic interneurons were viable 3 – 7 days after ischemia (Kirino, 1982; Pulsinelli et al., 1982). At this time point, no tissue shrinkage in the CA1 and CA3 sectors and dentate gyrus was observed. In addition, no visible damage of the pyramidal cells in the CA3 and granule cells in the dentate gyrus was noticed.

Long-term alteration

In contrast to the limited damage in CA1 and hilus after short-term observation, animals killed 100 days after ischemia confirmed marked shrinkage of bilateral CA1, which resulted in distortion of the cerebral cortex facing the CA1 regions as well as the hippocampal formation, with a general decrease in the size of the ischemic hippocampus. The thickness of the CA1 sector had decreased by 77% 100 days after ischemia. Some ischemic animals exhibited enlargement of lateral ventricles (*hydrocephalus*). CA2 and CA3 pyramidal cells were destroyed along with CA1 neurons in 80% of animals and neuronal injury spread from CA2 into CA3 sectors (Onodera et al., 1990a). Interestingly, the animals with CA2 and CA3 damage on one side exhibited a similar degree of neuronal damage on the other side. In the most severe cases, CA3a appeared to be depopulated of neurons. The number of neurons located in the stratum pyramidale of the CA3b had decreased by 35% 100 days after ischemia. In the most severe case, the number of neurons in the CA3b had decreased to 45% of those of the control group. The thickness of the CA3b region was not different from that in the control group. The neurons in the hilus were severely injured as reported previously. The dentate granule cells appeared normal and the thickness of the strata moleculare of both dorsal and ventral blades was not different from that of the control. As stated above, the reduction of neuronal density was most prominent in the CA3a subregion contiguous to CA1 rather than in the CA3b subregion. Limited but significant ischemic damage to CA3 neurons was reported after a relatively short observation period. Although their ischemic model was different, Smith et al. (1984) reported that 6 – 10 min of transient ischemia resulted in CA3 neuronal damage seven days after ischemia.

Schmidt-Kastner and Hossmann (1988) reported that CA3 pyramidal cells at the septal extreme were damaged after 30 min of forebrain ischemia in the rat, although they used much more severe ischemic conditions than those used in the present study. However, they failed to observe CA3 damage at mid-dorsal levels, where the estimation of neuronal damage and synaptic sprouting occurred in the present report. Thus, damage to CA3 pyramidal cells after prolonged post-ischemic survival could be produced by a different mechanism from that observed after a short observation period. Although discussion of the mechanism of CA3 damage is beyond the scope of the present study, deprivation of the target CA1 pyramidal cells could play a critical role in CA3 pyramidal cell damage because most CA3 pyramidal cells project to the CA1 pyramidal cells via Schaffer's collateral and commissural fibers. We cannot rule out the possibility that depletion of an unknown neurotrophic substance produced by CA1 neurons contributes to the CA3 damage. Another possibility is that CA1 pyramidal cell depletion alters neuronal circuits and enhances granule cell activity enough to cause excitotoxic damage to CA3 pyramidal cells.

The marked decrease in CA1 thickness cannot be explained solely by the depletion of CA1 pyramidal cells (Mudrick and Baimbridge, 1989). Since presynaptic components that terminate on the CA1 neurons occupy a considerable volume of the normal CA1 subfield, the decreased volume of the CA1 subfield 100 days after ischemia could result from

TABLE I

Neuronal density in the stratum pyramidale of the CA3b and Timm's scoring of hippocampal sections 100 days after transient forebrain ischemia

Timm's score	0	1	2	3
Neuronal density in the CA3b (cells/mm)				
< 25	0	0	0	0
25 – 50	1	2	0	0
50 – 75	1	1	2	0
75 – 100	1	0	1	0

Number of animals: $n = 9$. Scoring criteria are as described by Tauck and Nadler (1985).

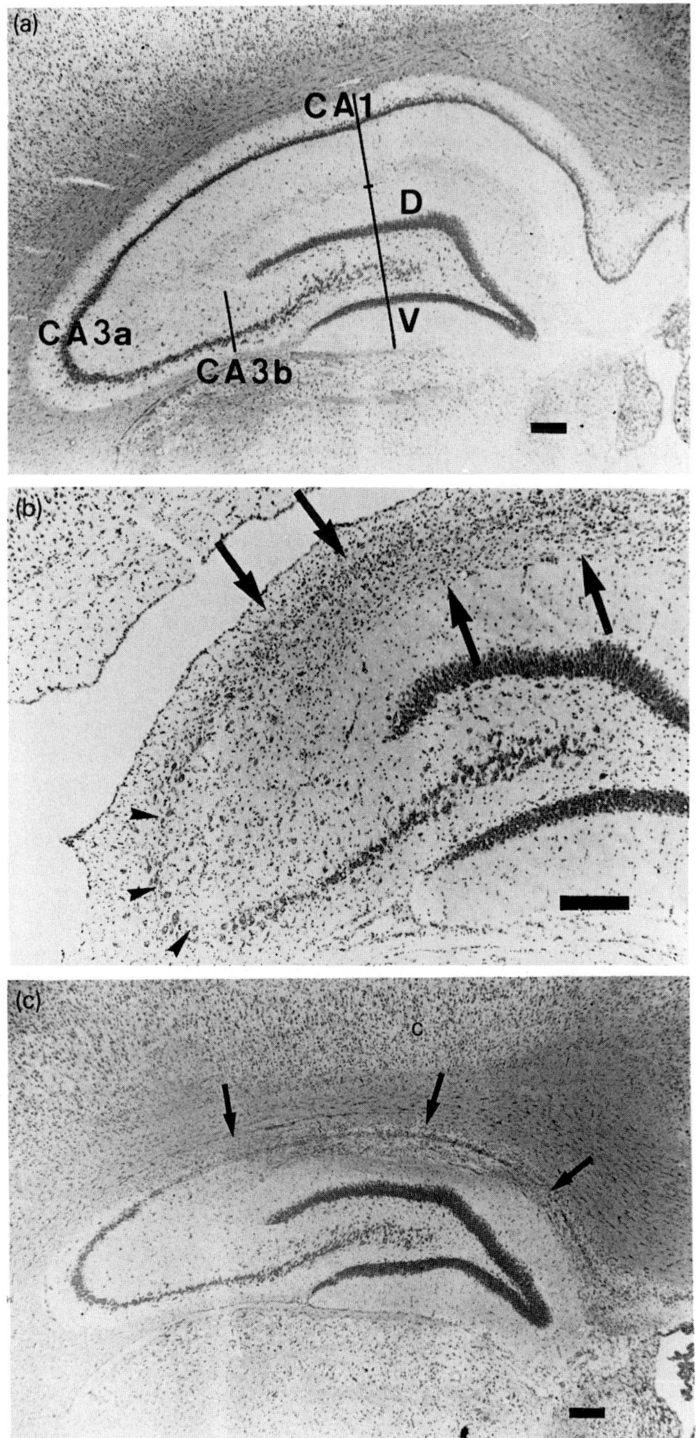

Fig. 1. Cresyl violet-stained sections of the hippocampi of rat brains; control and after 20 min of transient forebrain ischemia by the four-vessel-occlusion model. *a*. Control animal. *b*. One-hundred days after ischemia. Note marked shrinkage of CA1 region (arrows). Neuronal cell loss was more pronounced in the CA2/CA3a subdivisions (arrowheads). Bars, 250 μm.

the degeneration of presynaptic fibers and/or decrease in synaptic density (e.g., CA3 pyramidal cells and septal cholinergic neurons).

Histochemistry

Timm's stain (Table I, Figs. 1, 2)

As reported, the regions with the highest degree of Timm's staining in normal animals were the terminal zones of granule cell axons, namely, the hilus and the stratum lucidum of the CA3 subfield. Aberrantly located Timm granules were noticed in the supragranular molecular layer in 70% of animals 100 days after ischemia (Onodera et al., 1990a). Mossy fiber sprouting was observed only around the tips of the supragranular layer. Neuronal loss in the CA3 did not correlate with mossy fiber sprouting. No Timm's deposits were visible in the infrapyramidal layer of the CA3 subfield. Animals killed 7 – 30 days after ischemia had no aberrant mossy fiber sprouting. The loss of entorhinal output to CA1 pyramidal cells may cause increased input to the dentate granule cells resulting in aberrant mossy fiber sprouting. It is well known that selective lesioning of CA3 neurons with kainic acid induces marked mossy fiber sprouting in the CA3 and in the dentate supragranular layer (Tauck and Nadler, 1985). In contrast, rats kindled by stimulation of the amygdala or the entorhinal cortex and hyperthyroid animals showed aberrant mossy fiber sprouting to the supragranular zone of the dentate gyrus in the absence of CA3 lesions. Although no correlation was observed between Timm's score and CA3 neuronal loss, we cannot rule out the possibility that supragranular mossy fiber sprouting was induced by the CA3 damage, which could not be detected in the present light microscopic study.

Acetylcholinesterase histochemistry

The major source of cholinergic innervation of the hippocampus arises from the medial septal nucleus and diagonal band, although a small population of cholinergic neurons intrinsic to the hippocampus has been identified.

Animals killed seven days after ischemia showed no visible changes in AChE histochemistry. One-hundred days after recirculation, a high density-band of septohippocampal fibers in the CA1, which are restricted to the stratum pyramidale in normal animals, was broadened into whole sublayers and no stratal difference was apparent (Onodera et al., 1990a). In contrast, the AChE activity of animals killed 1 – 30 days after ischemia was not different from that of the control. The CA3 and dentate gyrus showed no visible changes in the AChE staining even in the animals with marked CA3 pyramidal cell loss. High AChE activity bands in supra- and infragranular layers of the dentate gyrus did not invade areas that are normally devoid of dense innervations.

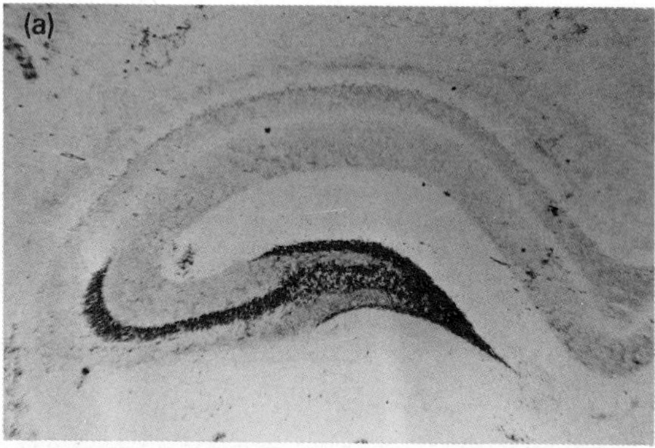

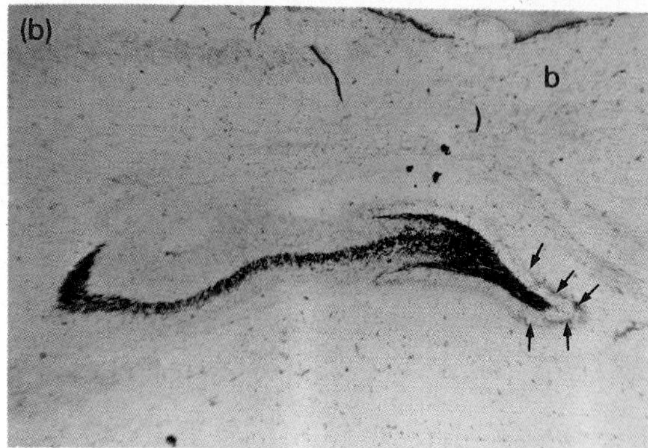

Fig. 2. The distribution of Timm-stained mossy fiber terminals in the hippocampus. *a*. Control animal. *b*. Animal killed 100 days after ischemia. Note the supragranular sprouting of mossy fibers in the fascia dentata of the ischemic animal (arrows).

SDH histochemistry (Fig. 3)

SDH histochemistry was employed to estimate neuronal activity in ischemic-damaged hippocampus. This mitochondrial enzyme involved in energy metabolism exhibits high activity in fields rich in synapses, reflecting high neuronal activity. In normal animals, SDH activity showed regional differences within the hippocampus. The dendritic fields have high SDH activity with the highest activity in the stratum moleculare of the dentate gyrus and to a lesser degree in the strata oriens and radiatum of the CA1 (Wolf et al., 1984; Onodera et al., 1990a). The CA3 also exhibited high SDH activity. In contrast to a moderate decrease in SDH activity and preserved stratal distinction of enzyme activity in the CA1 of animals killed seven days after ischemia, when CA1 pyramidal cells were necrotic, SDH activity in this subfield was depleted 100 days after ischemia in all animals studied. In the CA3 subfield, 100 days after ischemia, animals with decreased CA3 pyramidal cell density lost SDH activity and stratal differences in the CA3, whereas animals without CA3 damage exhibited near normal SDH activity in the CA3. SDH activity was unaltered in the dentate gyrus. Although significant SDH activity was noted in the CA1 seven days after ischemia, all animals studied were devoid of SDH activity in the CA1 100 days after ischemia, irrespective of CA3 pyramidal cell damage. Inputs to CA1 neurons is a major determinant of SDH activity in the CA1. Wolf et al. (1984) also reported that lesions of CA3 axons reduced SDH activity in the CA1 20 days after operation. A marked reduction of SDH activity in the CA3 in animals with CA3 pyramidal cell loss may also reflect similar phenomena observed in the CA1 subfield.

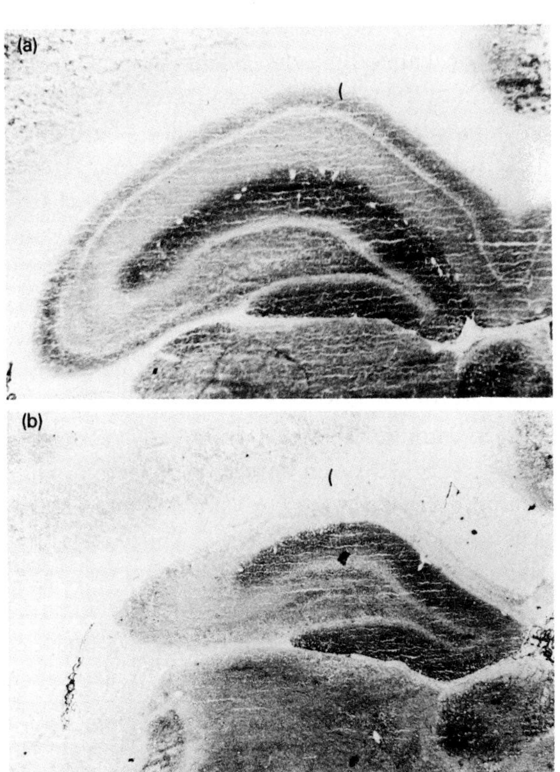

Fig. 3. Histochemical demonstration of succinic dehydrogenase (SDH) in the rat hippocampus. *a*. Control. *b*. SDH activity in the CA1 was severely reduced 100 days after ischemia.

Immunohistochemistry

Post-ischemic changes in the expression of certain proteins have been studied by means of immunohistochemistry. Ischemia induces marked alteration of protein metabolism both at the transcriptional and the translational level (see Hossmann, this volume). In spite of gradual recovery of the total protein synthesis level in ischemia-resistant neurons, estimated by means of radiolabeled amino acid incorporation, the CA1 pyramidal cells could not reconstitute intracellular systems for protein metabolism. Fos and Jun, which are proto-oncogene c-*fos* and c-*jun* products, respectively, are well known proteins as immediate early genes, and they are transiently expressed after ischemia (Onodera et al., 1989b). However, their expression level and temporal profiles are different among brain areas. For instance, most neurons show transient and marked Fos synthesis immediately after ischemia (0.5 – 3 h). In the hippocampus, however, c-*fos* mRNA increase was not marked in the CA1 pyramidal cells compared with the CA3 pyramidal cells and dentate granule cells. Similarly, increase in the expression of heat shock protein 70 (hsp70), another stress response protein, in the CA1 pyramidal neurons was minimal in spite of enhanced induction in the CA3 and dentate gyrus. At present, target molecules of these early gene products and stress proteins are not clear. In the model of epilepsy, c-*fos* and c-*jun* complexes have been reported to interact with the promoter area of opioid peptide DNA which in turn activates the transcription of opioid peptide mRNA. We also cannot rule out the possibility of non-specific induction of these early genes after energy failure.

Calcium/calmodulin-regulated proteins

Accumulating data indicate that abnormal regulation of neurotransmission plays a critical role in CA1 pyramidal cell death. Although involvement of excitatory amino acid (glutamate) in mediating CA1 pyramidal cell death is still controversial, NMDA and non-NMDA receptor antagonists have been reported to modify the fate of vulnerable CA1 neurons. Calcium ion is the most relevant intracellular messenger in the regulation of neurotransmission and neuronal plasticity and calcium also plays a critical role in ischemic neuronal death. Calcium-binding protein, calmodulin, regulates cellular functions. Immunostaining revealed decreased calmodulin-like immunoreactivity in the ischemic CA1 and CA3 subfields one day after ischemia in the rat forebrain ischemia model. Massive calcium influx in the ischemic cells also modulates cellular functions controlled by calcium-calmodulin systems.

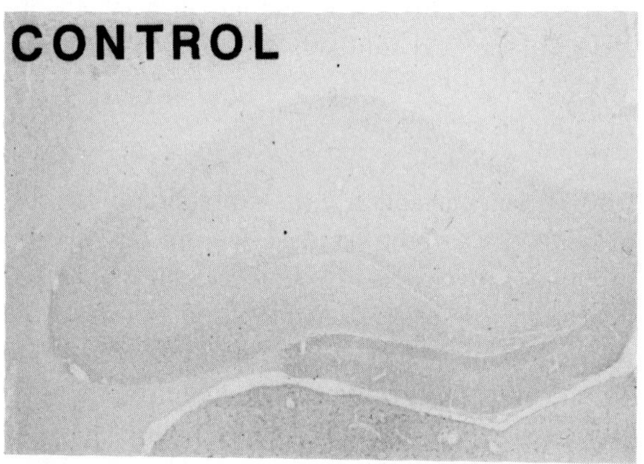

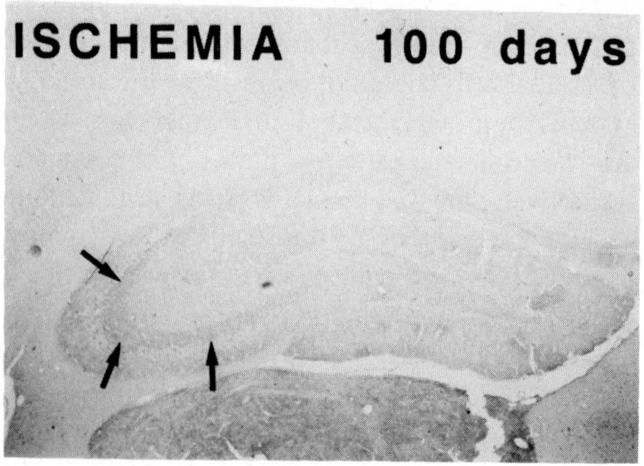

Fig. 4. Calcium/calmodulin-dependent protein kinase II immunoreactivity in the hippocampus. Immunoreactivity in the CA1 subfield was markedly reduced 100 days after ischemia. The mossy fibers showed enhanced immunoreactivity after long-term survival.

Calcium/calmodulin-dependent protein kinase II (Fig. 4)

Calcium/calmodulin-dependent protein kinase II (CaM kinase II) is highly concentrated in the brain and hippocampal CA1 neurons have the highest kinase II level in the brain. In normal animals, the CA1 pyramidal cells and the dentate granule cells exhibited strong CaM kinase II immunoreactivity and neuronal somata had higher immunoreactivity than dendrites (Onodera et al., 1990b). The CA3 pyramidal cells exhibited moderate immunoreactivity and the CA3 stratum lucidum, where mossy fibers terminate, was also immunopositive. CaM kinase II immunoreactivity was greatly reduced in the CA1 subfield seven days after ischemia, while immunoreactivity in the CA3 subfield and dentate gyrus was not consistently altered. Thirty days after ischemia, although CaM kinase II immunoreactivity was minimal in the CA1 subfield, the remaining CA1 pyramidal cells had enhanced CaM kinase II staining intensity with higher immunoreactivity in their apical and basal dendrites than in perikarya. At this time point, enhanced CaM kinase II immunoreactivity was also observed in the stratum lucidum of the CA3 subfield, where mossy fibers from the dentate granule cells terminate. One-hundred days after ischemia, CaM kinase II immunoreactivity remained depressed in the CA1 subfield. At this time point, mossy fibers also had higher CaM kinase II immunoreactivity as was observed 30 days after ischemia. Staining intensity in the CA3 neurons and dentate granule cells was visibly unaltered. CaM kinase II immunoreactivity of GABAergic interneurons in the CA1, which are resistant to ischemia, remained unchanged throughout the observation period. Astrocytes with glial fibrillary acidic protein (GFAP) immunoreactivity had traces of CaM II immunoreactivity.

Interestingly, normal CA1 pyramidal cells exhibit higher CaM kinase II immunoreactivity in perikarya than in dendrites; increased CaM kinase II immunoreactivity in surviving neurons may reflect the reconstruction of signal transduction systems in the ischemic-damaged CA1 subfield. Interestingly, McKee et al. (1990) reported that CaM kinase II immunoreactivity in the CA1 and subicular pyramidal neurons were markedly increased in Alzheimer's disease. They also reported a shift in immunoreactivity to the distal dendritic tree creating a dense network of finely interlacing stained fibers in the neurpil, as was observed in the present study. Taken together, enhancement and redistribution of CaM kinase II activity may be a common phenomenon of surviving neurons in vulnerable areas. Similarly, deafferentation also enhanced CaM kinase II immunoreactivity and CaM kinase II mRNA levels in monkey visual cortex (Hendry and Kennedy, 1989; Benson et al., 1991) after monocular deprivation. Since CaM kinase II phosphorylates components of neuronal cytoskeletal protein (e.g., tubulin, microtubule associated protein 2 (MAP2) and tau factor) and is highly concentrated in cytoskeletal fractions and in postsynaptic density, the disruption of CaM kinase II systems could affect transport of materials through neuronal processes, the shape of neurites and/or membrane-bound receptor signaling. Alteration of an entire cascade of second messenger systems should also be considered. Another important finding was enhanced CaM kinase II immunoreactivity in the terminal zones of dentate granule cell axons (the hilus and the stratum lucidum of the CA3 subfield) 30 and 100 days after ischemia. Although we reported mossy fiber sprouting in the supragranular layer in the dentate gyrus 100 days after ischemia (Onodera et al., 1990a), we failed to observe aberrant CaM kinase II immunoreactivity in the supragranular layer, where aberrant mossy fibers sprouted after long-term survival. Interestingly, dystrophic neurites in the hippocampus of Alzheimer's disease were not CaM kinase II immunoreactive (McKee et al., 1990). Thus expression of CaM kinase II may be restricted to functioning neurites.

Autoradiographic analysis of second messengers

Protein kinase C; phorbol ester binding sites (Fig. 5)

After transient forebrain ischemia, phorbol ester binding sites in the CA1 subfield increased 3 – 12 h after ischemia followed by a 50% loss seven days after ischemia. However, the CA1 subfield regained a subnormal level of [^{3}H]phorbol 12, 13-dibutyrate binding 100 days after ischemia (Onodera et al., 1989a). [^{3}H]PDBu binding in the CA3 was not different from that in the control group even after 100 days following ischemia. In the dentate gyrus, phorbol ester binding sites in the molecular layer increased by 30% seven days after ischemia. One-hundred days after ischemia [^{3}H]PDBu binding was not different from the control group in this sublayer, although grain density in the inner region of the stratum moleculare was slightly increased in animals with CA3 pyramidal cell loss. No abberant increase of [^{3}H]PDBu binding was observed in the hippocampal formation. We observed a 33% increase of [^{3}H]PDBu binding in the stratum moleculare of the dentate gyrus seven days after ischemia, while the inner region of the stratum moleculare (supragranular layer) gained a higher grain density compared to the outer region. However, 100 days after CA1 damage, [^{3}H]PDBu binding in this region was not significantly different from that in the control group, since only animals with CA3 neuronal loss exhibited a small increase in [^{3}H]PDBu binding in the supragranular layer.

Forskolin binding sites (Fig. 5)

[^{3}H]Forskolin binding sites in the CA1 were relatively low, whereas CA3 and hilus had a very high density of [^{3}H]forskolin binding sites (Onodera and Kogure, 1989). Until seven days after ischemia, forskolin binding sites in the CA1 were depleted and binding in the CA3 showed no significant changes. One-hundred days after ischemia, [^{3}H]forskolin binding in the CA1 had decreased by only 20%. Although [^{3}H]forskolin binding in the stratum lucidum of the CA3 and in the stratum moleculare of the dentate gyrus was not altered, binding in the hilus had increased by 62% 100 days after ischemia. The cell density in the CA3 did not influence the hilar increase in [^{3}H]forskolin binding. No visible supragranular increase in [^{3}H]forskolin binding was observed. [^{3}H]forskolin binding cannot be interpreted solely on the basis of adenylate cyclase activity. In contrast to very low [^{3}H]forskolin receptor density in the CA1, the distribution of G protein, estimated by autoradiographic localization and by immunohistochemistry, were highly concentrated in the strata oriens and radiatum of the CA1. Moreover, the hippocampus has exhibited no enhancement of adenylate cyclase activity by GTP analogue nor Mg^{2+}. Taken together, most forskolin binding sites in the CA1 appear not to be regulated by G proteins. Forskolin also labels glucose transporter protein and inhibits glucose transport by a mechanism other than stimulation by adenylate cyclase. Furthermore, forskolin directly alters the gating of voltage-dependent ion channels independent of the activation of adenylate cyclase.

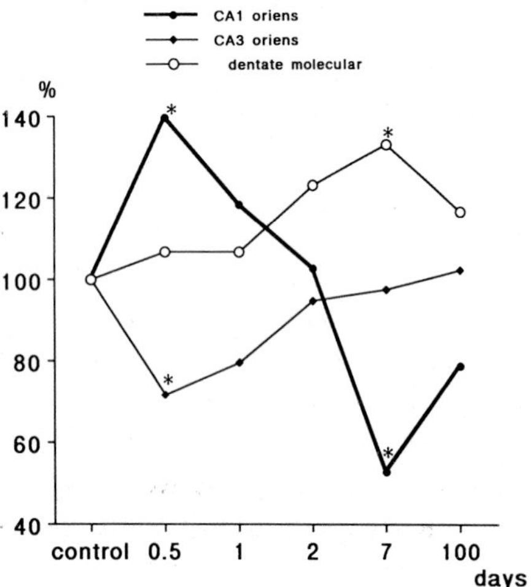

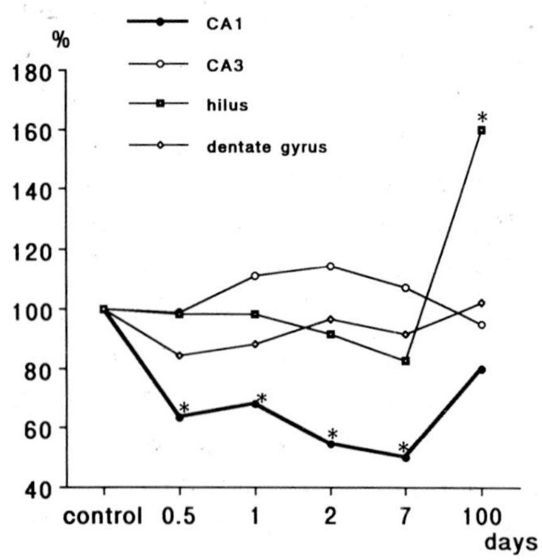

Fig. 5. Graphs of typical time courses of (*a*) phorbol ester binding sites and (*b*) forskolin binding sites in the hippocampal formation after 20 min of transient forebrain ischemia. Binding activities are expressed as percentage of control. * $P < 0.01$.

"Recovered" binding 100 days after CA1 pyramidal cell death may not reflect [^{3}H]PDBu and [^{3}H]forskolin binding sites on neuronal components (interneurons and/or fibers from the CA3 or the entorhinal cortex). Contribution of glial cells and blood vessels after marked CA1 shrinkage to residual binding should also be considered. In contrast to unaltered [^{3}H]forskolin binding in the stratum lucidum of the CA3 and in the stratum moleculare of the dentate gyrus, a marked increase in [^{3}H]forskolin binding (62%) was observed in the hilus. We previously reported that [^{3}H]forskolin binding in the hilus decreased by 17% seven days after recirculation. Johansen et al. (1987) observed, using the same ischemic model, a 70% loss of hilar somatostatin-immunopositive neurons. Although supplementary response after the loss of somatostatin-immunopositive neurons may affect hilar [^{3}H]forskolin binding after long-term survival, further investigations are needed to elucidate increased [^{3}H]forskolin binding.

Inositol 1,4,5-trisphosphate binding (IP_3 receptor)

[^{3}H]Inositol 1,4,5-trisphosphate presumably binds to the endoplasmic reticulum, but may also label its own metabolizing enzyme and ion channels in the plasma membrane. In the central nervous system, the CA1 pyramidal cells and cerebellar Purkinje cells have a very high density of IP_3 receptors. The CA3 region and dentate gyrus have a very low density of binding sites. In the early post-ischemic period, IP_3 binding sites decreased only 3 h after ischemia in the dendritic fields of the CA1 (strata oriens and radiatum), although IP_3 binding in the stratum pyramidale remained unaltered until the death of the CA1 pyramidal cells. IP_3 binding sites in the CA1 were depleted seven days after ischemia. These data clearly indicate the location of IP_3 receptors in the CA1 pyramidal cells. In situ hybridization study also showed predominant localization of IP_3 receptor mRNAs in the CA1 pyramidal cells. One-hundred days after ischemia, IP_3 binding in the CA1 remained depleted and that in other hippocampal subregions remained unaltered.

Reconstruction of hippocampal function by means of fetal hippocampal transplants

Fetal brain transplants have been used extensively in studies of neuronal plasticity and repair of damaged circuits. Functional synaptic connections between grafts and hosts have been demonstrated by means of morphological and electrophysiological studies. The CA1 pyramidal cells receive Schaffer/commissural fibers from CA3 pyramidal cells, and fibers from entorhinal cortex. As stated above, ectopic mossy fiber sprouting was observed in the dentate gyrus after ischemia. However, fetal hippocampal transplants stereotaxically placed into the ischemic-damaged CA1 reduced aberrant mossy fiber sprouting in the dentate gyrus. Thus, synaptic connection between host CA3 pyramidal cells and fetal hippocampal graft modulated CA3 neuronal activity, which in turn influenced granule cell activity and inhibited aberrant mossy fiber sprouting. We also observed a beneficial effect of transplantation of fetal hippocampus on the recovery of post-ischemic impairment of learning by the T-shaped maze test. Therefore, integration of the grafted neurons with the host hippocampus has been estimated by histochemical techniques and by observing the amelioration of spatial memory performance deficit. Restoration of neuronal function after ischemia could not solely be interpreted as reconstruction of damaged neuronal circuits. Neurotrophic factors supplied by transplanted neurons, which are normally secreted by CA1 pyramidal cells, could play a beneficial role for the cellular function of neurons that have connections with CA1 pyramidal cells.

Conclusions

Long-term survival after ischemia induces synaptic rearrangements in the whole hippocampal formation. Marked shrinkage of ischemic-damaged CA1 subfield also reflects the changes in presynaptic components after long-term survival. Limited but significant neuronal loss in the CA3 subfield may be caused partly by the depletion of neurotrophic factors for the CA3 pyramidal cells supplied by the CA1 pyramidal cells. Modulation of neuronal acitivities in the CA3 neurons can induce a plastic response of dentate granule neurons (ectopic mossy fiber sprouting). These changes may be beneficial to the reorganization of hippocampal functions after the loss of CA1 pyramidal cells and hilar neurons, because several studies have shown gradual recovery of post-ischemic impairment of learning activities characteristic of hippocampal damage. However, in the case of selective CA3/4 neuronal depletion by kainic acid, aberrant mossy fiber sprouting leads to a reduction in the seizure threshold and correlates well with abnormal excitability. The critical question that remains is whether the rearrangement of the neuronal network after neuronal damage is beneficial to the reinstitution of normal functions.

References

Benson, D.L., Isackson, P.J., Gall, C.M. and Jones, E.G. (1991) Differential effects of monocular deprivation on glutamic acid decarboxylase and type II calcium-calmodulin-dependent protein kinase gene expression in the adult monkey visual cortex. *J. Neurosci.*, 11: 31 – 47.

Hendry, S.H. and Kennedy, M.B. (1989) Immunoreactivity for a calmodulin-dependent protein kinase is selectively increased in macaque striate cortex after monocular deprivation. *Proc. Natl. Acad. Sci. U.S.A.*, 83: 1536 – 1540.

Johansen, F.F., Zimmer, J. and Diemer, N.H. (1987) Early loss of somatostatin neurons in dentate hilus after cerebral ischemia in the rat precedes CA-1 pyramidal cell loss. *Acta Neuropathol. (Berl.)*, 73: 110 – 114.

Kirino, T. (1982) Delayed neuronal death in the gerbil hippocampus following ischemia. *Brain Res.*, 239: 57 – 69.

McKee, A.C., Kosik, K.S., Kennedy, M.B. and Kowall, N.W. (1990) Hippocampal neurons predisposed to neurofibrillary tangle formation are enriched in type II calcium/calmodulin-dependent protein kinase. *J. Neuropathol. Exp. Neurol.*, 49: 49 – 63.

Mudrick, L.A. and Baimbridge, K.G. (1989) Long-term structural changes in the rat hippocampal formation following cerebral ischemia. *Brain Res.*, 493: 179 – 184.

Onodera, H. and Kogure, K. (1989) Mapping second messenger systems in the rat hippocampus after transient forebrain ischemia: in vitro [^{3}H]forskolin and [^{3}H]inositol 1,4,5-trisphosphate binding. *Brain Res.*, 487: 343 – 349.

Onodera, K., Kogure, K., Ono, Y., Igarashi, K., Kiyota, Y. and Nagaoka, A. (1989b) Proto-oncogene c-*fos* is transiently induced in the rat cerebral cortex after forebrain ischemia. *Neurosci. Lett.*, 98: 101 – 104.

Onodera, H., Araki, T. and Kogure, K. (1989a) Protein kinase C activity in the rat hippocampus after forebrain ischemia: autoradiographic analysis by [^{3}H]phorbol 12,13-dibutyrate *Brain Res.*, 481: 1 – 7.

Onodera, H., Aoki, H., Yae, T. and Kogure, K. (1990a) Post-ischemic synaptic plasticity in the rat hippocampus after long-term survival: a histochemical and autoradiographic study. *Neuroscience*, 38: 125 – 136.

Onodera, H., Hara, H., Kogure, K., Fukunaga, K., Ohta, Y. and Miyamoto, E. (1990b) Calcium/calmodulin-dependent protein kinase II immunoreactivity in the rat hippocampus after forebrain ischemia. *Neurosci. Lett.*, 113: 134 – 138.

Pulsinelli, W.A. and Brierley, J.B. (1979) A new model of bilateral hemispheric ischemia in the unanaesthetized rat. *Stroke*, 10: 262 – 272.

Pulsinelli, W.A., Brierley, J.B. and Plum, F. (1982) Temporal profile of neuronal damage in a model of transient forebrain ischemia. *Ann. Neurol.*, 11: 491 – 498.

Schmidt-Kastner, G. and Hossmann, K.A. (1988) Distribution of ischemic neuronal damage in the dorsal hippocampus of rat. *Acta Neuropathol. (Berl.)*, 76: 411 – 421.

Smith, M.L., Auer, R.N. and Siesjö, B.K. (1984) The density and distribution of ischemic brain injury in the rat following 2 – 10 min of forebrain ischemia. *Acta Neuropathol. (Berl.)*, 64: 319 – 332.

Suga, S. and Nowak, T.S. (1991) Localization of immunoreactive fos and jun proteins in gerbil brain: effect of transient ischemia. *J. Cereb. Blood Flow Metab.*, 11 (Suppl. 2): 352.

Tauck, D.L. and Nadler, J.V. (1985) Evidence of functional mossy fiber sprouting in hippocampal formation of kainic acid-treated rats. *J. Neurosci.*, 5: 1016 – 1022.

Wolf, G., Schunzel, G. and Mathisen, S. (1984) Lesions of Schaffer's collaterals in the rat hippocampus affecting glutamate dehydrogenase and succinate dehydrogenase activity in the stratum radiatum of CA1. A study with special reference to glutamate transmitter metabolism. *J. Hirnforsch.*, 25: 149 – 153.

Subject Index